चरक संहिता - II

ENGLISH TRANSLATION

डा. जनार्धन वि हेब्बार

|| Jai Guruji ||

I, Dr. Janardhana V. Hebbar, dedicate this book at the holy feet of Sri Guruji – Swami Vivekananda and my spiritual Guru, Dr. A. Chandrashekhara Udupa MBBS, F.A.G.E, Managing Director, Divine Park Trust (R), Saligrama, Udupi. (www.divinepark.org)

He guides, He energizes, He shows the path,
He holds my hand and makes me walk!Charaka Jwara Nidana: 1st Chapter

क्रम-सूची

पावती (स्वीकृति)   vii

भूमिका   ix

निदान स्थानम् Nidana Sthanam

1. Nidanasthana Chapter 1 Jwara Nidanam   3
2. Nidanasthana Chapter 2 Raktapitta Nidanam   16
3. Nidanasthana Chapter 3 Gulma Nidanam   22
4. Nidanasthana Chapter 4 Prameha Nidanam   29
5. Nidanasthana Chapter 5 Kushta Nidanam   38
6. Nidanasthana Chapter 6 Shosha Nidanam   45
7. Nidanasthana Chapter 7 Unmada Nidanam   52
8. Nidanasthana Chapter 8 Apasmara Nidanam   60

विमानस्थानम् Vimana Sthanam

9. Vimanasthana Chapter 1 Rasa Vimanam   71
10. Vimanasthana Chapter 2 Trividhakukshiya Vimanam   81
11. Vimanasthana Chapter 3 Janapadoddhvamsaniyam Vimanam   87
12. Vimanasthana Chapter 4 Trividha Roga Vishesha Vijnaniya Vimanam   99
13. Vimanasthana Chapter 5 Srotasam Vimanam   104
14. Vimanasthana Chapter 6 Roganikam Vimanam   111
15. Vimanasthana Chapter 7 Vyadhita Rupiya Vimanam   120
16. Vimanasthana Chapter 8 Roga Bhishagjiteeya Vimanam   131

शारीरस्थानम् Shareera Sthanam

17. Shareerasthana Chapter 1 Katidha Purusheeyam   187
18. Shareerasthana Chapter 2 Atulya Gotreeya Shareeram   209
19. Shareerasthana Chapter 3 Khuddika Garbhavakranti Shareeram   217
20. Shareerasthana Chapter 4 Mahatim Garbhavakranti Shareeram   227
21. Shareerasthana Chapter 5 Purusha Vichayam Shareeram   239
22. Shareerasthana Chapter 6 Shareera Vichayam Shareeram   246
23. Shareerasthana Chapter 7 Shareera Samkhya Shareeram   255
24. Shareerasthana Chapter 8 Jatisutreeyam Shareeram   262

इन्द्रियस्थानम् Indriya Sthanam

25. Indriyasthana Chapter 1 Varna Swareeyam Indriyam   293
26. Indriyasthana Chapter 2 Pushpitakam Indriyam   300
27. Indriyasthana Chapter 3 Parimarshaneeyam Indriyam   303
28. Indriyasthana Chapter 4 Indriyaneekam Indriyam   306
29. Indriyasthana Chapter 5 Purvaroopeeyam Indriyam   310

क्रम-सूची

30. Indriyasthana Chapter 6 Katamani Shareereeyam Indriyam — 316

31. Indriyasthana Chapter 7 Pannaroopeeyam Indriyam — 319

32. Indriyasthana Chapter 8 Avak Shiraseeyam Indriyam — 323

33. Indriyasthana Chapter 9 Yasya Shyava Nimitteeyam Indriyam — 327

34. Indriyasthana Chapter 10 Sadyo Maraneeyasm Indriyam — 330

35. Indriyasthana Chapter 11 Anu Jyoteeyam Indriyam — 333

36. Indriyasthana Chapter 12 Gomaya Choorneeyam Indriyam — 337

Easy Ayurveda Publications — 349

पावती (स्वीकृति)

Special thanks to Dr Raghuram YS for painstakingly editing the entire book.
Special thanks to my family members who have been supporting me unconditionally throughout this journey of Easy Ayurveda. Thank you for tolerating all the pains.
Smt. Padmakshamma (mother), Karthyayini (wife and staff), Smt. Vanamala (mother-in-law).
Daughters – Sadhvi & Chinmayi
     Sister Sharada, brother-in-law Mr ShashiKumar, Tushar, Ms Sharada.
All my staff who make Easy Ayurveda possible, everyday.
Dr Sudarshan CH, Dr Shilpa Ramdas, Dr Renita D'Souza,
Mr Sachidananda Bhat, Smt. Nayana, Mr Nikhil and Smt. Sumangala.
My mentors - Dr MB Gururaja, Dr MS Krishnamurthy and Dr Prashanth BK

भूमिका

This book covers the 8 chapters of Nidanasthana, 8 chapters of Vimanasthana, 8 chapters of Shareerasthana and 12 chapters of Indriyasthana of Charaka Samhita.

Charaka Samhita is a popular Ayurvedic treatise. As the name indicates, it is a compilation of Ayurveda lessons comprising of various aspects including basic concepts (Sutra sthana), diagnosis of diseases (Nidana sthana), treatment concepts (Chikitsa sthana) etc. and is written by Charaka. (Charaka Samhita means 'treatise written by Charaka).

Acharya Charaka redacted the treatise 'Agnivesha Tantra' which has become popular in the name of 'Charaka Samhita'. This means to tell that the text 'Agnivesha Tantra' written by Agnivesha was re-modulated by Charaka, which later came to be called as 'Charaka Samhita'.

Charaka Samhita is the first and foremost authentic treatise of Ayurveda and is one of the 'greatest trio' (Brihat-Trayee).

Master Charaka was so keen to help people with Ayurveda that he used to roam from one place to the other continuously. Hence he got the name Charaka.

Charati iti Charakaha – One who moves continuously.

Charaka Samhita

Charaka Samhita, a part of Brihat Trayi or greater trio of Ayurveda occupies a significant place in the history of world's medical science.

Atreya Punarvasu has many intelligent students. Punarvasu was the most respected, learned Guru (teacher) and preacher of Ayurveda. Among the clan of his elite students Agnivesha was the best.

According to the directions and teachings of his teacher Punarvasu Atreya, Agnivesha recorded, documented and composed his work on Ayurveda.

It was called as Agnivesha Tantra. It was subsequently redacted by Charaka which in due course of time got popular in the name 'Charaka Samhita'. This Charaka Samhita was further redacted by Dridhabala.

In Charaka Samhita, we can find that the justice has been done in covering all the aspects and 8 branches of Ayurveda. But the emphasis has been given in covering the concepts of Kaya Chikitsa (General medicine) in detail. That is why, Charaka Samhita is considered to be the best reference and authentic text of Kaya Chikitsa.

More than 40 commentaries are written on Charaka Samhita. It is translated into all the Indian languages. It is also translated into many foreign languages including Persian, Simhali, Nepali, Arabic etc.

Sections and Chapters of Charaka Samhita:

Charaka Samhita has been dealt with in 8 sections and 120 chapters.

Sutrasthana – Basic Principles – 30 chapters, 1952 Verses.

Nidana Sthana – Pathology – 8 chapters, 247 verses

Vimana Sthana – Specific determination – 8 chapters, 354 verses

Shareera Sthana – Anatomy – 8 chapters , 382 verses

Indriya Sthana – Sensory organ based prognosis – 12 chapters, 378 verses

Chikitsa Sthana – Therapeutics – 30 chapters, 4904 verses

Kalpasthana – Pharmaceutics and toxicology – 12 chapters – 378 verses

Siddhi Sthana – Success in treatment – 12 chapters – 700 verses

Total – 9295 verses (Sutras)

Sutra sthana

Deals with fundamental principles of Ayurveda covered in 30 chapters

Sutra Sthana is sub-divided into Sapta Chatushkas (7 quadrates), having 4 chapters each.

They are:

Bheshaja Chatushka – quadrate on drugs

Swasta Chatushka – quadrate on regimen for the maintenance of health

Nirdesha Chatushka – quadrate on various instructions

Kalpana Chatushka – quadrate on description of therapeutic procedures

Roga Chatushka – quadrate on description of diseases

Yojana Chatushka – quadrate on administration of various therapies

Annapana Chatushka – quadrate on description of diet and drinks

Sangraha adhyaya – 2 chapters at the end of Sutra Sthana are known by the name Sangraha Adhyaya, the concluding chapters

Vimana Sthana

Deals with the principles governing the bodily factors that cause diseases – drugs and medicaments covered in 8 chapters

a. In Rasa Vimana chapter, sweet, sour etc tastes, qualities, functions, effect on Dosha, oils, ghee, honey etc, their effect on health and asta vidha vishesha Ayatana are explained.

b. In Trividha Kuksheeya Vimana, GI tract, quantity of food to be taken, what happens if the food is taken excessively or in low quantities, Visuchika, Alasaka etc digestive tract disorders are mentioned.

c. In Janapadodhvamsaneeya chapter – communicable disorders, endemic diseases, reasons, preventive measures are mentioned.

d. In Trividha Roga VIshesha Vijnaneeya chapter, Pratyaksha – direct observation, Anumana, Aptaopadesha – means of knowledge, etc are explained.

e. In Sroto Vimana chapter, all the body channels, causes, symptoms and treatment of vitiation of body channels are mentioned.

f. In Roganeeka Vimana – types of diseases – mental, physical, types of Agni, Prakriti – body types etc are mentioned.

g. In Vyadhita Rupeeya Vimana – Guru, Laghu etc patient features, Krumi causes and treatment are mentioned.

h. In Roga Bhishag Jiteeya chapter, causes for diseases, sambhasha – discussion, 10 types of patient examination etc are explained.

Nidana Sthana

Deals with aetiology, pathogenesis and diagnosis of diseases covered in 8 chapters.

For each disease, causative factors, prodromal symptoms, signs and symptoms, pathogenesis, prognosis are explained in detail.

Jwara, Rakthapitha, Gulma, Prameha, Kushta etc diseases are explained in detail.

Shareera Sthana

Deals with embryology, anatomy and physiology covered in 8 chapters. This section gives detail discription about Human Anatomy and its application in treatment, panchamahabhutha (Basic 5 elements of earth), conception, embryology, signs of pregnancy, monthwise fetal development, manas prakruti (constitution of mind), determination of prakruti in the fetus, procedure of labour, diseases of children, bala samskara (Agewise ceremony), child nutrition and treatment of child disease.

Indriya Sthana

Deals with prognostic signs and symptoms covered in 12 chapters

In this section signs and symptoms of bad prognosis, inauspicious symptoms pertaining to skin complexion, voice, odour, taste, touch, sight, sound, mind, tongue, nose, fire, hygiene, behavioural activities, memory, tolerance capacity of patient, strength, structure of body, dryness, unctuousness, heaviness, digestion of food etc

Importance of inauspicious symptoms in the origin of disease, pain, advice, shadow, dreams, to see inauspicious signs on the road, auspicious and inauspicious signs related to sense organs and its perceived senses, curable and incurable signs of disease and patients life span are mentioned.

Chikitsa Sthana

Deals with treatment of various diseases covered in 30 chapters

This section explains in detail under Rasayana chapters – Rasayana medicines, intake procedure of rasayana, types of rasayana, rasayana properties of hareethaki and amalaki, procedure of its preparation, intake and its doses. It also deals with acharya rasayana.

Vachikarana chapters deals with – causes, types and treatment of infertility, use of vajikaran medicines, its method of preparation and intake.

Causes, signs and symptoms, types and treatment of various disease beginning from jwara, rakthapitha, gulma, prameha, doshagatha diseases, mental disorders, alcoholism,poisoning etc are mentioned here.

Kalpa Sthana

Deals with formulations for vamana (emesis), virechana (purgation) etc covered in 12 chapters.

This section deals with various medicinal formulations of madanaphala, jeemuthaka, dhamargava, krethavedhana, trivruth, aaragvadha, bilva, sapthala, danthi, dravathi etc, its origin, collection, types and properties are also mentioned here.

Siddhi Sthana

Deals with principles governing the administration of elimination therapies covered in 12 chapters

This section explains in detail – procedure of administration of elimination therapies(panchakarma), its indication and contraindications, complications developed due to improper administration of elimination therapy and its treatment. It also explains signs and symptoms produced due to excess, improper and proper administration of elimination therapy.

The three stages of Panchakarma – priliminary therapy (purvakarma), main therapy (pradhanakarma), post therapy procedures (paschathkarma) are explained orderly.

Persons indicated and contraindicated for elimination therapy and purificatory procedure for contraindicated person is also explained here.

Salient features of Charaka Samhita –

The titles of some chapters are based on the first word occurring in the chapter and others are based on the subject matter discussed in that particular chapter

4 types of Sutras are found in Charaka Samhita such as:

Guru Sutra – statements made by the teacher

Shishya Sutra – statements / enquires made by the disciple

Pratisamskarta Sutra – Statement of the redactor

Ekiya Sutra – statements made by individual scholars

Subject matter of each chapter is described as Uddeshya (brief statement and intention of chapter) followed by Nirdesha (detailed expansion of the above statement) and Lakshana (definition)

The colophons give the information of the author's name, name of redactor, title of the section and chapter and also the serial number of the chapter

The explanation of topics like Swabhavoparama vada highlights the influence of Buddhism on Charaka Samhita

Scientific explanation of the Ayurvedic fundamental principles like Tridoshas, Pancha Mahabhutas and Rasa Panchakas etc can be seen

Importance of Roga and Rogi Pareeksha (examination of disease and the diseased) has been emphasised

At the end of each chapter, the complete contents of the chapter are enlisted

Commentaries

More than 40 Sanskrit Commentaries were written on Charaka Samhita. Out of them the following are available partly or in full form.

Charakanyasa – By Bhattara Harishchandra in 4th century AD

Charaka Panjika – By Swami Kumara after 4th century AD

Nirantarapada Vyakhya – By Jejjata in 6th century AD

Ayurveda Deepika – By Chakrapani in 11th century AD

Tatwa Chandrika – By Shivadas Sen in 15th century AD

Jalpakalpataru – By Gangadhar Sen in 19th century AD

Charakopaskara – By Yogendranath Sen in 20th century AD

Charaka Pradipika – By Jyotishchandra Saraswati in 20th century AD

Charaka, the highly valued

Since 4th century A.D. onwards great scholars of Ayurveda, authors, scientists, commentators etc gave utmost respect to the sage 'Charaka'.

Famous commentators like Bhattara Harischandra, Swami Kumara, Yogendranatha Sen etc, paid their tributes to Acharya Charaka by naming their works as Charakanyasa, Charaka Panjika and Charakopaskara respectively. There are as many as 43 Sanskrit commentaries on this work.

In the beginning of 8th century AD Charaka Samhita was translated into Arabic language.

According to the Colophon, Agnivesha, on the advice of his preceptor Punarvasu Atreya, composed this work which was subsequently redacted by Charaka and Dridhabala

Charaka's Club – It is a medical organization which was established in New York in November 1898. It was founded by a group of 4 doctors Charles. L. Dana, Joseph Colliers, Fredrick Peterson and Barnad Sachs. This club discussed a wide array of subjects involving fields like medical, medical history, literature, poetry etc.

निदान स्थानम् Nidana Sthanam

1

Nidanasthana Chapter 1 Jwara Nidanam

The 1st Chapter of Charaka Samhita Nidana Sthana is called Jwara Nidana. It deals with causes, pathology, types and symptoms of Jwara – fever, as per Ayurveda.

Chapter -1
Diagnosis of Fever (Jwara Nidana)
अथातो ज्वर निदानं व्याख्यास्यामः||१||
इति ह स्माह भगवानात्रेयः||२||
We shall now explore the chapter on the "diagnosis of Jvara (fever)" [1]
Thus said Lord Atreya [2]

Synonyms of Nidana – Causative factors and its Categories:
इह खलु हेतु निमित्तमायतनं कर्ता कारणं प्रत्ययः समुत्थानं निदानमित्यनर्थान्तरम्|
तत्त्रिविधम्- असात्म्येन्द्रियार्थसंयोगः, प्रज्ञापराधः, परिणामश्चेति||३||
Synonyms of Nidana (Causative factor) in the present context
Hetu
Nimitta
Ayatana
Karta
Karana
Pratyaya and
Samutthana
Causative factors are of the following 3 categories:
Asatmyendriyartha samyogah - Unwholesome contacts of the sense organs with their objects
Prajnaparadah — intellectual blasphemy
Parinama — seasonal vagaries [3]

Dual classification of disease:
अतस्त्रिविधा व्याधयः प्रादुर्भवन्ति- आग्नेयाः, सौम्याः,
वायव्याश्च; द्विविधाश्चापरे- राजसाः, तामसाश्च||४||
Diseases so caused are primarily of 3 types Viz.,
Agneya (Paittika)
Saumya (Slaismika)
Vayavya (Vatika)

Some others, that is minor ones, are of 2 types viz,
Rajasa
Tamasa. [4]

Synonyms of Roga – Disease:
तत्र व्याधिरामयो गद आतङ्को यक्ष्मा ज्वरो विकारो रोग इत्यनर्थान्तरम्||५||
Below mentioned are the synonyms of Roga (disease):
Vyadhi
Amaya
Gada
Atanka
Yaksma
Jvara
Vikara [5]

Means of diseases:
तस्योपलब्धि निंदान पूर्वरूप लिङ्गोपशय सम्प्राप्तितः||६||
Diseases can be diagnosed by the study of
Nidana (etiology)
Purvarupa (premonitory symptoms)
Linga (actual symptoms)
Upashaya (exploratory therapy)
Samprapti (Pathogenesis). [6]

Definition of Nidana – causative factor:
तत्र निदानं कारणमित्युक्तमग्रे||७||
Nidana is already described to constitute the causative factors of diseases [7]

Definition of Purvarupa – Premonitory Symptoms:
पूर्वरूपं प्रागुत्पत्ति लक्षणं व्याधेः||८||
Symptoms which manifest themselves before the appearance of the disease (premonitory symptoms) are known as
Purva-Rupa [8]

Features of Lakshana:
प्रादुर्भूत लक्षणं पुनर्लिङ्गम्|
तत्र लिङ्गमाकृतिर्लक्षणं चिह्नं संस्थानं व्यञ्जनं रूपमित्यनर्थान्तरम्||९||
Symptoms when fully manifested are called Linga (Rupa).
Below mentioned are its synonyms –
Akrti
Lakshana
Chihna
Samsthana
Vyanjana
Rupa [9]

Definition of exploratory therapy:

उपशयः पुनर्हेतु व्याधि विपरीतानां विपरीतार्थकारिणां चौषधाहार विहाराणामुपयोगः सुखानुबन्धः||१०||

Such medicines, diets and regimens which bring about happiness (relief from disease) either by acting directly against the cause of the diseases, and or the disease itself or by producing such effects indirectly are called Upashaya (exploratory therapy). [10]

Synonyms of Pathogenesis:

सम्प्राप्तिर्जातिरागतिरित्यनर्थान्तरं व्याधे:||११||

These words are synonymous with the pathogenesis of a disease:

Samprapti

Jati

Agati [11]

Classification of Samprapti – pathogenesis:

सा सङ्ख्या प्राधान्य विधि विकल्प बल काल विशेषैर्भिद्यते|१२|

Samprapti is further classified depending upon certain specific characteristics like

Sankhya – the number of the types of disease,

Pradhanya – dominance of the other attributes of Doshas

Vidhi – variety of diseases

Vikalpa – predominance of one or the other fraction of the dosha / doshas in the (manifestation) of the disease.

Bala kala – the time of manifestation or aggravation of the disease [(1)]

Enumeration of disease:

सङ्ख्या तावद्यथा- अष्टौ ज्वराः, पञ्च गुल्माः, सप्त कुष्ठान्येवमादि:|१२|

The number of the (types of the) disease is responsible for the variation of the Samprapti for example-

8 types of Jvara (fever),

5 types of Gulma (abdominal tumour),

7 types of Kushta (obstinate skin diseases including leprosy) [(2)]

Degree of Doshic- vitiation:

प्राधान्यं पुनर्दोषाणां तरतमाभ्यामुपलभ्यते|

तत्र द्वयोस्तरः, त्रिषु तम इति|१२|

If 2 out of the 3 Doshas get vitiated, the comparative term, that is 'Tara'; is used to indicate the predominant one. If, however, all the 3 Doshas get vitiated then the superlative term 'Tama' is used to indicate the most predominant one. [(3)]

Variety of diseases:

विधिर्नाम- द्विविधा व्याधयो निजागन्तु भेदेन, त्रिविधास्त्रिदोषभेदेन, चतुर्विधाः साध्यासाध्यमृदुदारुणभेदेन|१२|

Vidhi or variety of diseases can be illustrated as below: - diseases are 2 varieties, they are –

Nija – exogenous or

Aagantu – endogenous;

On the basis of vitiation of Doshas they are of four varieties, they are –

Sadhya – curable

Asadhya – incurable

Mrudu – mild and

Daruna – acute. [(4)]

Definition of Vikalpa:

समवेतानां पुनर्दोषाणामंशांशबलविकल्पो विकल्पोऽस्मिन्नर्थे||१२|

Predominance of one or the other fraction of the 3 Doshas (in the manifestation of a disease) is known as Vikalpa in the present context. [5]

Time of manifestation of disease:

बल काल विशेषः पुन व्याधीनामृत्वहोरात्राहार काल विधि विनियतो भवति||१२||

Specific time for the aggravation and manifestation of diseases is determined on the basic of the variations in seasons, timings of the day, night and intake of food. [12]

Properly understanding of disease by the physician:

तस्माद्व्याधीन् भिषगनुपहत सत्व बुद्धिर्हेत्वादिभिर्भावैर्यथावदनुबुद्ध्येत||१३||

On the basis of these factors, the physician with the peace of mind and unimpaired intellect should understand the disease properly. [13]

Topics dealt within the section:

इत्यर्थ सङ्ग्रहो निदान स्थानस्योदिदिष्टो भवति|
तं विस्तरेणोपदिशन्तो भूयस्तरमतोऽनुव्याख्यास्यामः||१४||

The above are in brief the topics to be dealt with in this section 'Diagnosis of diseases' (Nidana sthana). They will again be elaborately discussed hereafter. [14]

Diagnosis and line of treatment of eight diseases:

तत्र प्रथमत एव तावदाद्याँल्लोभाभिद्रोह कोप प्रभवानष्टौ व्याधीन्निदानपूर्वेण क्रमेण व्याख्यास्यामः, तथा सूत्र सङ्ग्रहमात्रं चिकित्सायाः|
चिकित्सितेषु चोतरकालं यथोपचित विकाराननुव्याख्यास्यामः ||१५||

In the following paragraphs, we shall describe the diagnosis as well as the time of treatment of 8 diseases (of ancient times) which are manifested as a result of greed, enemity and anger in the order of the Nidana (causative factors etc.) Later, other diseases (along with those of this section) will be described. [15]

Priority of fever:

इह खलु ज्वर एवादौ विकाराणामुपदिश्यते, तत्प्रथमत्वाच्छारीराणाम्||१६||

Among the somatic diseases, Jvara (fever) appeared in the beginning: hence it is being described first. [16]

Jwara Nidana – Causative factors of fever:

अथ खल्वष्टाभ्यः कारणेभ्यो ज्वरः सञ्जायते मनुष्याणां; तद्यथा- वातात्, पित्तात्, कफात्, वातपित्ताभ्यां, वातकफाभ्यां, पित्तकफाभ्यां, वातपित्तकफेभ्यः, आगन्तोरष्टमात् कारणात्||१७||

The 8 factors responsible for the causation of fever in human beings are

Vata

Pitta

Kapha

Vata pitta

Vata-kapha

Pitta kapha

Vata pitta kapha and

Aagantuja – Extrinsic factors [17]

Specific factors of diseases:

तस्य निदान पूर्वरूप लिङ्गोपशय विशेषाननुव्याख्यास्यामः ||१८||

We shall now explain the Nidana (etiology), Purvarupa (premonitory symptoms), Linga (actual symptoms) and Upashaya (exploratory therapy) – all these factors as specific to the various types of this disease (jvara or fever). [18]

Causes of aggravation of vata:

रूक्ष लघु शीत वमन विरेचनास्थापन शिरोविरेचनातियोग व्यायाम वेगसन्धारणानशनाभिघात- व्यवायोद्वेग शोक शोणितातिषेकजागरण विषम शरीरन्यासेभ्योऽतिसेवितेभ्यो वायुः प्रकोपमापद्यते॥१९॥

Vata gets aggravated by the

Ruksha aahara – over indulgence and the intake of ununctuous

Laghu shita aahara – light and cold things

Ati vamana – over administration of emesis

Ati virechana – purgation

Asthapana type of enema

Ati shiro virechana – errhines

Vyayama – physical exercise

Vega sandharana – suppression of the natural urges

Anashana – fasting

Abhighata – assault

Vyavaya – sexual indulgence

Udvega – anxiety

Shoka – grief

Shonita atisheka – bloodletting in excess

Jagarana -vigil during the night and

Vishama sharira – by maintaining irregular posture. [19]

Pathogenesis of fever:

स यदा प्रकुपितः प्रविश्यामाशयमूष्मणा सह मिश्रीभूयाद्यमाहार परिणाम धातुं रसनामानमन्ववेत्य रसस्वेदवहानि स्रोतांसि पिधायाग्निमुपहत्य पक्तिस्थानादूष्माणं बहिर्निरस्य केवलं शरीरमनुप्रपद्यते, तदा ज्वरमभिनिर्वर्तयति॥२०॥

This aggravated Vata afflicts Amashaya (stomach including small intestine), gets mixed with Agni (enzymes responsible for digestion), follows the course of Rasa which is the first product after the transformation of food, obstructs the channels of Rasa and sweat, suppresses the activity of Agni (enzymes responsible for tissue metabolism), extradites the heat from the site of digestion and spreads it all over the body, thus causing Jvara (fever). [20]

Symptoms of Vataja Fever:

तस्येमानि लिङ्गानि भवन्ति; तद्यथा- विषमारम्भ विसर्गित्वम्, ऊष्मणो वैषम्यं, तीव्र तनुभावानवस्थानानि ज्वरस्य, जरणान्ते दिवसान्ते निशान्ते घर्मान्ते वा ज्वरस्याभ्यागमनमभिवृद्धिर्वा, विशेषेण परुषारुणवर्णत्वं नख नयन वदन मूत्र पुरीष त्वचामत्यर्थ क्लृप्तीभावश्च; अनेक विधोपमाश्चलाचलाश्च वेदनास्तेषां तेषामङ्गावयवानां; तद्यथा- पादयोः सुप्तता, पिण्डिकयोरुद्वेष्टनं, जानुनोः केवलानां च सन्धीनां विश्लेषणम्, ऊर्वोः सादः, कटी पार्श्व पृष्ठ स्कन्ध बाह्वंसोरसां च भग्न रुग्णमृदितमथितचटिताववपाटितावनुन्नत्वमिव, हन्वोश्चाप्रसिद्धिः, स्वनश्च कर्णयोः, शङ्खयोर्निस्तोदः, कषायास्यता आस्यवैरस्यं वा, मुख तालु कण्ठ शोषः, पिपासा, हृदयग्रहः, शुष्कच्छर्दिः, शुष्ककासः, क्षवथूद्गारविनिग्रहः, अन्नरसखेदः, प्रसेकारोचकविपाकाः, विषाद जृम्भा विनाम वेपथु श्रम भ्रम प्रलाप प्रजागर रोमहर्ष दन्तहर्षाः, उष्णाभिप्रायता, निदानोक्तानामनुपशयो विपरीतोपशयश्चेति वातज्वरस्य लिङ्गानि भवन्ति॥२१॥

Following are the symptoms of this type of fever:-

Vishamarambha visargitvam – Irregularity in onset and alleviation

Ushmano vaishamyam – Irregularity in temperature

Tīvra tanubhāvānavasthanāni jvarasya – Irregularity in the acuteness and mildness of fever

Jaraṇānte divasānte niśānte gharmānte vā jvarasyābhyāgamanamabhivṛddhirvā – Occurrence or aggravation of fever after the digestion of food in the afternoon during dawn or at the end of summer season

Viśeṣeṇa paruṣāruṇavarṇatvaṃ nakha nayana vadana mūtra purīṣa tvacāmatyarthaṃ klṛptībhāvaśca – Excessive roughness and reddishness of nail, eyes, face, urine, stool and skin.

Excessive retention of urine and stool

Occurrence of different types of fixed or shifting pain in various organs of the body.

For example

pādayoḥ suptatā -numbness in feet and piṇḍikayorudveṣṭanaṃ – cramps in calf

Jānunoḥ kevalānāṃ ca sandhīnāṃ viśleṣaṇam – feeling of looseness in knee joints as also in other joints

Urvoḥ sādaḥ – inactivity of thigh

kaṭī pārśva pṛṣṭha skandha bāhvaṃsorasāṃ ca bhagna rugṇamṛditamathitacaṭitāvapāṭitāvanunnatvamiva – Breaking, brushing, grinding, churning, cracking, bursting and twisting pain in waist, side, back, shoulder, arms, scapular region and chest

hanvoścāprasiddhiḥ – Stiffness of jaws

svanaśca karṇayoḥ – Noise in the ears

śaṅkhayornistodaḥ – Pain in temples

kaṣāyāsyatā āsyavairasyaṃ vā – Astringent taste in the mouth or dyspepsia

mukha tālu kaṇṭha śoṣaḥ – Dryness of mouth, palate and throat

pipāsā -Thirst

hṛdayagrahaḥ – Impairment of the functions of heart

śuṣkacchardiḥ – Dry vomiting

śuṣkakāsaḥ – Dry cough

kṣavathūdgāravinigrahaḥ – Suppression of sneezing and eructation

annarasakhedaḥ – Aversion to the taste of food

prasekārocakāvipākāḥ – Salivation, anorexia and indigestion

viṣāda jṛmbhā vināma vepathu śrama bhrama pralāpa prajāgara romaharṣa dantaharṣāḥ – Depression, yawning, flexion of the body, trembling, exhaustion, giddiness, delirium, sleeplessness, horripilation, tingling of the teeth

uṣṇābhiprāyatā – Liking for hot things

nidānoktānāmanupaśayo viparītopaśayaśceti – Aggravation of the condition by the administration of such things as are described to be its etiological factors and

Alleviation of the condition by the administration of such things is of opposite qualities to its etiological factors. [21]

Aggravation of Pitta, pathogenesis and symptoms of Paittika fever:

उष्णाम्ल लवण क्षार कटुकाजीर्णभोजनेभ्योऽतिसेवितेभ्यस्तथा तीक्ष्णातपाग्नि सन्ताप श्रम क्रोध विषमाहारेभ्यश्च पित्तं प्रकोपमापद्यते||२२||

तद्यदा प्रकुपितमामाशयादूष्माणमुपसृज्याद्यमाहार परिणाम धातुं रसनामानमन्ववेत्य रसस्वेदवहानि स्रोतांसि पिधाय द्रवत्वादग्निमुपहत्य पक्तिस्थानादूष्माणं बहिर्निरस्य प्रपीडयत् केवलं शरीरमनुप्रपद्यते, तदा ज्वरमभिनिर्वर्तयति||२३||

तस्येमानि लिङ्गानि भवन्ति; तद्यथा- युगपदेव केवले शरीरे ज्वरस्याभ्यागमनमभिवृद्धिर्वा भुक्तस्य विदाहकाले मध्यन्दिनेऽर्धरात्रे शरदि वा विशेषेण, कटुकास्यता, घ्राण मुख कण्ठौष्ठ तालु पाकः, तृष्णा, मदो, भ्रमो, मूर्च्छा, पित्तच्छर्दनम्, अतीसारः, अन्नद्वेषः, सदनं, खेदः, प्रलापः, रक्तकोठाभि निर्वृत्तिः शरीरे, हरितहारिद्रत्वं नख नयन वदन मूत्र पुरीष त्वचाम्, अत्यर्थमूष्मणस्तीव्रभावः, अतिमात्रं दाहः, शीताभिप्रायता, निदानोक्तानुपशयो विपरीतोपशयश्चेति पित्त ज्वर लिङ्गानि भवन्ति||२४||

Pitta gets aggravated by the excessive intake of

Ushna (hot),

Amla (sour),

Lavana (saline)

Ksara (alkaline)

Katu (pungent) food,

ājīrṇabhojanebhyo'tisevitebhyastathā – intake of meals while suffering from indigestion and exposure to scorching sun, heat of fire, exhaustion, anger and irregular dieting. This aggravated Pitta approaches the site of Agni in the Amashaya (stomach including small intestine), follows the path of Rasa which is the first product of food after transformation, obstructs the channels of circulation of Rasa and sweet, impairs Agni due to its liquidity, extradites Agni from the site of digestion, inflicts pressure and spreads all over the body, thus causing Jvara (fever).

Following are the symptoms of this type of fever (Pitta Jvara):

jvarasyābhyāgamanamabhivṛddhirvā bhuktasya vidāhakāle madhyandine'rdharātre śaradi vā viśeṣeṇa – Simultaneous manifestation or aggravation of fever in process of digestion, during the mid-day, mid-night and in the autumn

kaṭukāsyatā – Pungent taste in the mouth

ghrāṇa mukha kaṇṭhauṣṭha tālu pākaḥ – Inflammation of nose, mouth, throat, lips and Palate

tṛṣṇā – Thirst

Mada – intoxication

Bhrama -giddiness and

Murccha – fainting

pittacchardanam – Bilious vomiting

atīsāraḥ – diarrhoea

annadveṣaḥ – aversion for food

khedaḥ – Lassitude

Pralap – delirium

raktakoṭhābhi nirvṛttiḥ śarīre – Appearance of rashes urticaria in the body

haritahāridratvaṃ nakha nayana vadana mūtra purīṣa tvacām – Greenish or yellowish color of nails, eyes, face, urine, stool and skin

atyarthamūṣmaṇastīvrabhāvaḥ – Hyper pyrexia

atimātraṃ dāhaḥ – Excessive burning sensation

śītābhiprāyatā – Liking for cold things

nidānoktānupaśayo viparītopaśayaśceti – Aggravation of the condition by the administration of such things which are described to be its etiological factors and alleviation of the condition by the administration of such things which have opposite qualities to its etiological factors. [22-24]

Aggravation of Kaphaand Pathogenesis of Kaphajafever:

स्निग्ध गुरु मधुर पिच्छिल शीताम्ल लवण दिवास्वप्न हर्ष व्यायामेभ्योऽतिसेवितेभ्यः श्लेष्मा प्रकोपमापद्यते||२५||

स यदा प्रकुपितः प्रविश्यामाशयमूष्मणा सह मिश्रीभूयाद्यमाहार परिणामधातुं रसनामानमन्ववेत्य रस स्वेदवहानि सोतांसि पिधायाग्निमुपहत्य पक्तिस्थानादूष्माणं बहिर्निरस्य प्रपीडयन् केवलं शरीरमनुप्रपद्यते, तदा ज्वरमभिनिर्वर्तयति||२६||

Kapha gets aggravated by the excessive intake of

Snigdha (unctuous)

Guru (heavy)

Madhura (sweet)

Picchila (slimy)

Shita (cold)

Amla (sour) and

Lavana (saline) food

Diva svapna (sleep during day time)

Harsha (merriment) and

Avyayama (lack of physical exercise)

This aggravated Kapha enters the Amashaya (stomach including small intestine), gets mixed up with Agni (enzymes responsible for digestion), follows the course of Rasa which is the first product of food after transformation, obstructs the channels of circulation of Rasa and sweet, suppresses the activity of Agni (enzymes responsible for tissue metabolism) extradites heat from the site of digestion, inflicts pressure and spreads it all over the body thus causing Jvara (fever). [25-26]

Symptoms of Kaphaja fever:

तस्येमानि लिङ्गानि भवन्ति; तद्यथा- युगपदेव केवले शरीरे ज्वरस्याभ्यागमनमभिवृद्धिर्वा भुक्तमात्रे पूर्वाह्णे पूर्वरात्रे वसन्तकाले वा विशेषेण, गुरुगात्रत्वम्, अनन्नाभिलाषः, श्लेष्मप्रसेकः, मुखमाधुर्य, हल्लासः, हृदयोपलेपः, स्तिमितत्वं, छर्दिः, मृद्वग्निता, निद्राधिक्यं, स्तम्भः, तन्द्रा, कासः, श्वासः, प्रतिश्यायः, शैत्यं, श्वैत्यं च नख नयन वदन मूत्र पुरीषत्वचाम्, अत्यर्थं च शीत पिडका भृशमङ्गेभ्य उतिष्ठन्ति, उष्णाभिप्रायता, निदानोक्तानुपशयो विपरीतोपशयश्च; इति (श्लेष्मज्वरलिङ्गानि भवन्ति)||२७||

Following are the symptoms of Kapha Jvara:

yugapadeva kevale śarīre jvarasyābhyāgamanamabhivṛddhirvā bhuktamātre pūrvāhṇe pūrvarātre vasantakāle vā viśeṣeṇa – Simultaneous manifestation or aggravation of fever in the entire body specifically immediately after- food, during the fore-noon, in the evening and during the spring season.

Guru gātratvam – Heaviness of the body

Anannābhilāṣaḥ – loss of appetite

śleṣma prasekaḥ – salivation

Mukha mādhuryam – sweet taste in the mouth

Hṛllāsaḥ – nausea

Hṛdayopalepaḥ – bradycardia

Stimitatvam – timidness and

Chardiḥ – vomiting

Mṛdvagnitā – Reduced power of digestion

Nidrādhikyam – excessive sleep

Stambhaḥ – stiffness

Tandra – drowsiness

Kāsaḥ – cough

Svasah – dysponea and

Pratishyaya – coryza

Shaitya – Feeling of cold

śvaityam ca nakha nayana vadana mūtra purīṣatvacām – White color of nails, eyes, face, urine, stool and skin

atyartham ca śīta piḍakā bhṛṣamaṅgebhya uttiṣṭhanti – Frequent appearance of large number of cold pimples in the body.

uṣṇābhiprāyatā – Liking for hot things

nidānoktānupaśayo viparītopaśayaśca – Aggravation of the condition by the administration of such things which are described to be its etiological factors and alleviation of the condition by the administration of such things which have qualities opposite to its etiological factors [27]

Etiological factors to aggravate all the Doshas:

विषमाशनादनशनादन्न परिवर्तादृतुव्यापत्तेर सात्म्य गन्धोपघ्राणादिविषोपहतस्य चोदकस्योपयोगाद्गरेभ्यो गिरीणां चोपश्लेषात् स्नेह स्वेद वमन विरेचनास्थापनानुवासन शिरोविरेचनानामयथावत्प्रयोगात् मिथ्यासंसर्जनाद्वा स्त्रीणां च विषम प्रजननात् प्रजातानां च मिथ्योपचाराद् यथोक्तानां च हेतूनां मिश्रीभावाद्यथानिदानं द्वन्द्वानामन्यतमः सर्वे वा त्रयो दोषा युगपत् प्रकोपमापद्यन्ते, ते प्रकुपितास्तयैवानुपूर्व्या ज्वरमभिनिर्वर्तयन्ति||२८||

Either 2 or all 3 Doshas in the body get aggravated all at a time- because of the combination of the etiological factors described earlier (paragraph nos 21, 24, 27) or due to the following :

Vishamashana – irregular dieting

Anashana -fasting sudden change in the food habit without following the proper procedure prescribed for it, seasonal vagaries,

Gandhopa ghrana advisho apahatasya – inhalation of substances having unwholesome smell, intake of poisonous water, habitation near poisonous (artificial) material or mountain, improper administration of oleation , fomentation, Emesis, Purgation, Asthapana, and Anuvasana types of enema and errhines,

giving improper diet after the administration of Panchakarma therapy, improper child delivery and resorting, to the aggravated Doshas manifest Jvaras due to the simultaneous vitiation of 2 Doshas or all 3 doshas. [28]

Simultaneous vitiation of doshas:

तत्र तथोक्तानां ज्वर लिङ्गानां मिश्रीभाव विशेष दर्शनाद्द्वान्दिवकमन्यतमं ज्वरं सान्निपातिकं वा विद्यात्||२९||

Symptoms of fever-due to simultaneous vitiation of the 3 doshas (as described in Para 21, 21& 27) combine in different modes to constitute the symptoms of fever due to the simultaneous vitiation of 2 Doshas, viz,Vatapitta Vatakapha and Kaphapitta or Sannipata (3 Doshas) [29]

Causes of exogenous fever:

अभिघाताभिषङ्गाभिचाराभिशापेभ्य आगन्तुर्हि व्यथापूर्वोऽष्टमो ज्वरो भवति|

स किञ्चित्कालमागन्तुः केवलो भूत्वा पश्चाद्दोषैरनुबध्यते|

तत्राभिघातजो वायुना दुष्ट शोणिताधिष्ठानेन, अभिषङ्गजः पुनर्वातपित्ताभ्याम्, अभिचाराभिशापजौ तु सन्निपातेनानुबध्येते||३०||

The exogenenous one (Agantu) caused due to assault (by staff etc) emotions, (like libido etc.) spell, (by the incantations prescribed by the Atharvan etc) and imprecations (of preceptors and those who have attained spiritual perfection) are the 8 types of fever. These are preceded with pain. For some time, it remains exclusively exogenous and afterwards becomes associated with Doshas. The exogenous fever caused by assault is associated with Vata having its abode in the vitiated Vata and Pitta. The exogenous type of fever caused by spell and imprecation is associated with the vitiated Vata, Pitta and Kapha- all the 3 Doshas. [30]

Characteristic of exogenous fever and line of treatment:

स सप्तविधाज्ज्वरादिविशिष्ट लिङ्गोपक्रम समुत्थानत्वादिविशिष्टो वेदितव्यः, कर्मणा साधारणेन चोपचर्यते |

इत्यष्टविधा ज्वर प्रकृतिरुक्ता||३१||

The exogenous type of fever is different from the other 7 types because of its specific symptoms, line of treatment and aetiology. This is treated with spiritual therapy like oblation, auspicious acts and Yajna, and other forms of rational therapy like fasting, intake of light diet, gruel and decoction. Thus, the characteristic features of 8 types of fever are described. [31]

Various types of Fever:

ज्वरस्त्वेक एव सन्ताप लक्षणः|

तमेवाभिप्रायविशेषादिद्विविधमाचक्षते, निजागन्तु विशेषाच्च|

तत्र निजं द्विविधं त्रिविधं चतुर्विधं सप्त विधं चाहुर्भिषजो वातादिविकल्पात्||३२||

Jvara (fever) is of 1 type only characterized by Hyperpyrexia.

They are of 2 types depending upon the craving of the patient for hot or cold things.

Similarly as exogenous and endogenous it is of 2 types. In an endogenous type of fever only 1 Dosha or a combination of Doshas may take part in the pathogenesis and as such it is of 2 types. This is also of 2 types depending upon the craving of the patient for hot or cold things. This is of 3 types with Doshas viz. Vata, Pitta, Kapha taking part in the pathogenesis of the disease.

This is once again of 4 types viz – Vatika, Paittika, Slaishmika and Sannipatika (combination of all 3 Dosha)

This is also of 7 types, Viz

Vatika

Paittika

Slasimika
Vata paittika
Pitta slaismika
Vata slaismika
Sannipatika.
All these classifications are based on the permutation and combination of various Doshas. [32]

Jwara Poorva Roopa :

तस्येमानि पूर्वरूपाणि भवन्ति; तद्यथा- मुखवैरस्यं, गुरुगात्रत्वम्, अनन्नाभिलाषः, चक्षुषोराकुलत्वम्, अश्रवागमनं, निद्राधिक्यम्, अरतिः, जृम्भा, विनामः, वेपथुः, श्रम भ्रम प्रलाप जागरणरोमहर्ष दन्तहर्षाः, शब्द शीत वातातप सहत्वासहत्वम्, अरोचकाविपाकौ, दौर्बल्यम्, अङ्गमर्दः, सदनम्, अल्पप्राणता, दीर्घसूत्रता, आलस्यम्, उचितस्य कर्मणो हानिः, प्रतीपता स्वकार्येषु, गुरूणां वाक्येष्वभ्यसूया, बालेभ्यः प्रद्वेषः, स्वधर्मेष्वचिन्ता, माल्यानुलेपनभोजन परिक्लेशनं, मधुरेभ्यश्च भक्षेभ्यः प्रद्वेषः, अम्ल लवण कटुक प्रियता च, इति ज्वरस्य पूर्वरूपाणि भवन्ति प्राक्सन्तापात्; अपि चैनं सन्तापार्तमनुबध्नन्ति॥३३॥

Premonitory symptoms of fever:
The premonitory symptoms of Jvara (fever) are
Mukha vairasyam – dyspepsia
Guru gatratvam – heaviness in body
Anannābhilāṣaḥ – loss of appetite
Cakṣuṣorākulatvam – congestion in the eyes
Aśrvāgamanaṃ – Lacrimation
Nidrādhikyam – excessive sleep
Aratiḥ – disliking for work
Jrmbha – yawning
Vināmaḥ – flexion
Vepathuḥ – tremors
Shrama – exhaustion
Bhrama – giddiness
Pralapa – delirium
Jagarana – sleeplessness
Roma harsha – horripilation
Dantaharṣāḥ – sensitiveness / tingling of the teeth
Sabda śīta vātātapa sahatvāsahatvam – wavering liking and disliking of sound , cold, wind and sun;
Arochaka – anorexia
Vipaka – indigestion
Daurbalya – weakness
Anga marda – malaise
Sadanam – lassitude
Alpa pranata – low-vitality
Dīrghasūtratā – dilatory tendency
Ālasyam – laziness
Ucitasya karmaṇo hāniḥ – loss of regular functions
Pratīpatā svakāryeṣu – aversion to work
Gurūṇāṃ vākyeṣvabhyasūyā – disregard for instructions of preceptors (superiors)
Mālyānulepanabhojana parikleśanaṃ – disliking for the use of garland, ointment and food
Madhurebhyaśca bhakṣebhyaḥ pradveṣaḥ – aversion to sweet food, liking four sour, saline and pungent foods.
All these premonitory symptoms appear before the onset of hyperpyrexia. Some of these symptoms also continue to

exist during the period of hyperpyrexia. [33]

Brief description of fever:

इत्येतान्येकैकशो ज्वर लिङ्गानि व्याख्यातानि भवन्ति विस्तर समासाभ्याम्||३४||

Thus the etiology, premonitory symptoms, symptoms, pathogenesis etc. of Vatika, Paittika and Slaismika type of Jvara have been described in detail: those of Dvandvaja (due to the simultaneous vitiation of 2 dosha) and Sannipatika (due to the simultaneous vitiation of 3 Doshas) are also described in brief. [34]

Mythological origin of fever and its effects:

ज्वरस्तु खलु महेश्वरकोपप्रभवः, सर्वप्राणभृतां प्राणहरो, देहेन्द्रियमनस्तापकरः, प्रज्ञा बल वर्ण हर्षोत्साह ह्रासकरः, श्रम क्लम मोहाहारोपरोध सञ्जननः; ज्वरयति शरीराणीति ज्वरः, नान्ये व्याधयस्तथा दारुणा बहूपद्रवा दुश्चिकित्स्याश्च यथाऽयम्|

स सर्वरोगाधिपतिः, नानातिर्यग्योनिषु च बहुविधैः शब्दैरभिधीयते|

सर्वे प्राणभृतः सज्वरा एव जायन्ते सज्वरा एव म्रियन्ते च; स महामोहः, तेनाभिभूताः प्राग्दैहिकं देहिनः कर्म किञ्चिदपि न स्मरन्ति, सर्वप्राणभृतां च ज्वर एवान्ते प्राणानादत्ते||३५||

Jvara (fever) is an outcome of the wrath of Mahesvara. It leads to the death of all living beings. It afflicts with misery the body (by producing heat), senses and mind.

It diminishes the

Prajna – intelligence

Bala -strength

Varna – complexion

Harsha – joyfulness and

Utsaha – enthusiasm

It produces

Shrama – exhaustion

Klama – exertion

Moha – unconsciousness

Aparodha – obstruction to food.

It is known as jvara because it brings miseries to the body (jvarayati= to bring misery). No other disease is so serious, so complicated and as difficult to cure as Jvara (fever). This is the king of all diseases and in animals it is known differently (by different names). All living beings are unable to remember anything of their past life. In the end, it is Jvara who takes away life. [35]

Jwara Chikitsa Sutra – Line of treatment:

तत्र पूर्वरूप दर्शने ज्वरादौ वा हितं लघ्वशनमपतर्पणं वा, ज्वरस्यामाशयसमुत्थत्वात्; ततः कषायपानाभ्यङ्ग स्नेह स्वेद प्रदेह परिषेकानुलेपन वमन विरेचनास्थापनानुवासनोपशमन- नस्तःकर्म धूप धूमपानाञ्जन क्षीरभोजन विधानं च यथास्वं युक्त्या प्रयोज्यम्||३६||

During the stage of Purvarupa (premonitory symptoms) or in the primary stage of Jvara (fever), intake of Laghvashana (light food) or Apartarpanam (fasting) is useful because Amashaya (stomach including small intestine) is the site of the origin of this disease. Thereafter, depending upon the Dosha involved and the therapeutic property, the patient is administered

Kashaya – decoction

Pana – drink

Abhyanga – unction

Sneha – oleation (therapy)

Sveda – fomentation

Pradeha – ointment

Parisheka – bath

Anulepana – application of pasted medicine

Vamana – emesis
Virechana – purgation
Asthapana type of enema
Shamana – alleviation therapy
Nasya karma – inhalation
Dhupana -smoking
Anjana – collyrium
Kshira bhojana – milk preparations [36]

Use of ghee in fever:
जीर्णज्वरेषु तु सर्वेष्वेव सर्पिषः पानं प्रशस्यते यथास्वौषधसिद्धस्य; सर्पिर्हि स्नेहाद्वातं शमयति, संस्कारात् कफं, शैत्यात् पितमूष्माणं च; तस्माज्जीर्णज्वरेषु सर्वेष्वेव सर्पिर्हितमुदकमिवाग्निप्लुष्टेषु द्रव्येष्विति||३७||
भवन्ति चात्र- यथा प्रज्वलितं वेश्म परिषिञ्चन्ति वारिणा|
नराः शान्तिमभिप्रेत्य तथा जीर्णज्वरे घृतम्||३८||
स्नेहाद्वातं शमयति, शैत्यात् पित्तं नियच्छति|
घृतं तुल्यगुणं दोषं संस्कारात् जयेत् कफम्||३९||
नान्यः स्नेहस्तथा कश्चित् संस्कारमनुवर्तते|
यथा सर्पिरतः सर्पिः सर्वस्नेहोत्तमं मतम्||४०||
In all the types of chronic fever, intake of ghee is beneficial. This ghee may however, be prepared by boiling with such drugs as would help alleviatethe particular Dosha(s) involved. Vata is alleviated by ghee due to the latter's unctuousness, Kapha due to the method of preparation (with drugs like those having pungent and bitter taste, which alleviate Kapha) and Pitta and hyperpyrexia due to coldness, thus, as water is useful for things burnt with fire, so also ghee is beneficial in all types of chronic fever (because it acts both against disease as well as the Doshas involved).

Thus it is said: – as people spray water over a house set on fire, so also ghee is used with a view to alleviate chronic jvara.

Vata is alleviated due to the latter's unctuousness, Pitta due to coldness and even Kapha which has identical properties (with ghee) due to suitable method of preparation. No other thing so carries the properties of drugs with which it is processed as ghee, hence ghee is considered to be the fat par excellence. [37- 40]

Clarification regarding repetition:
गद्योक्तो यः पुनः श्लोकैरर्थः समनुगीयते|
तद्व्यक्तिव्यवसायार्थं द्विरुक्तं तन्न गर्ह्यते||४१||
It is only for the clarity that something already stated in prose is again repeated in verse. This kind of repetition does not constitute any defect. [41]

Brief description:
तत्र श्लोकाः:- त्रिविधं नामपर्यायैर्हेतुं पञ्चविधं गदम्|
गदलक्षणपर्यायान् व्याधेः पञ्चविधं ग्रहम्||४२||
ज्वरमष्टविधं तस्य प्रकृष्टासन्नकारणम्|
पूर्वरूपं च रूपं च भेषजं सङ्ग्रहेण च||४३||
व्याजहार ज्वरस्याग्रे निदाने विगतज्वरः|
भगवानग्निवेशाय प्रणताय पुनर्वसुः||४४||
The varieties of etiological factors and their synonyms, the 5-fold classification of disease and its synonyms, 5 factors for the diagnosis of diseases, 8 types of fever, its distant and immediate causes, its premonitory symptoms,

actual symptoms, and treatment in brief- all these were explained to Lord Agnivesha by the enlightened one-Lord Punarvasu. [42- 44]

इत्यग्निवेशकृते तन्त्रे चरक प्रतिसंस्कृते निदान स्थाने ज्वरनिदानं नाम प्रथमोऽध्यायः||१||
Thus ends the first chapter on the "Diagnosis of fever" of the Nidana section of Agnivesha's work as redacted by Charaka.

इत्यग्निवेशकृते तन्त्रे चरक प्रतिसंस्कृते निदान स्थाने ज्वरनिदानं नाम प्रथमोऽध्यायः||१||

2

Nidanasthana Chapter 2 Raktapitta Nidanam

The 2nd chapter of Charaka Samhita Nidana Sthana is called Raktapitta Nidana. It deals with causes, pathology, types and symptoms of Rakthapitta as per Ayurveda.

अथातो रक्तपित्त निदानं व्याख्यास्यामः||१||

इति ह स्माह भगवानात्रेयः||२||

We shall now explore the chapter on the "diagnosis of raktapitta" (a disease characterized by bleeding from various parts of the body). Thus said Lord Atreya [1-2]

Pathology responsible for Rakthapitta:

पित्तं यथाभूतं लोहित पित्तमिति सञ्ज्ञां लभते, तद् व्याख्यास्यामः||३||

We shall now explain the pathological changes of Pitta in the manifestation of raktha pitta [3]

Raktapitta Nidana and Samprapti:

यदा जन्तुर्यव कोद्दालक कोरदूष प्रायाण्यन्नानि भुङ्क्ते, भृशोष्ण तीक्ष्णमपि चान्यदन्नजातं निष्पाव माष कुलत्थ सूप क्षारोपसंहितं, दधि दधिमण्डोदश्वित्कट्वराम्ल काञ्जिकोपसेकं वा, वाराह माहिषाविक मात्स्य गव्य पिशितं, पिण्याक पिण्डालु शुष्क शाकोपहितं, मूलक सर्षप लशुन करञ्ज शिग्रु मधुशिग्रु(खडयूष) भूस्तृण सुमुख सुरस कुठेरक गण्डीरकालमालकपर्णास क्षवक फणिज्झकोपदंशं, सुरा सौवीर तुषोदक मैरेय मेदक मधूलक शुक्त कुवल बदराम्ल प्रायानुपानं वा, पिष्टान्नोत्तरभूयिष्ठम्; उष्णाभितप्तो वातिमात्रमतिवेलं वाऽऽमं पयः पिबति, पयसा समश्नाति रौहिणीकं, काण कपोतं वा सर्षप तैल क्षार सिद्धं, कुलत्थ पिण्याक जाम्ब वलकुचपक्वैः शौक्तिकैर्वा सह क्षीरं पिबत्युष्णाभितप्तः; तस्यैवमाचरतः पित्तं प्रकोपमापद्यते, लोहितं चस्वप्रमाणमतिवर्तते|

तस्मिन् प्रमाणातिवृत्ते पित्तं प्रकुपितं शरीरमनुसर्पद्येव यकृत्प्लीह प्रभवाणां लोहितवहानां च स्रोतसां लोहिताभिष्यन्दगुरूणि मुखान्यासाद्य प्रतिरुन्ध्यात् तदेव लोहितं दूषयति||४||

Causes and pathogenesis of Rakthapitta:

Pitta gets aggravated and Rakta (blood) exceeds its normal quantity due to the following:

Intake of food mostly containing yavaka (a type of hordeum vulgare linn).

Uddalaka and koradusa (paspalum scrobiculalum linn) and such other food products as par excessively hot and sharp along with foods like nispava (a type of dolichos trilobus linn), masha (phaseolus rasiatus linn),

Kulattha – horse gram and alkalies or mixed with curd, whey, udasvit (a mixture of water and butter milk in equal quantity), katvara (sour butter milk) and sour congee:

vārāha māhiṣāvika mātsya gavya piśitaṃ – Intake of the meat of pig, buffalo, sheep, fish and cow, mixed with oil cake, piṇyāka piṇḍālu śuṣka śākopahitaṃ – pindalu (a tuber), dry vegetable or

– taking radish, mustard, garlic, karanja (Pongamia pinnata), sigru (Moringa oleifera lam), madhusigru (a type of Moringa oleifera lam), khabadayusa (vide commentary), bhustrna (Cymbopogom citratuus stapf), varieties of basil, viz sumukha, sarosa, kutheraka gandiraka, alamala, parnasa, phanijjhaka or followed by sura, sauvira, tusodaka, maireya, madhulaka and sukta types of wine, sour preparations of kuvala (Zizyphus sativa gaertn) and badara (Zizyphus jujuba)

piṣṭānnottarabhūyiṣṭham – Intake of pastries in excess after food.
Frequent intake of un-boiled milk in excess while getting exposed to heat
payasā samaśnāti rauhiṇīkam – Intake of vegetable of rohinika (Picrorhiza kurroa royle ex benth) with milk
kāṇa kapotaṃ vā sarṣapa taila kṣāra siddhaṃ – Intake of small pigeon boiled with mustard oil or alkalies and
Intake of milk with kulattha (Dolichos biflorus linn) oil cake ripe fruit of jambu (Syzygium cumini skeels) lakuca (Artocarpus lakoocha roxb) or badara (Zizyphus jujuba) while exposed to heat.

Raktapit Samprapti:
When the rakta exceeds its normal quantity, it results in the opening of the entrances of channels of circulation which originate from spleen and liver. The aggravated fraction of pitta enters into these channels while circulating in the body and obstructs them resulting in the vitiation of blood. [4]

Definitions of Raktapitta:
संसर्गाल्लोहित प्रदूषणाल्लोहित गन्धवर्णानुविधानाच्च पितं लोहित पित्तमित्याचक्षते॥७॥
The disease is called rakthapitta because pitta comes into contact with and vitiates rakta and also because it acquires the smell and color of the latter (blood). [5]

Raktapitta – Poorvaroopa –
तस्येमानि पूर्वरूपाणि भवन्ति; तद्यथा- अनन्नाभिलाषः, भुक्तस्य विदाहः, शुक्ताम्ल गन्ध रस उद्गारः, छर्देरभीक्ष्णमागमनं, छर्दितस्य बीभत्सता, स्वरभेदो, गात्राणां सदनं, परिदाहः, मुखाद्धूमागम इव, लोह लोहित मत्स्यामगन्धित्वमिव चास्यस्य, रक्त हरित हारिद्रत्वमङ्गाव यव शकृन्मूत्रस्वेद लाला सिङ्घाणकास्य कर्ण मल पिडकोलिका पिडकानाम्, अङ्गवेदना, लोहित नील पीत श्यावानामर्चिष्मतां च रूपाणां स्वप्ने दर्शनमभीक्ष्णमिति (लोहितपित्तपूर्वरूपाणि भवन्ति) ॥६॥

Premonitory symptoms of Raktapitta are:
Anannābhilāṣaḥ – loss of appetite
Bhuktasya vidāhaḥ – improper digestion of food resulting in the burning sensation in chest
Shuktāmla gandha rasa udgāraḥ – eructation having sour taste and smell like vinegar
Charderabhīkṣṇamāgamanaṃ – frequent urge for vomiting
Charditasya bībhatsatā – discoloration and foul smell of vomited material
Svarabhedo – hoarseness of voice
Gātrāṇāṃ sadanaṃ – prostration of the body
Mukhāddhūmāgama iva – burning sensation all over the body, a sensation as if smoke is coming out of the mouth;
Loha lohita matsyāmagandhitvamiva cāsyasya – smell of meal, blood, fish and raw flesh in the mouth
Rakta harita hāridratvamaṅgāva yava śakṛnmūtrasveda lālā siṅghāṇakāsya karṇa mala piḍakolikā piḍakānām – Red, green and yellow coloration of different organs of the body, stool, urine, saliva, excreta from nose, mouth, ear and eyes and appearance of pimples;
Anga vedanam – Body ache,
Lohita nīla pīta śyāvānāmarciṣmatāṃ ca rūpāṇāṃ svapne darśanamabhīkṣṇamiti lohitapittapūrvarūpāṇi – frequent dreams of such objects as are red, blue, yellow and brown in color and dazzling.
These are the premonitory symptoms of Raktha pitta [6]

Complication of Rakthapitta:

उपद्रवास्तु खलु दौर्बल्यारोचकाविपाक श्वास कास ज्वरातीसार शोफ शोष पाण्डुरोगाः स्वरभेदश्च||७||

Complications of rakthapitta are

Daurbalya – weakness

Arochaka – anorexia

Avipaka – indigestion

Shvasa – dyspnoea

Kasa – cough

Jvara – fever

Atisara – diarrhea

Sopha – oedema

Sosha – consumption

Pandu – anemia and

Svara bheda – hoarseness of voice [7]

Pathways of disease of its prognosis:

मार्गौ पुनरस्य द्वौ ऊर्ध्व, चाधश्च|

तद्बहुश्लेष्मणि शरीरे श्लेष्म संसर्गादूर्ध्व प्रतिपद्यमानं कर्ण नासिका नेत्रास्येभ्यः प्रच्यवते, बहुवाते तु शरीरे वात संसर्गादधः प्रतिपद्यमानं मूत्र पुरीष मार्गाभ्यां प्रच्यवते, बहुश्लेष्मवाते तु शरीरे श्लेष्म वात संसर्गाद्द्वावपि मार्गौ प्रतिपद्यते, तौ मार्गौ प्रतिपद्यमानं सर्वेभ्य एव यथोक्तेभ्यः खेभ्यः प्रच्यवते शरीरस्य||८||

तत्र यदूर्ध्वभागं तत् साध्यं, विरेचनोपक्रमणीयत्वाद्बह्वौषधत्वाच्च; यदधोभागं तद्याप्यं, वमनोपक्रमणीयत्वादल्पौषधत्वाच्च; यदुभयभागं तदसाध्यं, वमन विरेचनायोगित्वादनौषधत्वाच्चेति||९||

This disease manifests itself in 2 ways –

Urdhvaṃ – Either through upper tracks or

Adhah – Through the lower tracks

tadbahuśleṣmaṇi śarīre śleṣma saṃsargādūrdhvaṃ pratipadyamānaṃ karṇa nāsikā netrāsyebhyaḥ pracyavate – In a patient having the dominance of kapha in his body, the disease manifests itself in (blood come out through) the upper tracks, viz, ear, nose, eyes and mouth due to the contact with kapha.

bahuvāte tu śarīre vāta saṃsargādadhaḥ pratipadyamānaṃ mūtra purīṣa mārgābhyāṃ pracyavate – In a patient whose body is dominated by vata, the disease manifests itself in (blood comes out through) the lower tracks, viz, the urethra and anus due to the contact with vata.

bahuśleṣmavāte tu śarīre śleṣma vāta saṃsargāddvāvapi mārgau pratipadyate – In a patient whose body is dominated with both by kapha and vata, the disease manifests itself through both the tracks enumerated above due to the contact with both kapha and vata.

Urdhvaga Raktapitta – where the upper tracks are afflicted is curable because of its amenability to purgation therapy and also because varieties of drugs available for the treatment of this condition.

Adhoga Raktapitta – where the lower tracks are afflicted are palliable because of its amenability to emetic therapy and also because of the limited varieties of drugs are available for the treatment of this condition.

Ubhayaga Raktapitta – The third type where both the upper and lower tracks are afflicted is incurable because it is neither amenable to purgation nor to emetic therapy and no medicine is suitable for the treatment of this condition. [8-9]

Episode regarding the manifestation of disease:

रक्त पित्त प्रकोपस्तु खलु पुरा दक्ष यज्ञोद्ध्वंसे रुद्र कोपामर्षाग्निना प्राणिनां परिगत शरीर प्राणानामभवज्ज्वरमनु||१०||

In times of yore, here arose the fire of wrath of lord Rudra during the destruction of Dakshas sacrifice. The body and Prana of living beings got heated by this fire. This resulted in the manifestation of jvara followed by raktha pitta. [10]

Raktapitta Chikitsa based on chronicity:
तस्याशुकारिणो दावाग्नेरिवापतितस्यात्ययिकस्याशु प्रशान्त्यै प्रयतितव्यं मात्रां देशं कालं चाभिसमीक्ष्य सन्तर्पणेनापतर्पणेन वा मृदु मधुर शिशिर तिक्त कषायैरभ्यवहार्यैः प्रदेह परिषेकावगाह संस्पर्शनैर्वमनाद्यैर्वा तत्रावहितेनेति॥११॥

This acute disease which spreads like forest fire is treated immediately and carefully, keeping in view the locality and time, with diets which are nourishing or depleting, soft, sweet, cold, bitter and astringent and also with such therapies like anointment, affusion, touch (of pearls etc.,) or emesis etc. [11]

Therapy-wise prognosis:
भवन्ति चात्र- साध्यं लोहित पित्तं तद्यद्यूर्ध्वं प्रतिपद्यते।
विरेचनस्य योगित्वाद्बहुत्वाद्भेषजस्य च॥१२॥
विरेचनं तु पित्तस्य जयार्थे परमौषधम्।
यश्च तत्रान्वयः श्लेष्मा तस्य चानधमं स्मृतम्॥१३॥
भवेद्योगावहं तत्र मधुरं चैव भेषजम्।
तस्मात् साध्यं मतं रक्तं यदूर्ध्वं प्रतिपद्यते॥१४॥

Thus, it is said:
Raktapitta afflicting the upper tracks is curable because it is amenable to purgation therapy and also because there are varieties of drugs available for its treatment.
Purgation is the best therapy for alleviating pitta and it also alleviates kapha.
Purgation further is an appropriate therapy for the cure of this disease. Drugs having sweet taste are also useful for this condition; hence this type of raktha pitta is curable. [12-14]

Nature of prognosis:
रक्तं तु यदधोभागं तद्याप्यमिति निश्चितम्।
वमनस्याल्पयोगित्वादल्पत्वाद्भेषजस्य च॥१५॥
वमनं हि न पित्तस्य हरणे श्रेष्ठमुच्यते।
यश्च तत्रान्वयो वायुस्तच्छान्तौ चावरं स्मृतम्॥१६॥
तच्चायोगावहं तत्र कषायं तिक्तकानि च।
तस्माद्याप्यं समाख्यातं यदुक्तमनुलोमगम्॥१७॥

Nature of prognosis: Rakthapitta affecting the lower tracks is certainly palliable because emetic (which is otherwise useful for alleviating this type of disease) is not very useful (because of certain reasons) and there are only limited types of drugs which are useful for the treatment of this condition. Emesis is not a very effective therapy for alleviation of the vitiated pitta. For the vitiated vata which is also associated with pitta in the pathogenesis of this disease, emetic therapy is least useful. Along with emesis drugs having astringent and bitter tastes are also not useful since they also vitiate vata. Therefore, rakthapitta affecting the lower tracks of the body is considered to be palliable. [15-17]

Prognosis of raktapitta depending upon affected channels:
रक्तपित्तं तु यन्मार्गौ द्वावपि प्रतिपद्यते।
असाध्यमिति तज्ज्ञेयं पूर्वोक्तादेव कारणात्॥१८॥
नहि संशोधनं किञ्चिदस्त्यस्य प्रतिमार्गगम्।
प्रतिमार्ग च हरणं रक्तपित्ते विधीयते॥१९॥

एवमेवोपशमनं सर्वशो नास्य विद्यते।
संसृष्टेषु च दोषेषु सर्वजिच्छमनं मतम्॥२०॥
इत्युक्तं त्रिविधोदर्कं रक्तं मार्गविशेषतः।२१।

Because of the reason mentioned before, rakthapitta affecting both the upward and downward tracks is incurable. The principle of treatment of raktapitta is to administer such therapies as would counteract the direction of bleeding. There is no such elimination therapy as the world produces such action in this type of rakthapitta. Further, in this type, all the 3 doshas are vitiated and there is little medicine which will alleviate all the 3 doshas. Thus, the prognosis of rakthapitta depending upon the channels affected is described. [18-20]

Causes of incurability of diseases:

एभ्यस्तु खलु हेतुभ्यः किञ्चित्साध्यं न सिध्यति॥२१॥
प्रेष्योपकरणाभावाद्दौरात्म्याद्वैद्यदोषतः।
अकर्मतश्च साध्यत्वं कश्चिद्रोगोऽतिवर्तते॥२२॥
तत्रासाध्यत्वमेकं स्यात् साध्ययाप्यपरिक्रमात्॥२३।

Causes of incurability of diseases: even same of the curable disease become incurable due to the following:

Lack of proper attendance and equipment

Lack of self- control in the patient

Incompetence of the physician

Lack of proper treatment or existence of past sinful acts of the patient which leads to the incurability of diseases

Besides, change in the course of the disease is the symptom par excellence indicative of the incurability of raktapitta. [21-22]

Asadhya Raktapitta:

रक्तपित्तस्य विज्ञानमिदं तस्योपदिश्यते॥२३॥
यत् कृष्णमथवा नीलं यद्वा शक्रधनुष्प्रभम्।
रक्तपित्तमसाध्यं तद्वाससो रञ्जनं च यत्॥२४॥
भृशं पूत्यतिमात्रं च सर्वोपद्रववच्च यत्।
बलमांसक्षये यच्च तच्च रक्तमसिद्धिमत्॥२५॥
येन चोपहतो रक्तं रक्तपित्तेन मानवः।
पश्येद्दृश्यं वियच्चापि तच्चासाध्यं न संशयः॥२६॥

The following signs and symptoms of incurable raktha pitta:

kṛṣṇamathavā nīlaṃ yadvā śakradhanuṣprabham – Discharge of blood having black, blue or rainbow colour whose stain on cloth does not get cleaned even after washing

Discharge of putrefied blood in excess

Excessive manifestation of all the complications

Diminution of strength and muscle tissue and

paśyeddṛśyaṃ viyaccāpi taccāsādhyaṃ na saṃśayaḥ- red vision in relation to sights in general and sky in particular [23-26]

Principles of treatment:

तत्रासाध्यं परित्याज्यं, याप्यं यत्नेन यापयेत्।
साध्यं चावहितः सिद्धैर्भेषजैः साधयेद्भिषक्॥२७॥

The enlightened physicians should not take the incurable patient in hand. The palliable condition is maintained with appropriate therapy. The curable one is treated carefully with proper medicine leading to cure. [27]

Conclusion:

तत्र श्लोकौ- कारणं नाम निर्वृतिं पूर्वरूपाण्युपद्रवान्|
मार्गौ दोषानुबन्धं च साध्यत्वं न च हेतुमत्||२८||
निदाने रक्तपितस्य व्याजहार पुनर्वसुः|
वीत मोह रजो दोष लोभ मान मद स्पृहः||२९||

Summary:
Etiology, derivation of the name of the disease, purvarupa (premonitory symptoms), complications, course, association of doshas, curability and otherwise with reasoning – all these are described in this chapter on the "diagnosis of rakthapitta" by lord Punarvasu who is devoid of passion, rajoguna, greed, vanity pride and treatment. [28-29]

इत्यग्निवेशकृते तन्त्रे चरक प्रतिसंस्कृते निदान स्थाने रक्तपित निदानं नाम दिवतीयोऽध्यायः||२||
Thus ends the 2nd chapter on the "Raktapitta Nidana" of the section on diagnosis of diseases of Agnivesha's work as redacted by Charaka.

3

Nidanasthana Chapter 3 Gulma Nidanam

The 3rd chapter of Charaka Samhita Nidana Sthana is called Gulma Nidana. It deals with causes, pathology, types, symptoms of Gulma, as per ayurveda.

अथातो गुल्म निदानं व्याख्यास्यामः||१||

इति ह स्माह भगवानात्रेयः||२||

We shall now explore the chapter on the Diagnosis of Gulma. Thus said Lord Atreya [1-2]

Types of Gulma:

इह खलु पञ्च गुल्मा भवन्ति; तद्यथा- वातगुल्मः, पित्तगुल्मः, श्लेष्मगुल्मो, निचयगुल्मः, शोणितगुल्म इति||३||

There are 5 types of Gulma viz

Vata gulma

Pitta gulma

Slesma/Kapha gulma

Nichaya Gulma – Gulma due to the simultaneous vitiation of all the 3 Doshas and

Shonita gulma – Gulma due to the affliction of blood [3]

Means to understand specific features of Gulma:

एवंवादिनं भगवन्तमात्रेयमग्निवेश उवाच- कथमिह भगवन् पञ्चानां गुल्मानां विशेषमभिजानीमहे; नह्य विशेषविद्रोगाणामौषधविदपि भिषक् प्रशमनसमर्थो भवतीति||४||

तमुवाच भगवानात्रेयः- समुत्थान पूर्वरूप लिङ्ग वेदनोपशय विशेषेभ्यो विशेष विज्ञानं गुल्मानां भवत्यन्येषां च रोगाणामग्निवेश! तत्तु खलु गुल्मेषूच्यमानं निबोध||५||

Agnivesha asked Lord Atreya, "How to understand the specific features of these 5 types of Gulma? Without this knowledge such patients cannot be successfully treated by a physician even though he is well versed in the selection of drugs".

Lord Atreya versed in the specific features of Gulma as of others diseases can be ascertained from

Nidana (etiology)

Purvarupa (premonitory symptoms)

Linga (symptomatology)

Vedana (various types of pain) and

Upashaya (exploratory therapy)

The following are the characteristic feature of different types of Gulma. [4-5]

Vataja Gulma Nidana:

यदा पुरुषो वातलो विशेषेण ज्वर वमन विरेचनातीसाराणामन्यतमेन कर्शनेन कर्शितो वातलमाहारमाहरति, शीतं वा विशेषेणातिमात्रम् , अस्नेह पूर्वे वा वमन विरेचने पिबति, अनुदीर्णा वा छर्दिमुदीरयति, उदीर्णान् वात मूत्र पुरीष वेगान्निरुणद्धि, अत्यशितो वा पिबति नवोदकमतिमात्रम्, अतिसङ्क्षोभिणा वा यानेन याति, अतिव्यवाय व्यायाम मद्य शोकरुचिर्वा, अभिघातमृच्छति वा, विषमासन शयन स्थान चङ्क्रमणसेवी वा भवति, अन्यद्वा किञ्चिदेवंविधं विषममतिमात्रं व्यायामजातमारभते, तस्यापचाराद्वातः प्रकोपमापद्यते||६||

Factors aggravating Vata in Gulma:

In the body of an individual who is of Vatika type of constitution and who is exceedingly emaciated due to Jvara (fever), Vamana (emesis), Virechana (purgation) or Atisara (diarrhea).

Vatala aahara sevana – Intake of Vata aggravating food

śītaṃ vā viśeṣeṇātimātram – Adoption of regimens which are exceedingly cold

Asneha pūrve vā vamana virecane pibati – Administration of emetic or purgation therapy without oleation

Anudīrṇāṃ vā chardimudīrayati – Vomiting without manifested urge

Udīrṇān vāta mūtra purīṣa vegānniruṇaddhi – Suppression of the manifested urge for passing flatus, urine and stool

Atyaśito vā pibati navodakamatimātram – Intake of fresh water in excess specially after heavy food

Atisaṅkṣobhiṇā vā yānena yāti – Travel in exceedingly jolting vehicles

Ativyavāya vyāyāma madya śokarucirvā – Excessive indulgence in sexual act, physical exercise, drink and anxiety

Abhighātamṛcchati vā – Assault

Viṣamāsana śayana sthāna caṅkramaṇasevī vā bhavati – Sitting, sleeping, standing or moving in irregular posture and

Anyadvā kiñcidevaṃvidhaṃ viṣamamatimātraṃ vyāyāmajātamārabhate – Indulgence in physical exercise of this sort in irregular posture [6]

Vataja Gulma Samprapti, Lakshana, Chikitsa:

स प्रकुपितो वायुर्महास्रोतोऽनुप्रविश्य रौक्ष्यात् कठिनीभूतमाप्लुत्य पिण्डितोऽवस्थानं करोति हृदि बस्तौ पार्श्वयोर्नाभ्यां वा; स शूलमुपजनयति ग्रन्थींश्चानेकविधान्, पिण्डितश्चावतिष्ठते, स पिण्डितत्वाद् 'गुल्म' इत्यभिधीयते; स मुहुराधमति , मुहुरल्पत्वमापद्यते; अनियत विपुलाण्वेदनश्च भवति चलत्वाद्वायोः, मुहुः पिपीलिका सम्प्रचार इवाङ्गेषु, तोद भेद स्फुरणायाम सङ्कोच सुप्ति हर्ष प्रलयोदय बहुलः; तदातुरः सूच्येव शङ्कुनेव चाभिसंविद्धमात्मानं मन्यते, अपि च दिवसान्ते ज्वर्यते , शुष्यति चास्यास्यम्, उच्छ्वासश्चोपरुध्यते, हृष्यन्ति चास्य रोमाणि वेदनायाः प्रादुर्भावे; प्लीहाटोपान्त्रकूजनाविपाकोदावर्ताङ्गमर्द मन्याशिरः शङ्ख शूल ब्रध्नरोगाश्चैनमुपद्रवन्ति; कृष्णारुण परुष त्वङ्नख नयन वदन मूत्र पुरीषश्च भवति, निदानोक्तानि चास्य नोपशेरते, विपरीतानि चोपशेरत इति वातगुल्मः||७||

Pathogenesis, Symptoms and exploratory therapy of Vataja Gulma:

Vata, thus aggravated, enters the alimentary tract (Maha srotas) which latter has become hard and round due to un-unctousness, then spreads and gets localized in heart, bladder, sides of the chest or umbilical region.

It produces colic pain and various types of nodules and remains in a round form. It is because of this round shape that the disease is known as 'Gulma'. This round mass at times increases and at times decreases. Because of the instability (Chalatva) of Vata there is irregularly acute and mild pain.

Often there is a

pipīlikā sampracāra ivāṅgeṣu – feeling as if ants are crawling on the limbs.

There is frequent disappearance and appearance of piercing, breaking and throbbing types of pain. The patient feels as if he is pierced with a needle or a nail.

api ca divasānte jvaryate -There is fever during the afternoon.

There is

śuṣyati cāsyāsyam – dryness of mouth

ucchvāsaścoparudhyate – obstruction to respiration and

hṛṣyanti cāsya romāṇi vedanāyāḥ prādurbhāve – horrification during the onset of pain.

Complications of these types of Gulma are

Plīhāṭopāntrakūjanā – affliction of spleen

Avipaka – metorism

Udavarta – intestinal gurgling / retrograde – reverse movement (abnormal course) of vata

Avipaka – loss of the power of digestion

Anga marda – malaise

manyāśiraḥ śaṅkha śūla bradhnarogāścainamupadravanti – pain in head, sterno-mastoid and temporal region, and swelling in the inguinal lymph glands

kṛṣṇāruṇa paruṣa tvaṅnakha nayana vadana mūtra purīṣaśca bhavati – blackness, reddishness and roughness in the skin, nails, eyes, faces, urine and stool.

Etiological factors enumerated above aggravate the condition whereas things having opposite qualities give relief to the patient. This is about the Vatika type of Gulma. [7]

Pittaja Gulma Nidana, Samprapti, Lakshana:
तैरेव तु कर्शनैः कर्शितस्याम्ल लवण कटुक क्षारोष्ण तीक्ष्ण शुक्त व्यापन्न मद्य हरितकफलाम्लानां विदाहिनां च शाकधान्यमांसादीनामुपयोगादजीर्णाध्यशनाद्रौक्ष्यानुगते चामाशये वमनमतिवेलं सन्धारणं वातातपौ चातिसेवमानस्य पित्तं सह मारुतेन प्रकोपमापद्यते||८||
तत् प्रकुपितं मारुत आमाशयैकदेशे संवर्त्य तानेव वेदनाप्रकारानुपजनयति, य उक्ता वातगुल्मे; पित्तं त्वेनं विदहति कुक्षौ हृद्युरसि कण्ठे च; स विदह्यमानः स धूममिवोद्गारमुदिगरत्यम्लान्वितं, गुल्मावकाशश्चास्य दह्यते दूयते धूप्यते ऊष्मायते स्विद्यति क्लिद्यति शिथिल इव स्पर्शासहोऽल्परोमाञ्चश्च भवति; ज्वर भ्रम दवथु पिपासा गलतालुमुखशोष प्रमोह विड्भेदाश्चैनमुपद्रवन्ति; हरित हारिद्र त्वङ्नख नयन वदन मूत्र पुरीषश्च भवति; निदानोक्तानि चास्य नोपशेरते, विपरीतान्युपशेरत इति पित्तगुल्मः||९||

Factors aggravating Pitta in Gulma – Pathogenesis and Symptoms:
The following factors aggravate Pitta along with Vata in an individual emaciated due either to fever, emesis, purgation or diarrhea.

karṣitasyāmla lavaṇa kaṭuka kṣāroṣṇa tīkṣṇa śukta vyāpanna madya haritakaphalāmlānām vidāhinām ca śākadhānyamāmsādīnāmupayogād – Intake of food articles which cause burning sensation like Amla (sour), Lavana (saline), Katu (pungent), Ksara (alkaline), Ushna (hot), Tikshna (sharp) and fermented diet, deteriorated wine, salads, sour fruits, vegetables, corns and flesh.

Ajīrṇādhyaśanādraukṣyānugate – Frequent meals even before the previous food is digested

Amashaye vamanamativelam – Administration of emesis therapy when the stomach is dry

Sandharanam – Suppression of manifested urges for a long time and

Vātātapau cātisevamānasya – Excessive exposure to wind and the sun. This aggravated Vata gets localized in a part of Amashaya (stomach including small intestine) and produces such pains which have been described to manifest in Vata gulma (in Para 7 above).

There is pittam tvenam vidahati kukṣau hṛdyurasi kaṇṭhe ca – Burning sensation in the pelvic region, heart region, chest and throat due to vitiated Pitta.

sa vidahyamānaḥ sa dhūmamivodgāramudgiratyamlānvitam – Due to this burning sensation there is eructation of sour taste and there is a feeling as if smoke is coming out through it.

In the region of Gulma there is

Dahyate – burning sensation

Duyate – pain

Dhupyate – feeling of fumigation

Ushmayate – heat

Svidyati iva bhavati – sweating

Klidyati – softening

śithila – looseness

Sparśāsaho'lparomāñcaśca – tenderness and slight horrification.

Complications of this type of Gulma are

Jvara – fever

Bhrama – giddiness

Davathu – throbbing pain

Pipāsā – thirst

Gala tālu mukha śoṣa – dryness of throat, palate and mouth

Pramoha – unconsciousness and

Vidbheda – diarrhea

Harita hāridra tvaṅnakha nayana vadana mūtra purīṣaśca bhavati – There is greenish discoloration and yellowness of the skin, nails, eyes, face, urine and stool.

Etiological factors enumerated above aggravate the condition whereas things having opposite qualities give relief to the patient. This is about Paittika type of Gulma. [8-9]

Kaphaja Gulma Nidana, Samprapti, Lakshana:

तैरेव तु कर्शनैः कर्शितस्यात्यशनादतिस्निग्ध गुरु मधुर शीताशनात् पिष्टेक्षुक्षीर तिल माष गुड विकृति सेवनान्मन्दक मद्यातिपानाद्धरितकातिप्रणनयादानूपौदक ग्राम्य मांसातिभक्षणात् सन्धारणादबुभुक्षस्य चातिप्रगाढमुदपानात् सङ्क्षोभणाद्वा शरीरस्य श्लेष्मा सह मारुतेन प्रकोपमापद्यते||१०||

तं प्रकुपितं मारुत आमाशयैकदेशे संवर्त्य तानेव वेदनाप्रकारानुपजनयति य उक्ता वातगुल्मे; श्लेष्मा त्वस्य शीत ज्वरारोचकाविपाकाङ्गमर्द हर्ष हृद्रोग च्छर्दि निद्रालस्य स्तैमित्य गौरव शिरोभितापानुपजनयति, अपि च गुल्मस्य स्थैर्य गौरव काठिन्यावगाढ सुप्तताः, तथा कास श्वास प्रतिश्यायान् राजयक्ष्माणं चातिप्रवृद्धः, श्वैत्यं त्वङ्नख नयन वदन मूत्र पुरीषेषूपजनयति, निदानोक्तानि चास्य नोपशेरते, विपरीतानि चोपशेरत इति श्लेष्म गुल्मः||११||

Factors aggravating Kapha-Pathogenesis and symptoms of Kapha:

The following factors aggravate Kapha along with Vata in an individual emaciated due to the Jwara (fever), Vamana (emesis), Virechana (purgation) and Atisara (diarrhoea).

Ati snigdha guru madhura shita aahara – Intake of excessively unctuous, heavy, sweet and cold food

Piṣṭekṣukṣīra tila māṣa guḍa vikṛti sevanā – Intake of pastry, preparations of sugarcane juice, milk, tila (Sesamum indicum Linn) Masha (Phaseolus rediatus Linn) and Sugar Candy.

Mandaka madya atipana – Intake of immature curd and wine in excess

Haritakātipraṇanayādānūpaudaka grāmya māṃsātibhakṣaṇāt – Intake of Haritaka (salads), the flesh of marshy, aquatic and domestic animals in excess

Sandharana – Suppression of the manifested natural urges

Bubhukṣasya cātipragāḍhamudapānāt – Intake of large quantity of water in the absence of appetite and

Saṅkṣobhaṇādvā śarīrasya – Physical assault.

This aggravated Vata gets localized in a part of Amashaya (stomach including small in instance) and produces such pains as are described to appear in Vatika gulma (in para 7 above).

The Vitiated Kapha produces

śleṣmā tvasya śīta tam jvara – fever beginning with cold

Arochaka – anorexia

Avipaka – indigestion

Angamarda – malaise

Harsha – horrification

Hrdroga – heart disease

Chardi – emesis

Ati-nidra – excessive sleep

Aalasya – Laziness

Staimitya – timidity

Gaurava – heaviness and

Shiro abhitapa – pain in the head.

The gulma remains stable (fixed), heavy, hard, deep seated and there is a feeling of numbness, when aggravated in excess, there is

Kasa – cough

Shvasa – dyspnoea

Pratishyaya – coryza and

Raja Yakshma – tuberculosis

śvaityaṃ tvaṅnakha nayana vadana mūtra purīṣeṣūpajanayati – Skin, nails, eyes, face, urine and stool-all become white.

Etiological factors enumerated above aggravate the condition whereas things having opposite qualities give relief to the patient. This is about the Slaismika/Kaphaja type of Gulma. [10-11]

Asadhya Gulma:

त्रिदोष हेतु लिङ्ग सन्निपाते तु सान्निपातिकं गुल्ममुपदिशन्ति कुशलाः|

स विप्रतिषिद्धोपक्रमत्वादसाध्यो निचय गुल्मः||१२||

Incurable Gulma:

Sannipatika type of Gulma is caused by the etiological factors responsible for the vitiation of all the 3 Doshas and it shares the symptoms of all the 3 types of Gulma, viz,

Vatika

Paittika and

Slaismika / Kaphaja

This type of Gulma is incurable because of the mutual contradiction involved in its treatment. [12]

Rakta gulma:

शोणित गुल्मस्तु खलु स्त्रिया एव भवति न पुरुषस्य, गर्भ कोष्ठार्तवागमनवैशेष्यात्|

पारतन्त्र्यादवैशारद्यात् सततमुपचारानुरोधाद्वा वेगानुदीर्णानुपरुन्धत्या आमगर्भे वाऽप्यचिरपतितेऽथवाऽप्यचिरप्रजातया ऋतौ वा वातप्रकोपणान्यासेवमानायाः क्षिप्रं वातः प्रकोपमापद्यते||१३||

स प्रकुपितो योनि मुखमनुप्रविश्यार्तवमुपरुणद्धि, मासि मासि तदार्तवमुपरुध्यमानं कुक्षिमभिवर्धयति|

तस्याः शूल कासातीसार च्छर्द्यरोचकाविपाकाङ्गमर्द निद्रालस्य स्तैमित्य कफप्रसेकाः समुपजायन्ते, स्तनयोश्च स्तन्यम्, ओष्ठयोः स्तनमण्डलयोश्च काष्ण्यम्, अत्यर्थं ग्लानिश्चक्षुषोः, मूर्च्छा, हल्लासः, दोहदः, श्वयथुश्च पादयोः, ईषच्चोद्गमो रोमराज्याः, योन्याश्चाटालत्वम्, अपि च योन्या दौर्गन्ध्यमास्रावश्चोपजायते, केवलश्चास्या गुल्मः पिण्डित एव स्पन्दते, तामगर्भी गर्भिणीमित्याहुर्मूढाः||१४||

Raktaja gulma:

The Gulma due to the vitiation of blood occurs not in males but in females because of their characteristic feature to pass menstrual blood through the uterus.

Vata in them gets immediately aggravated because of the following: -

Suppression of natural urges due to their subordinate position in the family, ignorance and disposition to the service of others.

sa prakupito yoni mukhamanupraviśyārtavamuparuṇaddhi – Instant abortion or Intake of Vata aggravating things immediately after delivery or burning menstrual period. The aggravated Vata enters into the cervix of the uterus and obstructs the menstrual blood.

māsi māsi tadārtavamuparudhyamānaṃ kukṣimabhivardhayati – Such obstruction of the menstrual- blood- flow goes on every month and as a result of this there is distension of the lower abdomen.

There is
Shula – colic pain
Kasa – cough
Atīsāra – diarrhea
Chardi – vomiting
Arochaka – anorexia
Avipaka – indigestion
Anga marda – malaise
Ati nidra – excessive sleep
Aalasya – laziness
staimitya – timidity and
Kapha prasekāḥ – excessive salivation

There is
atyarthaṃ glāniścakṣuṣoḥ – excessive strain on eyes
Mūrcchā – fainting
Hṛllāsaḥ – Nausea
Dohadaḥ – longings for specific objects
śvayathuśca pādayoḥ – swelling in feet
īṣaccodgamo romarājyāḥ – appearance of small hairs in small quantity
Yonyāścāṭālatvam – dilatation of the vaginal orifice and
api ca yonyā daurgandhyamāsrāvaścopajāyate – foul smelling discharge from the uterus
Kevalaścāsyā gulmaḥ piṇḍita eva spandate – There is pulsation in the entire mass of Gulma which is round is shape.
Tāmagarbhāṃ garbhiṇīmityāhurmūḍhāḥ -The ignorant considers such a patient as a case of pregnancy even though there is actually no pregnancy. [13-14]

Gulma Purvaroopa:
एषां तु खलु पञ्चानां गुल्मानां प्रागभिनिर्वृत्तेरिमानि पूर्वरूपाणि भवन्ति; तद्यथा- अनन्नाभिलषणम्, अरोचकाविपाकौ, अग्निवैषम्यं, विदाहो भुक्तस्य, पाककाले चायुक्त्या छर्द्युद्गारौ, वात मूत्र पुरीष वेगानां चाप्रादुर्भावः, प्रादुर्भूतानां चाप्रवृत्तिरीषदागमनं वा, वात शूलाटोपान्त्रकूजनापरिहर्षणातिवृतपुरीषताः, अबुभुक्षा, दौर्बल्यं, सौहित्यस्य चासहत्वमिति॥१५॥

Premonitory symptoms of Gulma:
Anannābhilaṣaṇam – loss of desire to take food
Arochaka – anorexia
Avipaka – indigestion
Agnivaiṣamyaṃ – irregularity in the power of digestion
vidāho bhuktasya – incomplete digestion of food
Pākakāle cāyuktyā chardyudgārau – vomiting ,eructation during the process of digestion without any specific cause,
Vātamūtrapurīṣavegānāṃ cāprādurbhāvaḥ, prādurbhūtānāṃ cāpravṛttirīṣadāgamanaṃ vā – non- manifestation of the urges for flatus, urination and defecation, even if such urges are manifested there is no excretion or excretion only in small quantity
Shula – colic pain due to Vata

Aatopa – meteroism
Aantra kujana – intestinal gurgling
Pari harsha – horripilation
Ativrtta purishtah – mis-peristalsis
Abubhukṣā – loss of appetite
Daurbalyam – weakness and
Sauhityasya cāsahatvamiti – intolerance to heavy food. [15]

Gulma Chikitsa Sutra:
सर्वेष्वपि खल्वेतेषु गुल्मेषु न कश्चिद्वातादृते सम्भवति गुल्मः|
तेषां सान्निपातिकमसाध्यं ज्ञात्वा नैवोपक्रमेत, एकदोषजे तु यथास्वमारम्भं प्रणयेत्, संसृष्टांस्तु साधारणेन कर्मणोपचरेत्|
यच्चान्यदप्यविरुद्धं मन्येत तदप्यवचारयेद्विभज्य गुरु लाघवमुपद्रवाणां, गुरूनुपद्रवांस्त्वरमाणश्चिकित्सेज्जघन्यमितरान्|
त्वरमाणस्तु विशेषमनुपलभमानो गुल्मेष्वात्ययिके कर्मणि वातचिकित्सितं प्रणयेत्, स्नेहस्वेदौ वातहरौ स्नेहोपसंहितं च मृदु विरेचनं
बस्तींश्च; अम्ललवणमधुरांश्च रसान् युक्त्याऽवचारयेत्|
मारुते ह्युपशान्ते स्वल्पेनापि प्रयत्नेन शक्योऽन्योऽपि दोषो नियन्तुं गुल्मेष्विति||१६||
भवति चात्र- गुल्मिनामनिलशान्तिरुपायैः सर्वशो विधिवदाचरितव्या|
मारुते ह्यवजितेऽन्यमुदीर्ण दोषमल्पमपि कर्म निहन्यात्||१७||

Principle of treatment of Gulma:
Vitiated Vata is an invariable causative factor for all the types of Gulma. Of them the Sannipatika type caused by the vitiation of all Doshas should not be treated as it is incurable. Gulma caused by only one of these 3 Doshas is treated according to the vitiated dosha. The types of Gulma caused by the simultaneous vitiation of 2 these Doshas is treated by adapting the general line of treatment. Therapies which are not mutually contradictory are to be adopted for the treatment of complications, of course, according to their seriousness or lightness. The serious complications are attempted immediately whereas the other ones can be treated even after some time. Should it be considered necessary to treat the patient suffering from Gulma immediately, the therapy may begin with the treatment of vata even if no specific symptom indicative of the type of Gulma is discernible.

For this purpose, the physician should carefully administer oleation and fomentation therapies, including drugs having sour, saline, and sweet tastes. If Vata is alleviated, other doshas pertaining to Gulma can be brought to their normal state with slight effort.

Thus, it is said: -
For a patient suffering from Gulma, such therapies as would alleviate Vata are administered carefully. Once the Vata is alleviated, other aggravated Doshas would get subsidized even with slight effort. [16-17]

तत्र श्लोकः- सङ्ख्या निमित्तं रूपाणि पूर्वरूपमथापि च|
दिष्टं निदाने गुल्मानामेकदेशश्च कर्मणाम्||१८||

Conclusion:
To sum up: The number, aetiology, symptomatology, premonitory symptoms and the line of treatment in brief are described in this chapter on the "Diagnosis of Gulma" [18]

इत्यग्निवेशकृते तन्त्रे चरक प्रतिसंस्कृते निदानस्थाने गुल्म निदानं नाम तृतीयोऽध्यायः||३||
Thus ends the third chapter on the "Gulma Nidana" of the section on the "Diagnosis of diseases" of Agnivesha's work as redacted by Charaka.

4

Nidanasthana Chapter 4 Prameha Nidanam

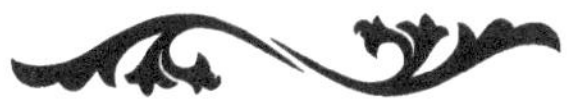

The 4th chapter of Charaka Samhita Nidana Sthana is called Prameha Nidana. It deals with causes, pathology, types and symptoms of Prameha – urinary disorder including Diabetes mellitus, as per Ayurveda.

अथातः प्रमेह निदानं व्याख्यास्यामः||१||

इति ह स्माह भगवानात्रेयः||२||

We shall now explore the chapter on the Diagnosis of Prameha (urinary disorder including Diabetes mellitus). Thus said Lord Atreya [1-2]

Types of Prameha:

त्रिदोष कोप निमिता विंशतिः प्रमेहा भवन्ति विकाराश्चापरेऽपरिसङ्ख्येयाः|

तत्र यथा त्रिदोष प्रकोपः प्रमेहानभिनिर्वर्तयति तथाऽनुव्याख्यास्यामः||३||

Due to the simultaneous vitiation of all the 3 Doshas, 20 types of Prameha as also innumerable other diseases are manifested. We shall now explain the way in which the vitiation of the 3 Doshas leads to the manifestation of the various types of Prameha. [3]

Specific features of etiological factors:

इह खलु निदान दोष दूष्य विशेषेऽयो विकार निग्रातभावाभाव प्रतिविशेषा भवन्ति|

यदा ह्येते त्रयो निदानादि विशेषाः परस्परं नानुबध्नन्त्यथवा काल प्रकर्षादबलीयांसोऽथवाऽनुबध्नन्ति न तदा विकाराऽभिनिर्वृतिः, चिराद्वाऽप्यभिनिर्वर्तन्ते, तनवो वा भवन्त्ययथोक्तसर्वलिङ्गा वा; विपर्यये विपरीताः; इति सर्व विकार विघात भावाभाव प्रति विशेषाभिनिर्वृतिहेतुर्भवत्युक्तः||४||

Specific features of causative factors, Doshas and Dhatus determine the bodily immunity or susceptibility to the manifestation of a disease. When they do not support each other or when they are weak due to temporal factors, then either the disease does not manifest itself or there is delay in manifestation or the disease is very mild or all its symptoms are not properly manifested. If the situations are contrary to what is mentioned above, the corresponding results will also be otherwise. Thus the specific factors which determine the ability or otherwise of the body to resist all types of diseases is described. [4]

Nidana – Causative factors of Kaphaja Prameha:

तत्रेमे त्रयो निदानादि विशेषाः श्लेष्म निमितानां प्रमेहाणामाश्वभि निर्वृतिकरा भवन्ति; तद्यथा- हायनक यव कचीन कोद्दालक नैषधैत्कट मुकुन्दक महाव्रीहि प्रमोदक सुगन्धकानां नवानामतिवेलमति प्रमाणेन चोपयोगः, तथा सर्पिष्मतां नव हरेणु माष सूप्यानां, ग्राम्यानूपौदकानां च मांसानां, शाक तिल पलल पिष्टान्न पायस कृशरा विलेपीक्षु विकाराणां, क्षीर नव मद्य मन्दक दधि द्रव मधुर तरुण प्रायाणां चोपयोगः, मृजा व्यायाम वर्जनं, स्वप्न शयनासन प्रसङ्गः, यश्च कश्चिद्विधिरन्योऽपि श्लेष्म मेदो मूत्र सञ्जननः, स सर्व निदान विशेषः||५||

बहुद्रवः श्लेष्मा दोष विशेषः||६||

बह्वबद्धं मेदो मांसं शरीरज क्लेदः शुक्रं शोणितं वसा मज्जा लसीका रसश्चौजःसङ्ख्यात इति दूष्य विशेषाः॥७॥

Pathogenic factors of Prameha:

The following factors help in the immediate manifestation of Prameha due to Kapha. Of these factors, the etiological factors are as follows:

hāyanaka yava kacīna koddālaka naiṣadhetkaṭa mukundaka mahāvrīhi pramodaka sugandhakānām navānāmativelamati pramāṇena copayogaḥ – Frequent and excessive intake of fresh corns like Hayanaka, Yavaka (a variety of Hordeum vulare Linne), Cinaka, Uddalaka (Cerbera odollam), Naisadha, Itkata, Mukundaka, Mahavrhi, Pramodaka and sugandhaka

tathā sarpiṣmatām nava hareṇu māṣa sūpyānām – Intake of Pulses like fresh Harenu (Pisum sativum Linn) and Masha (Phaseolus mungo) with ghee

grāmyānūpaudakānām ca māmsānām – Intake of the meat of domesticated, Marshy and aquatic animals
śāka tila palala piṣṭānna pāyasa kṛśarā vilepīkṣu vikārāṇām – Intake of vegetables, Tila – Sesame (Sesamum indicum), oil cake of Tila – Sesame (Sesamum indicum), Pastry (Milk preparation), Krsara (gruel prepared of Tila – Sesame (Sesamum indicum), rice and black gram, Vilepi (a type of gruel prepared with four times of water) and preparations of sugarcane

kṣīra nava madya mandaka dadhi drava madhura taruṇa prāyāṇām copayogaḥ – Intake of milk, fresh wine, immature curd and curd which are mostly liquid, sweet and immature in nature

mṛjā vyāyāma varjanam – Avoidance of unction and physical exercise

svapna śayanāsana prasaṅgaḥ – Indulgence in sleep, bed rest and sedentary habits

yaśca kaścidvidhiranyo'pi śleṣma medo mūtra sañjananaḥ – Resorting to even such other regimens which produce more of Kapha, fat and urine.

Kapha having liquidity in excess is the Dosha involved. Dhatus specially involved in this Prameha are:
Medas (fat)
Mamsa (muscle tissue)
Vasa (muscle fat)
Majja (marrow)
Kleda (body fluids)
Shukra (semen)
Rakta (blood)
Lasika (lymph) and
Rasa (Plasma) which later is also known as Ojas.
Of them, the first 4 Dhatus are of incurred quantity and decrease viscosity; remaining Dhatus are of increased quantity only. [5-7]

Samprapti – Pathogenesis of Kaphaja prameha:

त्रयाणामेषां निदानादि विशेषाणां सन्निपाते क्षिप्रं श्लेष्मा प्रकोपमापद्यते, प्रागति भूयस्त्वात्; स प्रकुपितः क्षिप्रमेव शरीरे विसृप्तिं लभते, शरीर शैथिल्यात्; स विसर्पत् शरीरे मेदसैवादितो मिश्रीभावं गच्छति, मेदसश्चैव बह्व बद्धत्वान्मेदसश्च गुणैः समान गुण भूयिष्ठत्वात्; स मेदसा मिश्रीभवन् दूषयत्येनत्, विकृतत्वात्; स विकृतो दुष्टेन मेदसोपहितः शरीर क्लेद मांसाभ्यां संसर्ग गच्छति, क्लेद मांसयोरतिप्रमाणाभिवृद्धत्वात्; स मांसे मांस प्रदोषात् पूति मांस पिडकाः शराविका कच्छपिकाद्याः सञ्जनयति, अप्रकृतिभूतत्वात्; शरीर

क्लेदं पुनर्दूषयन् मूत्रत्वेन परिणमयति, मूत्रवहानां च स्रोतसां वङ्क्षण बस्ति प्रभवाणां मेदःक्लेदोपहितानि गुरूणि मुखान्यासाद्य प्रतिरुध्यते; ततः प्रमेहांस्तेषां स्थैर्यमसाध्यतां वा जनयति, प्रकृति विकृति भूतत्वात्||८||

By the favourable combination of all 3 specific factors, viz causes, Doshas and Dhatus, Kapha gets immediately aggravated because of the excessiveness in quantity already attained by it and initiates the process of manifestation of Prameha. The aggravated Kapha spreads all over the body, it first of all gets mixed with Medas (fat) because there is an increase in the quantity and decrease in the viscosity of Medas. Kapha itself is vitiated; it vitiates Medas while getting mixed with the latter.

The vitiated Kapha along with vitiated Medas gets in as much as these 2 are supposed to have already exceeded their quantity. Vitiation of the muscle tissue provides a congenial atmosphere for the manifestation of putrefied carbuncles like Saravika and Kacchapika in the muscle.

The liquid Dhatus of the body are further vitiated and transformed into urine. Kidneys and bladder are the root (controlling organs) of the channels carrying urine and the openings of these channels obstruct them. This results in the manifestation of Prameha which becomes chronic or incurable due to the affection of all the qualities of kapha and also due to the simultaneous vitiation of homogeneous and heterogeneous Dhatus. [8]

Signs of Kaphaja Prameha, Varieties and Prognosis:

शरीरक्लेदस्तु श्लेष्म मेदो मिश्रः प्रविशन् मूत्राशयं मूत्रत्वमापद्यमानः श्लैष्मिकैरेभिर्दशभिर्गुणैरुपसृज्यते वैषम्य युक्तैः; तद्यथा- श्वेत शीत मूर्त पिच्छिलाच्छ स्निग्ध गुरु मधुर सान्द्र प्रसाद मन्दैः, तत्र येन गुणेनैकेनानेकेन वा भूयस्तरमुपसृज्यते तत्समाख्यं गौणं नाम विशेषं प्राप्नोति||९||

ते तु खल्विमे दश प्रमेहा नाम विशेषेण भवन्ति; तद्यथा- उदकमेहश्च, इक्षुवालिका रस मेहश्च, सान्द्र मेहश्च, सान्द्रप्रसाद मेहश्च, शुक्लमेहश्च, शुक्रमेहश्च, शीतमेहश्च, सिकतामेहश्च, शनैर्मेहश्च, आलालमेहश्चेति||१०||

ते दश प्रमेहाः साध्याः; समान गुण मेदःस्थानकत्वात्, कफस्य प्राधान्यात्, समक्रियत्वाच्च||११||

Signs of Kaphaja Prameha, Varieties and Prognosis:

Fluid Dhatus of the body along with Kapha and Medas (fat) enter into the kidneys and bladder and get transformed into urine. During this process they acquire the morbid qualities of Kapha, viz,

Śveta – whiteness

Śīta –coldness

Mūrta – viscosity

Picchilā – sliminess

Achha – transparency

Snigdha – unctuousness

Guru – heaviness

Madhura – sweetness

Sāndra prasāda – density combined with clarity and

Mandaiḥ – slowness

The morbid conditions are named after these qualities- many of which may dominate the process of pathogenesis.

Types of Kaphaja Prameha:

Udakameha (Hydruria)

Iksuvalikarasameha (glycosuria)

Sandrameha (Chyluria)

Sandraprasadameha (Bilirubinuria)

Suklameha (passing of white urine)

Sukrameha (spermaturia)

Sheetameha (Phosphaturia)

Sikatameha (Graveluria)

Sannairmeha (Slow micturition)

Alalameha (Pyuria)

These 10 types of Prameha are curable because:

The Medas (fat) having homogenous properties are affected

The Kapha is dominant and

Both these two factors are amenable to the same type of treatment [9-11]

Specific characteristic of Kaphaja Prameha:

तत्र श्लोकाः श्लेष्म प्रमेह विशेष विज्ञानार्था भवन्ति-||१२||

अच्छं बहु सितं शीतं निर्गन्धमुदकोपमम्|

श्लेष्मकोपान्नरो मूत्रमुदमेही प्रमेहति||१३||

अत्यर्थमधुरं शीतमीषत्पिच्छिलमाविलम्|

काण्डेक्षु रसमङ्काशं श्लेष्म कोपात् प्रमेहति||१४||

यस्य पर्युषितं मूत्रं सान्द्रीभवति भाजने|

पुरुषं कफ कोपेन तमाहुः सान्द्र मेहिनम्||१५||

यस्य संहन्यते मूत्रं किञ्चित् किञ्चित् प्रसीदति|

सान्द्र प्रसाद मेहीति तमाहुः श्लेष्मकोपतः||१६||

शुक्लं पिष्टनिभं मूत्रमभीक्ष्णं यः प्रमेहति|

पुरुषं कफकोपेन तमाहुः शुक्ल मेहिनम्||१७||

शुक्राभं शुक्रमिश्रं वा मुहुर्मेहति यो नरः|

शुक्रमेहिनमाहुस्तं पुरुषं श्लेष्म कोपतः||१८||

अत्यर्थमधुरं शीतं मूत्रं मेहति यो भृशम्|

शीत मेहिनमाहुस्तं पुरुषं श्लेष्म कोपतः||१९||

मूर्तान्मूत्रगतान् दोषानणून्मेहति यो नरः|

सिकतामेहिनं विद्यात्ं नरं श्लेष्म कोपतः||२०||

मन्दं मन्दमवेगं तु कृच्छ्रं यो मूत्रयेच्छनैः|

शनैर्मेहिनमाहुस्तं पुरुषं श्लेष्मकोपतः||२१||

तन्तु बद्धमिवालालं पिच्छिलं यः प्रमेहति|

आलालमेहिनं विद्यात्ं नरं श्लेष्म कोपतः||२२||

इत्येते दश प्रमेहाः श्लेष्म प्रकोप निमित्ता व्याख्याता भवन्ति||२३||

The features of different types of Prameha caused by Kapha are given below:

Accham bahu sitam śītam nirgandhamudakopamam –

In Udakameha (Hydruria) the individual passes a large quantity of water like urine which is transparent, white, cold and without any smell.

Atyarthamadhuram śītamīṣatpicchilamāvilam kāṇḍekṣu rasamaṅkāśam śleṣma kopāt pramehati – In **Iksuvalikarasameha (glycosuria)** the patient passes urine like the sugar cane juice which is exceedingly sweet, cold, slightly saline and turbid.

InSandrameha (Chyluria) the patient in whom there is aggravation of kapha passes urine which when kept in a vessel gets solidified after some time.

In Sandraprasada meha (Bilirubinuria) the urine of the patient becomes partly viscous and partly clear when kept overnight.

InShukla Meha the patient passes urine having white colour like that of pasted flour.

In Sukrameha (spermaturia) the patient passes urine which resembles semen or mixed with semen frequently.

In **Sheeta Meha** (Phosphaturia) the patient gets frequent maturation which is exceedingly sweet and cold

In **Sikata meha** (graveluria), the vitiated Doshas come through the urine in the form of gravel / small hard things.

Mandaṃ mandamavegaṃ tu kṛcchraṃ yo mūtrayecchanaiḥ| śanairmehinamāhustaṃ puruṣaṃ śleṣmakopataḥ -

In **Shanair meha,** the patient passes small quantity of urine with difficulty and very slowly

In Alalameha (pyuria), the patient passes urine which is like slime phlegm and as if full of threads.

Thus ends 10 types of Prameha due to the vitiation of Kapha are explained [12-23]

Nidana – Causes and types of Pittaja Prameha:

उष्णाम्ल लवण क्षार कटुकाजीर्ण भोजनोप सेविनस्तथाऽतितीक्ष्णातपाग्नि सन्तापश्रम क्रोध विषमाहारोप सेविनश्च तथाविधशरीरस्यैव क्षिप्रं पित्तं प्रकोपमापद्यते, तत्तु प्रकुपितं तयैवानुपूर्व्या प्रमेहानिमान् षट् क्षिप्रतरमभिनिर्वर्तयति||२४||

तेषामपि तु खलु पित्तगुण विशेषेणैव नामविशेषा भवन्ति; तद्यथा- क्षारमेहश्च, कालमेहश्च, नीलमेहश्च, लोहितमेहश्च, माञ्जिष्ठमेहश्च, हारिद्रमेहश्चेति||२५||

ते षड्भिरेव क्षाराम्ल लवण कटुक विस्रोष्णैः पित्तगुणैः पूर्ववद्युक्ता भवन्ति||२६||

Nidana – Causes and types of Pittaja Prameha:

Pitta gets immediately aggravated in an individual whose body is affected by conditions mentioned above (in para 7) due to the following:-

uṣṇāmla lavaṇa kṣāra kaṭukājīrṇa bhojanopa sevina – Intake of hot, sour, saline, alkaline and pungent food

stathā'titīkṣṇātapāgni – Intake of food before the digestion of the previous meal

santāpaśrama krodha sevinaśca – Exposure to excessively hot sun, heat of the fire, physical exertion and anger and

viṣhama aahara sevina – Intake of mutually contradictory food articles.

The aggravated Pitta following the same pathogenic process (as mentioned in para 8) manifests 6 types of Prameha. The process of manifestation here is quicker than that of the Kaphameha.

Types of Pittaja Meha:

Ksarameha (Alkalinuria)

Kalameha (Melanuria)

Nilameha (Indigouria)

Raktameha (Hematuria)

Manjisthameha (Hemoglobinuria)

Haridrameha (Urobilinuria)

As described before, these varieties of Prameha are also manifested due to the permutation and combination of the 6 qualities of Pitta which are sour, saline, pungent, hot and having smell like that of raw flesh. [24-26]

Pathological characteristics Pittaja Prameha:

सर्व एव ते याप्याः संसृष्ट दोष मेदःस्थानत्वादिवरुद्धोपक्रमत्वाच्चेति||२७||

तत्र श्लोकाः पित्त प्रमेह विशेष विज्ञानार्था भवन्ति-||२८||

गन्ध वर्ण रस स्पर्शैर्यथा क्षारस्तथाविधम्|

पित्तकोपान्नरो मूत्रं क्षारमेही प्रमेहति||२९||

मसी वर्ण मजसं यो मूत्रमुष्णं प्रमेहति|

पित्तस्य परिकोपेण तं विद्यात् काल मेहिनम्||३०||

चाषपक्षनिभं मूत्रमम्लं मेहति यो नरः|

पित्तस्य परिकोपेण तं विद्यान्नीलमेहिनम्||३१||

विस्रं लवणमुष्णं च रक्तं मेहति यो नरः|

पित्तस्य परिकोपेण तं विद्याद्रक्तमेहिनम्||३२||

मञ्जिष्ठोदक सङ्काशं भृशं विस्रं प्रमेहति|

पित्तस्य परिकोपातं विद्यान्माञ्जिष्ठमेहिनम्||३३||
हरिद्रोदक सङ्काशं कटुकं यः प्रमेहति|
पित्तस्य परिकोपातं विद्याद्धारिद्रमेहिनम्||३४||
इत्येते षट् प्रमेहाः पित्त प्रकोप निमिता व्याख्याता भवन्ति||३५||

Pathological characteristics Pittaja Prameha:

All these types of Prameha are palliable because the site Medas which is vitiated in the pathogenesis of this disease is closer to threat of the affected Dosha that is Pitta and also because the treatment of Pitta and Medas is involved in mutual contradiction.

The specific features of different types of Prameha caused by Pitta are as follows:

pitta prameha viśeṣa vijñānārthā bhavanti gandha varṇa rasa sparśairyathā kṣārastathāvidham –In **Ksarameha** (Alkalinuria) the patient passes urine having the smell, colour, taste and touch like those of alkaline.

In **Kalameha** (Melanuria) the patient passes a large quantity of black urine.

masī varṇa majasram yo mūtramuṣṇam pramehati – **In Neelameha (indigouria)** the patient passes urine having a sour taste and colour like that of the feather of the Casa Bird (blue jay).

visram lavaṇamuṣṇam ca raktam mehati yo naraḥ – In **Raktameha** (Hematuria) the patient passes urine having red colour, saline taste and smell like that of raw flesh.

mañjiṣṭhodaka saṅkāśam bhṛśam visram pramehati – In **Manjistha meha** (hemoglobinuria) the patient frequently passes urine having the smell like that of raw flesh and colour like that of the juice of Manjistha (Rubia cordifolia Linn).

haridrodaka saṅkāśam kaṭukam yaḥ pramehati – In **Haridra meha** (urobilinuria) the patient passes urine having pungent tastes and colour like that of the juice of Haridra (turmeric – Curcuma longa)

Thus 6 varieties of Prameha due to the vitiation of Pitta are explained. [27-35]

Nidana and Samprapti – Pathogenesis of Vataja Prameha:

कषाय कटु तिक्त रूक्ष लघु शीत व्यवाय व्यायाम वमन विरेचनास्थापन-शिरोविरेचनातियोग सन्धारणानशनाभिघातातपोद्वेगशोक शोणितातिषेक- जागरण विषम शरीरन्यासानुपसेवमानस्य तथा विध शरीरस्यैव क्षिप्रं वातः प्रकोपमापद्यते||३६||
स प्रकुपितस्तथाविधे शरीरे विसर्पन् यदा वसामादाय मूत्रवहानि स्रोतांसि प्रतिपद्यते तदा वसा मेहमभिनिर्वर्तयति; यदा पुनर्मज्जानं मूत्रबस्तावाकर्षति तदा मज्ज मेहमभिनिर्वर्तयति; यदा तु लसीकां मूत्राशयेऽभिवहन्मूत्रमनुबन्धं च्योतयति लसीकातिबहुत्वादिविक्षेपणाच्च वायोः खल्वस्यातिमूत्रप्रवृत्ति सङ्गं करोति, तदा स मत्त इव गजः क्षरत्यजस्रं मूत्रमवेगं, तं हस्तिमेहिनमाचक्षते; ओजः पुनर्मधुरस्वभावं, तद् यदा रौक्ष्याद्वायुः कषायत्वेनाभिसंसृज्य मूत्राशयेऽभिवहति तदा मधुमेहं करोति||३७||

Nidana and Samprapti – Pathogenesis of Vataja Prameha:

Vata gets immediately vitiated in an individual whose body is afflicted with the conditions mentioned above (in para 7) due the following: -

kaṣāya kaṭu tikta rūkṣa laghu śīta aahara – Excessive intake of astringent, pungent, bitter, rough light and credit things.

Ati vyavāya vyāyāma – Excessive indulgence in sex and physical exercise

vamana virecanāsthāpana-śirovirecanātiyoga – Excessive administration of emesis, purgation, Asthapana type of enema and Sirvovirecana (elimination of Doshas from the head)

sandhāraṇānaśanābhighātātapodvega śoka śoṇitātiṣeka jāgaraṇa viṣama śarīranyāsānupasevamānasya tathā vidha śarīrasyaiva kṣipram vātaḥ prakopamāpadyate – Resorting to suppression of the manifested urges, fasting, assault, exposure to sun, anxiety, grief, excessive bloodletting, keeping awake at night and irregular posture of the body.

Vasameha (Lipuria) - The aggravated Vata in that type of body spreads, and along with Vasa (muscle fat), enters into channels carrying urine leading to the manifestation of Vasameha (lipuria).

Majjameha (Myelouria) - When it carries marrow to the urinary bladder then it results in Majjameha (Myelouria).

Hastimeha (Diabetes insipidus) - Due to the excess in quality of Lasika (lymph) and also due to the property of Vata to dissipate things, when the lymph entering into the urinary bladder produces large quantity of urine, the patient feels continuous urge for micturation and passes large quantity of urine continuously (even) without any pressure like an elephant gone amuck. This is known as Hastimeha (diabetes insipidus).

Madhumeha (Diabetes Mellitus) - Ojas, by nature is of sweet taste. When due to the roughness, Vata converts it into that of astringent taste and takes it into the urinary bladder, due to its roughness, this causes Madhumeha (Diabetes mellitus) [36- 37]

Asadhyata – incurable characteristics of Vataja Prameha:
इमांश्चतुरः प्रमेहान् वातजानसाध्यानाचक्षते भिषजः, महात्ययिकत्वादिविरुद्धोपक्रमत्वाच्चेति||३८||
तेषामपि पूर्ववद्गुण विशेषेण नाम विशेषा भवन्ति; तद्यथा- वसामेहश्च, मज्जमेहश्च, हस्तिमेहश्च, मधुमेहश्चेति||३९||
तत्र श्लोका वात प्रमेह विशेष विज्ञानार्था भवन्ति||४०||
वसामिश्रं वसाभं वा मुहु र्मेहति यो नरः|
वसामेहिनमाहुस्तमसाध्यं वातकोपतः||४१||
मज्जानं सह मूत्रेण मुहुर्मेहति यो नरः|
मज्जमेहिनमाहुस्तमसाध्यं वातकोपतः||४२||
हस्ती मत्त इवाजस्रं मूत्रं क्षरति यो भृशम्|
हस्तिमेहिनमाहुस्तमसाध्यं वातकोपतः||४३||
कषाय मधुरं पाण्डु रूक्षं मेहति यो नरः|
वातकोपादसाध्यं तं प्रतीयान्मधुमेहिनम्||४४||
इत्येते चत्वारः प्रमेहा वात प्रकोप निमित्ता व्याख्याता भवन्ति||४५||
एवं त्रिदोष प्रकोप निमित्ता विंशतिः प्रमेहा व्याख्याता भवन्ति||४६||

These 4 varieties of Prameha due to the Vitiation of Vata are known to be incurable because of their seriousness and also because of the contradiction involved in their treatment. As in the case of other Pramehas, these varieties of Prameha are also named after the attributes involved in the pathogenesis.

Types of Vataja prameha:
Vasameha (Lipuria)
Majjameha (Myelo-Uria)
Hastimeha (Diabetes Insipidus) and
Madhumeha (Diabetes Mellitus).

The specific features of different of Prameha caused by Vata are given below:
In **Vasameha** (lipuria) which is incurable and caused by the aggravation of Vata the patient frequently passes urine mixed with Vasa (muscle fat) or having the appearance of Vasa

Majjānaṃ saha mūtreṇa muhurmehati yo naraḥ majjamehinamāhustamasādhyaṃ vātakopataḥ –
In**Majjameha**(myelo-Uria) which is incurable and caused by the aggravation of Vata the patient passes urine mixed with Majja (marrow)

Hastī matta ivājasraṃ mūtraṃ kṣarati yo bhṛśam –
In**Hastimeha** (Diabetes insipidus) which is incurable and caused by the aggravation of Vata, the patient passes large quantities of urine frequently like an elephant gone amuck.

Kaṣāya madhuraṃ pāṇḍu rūkṣaṃ mehati yo naraḥ –

In **Madhumeha** (Diabetes Mellitus) which is incurable and caused by the aggravation of Vata the patient passes large quantities of urine, sweet and astringent in taste, pale in colour and un-unctuous.

The 4 varieties of Prameha due to the aggravation of Vata are thus explained. Thus the 20 types of Prameha due to the aggravation of the 3 Doshas are explained. [38-46]

Prameha Poorvaroopa:

त्रयस्तु खलु दोषाः प्रकुपिताः प्रमेहानभिनिर्वर्तयिष्यन्त इमानि पूर्वरूपाणि दर्शयन्ति; तद्यथा- जटिलीभावं केशेषु, माधुर्यमास्यस्य, करपादयोः सुप्तता दाहौ, मुख तालु कण्ठ शोषं, पिपासाम्, आलस्यं, मलं काये, कायच्छिद्रेषूपदेहं, परिदाहं सुप्ततां चाङ्गेषु, षट्पद पिपीलिकाभिश्च शरीर मूत्राभिसरणं, मूत्रे च मूत्रदोषान्, विस्रं शरीरगन्धं, निद्रां, तन्द्रां च सर्वकालमिति||४७||

Premonitory symptoms of Prameha:

The 3 vitiated Doshas while initiating the process of manifestation of various types of Prameha produces the following premonitory symptoms:

Jaṭilībhāvaṃ keśeṣu – Matting of the hair

Mādhuryamāsyasya – Sweet taste in the mouth

Karapādayoḥ suptatā dāhau -Numbness and burning sensation in hands and feet

Mukha tālu kaṇṭha śoṣaṃ -Dryness in mouth, palate and throat

Pipāsām -Thirst

Aalasyaṃ – laziness

malaṃ kāye – Increased amount of excreta from the body

Kāyacchidreṣūpadehaṃ – Adherence of excreta in the orifices of the body

Paridāhaṃ suptatāṃ cāṅgeṣu – Burning sensation and numbness in various organs of the body

Shatpada pipīlikābhiśca śarīra mūtrābhisaraṇaṃ – Attraction of insects and by the body and urine

Mūtre ca mūtradoṣān – Appearance of abnormalities in the urine

Visraṃ śarīragandhaṃ – Smell of raw flesh in the urine and

Nidrāṃ, tandrāṃ ca sarvakālamiti – Excessive sleep and continuous drowsiness. [47]

Prameha Upadrava – Complications and line of treatment:

उपद्रवास्तु खलु प्रमेहिणां तृष्णातीसार ज्वर दाह दौर्बल्यारोचकाविपाकाः पूतिमांस पिडकालजी विद्रध्यादयश्च तत्प्रसङ्गादभवन्ति||४८||
तत्र साध्यान् प्रमेहान् संशोधनोपशमनैर्यथार्हमुपपादयंश्चिकित्सेदिति||४९||

Complications of Prameha are

Trshuna – thirst

Atisara – diarrhoea

Jvara – fever

Daha – burning sensation

Daurbalya – weakness

Arochaka – anorexia and

Avipaka – indigestion

pūtimāṃsa piḍakālajī vidradhyādayaśca tatprasaṅgādbhavanti – Carbuncles which putrefy the muscle tissues like Alaji and Vidradhi appear during the chronic stage of the disease. Of them the curable types of Prameha is treated with the appropriate elimination and alleviation therapies. [48-49]

Brief etiology:

भवन्ति चात्र- गृध्नुमभ्यवहार्येषु स्नान चङ्क्रमणादिवषम्|

प्रमेहः क्षिप्रमभ्येति नीडद्रुममिवाण्डजः||५०||
मन्दोत्साहमतिस्थूलमतिस्निग्धं महाशनम्|
मृत्युः प्रमेह रूपेण क्षिप्रमादाय गच्छति||५१||
यस्त्वाहारं शरीरस्य धातु साम्यकरं नरः|
सेवते विविधाश्चान्याश्चेष्टाः स सुखमश्नुते||५२||

Thus, it said:

As the birds are attracted towards the trees where it lays their nests similarly, Prameha affects people who are voracious eaters and have aversion to bath and physical exercises. Death immediately comes in the form of Prameha to those who are less enthusiastic, over-corpulent, over unctuous and gluttons. The individual who takes such diets and resorts to such regimens which bring about the normal state of the Dhatus in the body leads a happy life. [50-52]

Conclusion:

तत्र श्लोकाः- हेतु व्याधि विशेषाणां प्रमेहाणां च कारणम्|
दोष धातु समायोगो रूपं विविधमेव च||५३||
दश श्लेष्मकृता यस्मात् प्रमेहाः षट् च पित्तजाः|
यथा च वायुश्चतुरः प्रमेहान् कुरुते बली||५४||
साध्यासाध्य विशेषाश्च पूर्वरूपाण्युपद्रवाः|
प्रमेहाणां निदानेऽस्मिन् क्रियासूत्रं च भाषितम्||५५||

To sum up:

In this chapter of Prameha Nidana, following topics have been discussed: -

Causative factors of diseases and those (specially) pertaining to various types of Prameha

Combination of Doshas and Dhatus

Signs and symptoms (of different types of Prameha)

Process of manifestation of 10, 6 and 4 varieties of Prameha caused by Kapha, Pitta and Vata respectively

Their prognosis, premonitory symptoms and complications and

Their line of treatment [53- 55]

इत्यग्निवेशकृते तन्त्रे चरक प्रति संस्कृते निदान स्थाने प्रमेह निदानं नाम चतुर्थोऽध्यायः||४||

Thus ends the 4th chapter on the Diagnosis of Prameha of the section on Diagnosis of Diseases (Nidana sthana) of Agnivesha's work as redacted by Charaka.

5

Nidanasthana Chapter 5 Kushta Nidanam

The 5th chapter of Charaka Samhita Nidana Sthana is Kushta Nidana. It deals with causes, pathology, types and symptoms of Kushta – skin Diseases, as per Ayurveda.

अथातः कुष्ठ निदानं व्याख्यास्यामः||१||

इति ह स्माह भगवानात्रेयः||२||

We shall explore the chapter on the "Diagnosis of Kushta". Thus said Lord Atreya

Kushta Dravya – Morbid factors that are involved in Kushta:

सप्त द्रव्याणि कुष्ठानां प्रकृति विकृतिमापन्नानि भवन्ति|

तद्यथा- त्रयो दोषा वात पित्त श्लेष्माणः प्रकोपण विकृताः, दूष्याश्च शरीरधातवस्त्वङ्मांस शोणित लसीकाश्चतुर्धा दोषोपघातविकृता इति|

एतत् सप्तानां सप्तधातुकमेवङ्गतमाजननं कुष्ठानाम्, अतःप्रभवाण्यभिनिर्वर्तमानानि केवलं शरीरमुपतपन्ति||३||

Morbid factors that are involved in Kushta:

Kushta is caused by 7 factors. They are the 3 Doshas, Viz,

Vata

Pitta and

Kapha which get vitiated by causative factors and

4 Dhatus of the body, viz

Tvak (skin or rasa)

Mamsa (Muscle)

Shonita (blood) and

Lasika (lymph) which gets vitiated by the morbid Doshas.

Thus the 7 types of Kusthas are produced by the 7 morbid Dhatus (which include 3 Doshas). The Kushta so caused spreads to the entire body after its manifestation. [3]

Innumerable classification of Kushta:

न च किञ्चिदस्ति कुष्ठमेकदोष प्रकोप निमित्तम्, अस्ति तु खलु समान प्रकृतीनामपि कुष्ठानां दोषांशांश विकल्पानुबन्धस्थानविभागेन वेदना वर्ण संस्थान प्रभाव नाम चिकित्सित विशेषः|

स सप्तविधोऽष्टादशविधोऽपरिसङ्ख्येय विधो वा भवति|

दोषा हि विकल्पनैर्विकल्प्यमाना विकल्पयन्ति विकारान्, अन्यत्रासाध्यभावात्|

तेषां विकल्प विकार सङ्ख्यानेऽतिप्रसङ्गमभिसमीक्ष्य सप्तविधमेव कुष्ठ विशेषमुपदेक्ष्यामः||४||

Innumerable classification of Kushta:

No Kushta manifests itself due to the aggravation of only one Dosha.

Depending upon the permutation and combination of the various factors of Dosha and their location in the body, there is variation in the

Vedana (pain),

Varna (colour),

Samsthana (shape),

Prabhava (specific manifestations),

Nama (name) and

Chikitsa (treatment) of the various types of skin disorders.

They may be of 7 types and according to another classification, 18 types. But in general, Kushta are of innumerable types. Doshas due to various forms of permutation and combination bring about varieties in these diseases excepting those which are incurable. As all the variations of the disease are too exhaustive to be narrated here, only the 7 fold classification of Kushta will be explained here [4]

Specific nature of Kushta:

इह वातादिषु त्रिषु प्रकुपितेषु त्वगादींश्चतुरः प्रदूषयत्सु वातेऽधिकतरे कपालकुष्ठमभिनिर्वर्तते, पित्ते त्वौदुम्बरं, श्लेष्मणि मण्डलकुष्ठं, वात पित्तयोरृष्यजिह्वं, पित्तश्लेष्मणोः पुण्डरीकं, श्लेष्म मारुतयोः सिध्म कुष्ठं, सर्व दोषाभिवृद्धौ काकणकमभिनिर्वर्तते; एवमेष सप्तविधः कुष्ठविशेषो भवति। स चैष भूयस्तरतमतः प्रकृतौ विकल्प्यमानायां भूयसीं विकारविकल्पसङ्ख्यामापद्यते॥५॥

The specific nature of the 7 types of Kusthas manifested due to

vitiation of 4 Dhatus, viz, Tvak (skin on Rasa dhatu) etc.,

by the 3 Doshas, Viz, Vata etc., is as follows:

Kapala due to Vata

Audumbara due to Pitta

Mandala due to Kapha

Rushyajihva Kushta due to Vata and Pitta

Pundarika due to the Kapha and Pitta

Sidhma due to Kapha and Vata

Kakanaka due to the involvement of all the three Doshas.

Depending upon the degree of affliction of these etiological factors and their permutation and combinations, this disease is of innumerable types. [5]

Kushta Nidana: – Etiology

तत्रेदं सर्वकुष्ठनिदानं समासेनोपदेक्ष्यामः:- शीतोष्णव्यत्यासमनानुपूर्व्योपसेवमानस्य तथा सन्तर्पणापतर्पणाभ्यवहार्यव्यत्यासं, मधु फाणित मत्स्य लकुच मूलक काकमाचीः सततमतिमात्रमजीर्ण च समश्नतः, चिलिचिमं च पयसा, हायनक यवक चीन कोद्दालक कोरदूष प्रायाणि चान्नानि क्षीर दधि तक्र कोल कुलत्थ माषातसी कुसुम्भ स्नेहवन्ति, एतैरेवातिमात्रं सुहितस्य च व्यवाय व्यायाम सन्तापान्त्युपसेवमानस्य, भय श्रम सन्तापोपहतस्य च सहसा शीतोदकमवतरतः, विदग्धं चाहारजातमनुल्लिख्य विदाहिन्यभ्यवहरतः, छर्दि च प्रतिघ्नतः, स्नेहांश्चातिचरतः, त्रयो दोषाः युगपत् प्रकोपमापद्यन्ते; त्वगादयश्चत्वारः शैथिल्यमापद्यन्ते; तेषु शिथिलेषु दोषाः प्रकुपिता: स्थानमधिगम्य सन्तिष्ठमानास्तानेव त्वगादीन् दूषयन्तः कुष्ठान्यभिनिर्वर्तयन्ति॥६॥

Etiology of Kushta:

Now we shall describe the etiology of all types of Kusthas in brief. All the 3 Doshas get simultaneously vitiated by the following:

Shītoṣṇavyatyāsamanānupūrvyopasevamānasya tathā santarpaṇāpatarpaṇābhyavahāryavyatyāsam – Non –compliance of the prescribed rules with regard to the order of responding to hot and cold regimens and intake of nourishing and depleting diets:

Madhu phāṇita matsya lakuca mūla kakākamācīḥ satatam atimātramajīrṇe ca samaśnataḥ – Continuous intake of honey, pendium, fish, Lakucha (Artocarpus lakooch Roxb), Radish and Kakamachi (Solanum nigrum Linn) in large quantity while suffering from indigestion.

Chilicimaṃ ca payasā – Intake of Cilicima (fish) with milk

Intake of food mostly containing Hayanaka (Oryza sativa linn), Yavaka (a type of Hordeum vulgare Linn), Cinaka (Cucumis utilissimus), Uddalaka (Paspalum scrobiculatum) and Koradusa (Paspalum scrobiculatum Linn) along with milk, curd, butter, milk, Kola (Zizyphus radiatus Linn), Atasi (Linum usitatissimum Linn), Kusumbha (Carthamus tinctorius Linn), and unctuous substances

Etairevātimātraṃ suhitasya ca vyavāya vyāyāma santāpānatyupasevamānasya – Excessive indulgence in cohabitation, physical exercise and exposure to heat after taking the above mentioned food to one's satisfaction.

Bhaya śrama santāpopahatasya ca sahasā śītodakamavatarataḥ – Entering into cold water immediately after one is afflicted with Bhaya (fear), Shrama (exhaustion) and Santapa (grief)

Vidagdhaṃ cāhārajātamanullikhya vidāhīnyabhyavaharataḥ – Intake of such food as would cause burning sensation without vomiting out the undigested food (in the stomach)

Chardiṃ ca pratighnataḥ – Suppression of the urge for emesis and

Snehāṃścāticarataḥ – Excessive oleation

The above factors also loses the 4 Dhatus, viz. Tvak (skin or Rasa dhatu) etc. the aggravated Doshas localized in these Dhatus vitiate the latter due to their looseness and so produce Kusthas. [6]

Kushta Purvarupa: Premonitory symptoms:

तेषामिमानि पूर्वरूपाणि भवन्ति; तद्यथा- अस्वेदनमतिस्वेदनं पारुष्यमतिश्लक्ष्णता वैवर्ण्यं कण्डूर्निस्तोदः सुप्तता परिदाहः परिहर्षो लोमहर्षः खरत्वमूष्मायणं गौरवं श्वयथु वीसर्पागमनमभीक्ष्णं च काये कायच्छिद्रेषूपदेहः पक्व दग्ध दष्ट भग्न क्षतोपस्खलितेष्वतिमात्रं वेदना स्वल्पानामपि च व्रणानां दुष्टिरसंरोहणं चेति||७||

The premonitory symptoms of Kushta:

Asvedanamatisvedanaṃ – No sweating or more sweating

Pāruṣyamatiślakṣṇatā – Having rough edges, thin and slightly elevated

Vaivarṇyaṃ – Discoloration of the skin

Kandu – severe itching

Nistoda – Pricking sensation

Suptatā – There is excessive numbness

Paridaha – Burning sensation

Pariharṣo lomaharṣaḥ – They are covered with horrent hairs and associated with excessive pain

ūṣmāyaṇaṃ – There is less of discharge of pus and serous exudation.

Their causation, manifestation and ulceration are instantaneous.

They are infested with germs and appear like pieces of earthen pot having black or reddish colour.

Signs and symptoms of different types of Kushta:

ततोऽनन्तरं कुष्ठान्यभिनिर्वर्तन्ते, तेषामिदं वेदनावर्णसंस्थानप्रभावनामविशेषविज्ञानं भवति;

Hereafter, characteristic features, pain, colour, shape and specific manifestations of Kushtas are explained.

1. Kapala Kushta:

तद्यथा- रूक्षारुणपरुषाणि विषमविसृतानि खरपर्यन्तानि तनून्युद्वृत्तबहिस्तनूनिसुप्तवत्सुप्तानि हृषितलोमाचितानिनिस्तोदबहुलान्यल्पकण्डूदाहपूयलसीकान्याशुगतिसमुत्थानान्याशुभेदीनि जन्तुमन्तिकृष्णारुणकपालवर्णानि च कपालकुष्ठानीति विद्यात् (१)

Kapala Kushta:

Kapala type of Kushta is dry, red coloured, rough skin surface, uneven shape, with rough edges, thin, slightly elevated at the periphery. It is characterized by numbness. The affected skin patches are covered by erect hairs and are associated with severe pain. There is less itching, burning sensation, and pus discharge and serous exudation. They occur instantaneously. They are infected with microbes and appear like pieces of earthen pot with black or red colour, hence the name – Kapala Kushta.

2. Audumbara Kushta:

ताम्राणि ताम्र खर रोम राजीभिरवनद्धानि बहलानि बहु बहल पूय रक्त लसीकानि कण्डू क्लेद कोथ दाह पाकवन्त्याशुगति समुत्थान भेदीनि ससन्ताप क्रिमीणि पक्वोदुम्बर फल वर्णान्यौदुम्बर कुष्ठानीति विद्यात् ||

Audumbara type of Kushta is:

Tāmrāṇitāmra khara roma – Coppery color and they are covered with hair of coppery color.

Bahalāni bahu bahala pūya rakta lasīkāni – They are very thick and associated with thick pus, blood and serous exudation in large quantities.

Kaṇḍū kleda kotha dāha pākavantyāśugati – They are associated with Kandu (itching), Kleda (sticky exudation), Kotha (sloughing), Daha (burning sensation) and Paka (suppuration).

Samutthāna bhedīni sasantāpa krimīṇi – Their causation, manifestation and ulceration are instantaneous.

Pakvodumbara phala varṇānyaudumbara kuṣṭhānīti – They are like the ripe fruit of Udumbara (Ficus racemosa Linn), in colour.

3. Mandala Kushta:

शुक्ल रक्तावभासा निशुक्ल रोमराजी सन्तानानि बहु बहल शुक्ल पिच्छिल स्रावीणि बहु क्लेद कण्डू क्रिमीणि सक्तगति समुत्थान भेदीनि परिमण्डलानि मण्डल कुष्ठनि विद्यात् |

Mandala type of Kushta is

śukla raktāvabhāsā niśukla romarājī – They are white and red in colour and are covered with white hairs.

Bahu bahala śukla picchila srāvīṇi bahu kleda kaṇḍū krimīṇi – They are associated with excessive sticky exudation and itching, and infested with numerous germs.

Saktagati samutthāna bhedīni parimaṇḍalāni – Their causation, manifestation and ulceration are sluggish and they are round in shape.

4. Rushyajihva type of Kustha :

परुषाण्यरुण वर्णानि बहिरन्तःश्यावानि नील पीत ताम्रावभासान्याशुगति समुत्थानान्यल्प कण्डू क्लेद क्रिमीणि दाह भेद निस्तोद (पाक)बहुलानि शूकोपहतोपमवेदनान्युत्सन्नमध्यानि तनु पर्यन्तानि कर्कश पिडकाचितानि दीर्घ परिमण्डलान्यृष्यजिह्वाकृतीनि ऋष्यजिह्वानीति विद्यात् |

Rushyajihva type of Kustha is

Parushya – rough

aruṇa varṇāni bahirantaḥśyāvāni nīla pīta tāmrāvabhāsānyāśugati samutthānā – reddish in colour and dark brown in the centre as well as in the periphery. They are of blue, yellow and coppery shade.

Alpa kaṇḍū kleda krimīṇi – There is less of itching, sticky exudation and germs

Dāha bheda nistoda (pāka) bahulāni – They are associated with excessive burning sensation, cutting and piercing pain and suppuration.

śūkopahatopamavedanānyutsanna madhyāni tanu paryantāni karkaśa piḍakācitāni dīrgha parimaṇḍalānyṛṣyajihvākṛtīni ṛṣyajihvānīti – There is pain as if inflicted with bristles. In the centre they are elevated and their peripheries are thin. They are associated with rough pimples and are elongated and round in shape like the tongue of a deer.

5. Pundareeka Kushta:

शुक्ल रक्तावभासानि रक्त पर्यन्तानि रक्तराजी सिरासन्ततान्युत्सेधवन्ति बहु बहल रक्त पूय लसीकानि कण्डू क्रिमि दाह पाकवन्त्याशुगति समुत्थानभेदीनि पुण्डरीक पलाश सङ्काशानि पुण्डरीकाणीति विद्यात्।

Pundarika type of Kustha is of

Shukla raktāvabhāsāni rakta paryantāni raktarājī sirā – white and red shade. Their borders are red, and they are covered with red lines and blood vessels.

Santatānyutsedhavanti bahu bahala rakta pūya lasīkāni kaṇḍū krimi dāha pākavantyāśugati samutthāna bhedīni – There is swelling and discharge of thick blood, pus and serum in excessive quantity. There is itching, germ infestation, burning sensation and suppuration. Their causation, manifestation and ulceration are instantaneous.

Puṇḍarīka palāśa saṅkāśāni puṇḍarīkāṇīti vidyāt – They appear like the petals of lotus flower.

6. Sidhma Kushta:

परुषारुणानि विशीर्णबहिस्तनून्यन्तःस्निग्धानि शुक्ल रक्तावभासानि बहून्यल्पवेदनान्यल्प कण्डू दाह पूय लसीकानि लघु समुत्थानान्यल्प भेदक्रिमीण्यलाबु पुष्प सङ्काशानि सिध्मकुष्ठानीति विद्यात्।

Sidhma type of Kustha is:

Paruṣāruṇāni viśīrṇabahistanūnyantaḥsnigdhāni – rough and reddish in colour, in the periphery they are fissured and thin and, in the centre, they are smooth.

śukla raktāvabhāsāni – They are of white and red shade.

Bahūnyalpavedanānyalpa kaṇḍū dāha pūya lasīkāni laghu samutthānānyalpa bheda krimi — they appear in large number and there is less of pain, itching, burning sensation, pus and serous discharge. Their causation of ulceration is sluggish and there is less of germ infestation.

Alābu puṣpa saṅkāśāni – They appear like the flower of alabu (Lagenaria siceraria Standl).

7. Kakanika kushta:

काकणन्तिकावर्णान्यादौ पश्चात्तु सर्व कुष्ठलिङ्ग समन्वितानि पापीयसा सर्वकुष्ठलिङ्गसम्भवेनानेकवर्णानि काकणानीति विद्यात्। तान्यसाध्यानि, साध्यानि पुनरितराणि॥८॥

Kakana type of Kustha are the:

Kākaṇantikāvarṇānyādau paścāttu sarvakuṣṭhaliṅga – Colour of Kakanantika (Abrus precatorius Linn) in the beginning and subsequently symptoms of all types of Kusthas are manifested there

Pāpīyasā sarvakuṣṭhaliṅgasambhavenānekavarṇāni kākaṇānīti vidyāt – Because of the combination of these painful characteristics of all other types of Kushta those belonging to Kakanantika category are of many colours

Tānyasādhyāni, sādhyāni punaritarāṇi – Kusthas belonging to this category are incurable. Others are curable. [8]

Kushta Sadhya Asadhyata:

तत्र यदसाध्यं तदसाध्यतां नातिवर्तते, साध्यं पुनः किञ्चित् साध्यतामतिवर्तते कदाचिदपचारात्। साध्यानि हि षट् काकणकवर्ज्यान्यचिकित्स्यमानान्यपचारतो वा दोषैरभिष्यन्दमानान्यसाध्यतामुपयान्ति॥९॥

Prognosis of Kushta:

Curable Kushtas may become incurable if the patient indulges in unwholesome regimens even after the manifestation of the disease. Excluding Kakanantika, other types of Kusthas, which are normally curable, may become incurable in the event of the saturation of the vitiated Doshas due to the lack of proper regimen or resort to unwholesome regimen. [9]

Complications caused by Negligence:

साध्यानामपि ह्युपेक्ष्यमाणानां त्वङ्मांस शोणित लसीका कोथ क्लेद संस्वेदजाः क्रिमयोऽभिमूर्च्छन्ति; ते भक्षयन्तस्त्वगादीन् दोषाः

पुनर्दूषयन्त इमानुपद्रवान् पृथक् पृथगुत्पादयन्ति- तत्र वातः श्यावारुणवर्णं परुषतामपि च रौक्ष्य शूल शोष तोद वेपथु हर्ष सङ्कोचायास स्तम्भ सुप्तिभेदभङ्गान्, पित्तं दाह स्वेद क्लेद कोथ स्राव पाक रागान्, श्लेष्मा त्वस्य श्वैत्य शैत्य कण्डू स्थैर्य गौरवोत्सेधोपस्नेहोपलेपान्, क्रिमयस्तु त्वगादींश्चतुरः सिराः स्नायूश्चास्थीन्यपि च तरुणान्याददते ||१०||

अस्यां चैवावस्थायामुपद्रवाः कुष्ठिनं स्पृशन्ति; तद्यथा- प्रस्रवणमङ्गभेदः पतनान्यङ्गावयवानां तृष्णा ज्वरातीसार दाह दौर्बल्यारोचकविपाकाश्च, तथाविधमसाध्यं विद्यादिति||११||

The complications caused by negligence are:

Tvaṅmāṃsa śoṇita lasīkā kotha kleda saṃsvedajāḥ krimayo'bhimūrcchanti – Germs on the slough of the skin, muscle tissue, blood and serous exudation , other softened tissues and sweet, appear even in the curable types of Kusthas when their treatment is neglected.

krimayo'bhimūrcchanti – While infesting the skin etc. these germs further vitiate the Doshas leading to complications which are described below separately (for each Doshas and germs).

Vātaḥ śyāvāruṇavarṇaṃ paruṣatāmapi ca raukṣya śūla śoṣa toda vepathu harṣa saṅkocāyāsa stambha suptibhedabhaṅgān – Complications due to Vata are blackish brown or reddish colour, roughness, dryness, piercing pain, emaciation, pricking pain, trembling, horripilation, contraction, exhaustion, stiffness, numbness, ulceration and fissures.

Pittaṃ dāha sveda kleda kotha srāva pāka rāgān – Complications due to Pitta are burning sensation, sweating, softening of tissues, putrefaction, serous exudation, suppuration and redness.

Shleṣmā tvasya śvaitya śaitya kaṇḍū sthairya gauravotsedhopasnehopalepān – Complications due to Kapha are whiteness, coldness, itching, steadiness, heaviness, swelling, unctuousness and adhesion.

Krimayastu tvagādīṃścaturaḥ sirāḥ snāyūścāsthīnyapi ca taruṇānyādadate – Germs afflict (eat away) the 4 Dhatus viz, skin etc vessels, ligaments, bones and cartilages.

During this stage, the patient shares the following complications:-

A patient having such complications is incurable:

Prasravaṇam – Excessive exudation

Aṅgabhedaḥ – ulceration of organs

Patanānyaṅgāvayavānā – sequestration of the organs of the body

Tṛṣṇā – thirst

Jvara – fever

Atisara – diarrhoea

Daha – burning sensation

Daurbalya – weakness

Arochaka – anorexia and

Avipaka – indigestion [10-11]

Warning regarding treatment:

भवन्ति चात्र- साध्योऽयमिति यः पूर्वं नरो रोगमुपेक्षते| स किञ्चित्कालमासाद्य मृत एवावबुध्यते||१२||

यस्तु प्रागेव रोगेभ्यो रोगेषु तरुणेषु वा| भेषजं कुरुते सम्यक् स चिरं सुखमश्नुते||१३||

यथा ह्यल्पेन यत्नेन छिद्यते तरुणस्तरुः| स एवातिप्रवृद्धस्तु छिद्यतेऽतिप्रयत्नतः||१४||

एवमेव विकारोऽपि तरुणः साध्यते सुखम्| विवृद्धः साध्यते कृच्छ्रादसाध्यो वाऽपि जायते||१५||

Thus, it is said: -the individual, who neglects the disease in the beginning thinking it as curable, comes to know of the reality while approaching death after some time. The individual who resorts to proper treatment of the disease before it is manifested or in its early stage, enjoys happiness for long.

As a young tree can be cut very easily and its cutting involves excessive effort when the tree is well grown, so also, the disease is easily curable in its primary stage; it becomes incurable or difficult for cure as and when it reaches the advanced stage. [12-15]

Subject matter: -

तत्र श्लोकः- सङ्ख्या द्रव्याणि दोषाश्च हेतवः पूर्वलक्षणम्|

रूपाण्युपद्रवाश्चोक्ताः कुष्ठानां कौष्ठिके पृथक्||१६||

Number, materials, Doshas, causative factors, premonitory symptoms (actual) symptoms, complications of various types of Kusthas all these are described in this chapter. [16]

To sum up:

इत्यग्निवेशकृते तन्त्रे चरक प्रतिसंस्कृते निदानस्थाने कुष्ठ निदानं नाम पञ्चमोऽध्यायः||५||

Thus ends the 5th chapter on the Diagnosis of Kushta (obstinate skin diseases) of the section on the "Diagnosis of Diseases" (Nidanasthana) of Agnivesha's work as redacted by Charaka.

6

Nidanasthana Chapter 6 Shosha Nidanam

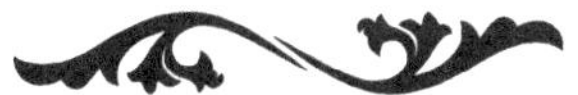

The 6th chapter of Charaka Samhita Nidana Sthana is called Shosha Nidana. It deals with causes, pathology, types and symptoms of Shosha – emaciation, fatigue as per Ayurveda.

अथातः शोष निदानं व्याख्यास्यामः||१||

इति ह स्माह भगवानात्रेयः||२||

We shall explore the chapter on the "Diagnosis of Consumption". Thus said Lord Atreya [1-2]

Nidana of Shosha (Etiology of consumption):

इह खलु चत्वारि शोषस्यायतनानि भवन्ति; तद्यथा- साहसं सन्धारणं क्षयो विषमाशनमिति||३||

There are 4 causative factors of Shosha viz.

Sāhasaṃ – excessive physical activities

Sandhāraṇaṃ – Suppression of the natural urges

Kshaya – Wasting and

Vishamashana – Irregular dieting [3]

Details of Sahasa Nidana for Shosha:

तत्र साहसं शोषस्यायतनगिति यदुक्तं तदनुत्याख्यास्यामः- यदा पुरुषो दुर्बलो हि सन् बलवता सह विगृह्णाति, अतिमहता वा धनुषा व्यायच्छति, जल्पति वाऽप्यतिमात्रम्, अतिमात्रं वा भारमुद्वहति, अप्सु वा प्लवते चातिदूरम्, उत्सादनपदाघातने वाऽतिप्रगाढमासंवते, अतिप्रकृष्टं वाऽध्वानं द्रुतमभिपतति, अभिहन्यते वा, अन्यद्वा किञ्चिदेवंविधं विषममतिमात्रं वा व्यायामजातमारभते, तस्यातिमात्रेण कर्मणोः क्षण्यते| तस्योरः क्षतमुपप्लवते वायुः| स तत्रावस्थितः श्लेष्माणमुरःस्थमुपसङ्गृह्य पित्तं च दूषयन् विहरत्यूर्ध्वमधस्तिर्यक् च| तस्य योंऽशः शरीरसन्धीनाविशति तेनास्य जृम्भाऽङ्गमर्दो ज्वरश्चोपजायते, यस्त्वामाशयमभ्युपैति तेन रोगा भवन्ति उरस्या अरोचकश्च, यः कण्ठमभिप्रपद्यते कण्ठस्तेनोद्ध्वंस्यते स्वरश्चावसीदति, यः प्राणवहानि स्रोतांस्यनेति तेन श्वासः प्रतिश्यायश्च जायते, यः शिरस्यवतिष्ठते शिरस्तेनोपहन्यते; ततः क्षणनाच्चैवोरसो विषमगतित्वाच्च वायोः कण्ठस्य चोद्ध्वंसनात् कासः सततमस्य सञ्जायते, स कास प्रसङ्गादुरसि क्षते शोणितं ष्ठीवति, शोणितागमनाच्चास्य दौर्बल्यमुपजायते; एवमेते साहस प्रभवाः साहसिकमुपद्रवाः स्पृशन्ति|

ततः स उपशोषणैरेतैरुपद्रवैरुपद्रुतः शनैः शनैरुपशुष्यति|

तस्मात् पुरुषो मतिमान् बलमात्मनः समीक्ष्य तदनुरूपाणि कर्माण्यारभेत कर्तुं; बलसमाधानं हि शरीरं, शरीरमूलश्च पुरुष इति||४||

भवति चात्र- साहसं वर्जयेत् कर्म रक्षञ्जीवितमात्मनः|

जीवन् हि पुरुषस्त्विष्टं कर्मणः फलमश्नुते||५||

Details of Sahasa Nidana for Shosha:

We shall now discuss "excess physical activity" as an etiological factor of Shosha. When a weak person fights with a stronger one or exerts with too big a bow or speaks too much, or carries too big a load or swims in water for long distance or resorts to forceful massage and application of pressure by feet or runs fast to cover a long distance or subjects himself to assault or indulges in such other irregular regimens and physical exercises in excess, his chest gets injured due to such excessive exercises. The injured chest of such a weak person is saturated with (vitiated) Vata. Being there, the vitiated vata would get mixed with the kapha located therein and also traverses upwards, downwards and side-wards after contaminating the pitta also.

The portion of that vitiated vata which affects the joints of the body causes
Jrumbha – yawning
Anga marda – malaise and
Jvara – fever
The portion which affects the Amashaya (stomach including small intestine) leads to
Arochaka – anorexia and
Urasya roga – The disease of the chest (like palpitation and cardiac pain)
The portion which affects throat causes
Kanthodhvamsa – irritation of the throat and
Svarabheda – hoarseness of voice

The portion which affects the head causes damage to that part. Thereafter, due to injury to the chest, irregular movement of Vata and irritation of the throat, the patient suffers from constant coughing.
Due to continued coughing there is further injury to the chest and the patient spits blood. These are the complications arising out of rash behaviour of an individual. These emaciating complications lead to cachexia. So a wise person should perform various activities with due regard to his own strength. The body is sustained by strength and the individual (Empirical self) by the body.
Thus it is said:-
The individual enjoys the desired fruit of his action only when he is alive. Therefore, one desirous of long life should avoid rash behaviour. [4-5]

Details of Sandharana – Suppression of natural urges as Nidana (etiological factor):
सन्धारणं शोषस्यायतनमिति यदुक्तं तदनुव्याख्यास्यामः- यदा पुरुषो राजसमीपे भर्तुः समीपे वा गुरोर्वा पाद मूले द्यूतसभमन्यं वा सतां समाजं स्त्रीमध्यं वा समनुप्रविश्य यानैर्वाऽप्युच्चावचैरभियान् भयात् प्रसङ्गादृधीमत्त्वादृधृणित्वाद्वा निरुणद्ध्यागतान् वात मूत्र पुरीष वेगान् तदा तस्य सन्धारणाद्वायुः प्रकोपमापद्यते, स प्रकुपितः पित्त श्लेष्माणौ समुदीर्योर्ध्वमधस्तिर्यक् च विहरति; ततश्चांश विशेषेण पूर्ववच्छरीरावयव विशेषं प्रविश्य शूलमुपजनयति, भिनत्ति पुरीषमुच्छोषयति वा, पार्श्वं चातिरुजति, अंसाववमृद्गति, कण्ठमुरश्चावधमति, शिरश्चोपहन्ति, कासं श्वासं ज्वरं स्वरभेदं प्रतिश्यायं चोपजनयति; ततः स उपशोषणैरेतैरुपद्रवैरुपद्रुतः शनैः शनैरुपशुष्यति।
तस्मात् पुरुषो मतिमानात्मनः शारीरेष्वेव योगक्षेमकरेषु प्रयतेत विशेषेण; शरीरं ह्यस्य मूलं, शरीरमूलश्च पुरुषो भवति॥६॥
भवति चात्र- सर्वमन्यत् परित्यज्य शरीरमनुपालयेत्।
तदभावे हि भावानां सर्वाभावः शरीरिणाम्॥७॥

Details of Sandharana – Suppression of natural urges as Nidana (etiological factor):
We shall now explain "Suppression of natural urges" as the etiological factor of Shosha.
When an individual suppresses the manifested urges of flatus, urine and stool because of apprehension, pre-occupation, bashfulness or hatred in front of the king or master or (while sitting) at the feet of the preceptor or while gambling or attending meetings of gentlemen or in the midst of women, or while travelling in high or low vehicles, then Vata in his body gets aggravated. This aggravated Vata carrying along with it provoked Pitta and kapha moves upwards, downwards and sideways.
Different portions of Vata enter into different parts of the body as described before (in para 4) and cause
Shula – colic pain
Purisha bhinna – diarrhoea

Parshva ati ruja – severe pain in the sides of the chest / flanks / shoulder region

Aṃsāvavamṛdgāti – increased respiratory movement in the chest and throat

Shiraścopahanti – damage to the head

Kasa – coughing

Shvasa – dyspnoea

Jvara – fever

Svarabhedaṃ – hoarseness of voice could make special efforts not to suppress the manifested urges with a view to sustaining his body.

The body constitutes the root cause of the wellbeing of the individual and the very production of the body is dependent upon the individual self.

Thus it is said:-

Leaving everything else, one should maintain the body. For if there is no body, there is nothing that can be made available to the individual. [6-7]

Details of Shosha (wasting) as Nidana (etiological factor):

क्षयः शोषस्यायतनमिति यदुक्तं तदनुव्याख्यास्यामः- यदा पुरुषोऽतिमात्रं शोक चिन्ता परिगत हृदयो भवति, ईर्ष्योत्कण्ठाभय क्रोधादिभिर्वा समाविश्यते, कृशो वा सन् रूक्षान्नपानसेवी भवति, दुर्बल प्रकृतिरनाहारोऽल्पाहारो वा भवति, तदा तस्य हृदय स्थायी रसः क्षयमुपैति; स तस्योपक्षयाच्छोषं प्राप्नोति, अप्रतीकाराच्चानुबध्यते यक्ष्मणा यथोपदेक्ष्यमाणरूपेण।८।

Details of Shosha (wasting) as Nidana (etiological factor):

We shall explain wasting 'as an etiological factor for Shosha' Rasa residing in the heart of an individual gets diminished due to the following-

Yadā puruṣo'timātraṃ śoka cintā parigata hṛdayo bhavati – Affliction of the heart of the individual, with excessive grief and worries.

īrṣyotkaṇṭhābhaya krodhādibhirvā samāviśyate – Affliction with jealousy, fear, anger etc. intake of un-unctuous diets and drinks by emaciated individuals.

Kṛśo vā san rūkṣānnapānasevī bhavati – Intake of food in lesser quantity or fasting by persons who are weak by nature.

Due to this diminution of Rasa, the individual is afflicted with Shosha and if this condition is not neutralized, it leads to the manifestation of tuberculosis in a manner to be described later. (1)

Loss of semen due to over-indulgence and its consequence:

यदा वा पुरुषोऽतिहर्षादति प्रसक्तभावः स्त्रीष्वतिप्रसङ्गमारभते, तस्यातिमात्र प्रसङ्गाद्रेतः क्षयमेति।

क्षयमपि चोपगच्छति रेतसि यदि मनः स्त्रीभ्यो नैवास्य निवर्तते, तस्य चाति प्रणीत सङ्कल्पस्य मैथुनमापद्यमानस्य न शुक्रं प्रवर्तेऽतिमात्रोपक्षीणरेतस्त्वात्, तथाऽस्य वायुर्व्यायच्छमानशरीरस्यैव धमनीरनुप्रविश्य शोणितवाहिनीस्ताभ्यः शोणितं प्रच्यावयति, तच्छुक्रक्षयादस्य पुनः शुक्रमार्गण शोणितं प्रवर्तते वातानुसृत लिङ्गम्।

अथास्य शुक्रक्षयाच्छोणित प्रवर्तनाच्च सन्धयः शिथिली भवन्ति, रौक्ष्यमुपजायते, भूयः शरीरं दौर्बल्यमाविशति, वायुः प्रकोपमापद्यते; स प्रकुपितो वशिकं शरीरमनुसर्पन्नुदीर्य श्लेष्मपित्ते परिशोषयति मांस शोणिते, प्रच्यावयति श्लेष्म पित्ते संरुजति पार्श्वे, अवमृद्गात्यंसौ, कण्ठमुद्ध्वंसति, शिरः श्लेष्माणमुपत्क्लेश्य प्रतिपूरयति श्लेष्मणा, सन्धींश्च प्रपीडयन् करोत्यङ्गमर्दमरोचकविपाकौ च, पित्तश्लेष्मोत्क्लेशात् प्रतिलोमगत्वाच्च वायुर्ज्वरं कासं श्वासं स्वरभेदं प्रतिश्यायं चोपजनयति; स कास प्रसङ्गादुरसि क्षते शोणितं ष्ठीवति, शोणित गमनाच्चास्य दौर्बल्यमुपजायते, ततः स उपशोषणेरेतैरुपद्रवैरुपद्रुतः शनैः शनैरुपशुष्यति।

तस्मात् पुरुषो मतिमानात्मनः शरीरमनुरक्षञ्छुक्रमनुरक्षेत्।

परा ह्येषा फल निर्वृतिराहारस्येति।।८।।

भवति चात्र- आहारस्य परं धाम शुक्रं तद्रक्ष्यमात्मनः।

क्षयो ह्यस्य बहून् रोगान्मरणं वा नियच्छति।।९।।

Loss of semen due to excess sex and its consequence:

When an individual due to excessive attachment borne out of excessive passion indulges in sexual act in excess, diminution of semen occurs due to his repeated indulgence in sex. If he is still determined to indulge in sexual act, he will have no ejaculation of semen during cohabitation because of his semen having been already exhausted.

During the process of coitus vata would enter the blood vessels. Vata would enter the blood vessels of this individual leading to the ejaculation of blood. The blood being vitiated by Vata, would then enter the seminal channels because of the diminution of semen. Due to the diminution of semen, and discharge of blood, the joints would become loose. There would be dryness and further weakness in the body and aggravation of Vata.

The vitiated Vata Dosha, while spreading all over the body from where semen is exhausted and aggravating Kapha and Pitta, would dry up (reduces) muscle tissues and blood, eliminate Kapha (Phlegm), grinding pain in the shoulders, irritate the throat, till up the head with Kapha, after vitiating the latter. It would also produce malaise, anorexia and indigestion after afflicting the joints.

Due to the vitiation of Pitta and kapha and adoption of opposite course, Vata would then produce

Jvara – fever

Kasa – cough

Shvasa – dyspnoea

Svara bheda – hoarseness of voice and

Pratishyaya – Coryza

Due to the injury in the chest because of continued coughing the patient would spit blood. Due to the loss of blood he would become weak. Later he would be afflicted by severe complications which would dry up the body (cachexia) gradually, day by day. Therefore, a wise person should protect his semen even as he puts all efforts to protect his body because it (semen) is the outcome par excellence of the food taken.

Thus it is said: – Semen is the outcome par excellence of food. One should preserve his own semen because its diminution leads to many diseases and even death. [8-9]

Vishamashana (irregular dieting) as etiological factor:

विषमाशनं शोषस्यायतनमिति यदुक्तं, तदनुव्याख्यास्यामः- यदा पुरुषः पानाशन भक्ष्यलेह्योपयोगान् प्रकृतिकरणसंयोगराशिदेशकालोपयोगसंस्थोपशयविषमानासेवते, तदा तस्य तेभ्यो वात पित्त श्लेष्माणो वैषम्यमापद्यन्ते; ते विषमाः शरीरमनुसृत्य यदा स्रोतसामयनमुखानि प्रतिवार्यावतिष्ठन्ते तदा जन्तुर्यद्यदाहारजातमाहरति तत्तदस्य मूत्रपुरीषमेवोपजायते भूयिष्ठं नान्यस्तथा शरीरधातुः; स पुरीषोपष्टम्भाद्वर्तयति, तस्माच्छुष्यतो विशेषेण पुरीषमनुरक्ष्यं तथान्येषामतिकृशदुर्बलानां; तस्यानाप्यायमानस्य विषमाशनोपचिता दोषाः पृथक् पृथग्पद्वैर्युञ्जन्तो भूयः शरीरमुपशोषयन्ति।

तत्र वातः शूलमङ्गमर्दं कण्ठोद्ध्वंसनं पार्श्व संरुजनंमंसावमर्दं स्वरभेदं प्रतिश्यायं चोपजनयति; पित्तं ज्वरमतीसारमन्तर्दाहं च; श्लेष्मा तु प्रतिश्यायं शिरसो गुरुत्वमरोचकं कासं च, स कास प्रसङ्गादुरसि क्षते शोणितं निष्ठीवति, शोणितगमनाच्चास्य दौर्बल्यमुपजायते।

एवमेते विषमाशनोपचितास्त्रयो दोषा राजयक्ष्याणमभिनिर्वर्तयन्ति।

स तैरुपशोषणैरुपद्रवैरुपद्रुतः शनैः शनैः शुष्यति।

तस्मात् पुरुषो मतिमान् प्रकृतिकरण संयोगराशिदेशकालोपयोग संस्थोपशयादविषममाहारमाहरेत्॥१०॥

भवति चात्र- हिताशी स्यान्मिताशी स्यात्कालभोजी जितेन्द्रियः।

पश्यन् रोगान् बहून् कष्टान् बुद्धिमान् विषमाशनात्॥११॥

Vishamashana (irregular dieting) as etiological factor:

We shall explain the "irregular dieting " as an etiological factor, viz drinkables, eatables, chewable and lickables without paying proper heed towards their nature, mode of preparation, combination, quantity, locality, time, dietetic rules and wholesomeness for the individual. Then Vata, Pitta and Kapha in his body get imbalanced due to this irregularity.

These imbalanced dosha spreads all over the body and when they get localized in view of the obstruction to the entrances of the channels of circulation, then whatever food is taken by the individual mostly gets converted into stool and urine rather than dhatus (tissue elements) of the body. The afflicted individual is sustained by the retention of the stool. Therefore, the fecal matter of individuals suffering from Shosha or others who are extremely emaciated or weak is retained. Doshas accumulated due to irregular dieting, produce severe complications and dries up the body.

Vata produces
Shula – colic pain
Angamarda – malaise
Antardaham – irritation in throat
Pārśva saṃrujanam – pain in the sides of the chest
Aṃsāvamardaṃ – grinding pain in the shoulders
Svara Bheda – hoarseness of voice and
Pratishyaya – Coryza
Pitta causes
Jvara – fever
Atisara – diarrhoea and
Antar daha – burning sensation inside the body, and
Kapha causes
Pratishyaya – coryza
Shiro gaurava – heaviness of head
Arochaka – anorexia and
Kasa – coughing
Due to excessive coughing there is injury to the chest (lungs) and the patient spits blood. Because of the discharge of blood he becomes weak. Thus the 3 Doshas accumulated due to irregular dieting manifest the disease Rajayakshma (Tuberculosis).

The emaciating complications lead to cachexia by and by. Therefore, a wise person should take such diets as are wholesome from the point of view of nature, mode of preparation, combination, quantity, locality, time, dietetic rules and the wholesomeness for the individual who takes them.

Thus, it is said: – In view of the association of painful diseases with irregular dieting, a wise man with good control over his senses should take wholesome food in proper quantity and in proper time [10-11]

Nomenclature of disease:
एतैश्चतुर्भिः शोषस्यायतनैरुपसेवितैर्वात पित्त श्लेष्माणः प्रकोपमापद्यन्ते|
ते प्रकुपिता नानाविधैरुपद्रवैः शरीरमुपशोषयन्ति|
तं सर्वरोगाणां कष्टतमत्वाद्राजयक्ष्माणमाचक्षते भिषजः; यस्माद्वा पूर्वमासीद्भगवतः सोमस्योडुराजस्य तस्माद्राजयक्ष्मेति||१२||
The 4 causative factors of Shosha, when resorted to lead to the aggravation of Vata, Pitta and Kapha
These aggravated Doshas deplete the body due to varieties of complications. This condition is known as Rajayakshma (lit. king of diseases or disease of the king) because of its most formidable nature among all the diseases and also because according to the mythological story, it afflicted the moon who is the king of stars [12]

Purva rupa of Shosha – Premonitory symptoms:

तस्येमानि पूर्वरूपाणि भवन्ति; तद्यथा- प्रतिश्यायः, क्षवथुरभीक्ष्णं, श्लेष्मप्रसेकः, मुख माधुर्यम्, अनन्नाभिलाषः, अन्नकाले चायासः, दोष दर्शनमदोषेष्वल्पदोषेषु वा भावेषु पात्रोदकान्नसूपापूपोपदंशपरिवेशकेषु, भुक्तवतश्चास्य हल्लासः, तथोल्लेखनमप्याहारस्यान्तरान्तरा, मुखस्य पादयोश्च शोफः, पाण्योश्चावेक्षणमत्यर्थम्, अक्ष्णोः श्वेतावभासता चातिमात्रं, बाह्वोश्च प्रमाणजिज्ञासा, स्त्रीकामता, निर्घृणित्वं, बीभत्स दर्शनता चास्य काये, स्वप्ने चाभीक्ष्णं दर्शनमनुदकानामुदकस्थानानां शून्यानां च ग्राम नगर निगम जनपदानां शुष्क दग्ध भग्नानां च वनानां कृकलास मयूर वानर शुक सर्पकाकोलूकादिभिः संस्पर्शनमधिरोहणं यानं वा श्वोष्ट्रखरवराहैः केशास्थिभस्मतुषाङ्गारराशीनां चाधिरोहणमिति (शोषपूर्वरूपाणि भवन्ति)।।१३।।

Shosha Purvaroopa:

Its premonitory symptoms are

Pratishyaya – Coryza

Kshavathu – frequent sneezing

Sleshma praseka – excessive salivation

Mukha madhuryam – sweet taste in the mouth

Anannābhilāṣaḥ – disinclination for food

Annakāle cāyāsaḥ – feeling of tiredness during the meal time

Doṣa darśanamadoṣeṣvalpadoṣeṣu vā bhāveṣu pātrodakānnasūpāpūpopadaṃśapariveśakeṣu – finding fault with such things as are without any fault or with negligible fault specially that of utensils, water, food soup, cake, Upadamsa (things which are chewed before taking food), and cateres,

Bhuktavataścāsya hṛllāsaḥ – Nausea after meals

Mukhasya pādayośca śophaḥ – swelling of the face and feet

Pāṇyoścāvekṣaṇamatyartham – frequent inspection of hands

Akṣṇoḥ śvetāvabhāsatā cātimātram – excessive whiteness of eyes

Bāhvośca pramāṇajijñāsā – enquiry about the measurement of arms

Strīkāmatā – passionate attachment with women

Nirghṛṇitvaṃ – cruel disposition, frightful appearance (discoloration and foul smell) in his body and

Bībhatsa darśanatā cāsya kāye – appearance of the following in dreams:

Svapne cābhīkṣṇaṃ darśanamanudakānāmudakasthānānām – Empty water reservoirs

Janapadānāṃ śuṣka bhagnānāṃ – villages, towns, cities and countries

Dagdha vanānāṃ – Dried, burnt and denuded forests

Kṛkalāsa mayūra vānara śuka sarpakākolūkādibhiḥ saṃsparśanamadhirohaṇaṃ – Coming into physical contact with chameleon, peacocks, monkey, parrots, serpents, crows, owls etc

Yānaṃ vā śvoṣṭrakharavarāhaiḥ – Riding over dogs, camels, donkeys and pigs or vehicles drawn by them

Keśāsthibhasmatuṣāṅgārarāśīnāṃ cādhirohaṇamiti – Climbing over heaps of hair, bones, ash chaff and fire brands [13]

Rupa – Eleven symptoms of Shosha:

अत ऊर्ध्वमेकादशरूपाणि तस्य भवन्ति; तद्यथा- शिरसः परिपूर्णत्वं, कासः, श्वासः, स्वरभेदः, श्लेष्मणश्छर्दनं, शोणितष्ठीवनं, पार्श्वसंरोजनम्, अंसावमर्दः, ज्वरः, अतीसारः, अरोचकश्चेति।।१४।।

Thereafter 11 symptoms of this disease are manifested they are

Shirasaḥ paripūrṇatvaṃ – Heaviness of head

Kāsaḥ – Cough

śvāsaḥ – Dyspnea

Svarabhedaḥ – Hoarseness of voice

śleṣmaṇaśchardanaṃ – Voiding of phlegm

śoṇitaṣṭhīvanaṃ – Spitting of blood

Pārśvasaṃrojanam – Pain in the sides of the chest

Aṃsāvamardaḥ – Grinding pain in the shoulder

Jvaraḥ – Fever

Atīsāraḥ – Diarrhea and

Arochaka – Anorexia [14]

Shosham Sadhya Asadhyata – Prognosis:

तत्रापरिक्षीण बल मांस शोणितो बलवानजातारिष्टः सर्वैरपि शोष लिङ्गैरुपद्रुतः साध्यो ज्ञेयः|

बलवानुपचितो हि सहत्वाद्व्याध्यौषधबलस्य कामं सुबहुलिङ्गोऽप्यल्पलिङ्ग एव मन्तव्यः||१५||

A patient whose strength, muscle tissues and blood have not undergone diminution, who is strong and, in whose body, bad prognostic symptoms have not appeared is curable even if all symptoms of the disease- Shosha- are manifested in his body. A strong and well-nourished patient can resist both the disease and medicines; hence even if all symptoms of the disease are manifested in his body, still he may be considered as having a few symptoms only i.e. easily curable. [15]

Asadhya Lakshana – Signs of incurable of Sosha:

दुर्बलं त्वतिक्षीण बल मांस शोणितमल्पलिङ्गमजातारिष्टमपि बहुलिङ्गं जातारिष्टं च विद्यात्, असहत्वाद्व्याध्यौषधबलस्य; तं परिवर्जयेत्, क्षणेनैव हि प्रादुर्भवन्त्यरिष्टानि, अनिमित्तश्चारिष्टप्रादुर्भाव इति||१६||

तत्र श्लोकः- समुत्थानं च लिङ्गं च यः शोषस्यावबुध्यते|

पूर्वरूपं च तत्त्वेन स राज्ञः कर्तुमर्हति||१७||

A patient even having a few symptoms of the disease and without bad prognostic signs is incurable (like the one having all symptoms and manifested bad prognostic signs) if he is weak and there is diminution of strength, muscle tissue and blood, because he will be unable to resist the effect of the diseases as well as the medicines. He should not be treated. Bad prognostic signs may appear in such patients in time and even without any causative factor. [16]

Merits of royal physician:

तत्र श्लोकः- समुत्थानं च लिङ्गं च यः शोषस्यावबुध्यते|

पूर्वरूपं च तत्त्वेन स राज्ञः कर्तुमर्हति||१७||

To sum up: - the physician who is well versed in the aetiology, symptomatology and premonitory symptoms of Shosha is verily competent to be a "Royal Physician". [17]

इत्यग्निवेशकृते तन्त्रे चरक प्रतिसंस्कृते निदान स्थाने शोष निदानं नाम षष्ठोऽध्यायः||६||

Thus ends the 6th chapter on "Shosha Nidana" of the section on the Diagnosis of Diseases (Nidana sthana) of Agniveshas work as redacted by Charaka.

7

Nidanasthana Chapter 7 Unmada Nidanam

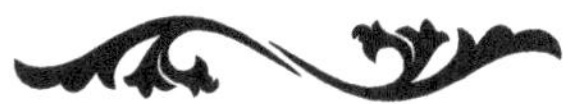

The 7th chapter of Charaka Samhitha Nidana Sthana is called Unmada Nidana. It deals with causes, pathology, types and symptoms of Unmada – Insanity, as per Ayurveda.

अथात उन्माद निदानं व्याख्यास्यामः||१||

इति ह स्माह भगवानात्रेयः||२||

We shall now explore the chapter on the "Diagnosis of Insanity". Thus said Lord Atreya [1-2]

Vidha (Types) of Unmada – Insanity:

इह खलु पञ्चोन्मादा भवन्ति; तद्यथा- वात पित्त कफ सन्निपातागन्तु निमित्ताः||३||

तत्र दोष निमित्ताश्चत्वारः पुरुषाणामेवंविधानां क्षिप्रमभिनिर्वर्तन्ते; तद्यथा- भीरूणामुपक्लिष्टसत्त्वानामुत्सन्न दोषाणां स मल विकृतोपहितान्यनुचितान्याहारजातानि वैषम्ययुक्तेनोपयोगविधिनोपयुञ्जानानां तन्त्रप्रयोगमपि विषममाचरतामन्याश्च शरीरचेष्टा विषमाः समाचरतामत्युपक्षीण देहानां व्याधि वेग समुद्भ्रमितानामुपहतमनसां वा काम क्रोध लोभ हर्ष भय मोहायास शोक चिन्तोद्वेगादिभिर्भूयोऽभिघाताभ्याहतानां वा मनस्युपहते बुद्धौ च प्रचलितायामभ्युदीर्णा दोषाः प्रकुपिता हृदयमुपसृत्य मनोवहानि स्रोतांस्यावृत्य जनयन्त्युन्मादम्||४||

Unmada (insanity) is of 5 types. They are due to:

Vata,

Pitta

Kapha and

Sannipata (combined vitiation of all the 3 Doshas) and

Aagantuja – exogenous.

The 4 types of Unmada caused by the vitiation of Doshas manifest themselves quickly in the following circumstances:

Bhīrūṇāmupakliṣṭa – When an individual is timid

Sattvānāmutsannadoṣāṇāṃ – When his mind is afflicted by the predominance of Rajas and Tamas

Mala vikṛtopahitānyanucitānyāhārajātāni- When Doshas in his body are aggravated and Vitiated

Vaiṣamyayuktenopayogavidhinopayuñjānānāṃ – When he takes food consisting of unwholesome and unclean ingredients possessing mutually contradictory properties or touched by unclean hands of persons suffering from contagious disease like leprosy, neglecting the prescribed dietetic rules, (viz. conformity with nature etc. of the ingredients)

Samācaratāmatyupakṣīṇadehānāṃ – When his body is exceedingly depleted

If he is not in a proper state of health due to other diseases

When his body is exceedingly depleted

If he is not in a proper state of health due to other diseases

Vyādhi vega samudbhramitānām upahata manasāṃ vā kāma krodha lobha harṣa bhaya mohs āyāsa śoka chinta udvegādibhir bhūyo abhighātābhyāhatānām – When his mind is afflicted over and over again by passion, anger, greed, excitement, fear, attachment, exertion, anxiety and grief and

Abhighātābhyāhatānām – When he is subjected to excessive physical assault

In the circumstances so enumerated above, the mind gets seriously affected and the intellect loses its balance. So the Doshas aggravated and vitiated enter the cardiac region and obstruct the channels of the mind resulting in Insanity. [3-4]

Definition of insanity:
उन्मादं पुनर्मनोबुद्धिसञ्ज्ञाज्ञान स्मृति भक्ति शील चेष्टाचार विभ्रमं विद्यात्||५||
Insanity is characterized by the:
Punar mano – pervasion of mind
Buddhi – intellect
Sanjna – consciousness
Jnana – knowledge
Smrti – memory
Sheela – desire
Chesta – manners
Achara – behavior and
Vibhrama – contact [5]

Unmada Purvarupa – Premonitory symptoms
तस्येमानि पूर्वरूपाणि; तद्यथा- शिरसः शून्यता, चक्षुषोराकुलता, स्वनः कर्णयोः, उच्छ्वासस्याधिक्यम्, आस्य संस्रवणम्, अनन्नाभिलाषारोचकाविपाकाः, हृद्ग्रहः, ध्यानायास सम्मोहोद्वेगाश्चास्थाने, सततं लोमहर्षः, ज्वरश्चाभीक्ष्णम्, उन्मत्त चित्तत्वम्, उदर्दित्वम्, अर्दिताकृतिकरणं च व्याधेः, स्वप्ने चाभीक्ष्णं दर्शनं भ्रान्तचलितानवस्थितानां रूपाणामप्रशस्तानां च तिलपीडकचक्राधिरोहणं वातकुण्डलिकाभिश्चोन्मथनं निमज्जनं च कलुषाणाम्भसामावर्ते चक्षुषोश्चापसर्पणमिति (दोषनिमित्तानामुन्मादानां पूर्वरूपाणि भवन्ति)||६||

Premonitory symptoms of insanity caused by the vitiation of Doshas:
Shirasaḥśūnyatā – Emptiness in head
Chakṣuṣorākulatā – Congestion in eyes
Svanaḥkarṇayoḥ – Noises in ears
Ucchvāsasyādhikyam – Hard breathing in excess
Aasya saṃsravaṇam – Excessive salivation in the mouth
Anannābhilāṣārocakāvipākāḥ – Absence of inclination for food, anorexia and indigestion
Hṛdgrahaḥ – Spasm in cardiac region
Dhyānāyāsasammohodvegāścāsthāne – Meditation, fatigue, unconsciousness and anxiety in improper situations
Satataṃlomaharṣaḥ – Continuous horripilation
Jvaraścābhīkṣṇam – Frequent pyrexia
Unmattacittatvam – Fickle mindedness
Udarditvam – Pain in the upper part of the body
Arditākṛtikaraṇaṃ ca vyādheḥ – Manifestation of symptoms of facial paralysis resulting in movement in one half of the face
Svapnecābhīkṣṇaṃdarśanam – Frequent appearance of the following in dreams
Bhrāntacalitānavasthitānāṃrūpāṇāmapraśastānām ca tilapīḍakacakrādhirohaṇaṃvātakuṇḍalikābhiśconmathanaṃ – Inauspicious objects that are wandering, moving and unstable
Nimajjanaṃ – Riding over the wheel of an oil press

Kaluṣāṇāmambhasāmāvarte – Being churned by whirl-winds
Sinking in fearful whirl pools and
Chakṣuṣoścāpasarpaṇamiti – Retraction of eyes.[6]

Distinctive features of insanity:

ततोऽनन्तरमेवमुन्मादाभिनिर्वृत्तिरेव।

तत्रेदमुन्मादविशेषविज्ञानं भवति; तद्यथा- परिसरणमजस्रम्, अक्षि भ्रुवौष्ठांसहन्वग्रहस्तपादाङ्ग विक्षेपणमकस्मात्, सततमनियतानां च गिरामुत्सर्गः, फेनागमनमास्यात्, अभीक्ष्णं स्मितहसितनृत्यगीतवादित्रसम्प्रयोगाश्चास्थाने, वीणावंश शङ्ख शम्या तालशब्दानुकरणमसाम्ना, यानमयानैः, अलङ्करणमनलङ्कारिकैर्द्रव्यैः, लोभश्चाभ्यवहार्येष्वलब्धेषु, लब्धेषु चावमानस्तीव्रमात्सर्यं च, कार्श्यं, पारुष्यम्, उत्पिण्डितारुणाक्षता, वातोपशयविपर्यासादनुपशयता च; इति वातोन्मादलिङ्गानि भवन्ति(१);

अमर्षः, क्रोधः, संरम्भश्चास्थाने, शस्त्रलोष्ट्रकशाकाष्ठमुष्टिभिरभिहननं स्वेषां परेषां वा, अभिद्रवणं, प्रच्छायशीतोदकान्नाभिलाषः, सन्तापश्चातिवेलं, ताम्रहरितहारिद्रसंरब्धाक्षता, पित्तोपशयविपर्यासादनुपशयता च; इति पित्तोन्मादलिङ्गानि भवन्ति(२);

स्थानमेकदेशे, तूष्णीम्भावः, अल्पशश्चङ्क्रमणं, लालासिङ्घाणकस्रवणम्, अनन्नाभिलाषः, रहस्कामता, बीभत्सत्वं, शौचद्वेषः, स्वप्ननित्यता, श्वयथुरानने, शुक्ल स्तिमितमलोपदिग्धाक्षत्वं, श्लेष्मोपशयविपर्यासादनुपशयता च; इति श्लेष्मोन्मादलिङ्गानि भवन्ति(३);

त्रिदोषलिङ्गसन्निपाते तु सान्निपातिकं विद्यात्; तमसाध्यमाचक्षते कुशलाः॥७॥

Clinical features of Unmada:

A) Vataja Unmad:

Parisaraṇamajasram – constant wandering

Akṣibhruvauṣṭhāṃsahanvagrahastapādāṅgavikṣepaṇamakasmāt – sudden spasm of eyes, eyebrows, lips, shoulder, jaws, fore-arms, and legs

Satatamaniyatānāṃ ca girāmutsargaḥ – constant and incoherent speech

Phenāgamanamāsyāt – froth coming out from the mouth

Abhīkṣṇaṃsmitahasitanṛtyagītavāditrasamprayogāścāsthāne – Always smiling, laughing, dancing, singing and playing with musical instruments in inappropriate situations

Vīṇāvaṃśaśaṅkhaśamyātālaśabdānukaraṇamasāmnā – Loudly imitating the sounds of flute, conch, Samya (cymbal played by right hand) and Tala (cymbal played by left hand)

Yānamayānaiḥ – Riding undesirable vehicles

Alaṅkaraṇamanalaṅkārikairdravyaiḥ – Getting decorated by things which are non-ornamental

Lobhaścābhyavahāryeṣvalabdheṣu – Longing for eatables not available

Labdheṣucāvamānastīvram mātsaryaṃ ca – Rejecting or insulting the eatables which are available, jealousy or hatred towards others

Kārśyaṃ, pāruṣyam – Emaciation and roughness

Utpiṇḍitāruṇākṣata – Projected and reddish eyes

Vātopaśayaviparyāsādanupaśayatā ca – Aggravation of the condition by such of the regimens which are not wholesome for Vata.

(B) Paittika Unmada:

Amarṣaḥ, krodhaḥ – Irritation and anger

Saṃrambhaścāsthāne – Excitement on inappropriate occasions

Shastraloṣṭrakaśākāṣṭhamuṣṭibhirabhihananaṃsveṣāṃpareṣāṃvāabhidravaṇam – Inflicting injury on own people or on others by weapons, brick, bats, whips, sticks and fist.

Pracchāyaśītodakānnabhilāṣaḥ – fleeing and desire for shade, cold water and food having cooling effect.

Santāpaścātivelaṃ – Continuous state of anguish

Tāmraharitahāridrasaṃrabdhākṣata – having ferocious eyes of coppery, green or yellow colour and

Pittopaśayaviparyāsādanupaśayatā ca – aggravation of the condition by such regimens which are not wholesome for Pitta.

(C) Slaismika Unmada:
Sthānamekadeśetūṣṇīmbhāvaḥ, alpaśaścaṅkramaṇam – Staying in one place and observance of silence
Lālāśiṅghāṇakasravaṇam – Discharge of saliva and nasal excretions
Anannābhilāṣaḥrahaskamata – disinclination for food and love for solitude
Bībhatsatvaṃ – Frightening appearance
śaucadveṣaḥ – Aversion for cleanliness
Svapnanityatā – Remaining always sleepy
śvayathurānane – oedema in the face
Shukla stimitamalopadigdhākṣatvaṃ – White and timid eyes with excreta adhered to them
Shleṣmopaśayaviparyāsādanupaśayatā ca – Aggravation of the condition by such regimens which are not wholesome for Kapha

(D) Sannipatika type: In the insanity caused by the combined vitiation of all the 3 Doshas, all the symptoms mentioned above are simultaneously manifested. This type of Insanity is considered to be incurable. [7]

Therapies as treatment:
साध्यानां तु त्रयाणां साधनानि- स्नेह स्वेद वमन विरेचनास्थापनानुवासनोपशमन नस्तःकर्म धूम धूपनाञ्जनावपीड प्रधमनाभ्यङ्ग प्रदेह परिषेकानुलेपनवधबन्धनावरोधन- वित्रासन विस्मापन विस्मारणापतर्पण सिराव्यधनानि, भोजन विधानं च यथास्वं युक्त्या, यच्चान्यदपि किञ्चिन्निदानविपरीतमौषधं कार्यं तदपि स्यादिति॥८॥
भवति चात्र- उन्मादान् दोषजान् साध्यान् साधयेद्भिषगुत्तमः।
अनेन विधियुक्तेन कर्मणा यत् प्रकीर्तितम्॥९॥
Therapies for treatment of the 3 types of insanity which are curable are
Snehana – oleation
Svedana – fomentation
Vamana – emesis
Virechana – purgation
Asthapana basti – type of enema wherein decoctions are used
Anuvasana basti – type of enema wherein medicated oils / ghee are used
Shamana – alleviation therapies
Nasya karma – ermines
Dhumapana - smoking
Dhupana – fumigation
Anjana – collyrium
Avapida and
Pradhamana types of Snuff
Abhyanga - massage
Pradeha – ointment
Parisheka – effusion
Anulepana – unction / anointment
Vadha – assault
Bandhana – tying
Avarodhana – confinement
Vitrasana – frightening
Vismapana – inducing astonishment and forgetfulness,

Vismarana – depletion and

Sira vyadhana – venesection

Suitable diets are given according to the requirements of the patient. Such other therapies as would work against the causative factors of the diseases are also given. Thus it is said: -Following the principles of treatment (to be detailed in Chikitsa 9) a competent physician should employ the above-mentioned therapies to treat the curable types of insanity caused by the vitiation of Doshas. [8-9]

Aagantuja unmada (Exogenous insanity):

यस्तु दोष निमित्तेभ्य उन्मादेभ्यः समुत्थान पूर्वरूप लिङ्ग वेदनोपशय विशेष समन्वितो भवत्युन्मादस्तमागन्तुकमाचक्षते|

केचित् पुनः पूर्वकृतं कर्माप्रशस्तमिच्छन्ति तस्य निमित्तम्|

तस्य च हेतुः प्रज्ञापराध एवेति भगवान् पुनर्वसुरात्रेयः|

प्रज्ञापराधाद्ध्ययं देवर्षिपितृ गन्धर्व यक्ष राक्षस पिशाच गुरुवृद्ध सिद्धाचार्यपूज्यानवमत्याहितान्याचरति, अन्यद्वा किञ्चिदेवंविधं कर्माप्रशस्तमारभते; तमात्मना हतमुपघ्नन्तो देवादयः कुर्वन्त्युन्मत्तम्||१०||

Aagantujaunmada (Exogenous insanity):

The type of insanity having aetiology, premonitory symptoms, actual symptoms, pain and homologation- (Upashaya) different from those of the types of insanity caused by the vitiation of Doshas is known as 'Exogenous'.

Some scholars hold the view that this type of insanity is caused by the effect of the sinful activities of the past life. Lord Punarvasu Atreya considered intellectual blasphemy as the causative factor of this condition.

Due to intellectual blasphemy the patient disregards the Gods, ascetics, ancestors, Gandharvas, Yaksas, Raksasas, Pisacas, Preceptors, elders, Adepts, teachers and the other respectable ones. He also resorts to undesirable and such other inauspicious activities. The Gods etc. cause insanity in him because of his own inauspicious activities. [10]

Purvarupa of Aagantuja Unmada

तत्र देवादिप्रकोपनिमित्तेनागन्तुकोन्मादेन पुरस्कृतस्येमानि पूर्वरूपाणि भवन्ति; तद्यथा- देव गो ब्राह्मण तपस्विनां हिंसारुचित्वं, कोपनत्वं, नृशंसाभिप्रायता, अरतिः, ओजो वर्ण च्छाया बलवपुषामुपतप्तिः, स्वप्ने च देवादिभिरभिभर्त्सनं प्रवर्तनं चेति; ततोऽनन्तरमुन्मादाभिनिर्वृतिः||११||

The premonitory symptoms of the exogenous type of insanity:

Deva go brāhmaṇatapasvināṃhiṃsārucitvaṃ – Desire for inflicting injury upon the gods, cows, Brahmins and ascetics'

Kopanatvaṃ, nṛśaṃsābhiprāyatā – Anger and liking for mischievous work

Aratiḥ, ojovarṇacchāyābalavapuṣāmupataptiḥ – Disliking attitude and impairment of Ojas, Colour complexion and physical strength and

Svapne ca devādibhirabhibhartsanaṃpravartanaṃ – Abuse and incitement by the gods etc.

Insanity manifests itself immediately after the occurrence of these premonitory symptoms. [11]

Agantuja Unmada Nidana – causative factors:

तत्रायमुन्मादकराणां भूतानामुन्मादयिष्यतामारम्भविशेषो भवति; तद्यथा- अवलोकयन्तो देवा जनयन्त्युन्मादं, गुरु वृद्ध सिद्धमहर्षयोऽभिशपन्तः, पितरो दर्शयन्तः, स्पृशन्तो गन्धर्वाः, समाविशन्तो यक्षाः, राक्षसास्त्वात्मगन्धमाघ्रापयन्तः, पिशाचाः पुनरारुह्य वाहयन्तः||१२||

Agantuja Unmada Nidana – causative factors:

The causative agents of the exogenous type of insanity and their action is as follows:-

Avalokayantodevājanayantyunmādaṃ – The gods produce insanity by their vision

Guru vṛddhasiddhamaharṣayo'bhiśapantaḥ – Preceptors, elders, adepts and ascetics by their curse

Pitarodarśayantaḥ – Ancestors by exhibiting themselves

Spṛśantogandharvāḥ – Gandharvas by their touch

Samāviśantoyakṣāḥ – Yakshas by seizure

Rākṣasāstvātmagandhamāghrāpayantaḥ – Raksasas by making the patient to smell the odour of their body

Piśācāḥpunarāruhyavāhayantaḥ – Pishacas by riding and driving their victims. [12]

Rupa – Symptoms of manifestations of disease:

तस्येमानि रूपाणि भवन्ति; तद्यथा- अत्यात्म बल वीर्य पौरुष पराक्रम ग्रहण धारण स्मरण ज्ञान वचन विज्ञानानि , अनियतश्चोन्मादकालः||१३||

Symptoms of this condition are the manifestations of:

Atyātma bala – superhuman strength

Vīrya – energy

Pauruṣa – manliness

Parākrama – enthusiasm

Grahaṇadhāraṇa – power of understanding and retention

Smaraṇa – memory

Jñānavacanavijñānāni – spiritual as well as artistic knowledge and

Aniyataśconmādakālaḥ – Power of speech in the patient himself.

There is no fixed time for manifestation of this insanity. [13]

Circumstances of victimization of the subject:

उन्मादयिष्यतामपि खलु देवर्षि पितृ गन्धर्व यक्ष राक्षस पिशाचानां गुरु वृद्ध सिद्धानां वा एष्वन्तरेष्वभिगमनीयाः पुरुषा भवन्ति; तद्यथा- पापस्य कर्मणः समारम्भे, पूर्वकृतस्य वा कर्मणः परिणामकाले, एकस्य वा शून्यगृहवासे चतुष्पथाधिष्ठाने वा, सन्ध्यावेलायाम्प्रयतभावे वा पर्वसन्धिषु वा मिथुनीभावे, रजस्वलाभिगमने वा, विगुणे वाऽध्ययन बलि मङ्गल होम प्रयोगे, नियम व्रत ब्रह्मचर्य भङ्गे वा, महाहवे वा, देश कुलपुरविनाशे वा, महाग्रहोपगमने वा, स्त्रिया वा प्रजननकाले, विविध भूताशुभा शुचि स्पर्शने वा, वमन विरेचन रुधिरस्रावे, अशुचेरप्रयतस्य वा चैत्यदेवायतनाभिगमने वा, मांस मधु तिल गुड मद्योच्छिष्टे वा, दिग्वाससि वा, निशि नगर निगम चतुष्पथो पवन श्मशानाघातनाभिगमने वा, द्विज गुरु सुरयतिपूज्याभिधर्षणे वा, धर्माख्यानव्यतिक्रमे वा, अन्यस्य वा कर्मणोऽप्रशस्तस्यारम्भे, इत्यभिघातकाला व्याख्याता भवन्ति||१४||

Human beings fall victims to the attack of insanity caused by the Gods, Ascetics, ancestors, Gandharvas, Yaksas, Rakshas, Pisacas, Preceptors, elders and adepts in the following circumstances:

Pāpasyakarmaṇaḥsamārambhe – In the beginning of sinful acts.

Pūrvakṛtasyavākarmaṇaḥpariṇāmakāle – When the (sinful) acts of the past life are matured enough to produce their effects

Ekasyavāśūnyagṛhavāsecatuṣpathādhiṣṭhāneva – Residing in a deserted house or going to cross roads alone.

Sandhyāvelāyāmaprayatabhāvevāparvasandhiṣuvāmithunībhāve – Sexual intercourse during the junctures of day and night or during the new moon and full moon days

Rajasvalābhigamaneva – Sexual intercourse with a lady during her menses

Viguṇevā'dhyayanabalimaṅgalahomaprayoge – Recitation of scriptures, religious offerings, auspicious rites and sacrifices in improper manner

Niyama vratabrahmacaryabhaṅgeva – Dishonouring a vow and discontinuing a religious duty or observance of celibacy

Mahāhaveva – Forceful battles

Deśakulapuravināśeva – Destruction of countries, communities and towns

Mahāgrahopagamaneva – Onset of inauspicious planets in the sky

Striyāvāprajananakāle – During the time of child- delivery of ladies

Vividhabhūtāśubhāśucisparśaneva – Coming in contact with different types of inauspicious and unclean creatures

Vamana virecanarudhirasrāve – Emesis, purgation and bleeding

Aśuceraprayatasyavācaityadevāyatanābhigamaneva – Visiting a Caitya (sacred tree) or temple when unclean and not following the prescribed rules

Māṃsamadhutilaguḍamadyocchiṣṭeva – Resorting to the remnants of meat, honey , till sugar candy and alcohol

Digvāsasivā – While naked

Niśi nagara nigamacatuṣpathopavanaśmaśānāghātanābhigamaneva – Visiting cities, towns, cross roads, gardens, cremation grounds, slaughter houses at night

Dvija guru surayatipūjyābhidharṣaṇeva – Insulting Dvija (twice born), preceptors, the Gods, ascetics and others who are respected.

Dharmākhyānavyatikrameva – Misinterpretation of religious scriptures and

Anyasyavākarmaṇo'praśastasyārambhe – Initiating such another inauspicious activities

Thus the circumstance in which a person is attached by an exogenous type of insanity is explained. [14]

Unmada Karana – 3 main causes:

त्रिविधं तु खलून्मादकराणां भूतानामुन्मादने प्रयोजनं भवति; तद्यथा- हिंसा, रतिः, अभ्यर्चनं चेति|

तेषां तं प्रयोजन विशेषमुन्मताचार विशेष लक्षणैर्विद्यात्|

तत्र हिंसार्थिनोन्माद्यमानोऽग्निं प्रविशति, अप्सु निमज्जति, स्थलाच्छवभ्रे वा पतति, शस्त्रकशाकाष्ठलोष्टमुष्टिभिर्हन्त्यात्मानम्, अन्यच्च प्राणवधार्थमारभते किञ्चित्, तमसाध्यं विद्यात्; साध्यौ पुनर्द्वावितरौ||१५||

Unmada Karana – 3 main causes:

Insanity is caused by these agents with 3 objectives,

Hiṃsā – To inflict injury

Ratiḥ – To play and

Abhyarcanaṃ – To offer prayer

Their intentions can be judged from the characteristic features of the patient:

Hiṃsārthinonmādyamāno'gnimpraviśati, apsunimajjati, sthalācchvabhrevāpatati, śastrakaśākāṣṭhaloṣṭamuṣṭibhirhantyātmānam – When the intention of the afflicted agents is to inflict injury, then the patient enters into fire sinks into water, falls into a pit, strikes himself with weapons, whips, sticks, brick bats, his own first etc.

Anyaccaprāṇavadhārthamārabhatekiñcit – he may also adopt such other means for killing himself. This type of insanity is incurable, if the intention of the causative agents is the remaining 2 i.e., to play or to offer prayer, then this is curable. [15]

Therapies:

तयोः साधनानि- मन्त्रौषधि मणि मङ्गल बल्युपहार होम नियम व्रत प्रायश्चित्तोपवास स्वस्त्ययनप्रणिपातगमनादीनि||१६||

एवमेते पञ्चोन्मादा व्याख्याता भवन्ति||१७||

Therapies for this type of insanity are incantation of Mantras, wearing of talisman and jewels, performance of auspicious rites, religious sacrifices, oblations and religious rites, taking a vow, performing religious duty, atonements, fasting, blessing, obeisance and pilgrimage. Thus the 5 types of insanity are explained. [16-17]

Classification and prognosis:

ते तु खलु निजागन्तुविशेषण साध्यासाध्य विशेषेण च प्रविभज्यमानाः पञ्च सन्तो द्वावेव भवतः|

तौ च परस्परमनुबध्नीतः कदाचिद्यथोक्तहेतुसंसर्गात्|

तयोः संसृष्टमेव पूर्वरूपं भवति, संसृष्टमेव च लिङ्गम्|

तत्रासाध्य संयोगं साध्यासाध्य संयोगं चासाध्यं विद्यात्, साध्यं तु साध्य संयोगम्|

तस्य साधनं साधनसंयोगमेव विद्यादिति||१८||

Insanity along with its 5 types, classified as endogenous or curable and incurable, are again grouped into 2. At times, due to the combination of etiological factors (of endogenous and exogenous types), they are manifested in a combined form. There is a combination in their premonitory as well as actual symptoms.

Combination of the incurable varieties or the curable and incurable varieties results in the incurability of the condition. Combination of the curable varieties, however, results in the curability of the condition. For the treatment of this (last mentioned) condition, there is the combination of therapies. [18]

Misdeeds as causes of insanity:

भवन्ति चात्र-

नैव देवा न गन्धर्वा न पिशाचा न राक्षसाः|

न चान्ये स्वयमक्लिष्टमुपक्लिश्नन्ति मानवम्||१९||

ये त्वेनमनुवर्तन्ते क्लिश्यमानं स्वकर्मणा|

न स तद्धेतुकः क्लेशो न ह्यस्ति कृतकृत्यता||२०||

Thus, it is said: -

Neither the gods, Nor Gandharvas nor Pisacas nor Rakshas afflict a person who himself is free from misdeeds. The primary causes of insanity in an individual are his own misdeeds and other agents like the gods etc. act only as the consequence of these misdeeds. There cannot be the manifestation of anything which is already manifested. Thus, verily the gods etc., are not causative factors of insanity in human beings. [19-20]

Causes and observance of wholesome regimens:

प्रज्ञापराधात् सम्भूते व्याधौ कर्मज आत्मनः|

नाभिशंसेद्बुधो देवान्न पितॄन्नापि राक्षसान्||२१||

आत्मानमेव मन्येत कर्तारं सुख दुःखयोः|

तस्माच्छ्रेयस्करं मार्गं प्रतिपद्येत नो त्रसेत्||२२||

देवादीनामपचितिर्हितानां चोपसेवनम्|

ते च तेभ्यो विरोधश्च सर्वमायतमात्मनि||२३||

तत्र श्लोकः- सङ्ख्या निमित्तं प्रागूपं लक्षणं साध्यता न च|

उन्मादानां निदानेऽस्मिन् क्रियासूत्रं च भाषितम्||२४||

Causes and observance of wholesome regimens:

The man should not blame the gods, ancestors or Rakshasa for diseases caused by his own misdeeds due to intellectual blasphemy. One should hold himself responsible for his happiness and miseries. Therefore, without apprehension one should follow the path of propitiousness. Prayer to the Gods etc and resorting to wholesome regimens act as antidotes to the misdeeds of the individual. Thus, the power either to avert or invite the attack of insanity rests with the individual himself [22-23]

Contents:

इत्यग्निवेशकृते तन्त्रे चरक प्रतिसंस्कृते निदान स्थाने उन्माद निदानं नाम सप्तमोऽध्यायः||७||

Number, aetiology, premonitory symptoms, curability or otherwise and the principles of treatment of various types of insanity are described in this chapter. [24]

Thus ends the 7th chapter on the "Unmada Nidana" of section of Nidana Sthana of Agnivesha's work as redacted by Charaka.

8

Nidanasthana Chapter 8 Apasmara Nidanam

The 8th chapter of Charaka Samhitha Nidana Sthana is called Apasmara Nidana. It deals with the causes, pathology, types and symptoms of Apasmara – Epilepsy, as per Ayurveda.

अथातोऽपस्मार निदानं व्याख्यास्यामः||१||

इति ह स्माह भगवानात्रेयः||२||

We shall now explore the chapter on the Apasmara – Diagnosis of Epilepsy. Thus said Lord Atreya [1-2]

Types of Apasmara (epilepsy):

इह खलु चत्वारोऽपस्मारा भवन्ति वात पित्त कफ सन्निपात निमित्ताः||३||

There are 4 types of epilepsy, viz,

Vataja

Pittaja

Kaphaja and

Sannipataja [3]

Subjects of epilepsy:

त एवंविधानां प्राणभृतां क्षिप्रमभिनिर्वर्तन्ते; तद्यथा- रजस्तमोभ्यामुपहतचेतसामुद्भ्रान्त विषम बहु दोषाणां स मल विकृतोपहितान्यशुचीन्यभ्यवहारजातानि वैषम्य युक्तेनोपयोग विधिनोपयुञ्जानानां तन्त्र प्रयोगमपि च विषममाचरतामन्याश्च शरीरचेष्टा विषमाः समाचरतामत्युपक्षयाद्वा दोषाः प्रकुपिता रजस्तमोभ्यामुपहतचेतसामन्तरात्मनः श्रेष्ठ तममायतनं हृदयमुपसृत्योपरि तिष्ठन्ते, तथेन्द्रियायतनानि च|

तत्र चावस्थिताः सन्तो यदा हृदयमिन्द्रियायतनानि चेरिताः काम क्रोध भय लोभ मोह हर्ष शोक चिन्तोद्वेगादिभिः सहसाऽभिपूरयन्ति, तदा जन्तुरपस्मरति||४||

Epilepsy manifests itself quickly in the following types of individuals:

Rajastamobhyāmupahata – When the mind of an individual is overshadowed by Rajas and Tamas

Chetasāmudbhrānta viṣama bahu doṣāṇāṃ – When the Doshas get exceedingly aggravated and their equilibrium is disturbed

Mala vikṛtopahitānyaśucīnyabhyavahārajātāni vaiṣamya yuktenopayoga vidhinopayuñjānānāṃ – When an individual takes food consisting of unclean and unwholesome ingredients possessing mutually contradictory (or touched by the unclean hands of persons suffering from contagious diseases like Leprosy), neglecting the prescribed deictic rules; when he resorts to unhealthy regimens and behaviour and when he suffers from excessive debility.

In the situations mentioned above, the Doshas get aggravated and attack the persons whose minds are overshadowed by Rajas and Tamas. The Doshas (so aggravated) permeate the heart, and organs. While staying there, the Doshas aggravated by force of etc, perturbation etc. all of a sudden, spread throughout the heart and the sense organs. Then an individual falls a victim to epilepsy. [4]

Definition of Epilepsy:
अपस्मारं पुनः स्मृति बुदि्ध सत्व सम्प्लवाद्बीभत्सचेष्टमावस्थिकं तमः प्रवेशमाचक्षते||५||
By occasional unconsciousness associated with loathsome activities (like vomiting of froth and abnormal postures of the body), due to the perversion of memory, intellect and other psychic faculties. [5]

Purvarupa (Premonitory symptoms) of Apasmara:
तस्येमानि पूर्वरूपाणि भवन्ति; तद्यथा- भ्रूव्युदासः सततमक्ष्णोर्वैकृतम शब्द श्रवणं लाला सिङ्घाण प्रस्रवणमनन्नाभिलषणमरोचकाविपाकौ हृदयग्रहः कुक्षेराटोपो दौर्बल्यमस्थिभेदोऽङ्गमर्दो मोहस्तमसो दर्शनं मूर्च्छा भ्रमश्चाभीक्ष्णं स्वप्ने च मदनर्तनव्यधनव्यथन वेपन पतनादीनीति||६||
ततोऽनन्तरमपस्माराभिनिर्वृतिरेव||७||

Purvarupa (Premonitory symptoms) of Apasmara:
The following are its Purvarupa (premonitory symptoms):-
Bhrūvyudāsaḥ – Contraction of eye- brows
Satatamakṣṇorvaikṛtama – Irregular movement of eyes constantly
Shabda śravaṇam – Hearing of such sounds which are non- existent
Lālā siṅghāṇa prasravaṇaman – Excessive discharge of saliva and nasal- excreta
Annābhilaṣaṇamarocakāvipākau hṛdayagrahaḥ – Disinclination for food, anorexia and indigestion, cardiac spasm
Kukṣeraṭopo – Distension of the lower abdomen with gurgling sound
Daurbalyam asthibhedo'ṅgamardo – Weakness, cracking pain in bones and malaise
Mohas tamaso darśanam mūrcchā bhrama – Unconsciousness, entering into darkness, fainting and giddiness
Abhīkṣṇam svapne ca madanartanavyadhanavyathana vepana patanādīnīti – Frequent appearance of scenes of intoxication, dancing, murdering, aching, shivering and falling in the dreams
Thereafter the epilepsy is manifested. [6-7]

Visesha rupa – Characteristic features of Apasmara (epilepsy):
तत्रेदमपस्मारविशेषविज्ञानं भवति; तद्यथा- अभीक्ष्णमपस्मरन्तं, क्षणेन सञ्ज्ञां प्रतिलभमानम्, उत्पिण्डिताक्षम्, असाम्ना विलपन्तम्, उद्वमन्तं फेनम्, अतीवाध्मातग्रीवम्, आविद्धशिरस्कं, विषमाविनताङ्गुलिम्, अनवस्थित पाणि पादम्, अरुण परुष श्याव नख नयन वदन त्वचम्, अनवस्थित चपल परुष रूक्ष रूप दर्शिनं, वातलानुपशयं, विपरीतोपशयं च वातेनापस्मरन्तं विद्यात् (१)||८||
अभीक्ष्णमपस्मरन्तं क्षणेन सञ्ज्ञां प्रतिलभमानम्, अवकूजन्तम्, आस्फालयन्तं भूमिं, हरित हारिद्र ताम नख नयन वदन त्वचं, रुधिरोक्षितोग्रभैरवादीप्तरुषितरूप दर्शिनं, पित्तलानुपशयं, विपरीतोपशयं च पित्तेनापस्मरन्तं विद्यात् (२)||८||
चिरादपस्मरन्तं, चिराच्च सञ्ज्ञां प्रतिलभमानं, पतन्तम्, अनतिविकृतचेष्टं, लालामुद्वमन्तं, शुक्ल नख नयन वदन त्वच्, शुक्ल गुरु स्निग्ध रूप दर्शिनं, श्लेष्मलानुपशयं, विपरीतोपशयं च श्लेष्मणाऽपस्मरन्तं विद्यात् (३)||८||
समवेत सर्वलिङ्गमपस्मारं सान्निपातिकं विद्यात्, तमसाध्यमाचक्षते (४)||८||
इति चत्वारोऽपस्मारा व्याख्याताः||८||

The following are the characteristic features of different types of epilepsy:
Vataja Apasmara Vishesha Rupa:
Abhīkṣṇamapasmarantaṃ – Losing and regaining consciousness instantaneously
Kṣaṇena sañjñāṃ pratilabhamānam utpiṇḍitākṣam – Projection of eye balls;
Asāmnā vilapantam – Incoherent speech
Udvamantaṃ phenam – Vomiting of frothy matter
Atīvādhmātagrīvam – Excessive heaviness and rigidity of neck

Aaviddhaśiraskaṃ – Bending of the head to one side
Viṣamavinatāṅgulim – Irregularly contracted fingers
Anavasthita pāṇi pādam – Instability of upper and lower limbs
Aruṇa paruṣa śyāva nakha nayana vadana tvacam – Reddishness, dryness and brownishness of nails, eyes, face and skin
Anavasthita capala paruṣa rūkṣa rūpa darśinaṃ – Vision (aura) of unstable, fickle, coarse and dry objects
Vātalānupaśayaṃ – Aggravation of the condition by such regimens as are aggravators of Vata and
Viparītopaśayaṃ ca vātenāpasmarantaṃ vidyāt – Alleviation of the condition by such regimens which alleviate Vata

Pittaja Apasmara Vishesha Rupa:

Abhīkṣṇamapasmarantaṃ kṣaṇena sañjñāṃ pratilabhamānam – Losing and regaining consciousness instantaneously
Avakūjantam – Sertorius breathing
Aasphālayantaṃ bhūmiṃ – Rubbing the earth
Harita hāridra tāmra nakha nayana vadana tvacam – Green, yellow or coppery colour of nails, eyes, face and skin
Rudhirokṣitograbhairavādīptaruṣitarūpa darśinaṃ – Vision (Aura) of bleeding, terrifying (which is also injurious), frightful, burning and angry looking objects
Pittalānupaśayaṃ,viparītopaśayaṃ ca pittenāpasmarantaṃ vidyāt – Aggravation of the condition by such regimens as are aggravators of pitta

Kaphaja Apasmara Vishesha Rupa:

Cirādapasmarantaṃ – Delay in losing and regaining consciousness
Cirācca sañjñāṃ pratilabhamānaṃ, patantam – falling down
Anativikṛtaceṣṭaṃ – Absence of much distortion of activities
Lālāmudvamantaṃ śukla nakha nayana vadana tvacam – Dribbling of saliva, white colour of nails, eyes, face and skin
Shukla guru snigdha rūpa darśinaṃ – Vision (aura) of white, heavy and unctuous objects
Shleṣmalānupaśayaṃ – Aggravation of the condition by such regimens as are aggravators of kapha and
Viparītopaśayaṃ ca śleṣmaṇā'pasmarantaṃ vidyāt – Alleviation of the condition by such regimens as alleviators of Kapha

Sannipatika Apasmara Vishesha Rupa:
Epilepsy of Sannipatika type (caused by the simultaneous vitiation of all the 3 Doshas) shares the symptoms of all the 3 Doshas (described above). This condition is incurable.
Thus the 4 types of epilepsy are explained. [8]

Extrinsic causative factors:
तेषामागन्तुरनुबन्धो भवत्येव कदाचित्, तमुत्तरकालमुपदेक्ष्यामः|
तस्य विशेष विज्ञानं यथोक्तलिङ्गैर्लिङ्गाधिक्यमदोषलिङ्गानुरूपं च किञ्चित्||९||
At times these conditions are associated with extrinsic causative factors which will be described later (in Chikitsa 10: 53). Their specific characteristics are the association of additional symptoms which are not manifested due to the various dosha already described. [9]

Types of treatment:
हितान्यपस्मारिभ्यस्तीक्ष्णानि संशोधनान्युपशमनानि च यथास्वं, मन्त्रादीनि चागन्तुसंयोगे||१०||
Strong elimination and alleviation therapies depending upon the specific requirements are useful for patients suffering from epilepsy. When this is associated with extrinsic causative factors, then Mantras etc., will be useful. [10]

Mythological origin of diseases, line of treatment and prognosis of epilepsy:
तस्मिन् हि दक्षाध्वरध्वंसे देहिनां नानादिक्षु विद्रवतामभिद्रवणतरण धावन प्लवन लङ्घनाद्यैर्देहविक्षोभणैः पुरा गुल्मोत्पतिरभूत्,
हविष्प्राशात् प्रमेहकुष्ठानां, भय त्रास शोकैरुन्मादानां, विविधभूता शुचिसंस्पर्शादपस्माराणां, ज्वरस्तु खलु महेश्वर ललाट प्रभवः ,
तत्सन्तापाद्रक्तपितम्, अतिव्यवायात् पुनर्नक्षत्रराजस्य राजयक्ष्मेति||११||
भवन्ति चात्र- अपस्मारो हि वातेन पित्तेन च कफेन च|
चतुर्थः सन्निपातेन प्रत्याख्येयस्तथाविधः||१२||
साध्यांस्तु भिषजः प्राज्ञाः साधयन्ति समाहिताः|
तीक्ष्णैः संशोधनैश्चैव यथास्वं शमनैरपि||१३||
यदा दोष निमित्तस्य भवत्यागन्तुरन्वयः|
तदा साधारणं कर्म प्रवदन्ति भिषग्विदः||१४||

Mythological origin:

During the destruction of Dakshas' sacrifice, Gulma manifested first due to the aggravation in their body because of fleeing, swimming, running, flying, jumping etc., Pramehas (obstinacy urinary disorders including diabetes) and Kusthas (obstinate skin diseases including leprosy) manifested themselves due to intake of ghee, various types of Unmada (insanity) due to fear, apprehension and grief, and Apasmara (epilepsy) due to coming into contact with various types of unclean objects. Fever came out of the forehead of Lord Shiva. Raktapitta (a condition characterized by bleeding from different parts of the body) due to its heat and Rajayaksma (Tuberculosis) occurred in the moon, the king of stars, due to excessive sexual indulgence.

Thus it is said: – epilepsy manifests itself due to the vitiation of Vata, Pitta and Kapha as well as due to Sannipata (combined vitiation of all the 3 Doshas). The last one is incurable. The curable varieties of epilepsy are carefully treated by the physician with strong elimination and alleviation therapies according to the Doshas vitiated.

When the epilepsy caused by the vitiation of Doshas gets associated with extrinsic causative factors then therapies as would bring the Doshas into normalcy and also correct the affection of extrinsic causative factors shall be done-say the wise physicians. [11-14]

Physician's merits:

सर्वरोग विशेषज्ञः सर्वौषध विशारदः|
भिषक् सर्वामयान् हन्ति न च मोहं निगच्छति ||१५||
The physician, well versed in the specific characteristics of all diseases and the properties of all medicines cures all diseases and does not get confused. [15]

इत्येतदखिलेनोक्तं निदान स्थानमुत्तमम्|१६|
Thus the section par excellence on the "Diagnosis of Diseases ' are described in its entirety.

Diseases as causative factors for other diseases:

निदानार्थिकरो रोगो रोगस्याप्युपलभ्यते||१६||
तद्यथा- ज्वर सन्तापाद्रक्तपितमुदीर्यते|
रक्तपिताज्ज्वरस्ताभ्यां शोषश्चाप्युपजायते ||१७||
प्लीहाभिवृद्ध्या जठरं जठराच्छोथ एव च|
अर्शोभ्यो जठरं दुःखं गुल्मश्चाप्युपजायते||१८||
प्रतिश्यायाद्भवेत् कासः कासात् सञ्जायते क्षयः|
क्षयो रोगस्य हेतुत्वे शोषस्याप्युपलभ्यते ||१९||

Diseases as causative factors for other diseases:

Diseases act as causative factors for other diseases as well; for example,

Raktapitta (the disease characterized by bleeding from different parts of the body) is produced by the heat of the Jvara (fever);

Jvara is also produced by Raktapitta

Ascitis is caused by the enlargement of spleen;

Shotha (General oedema) due to ascites, painful ascites and Gulma due to piles;

Kasa (coughing) due to Coryza;

Kshaya (Wasting) of tissue elements due to Kasa and

Sosha (Consumption) due to wasting of tissue elements. [16-19]

Causative factors as diseases in stages:

ते पूर्व केवला रोगाः पश्चाद्धेत्वर्थकारिणः।

उभयार्थकरा दृष्टास्तथैवैकार्थकारिणः ||२०||

These conditions in the primary stage manifest themselves as diseases and subsequently they act as causative factors of other diseases. They are found acting both as the disease and causative factor: some of them act in one way also –either as a disease or as a causative factor: [20]

Nature of disease:

कश्चिदिध रोगो रोगस्य हेतुर्भूत्वा प्रशाम्यति।

न प्रशाम्यति चाप्यन्यो हेत्वर्थं कुरुतेऽपि च||२१||

Some disease gets subsided after causing another disease and some others even after causing another disease do not subside.

For example, coryza may continue to exit along with Kasa (coughing) after causing the latter; and at times after causing Kasa, coryza itself may get subsided. In the former case, coryza is considered both as a disease as well as a causative factor, in the latter case it acts only as a causative factor. [21]

Difficulty in cure:

एवं कृच्छ्रतमा नृणां दृश्यन्ते व्याधि सङ्कराः।

प्रयोगापरिशुद्धत्वात्तथा चान्योन्यसम्भवात्||२२||

Such combination of diseases due to the incorrect administration of therapies or production of one disease out of the other, makes the condition difficult to cure. [22]

Correctness of therapy:

प्रयोगः शमयेद्व्याधिं योऽन्यमन्यमुदीरयेत्।

नासौ विशुद्धः, शुद्धस्तु शमयेद्यो न कोपयेत्||२३||

The therapy which while curing one disease provokes another is not the correct one. The correct therapy is the one which while curing a disease does not provoke the manifestation of other diseases. [23]

Productivity of Causative factors:

एको हेतुरनेकस्य तथैकस्यैक एव हि।

व्याधेरेकस्य चानेको बहूनां बहवोऽपि च||२४||

ज्वर भ्रम प्रलापाद्या दृश्यन्ते रूक्ष हेतुजाः।

रूक्षेणैकेन चाप्येको ज्वर एवोपजायते||२५||

हेतुभिर्बहुभिश्चैको ज्वरो रूक्षादिभिर्भवेत्।

रूक्षादिभिर्ज्वराद्याश्च व्याधयः सम्भवन्ति हि||२६||

One causative factor may produce many diseases. Similarly there may be only one causative factor for one disease.

There may be many causative factors for one disease. Similarly there may be many causative factors for many diseases. Example, due to dry causative factors many diseases like fever, and giddiness and delirium are manifested. Dry causative factors on the other hand can produce only one disease i.e. fevers. Similarly due to dryness etc many etiological / causative factors many diseases like fever, giddiness etc may get manifested. [24-26]

Relation of Symptoms with disease:

लिङ्गं चैकमनेकस्य तथैवैकस्य लक्ष्यते|
बहून्येकस्य च व्याधेर्बहूनां स्युर्बहूनि च||२७||
विषमारम्भमूलानां लिङ्गमेकं ज्वरो मतः|
ज्वरस्यैकस्य चाप्येकः सन्तापो लिङ्गमुच्यते||२८||
विषमारम्भमूलैश्च ज्वर एको निरुच्यते|
लिङ्गैरेतैर्ज्वर श्वास हिक्काद्याः सन्ति चामयाः||२९||

One symptom may be common to many diseases; e.g. fever may be the common symptom of many diseases having irregularity as their onset. One symptom may be related to only one disease. E.g. hyperpyrexia is the symptom of fever alone. Many symptoms may be common to many diseases, e.g. many symptoms like irregularity in onset may be common to many diseases, like fever, asthma and hiccup. [27-29]

Effect of therapy on disease:

एका शान्तिरनेकस्य तथैवैकस्य लक्ष्यते|
व्याधेरेकस्य चानेका बहूनां बह्व्य एव च||३०||
शान्तिरामाशयोत्थानां व्याधीनां लङ्घनक्रिया|
ज्वरस्यैकस्य चाप्येका शान्तिर्लङ्घनमुच्यते||३१||
तथा लघ्वशनाद्याश्च ज्वरस्यैकस्य शान्तयः|
एताश्चैव ज्वर श्वास हिक्कादीनां प्रशान्तयः||३२||

One single therapy may cure many diseases, e.g. diseases having their origin from Amashaya (stomach including small intestine) are cured by fasting. There may be one single therapy only for one disease e.g. fasting is a therapy for the cure of fever alone. There may be many therapies for one disease, e.g. intake of light diet etc., cures only one disease, viz fever. There may be many therapies for many diseases, e.g., intake of light diet etc. may cure many diseases viz, fever, asthma, hiccup etc. [30-32]

Definition of curable, Palliable and incurable diseases:

सुखसाध्यः सुखोपायः कालेनाल्पेन साध्यते|
साध्यते कृच्छ्रसाध्यस्तु यत्नेन महता चिरात्||३३||
याति नाशेषतां व्याधिरसाध्यो याप्यसञ्ज्ञितः|
परोऽसाध्यः क्रियाः सर्वाः प्रत्याख्येयोऽतिवर्तते||३४||
नासाध्यः साध्यतां याति साध्यो याति त्वसाध्यताम्|
पादापचाराद्दैवाद्वा यान्ति भावान्तरं गदाः||३५||

Easily curable diseases are cured by simple measures in a short time. Diseases which are difficult to cure involve much of effort and they take a long time for cure. The palliable variety of incurable diseases can never be eradicated from the root. The irremediable variety of an incurable disease is not amenable to any type of treatment. The incurable varieties never become curable; the curable variety may on the other hand become incurable. Due to the defects in the four agents of therapeutics or due to misfortune, the easily curable variety may become difficult to cure: diseases which are difficult to cure may become palliable and palliable variety may become irremediable. [33-35]

Observation on the states of disease:

वृद्धि स्थान क्षयावस्थां रोगाणामुपलक्षयेत्।
सुसूक्ष्मामपि च प्राज्ञो देहाग्नि बल चेतसाम्।।३६।।
व्याध्यवस्था विशेषान् हि ज्ञात्वा ज्ञात्वा विचक्षणः।
तस्यां तस्यामवस्थायां चतुःश्रेयः प्रपद्यते।।३७।।

A wise physician should closely observe the subtleties of aggravated, normal and diminished states of diseases, body, and power of digestion, strength and mental faculties. Having close acquaintance with the various states of the disease, an intelligent physician should prescribe for these difficult states such therapies as would help attainment of the four- fold blessings. [36-37]

Principles of treatment:

प्रायस्तिर्यग्गता दोषाः क्लेशयन्त्यातुरांश्चिरम्।
तेषु न त्वरया कुर्याद्देहाग्निबलवित् क्रियाम्।।३८।।
प्रयोगैः क्षपयेद्वा तान् सुखं वा कोष्ठमानयेत्।
ज्ञात्वा कोष्ठ प्रपन्नांस्तान् यथासन्नं हरेद्बुधः।।३९।।

If the aggravated Doshas spread sideward's then the patient continues to be afflicted with the disease for a long time. One acquainted with nature of the body, power of digestion and strength of the individual should not administer strong therapies for the treatment of this condition. By administering slow acting therapies in small Doshas, such diseases should either be suppressed or brought to the Kostha (alimentary tract) with ease. Having known of their arrival in the Kostha, the wise Physician should eliminate these Doshas from their respective abodes by the administration of appropriate therapies. [38-39]

Difference between symptoms and disease:

ज्ञानार्थं यानि चोक्तानि व्याधि लिङ्गानि सङ्ग्रहे।
व्याधयस्ते तदात्वे तु लिङ्गानीष्टानि नामयाः।।४०।।

In this section on the "Diagnosis of Diseases" Jvara (fever) etc., are described to have some symptoms, viz Aruchi (anorexia) etc. these symptoms in themselves also constitute diseases. But here, because of their subordinate nature, they are only symptoms and not diseases. [40]

Dependence of causes:

विकारः प्रकृतिश्चैव द्वयं सर्व समासतः।
तद्धेतुवशगं हेतोरभावान्नानुवर्तते।।४१।।

All manifestations relating to the body and soul can briefly be categorized into two, viz. normal and abnormal, and both of them are dependent upon causative agents- none of these manifestations can continue in the absence of these causative agents. [41]

Conclusion:

तत्र श्लोकाः- हेतवः पूर्वरूपाणि रूपाण्युपशयस्तथा।
सम्प्राप्तिः पूर्वमुत्पत्तिः सूत्रमात्रं चिकित्सितात्।।४२।।
ज्वरादीनां विकाराणामष्टानां साध्यता न च।
पृथगेकैकशश्चोक्ता हेतु लिङ्गोपशान्तयः।।४३।।
हेतु पर्याय नामानि व्याधीनां लक्षणस्य च।
निदान स्थानमेतावत् सङ्ग्रहेणोपदिश्यते।।४४।।

To sum up: Causes, premonitory, symptoms, actual symptoms, homologation, pathogenesis, first origin (mythological) and the brief line of treatment of epilepsy are described in this chapter. Curability or otherwise of the 8 diseases, viz fever etc., description of etiology, symptomatology including premonitory symptoms and treatment including homologation of all diseases in common and individually, symptoms of etiology, disease and symptoms-these are described in brief in this section on the Diagnosis of Diseases. [42-44]

इत्यग्निवेशकृते तन्त्रे चरक प्रति संस्कृते निदान स्थाने अपस्मार निदानं नामाष्टमोऽध्यायः||८||
इति चरकसंहितायां द्वितीयं निदानस्थानं समाप्तम्|

Thus ends the 8th chapter on the "diagnosis of Epilepsy "of the section on "Diagnosis of Diseases" (Nidana sthana) of Agnivesha' work as redacted by Charaka. Thus ends the "section on Diagnosis of Diseases".

विमानस्थानम् Vimana Sthanam

9

Vimanasthana Chapter 1 Rasa Vimanam

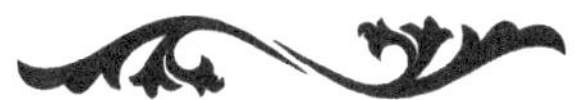

First Chapter of Charaka Samhitha Vimana Sthana is called Rasa Vimana. It deals with the knowledge of specific attributes of Rasa (taste), diet rules, three things that should not be taken for long periods of time etc.

अथातो रसविमानं व्याख्यास्यामः||१||
इति ह स्माह भगवानात्रेयः||२||
We shall now explore the chapter on the knowledge of specific qualities of Rasa (taste). Thus said Lord Atreya [1-2]

Measurement of Doshas etc.
इह खलु व्याधीनां निमित्तपूर्वरूपरूपोपशयसङ्ख्याप्राधान्यविधिविकल्प बलकालविशेषाननुप्रविश्यानन्तरं दोषभेषजदेशकालबलशरीरसाराहारसात्म्यसत्त्वप्रकृतिवयसां मानमवहितमनसा यथावज्ज्ञेयं भवति भिषजा, दोषादिमानज्ञानायतत्वात् क्रियायाः।
न ह्यमानज्ञो दोषादीनां भिषग् व्याधिनिग्रहसमर्थो भवति।
तस्माद्दोषादिमानज्ञानार्थं विमानस्थानमुपदेक्ष्यामोऽग्निवेश!||३||

After ascertaining the characteristic features, causes, premonitory symptoms, symptoms, curability, number, dominance, permutation and combination, and temporal strength, the physician should devote himself to a correct appraisal of the measurement and specific characteristics of Doshas, medicines, locality, season, strength, physique, and excellence of Dhatus, diet, homologation, mind, constitution and age.

Treatment of a disease depends upon the knowledge of the specific features of these factors, viz, Doshas etc., in the patient. A physician not acquainted with the specific features of Doshas etc., will not be able to cure the disease properly. Therefore, O! Agnivesha, we shall describe the section on the "Knowledge of Specific Attributes of Doshas Drugs" etc. [3]

Qualities, features of tastes
तत्रादौ रसद्रव्यदोषविकारप्रभावान् वक्ष्यामः।
रसास्तावत् षट्- मधुराम्ललवणकटुतिक्तकषायाः।
ते सम्यगुपयुज्यमानाः शरीरं यापयन्ति, मिथ्योपयुज्यमानास्तु खलु दोषप्रकोपायोपकल्पन्ते||४||

In the beginning, we shall describe the specific attributes of Rasa (taste), Dravya (substance), Doshas and Vikara (disease).

There are 6 Rasas (tastes), Viz

Madhura – sweet

Amla – sour

Lavana – Saline

Katu – Pungent

Tikta – bitter and

Kashaya – astringent

When employed properly, they maintain the body and their incorrect utilization result in the vitiation of Doshas [4]

Doshas :

दोषाः पुनस्त्रयो वातपित्तश्लेष्माणः|

ते प्रकृतिभूताः शरीरोपकारका भवन्ति, विकृतिमापन्नास्तु खलु नानाविधैर्विकारैः शरीरमुपतापयन्ति||५||

Doshas are 3, Viz,

Vata, Pitta and Kapha.

During their normal state, they sustain the body. When vitiated, they afflict the body with various types of diseases. [5]

Rasas and Doshas relationship

तत्र दोषमेकैकं त्रयस्त्रयो रसा जनयन्ति, त्रयस्त्रयश्चोपशमयन्ति|

तद्यथा- कटुतिक्तकषाया वातं जनयन्ति, मधुराम्ललवणास्त्वेनं शमयन्ति; कटुम्ललवणाः पित्तं जनयन्ति, मधुरतिक्तकषायास्त्वेनच्छमयन्ति; मधुराम्ललवणाः श्लेष्माणं जनयन्ति, कटुतिक्तकषायास्त्वेनं शमयन्ति||६||

Each Dosha is vitiated by the 3 Rasas (tastes) the remaining 3 Rasas alleviate particular Doshas as follows: -

Sweet, sour and salt taste increase Kapha and rest three decrease Kapha.

Pungent, bitter and astringent – increase Vata. The other three tastes decrease Vata.

Sweet, bitter and astringent tastes decrease Pitta Dosha and sour, salt and pungent tastes increase Kapha Dosha.

रसदोषसन्निपाते तु ये रसा यैर्दोषैः समानगुणाः समानगुणभूयिष्ठा वा भवन्ति ते तानभिवर्धयन्ति,

विपरीतगुणा विपरीतगुणभूयिष्ठा वा शमयन्त्यभ्यस्यमाना इति|

एतद्व्यवस्थाहेतोः षट्त्वमुपदिश्यते रसानां परस्परेणासंसृष्टानां, त्रित्वं च दोषाणाम्||७||

In the course or interaction between the Rasa (tastes) and Doshas inside the body, Doshas are aggravated by such of the Rasa which are entirely or considerably homologous with them.

On the other hand, Doshas get alleviated by the habitual utilization of the Rasas having contradictive properties entirely or considerably. It is with a view to indicating this mode of action that the six Rasa (tastes) and the 3 Doshas are described individually unmixed with each other. [7]

Innumerability of permutations and combinations of Rasas and Doshas:

संसर्गविकल्पविस्तरो ह्येषामपरिसङ्ख्येयो भवति, विकल्पभेदापरिसङ्ख्येयत्वात्||८||

Innumerable are the permutations and combinations of Rasas and Doshas, as the degrees of their combinations are innumerable. [8]

तत्र खल्वनेकरसेषु द्रव्येष्वनेकदोषात्मकेषु च विकारेषु रसदोषप्रभावमेकैकश्येनाभिसमीक्ष्य ततो द्रव्यविकारयोः प्रभावतत्त्वं व्यवस्येत्||९||

Substances are composed of many tastes. Similarly, diseases are caused by many Doshas. Therefore, the specific manifestations of drugs and diseases can be determined by taking into account the specific attributes of the tastes and determine the attributes of the Rasas (tastes) and Doshas (jointly and separately) [9]

न त्वेवं खलु सर्वत्र|

न हि विकृतिविषमसमवेतानां नानात्मकानां परस्परेण चोपहतानामन्यैश्च [विकल्पनैर्विकल्पितानामवयवप्रभावानुमानेनैव समुदायप्रभावतत्त्वमध्यवसातुं शक्यम्||१०||

The above statement (in Para- 9) does not hold good in all circumstances. Because of the variations in the curative effects of drugs, affections, of one property of the drug by another and method of their preparation which leads to prevention or irregularity in combination, it is not possible to determine the attributes of a substance having many tastes or the manifestation of a disease caused by many Doshas, simply by taking into account, the attributes of individual tastes and Doshas. [10]

Need for ascertaining the total effect:

तथायुक्ते हि समुदये समुदायप्रभावतत्त्वमेवमेवोपलभ्य ततो द्रव्यविकारप्रभावतत्त्वं व्यवस्येत्||११||

From that type of combination involving the manifestation of attributes which are contradictory to those normally present in the constituent factor, one should determine the specific attributes of compounds and thereafter proceed to ascertain the specific attributes/ manifestations of drugs and diseases. [11]

तस्माद्रसप्रभावतश्च द्रव्यप्रभावतश्च दोषप्रभावतश्च विकारप्रभावतश्च तत्त्वमुपदेक्ष्यामः||१२||

Therefore, we shall explain their specific attributes and manifestations on the basis of the specific attributes of tastes, specific attributes of drugs, specific manifestations of Doshas and diseases. [12]

Specific attributes of Rasas:

तत्रैष रसप्रभाव उपदिष्टो भवति|

द्रव्यप्रभावं पुनरुपदेक्ष्यामः|

Specific attributes of taste are described above (in Paras 4- 12) in brief. Specific attributes of drugs (already described in brief) will be further elaborated.

तैलसर्पिर्मधूनि वातपित्तश्लेष्मप्रशमनार्थानि द्रव्याणि भवन्ति||१३||

Oil, ghee and honey are alleviaters of Vata, pitta and Kapha respectively.

Oil for Vata Dosha balance

तत्र तैलं स्नेहौष्ण्यगौरवोपपन्नत्वाद्वातं जयति सततमभ्यस्यमानं; वातो हि रौक्ष्यशैत्यलाघवोपपन्नो विरुद्धगुणो भवति, विरुद्धगुणसन्निपाते हि भूयसाऽल्पमवजीयते, तस्मात्तैलं वातं जयति सततमभ्यस्यमानम्|

Continuous use of oil alleviates Vata, as oil is unctuous, hot and heavy; vata being dry, cold and light is of the opposite nature. When there is the interaction between substances having mutually opposite qualities, the stronger dominates over the weaker; therefore, continuous use of oil alleviates Vata.

सर्पिः खल्वेवमेव पित्तं जयति, माधुर्याच्छैत्यान्मन्दत्वाच्च ; पित्तं ह्यमधुरमुष्णं तीक्ष्णं च|

Similarly due to sweet taste, coldness and dullness, ghee alleviates Pitta; Pitta is pungent (other than sweet) in taste, hot and sharp.

मधु च श्लेष्माणं जयति, रौक्ष्यात्तैक्ष्ण्यात् कषायत्वाच्च; श्लेष्मा हि स्निग्धो मन्दो मधुरश्च |

Honey alleviates Kapha as it is dry, sharp and pungent in taste; Kapha is unctuous, dull and sweet.

यच्चान्यदपि किञ्चिद्द्रव्यमेवं वातपित्तकफेभ्यो गुणतो विपरीतं स्यात्तच्चैताञ्जयत्यभ्यस्यमानम्||१४||

Other substances having attributes opposite to those of the respective Dosha (i. e Vata, Pitta and kapha) also alleviate them when continuously used. [13-14]

Three Substances not to be used in excess

अथ खलु त्रीणि द्रव्याणि नात्युपयुञ्जीताधिकमन्येभ्यो द्रव्येभ्यः; तद्यथा- पिप्पली, क्षारः, लवणमिति||१५||

Of all the substances, one should not resort too much to the 3, Viz.

Pippali – Long pepper fruit – Piper longum.

Kshara – Alkali and

Lavana – Salt. [15]

Justification for not using Pippali in excess:

पिप्पल्यो हि कटुकाः सत्यो मधुरविपाका गुर्व्योनात्यर्थं स्निग्धोष्णाः प्रक्लेदिन्यो भेषजाभिमताश्चताः सद्यः; शुभाशुभकारिण्यो भवन्ति; आपातभद्राः, प्रयोगसमसाद्गुण्यात्; दोषसञ्चयानुबन्धाः;- सततमुपयुज्यमाना हि गुरुप्रक्लेदित्वाच्छ्लेष्माणमुत्क्लेशयन्ति, औष्ण्यात् पित्तं, न च वातप्रशमनायोपकल्पन्तेऽल्पस्नेहोष्णभावात्; योगवाहिन्यस्तु खलु भवन्ति; तस्मात् पिप्पलीर्नात्युपयुञ्जीत||१६||

Pippali in spite of their pungent taste are:

Madhura vipaka – sweet in Vipaka

Guru – heavy

Na Atyarthamsnigdhaushna – neither too unctuous nor too hot,

Prakledinyo – deliquescent and

bheṣajābhimatāścatāḥsadyaḥ – useful as medicine when administered afresh.

śubhāśubhakāriṇyobhavanti – Depending upon the frequency of use they are both useful and harmful.

prayogasamasādguṇyat; doṣasañcayānubandhāḥ – When properly used (in small dose for a short period) they produce good results instantaneously, otherwise, they are responsible for the accumulation of Doshas.

satatamupayujyamānā hi guru prakleditvācchleṣmāṇamutkleśayanti – When continuously used in large dose, they aggravate Pitta owing to their hot property.

auṣṇyātpittam, na ca vātapraśamanāyopakalpante'lpasnehoṣṇabhāvāt – They do not alleviate Vata because they are not adequately unctuous or hot.

Therefore, Pippali –Piper longum is not to be used in excess. [16]

Justification for not using Kshara in excess:

क्षारः पुनरौष्ण्यतैक्ष्ण्यलाघवोपपन्नः क्लेदयत्यादौ पश्चादि्वशोषयति, स पचनदहनभेदनार्थमुपयुज्यते; सोऽतिप्रयुज्यमानः केशाक्षिहृदयपुंस्त्वोपघातकरः सम्पद्यते|

ये ह्येनं ग्रामनगरनिगमजनपदाः सततमुपयुञ्जते त आन्ध्यषाण्ढ्यखालित्यपालित्यभाजो हृदयापकर्तिनश्च भवन्ति, तद्यथा- प्राच्याश्चीनाश्च; तस्मात् क्षारं नात्युपयुञ्जीत||१७||

Alkali is associated with these properties

Ushna – hot

Taikshna – sharp

Laghu – light.

In the beginning it works as a

Kledayati – deliquescent and

Vishoshana – afterwards as a desiccant.

It is used for

Pachana – suppuration

Dahana – cauterization and

Bhedana – penetration.

Excessive use of Kshara :

keśākṣihṛdayapuṃstvopaghātakaraḥsampadyate – injurious effects on hair, eyes, heart and variety.

ye hyenaṃgrāma nagara nigamajanapadāḥsatatamupayuñjate ta āndhyaṣāṇḍhyakhālityapālityabhājohṛdayāpakartinaścabhavanti – People of villages, towns, cities and countries, where this is continuously used in excess, suffer from blindness, impotency, baldness, grey hair and heart diseases characterized by sawing pain.

They are the people of the Eastern side and Chinese. Therefore, alkali should not be used in excess. [17]

Justification for not using salt in excess:

लवणं पुनरौष्ण्यतैक्ष्ण्योपपन्नम्, अनतिगुरु, अनतिस्निग्धम्, उपक्लेदि, विस्रंसनसमर्थम्, अन्नद्रव्यरुचिकरम्, आपातभद्रं प्रयोगसमसाद्गुण्यात्, दोषसञ्चयानुबन्धं, तद्रोचनपाचनोपक्लेदनविस्रंसनार्थमुपयुज्यते|

तदत्यर्थमुपयुज्यमानं ग्लानिशैथिल्यदौर्बल्याभिनिर्वृतिकरं शरीरस्य भवति|

ये ह्येनद्ग्रामनगरनिगमजनपदाः सततमुपयुञ्जते, ते भूयिष्ठं ग्लास्नवः शिथिलमांसशोणिता अपरिक्लेशसहाश्च भवन्ति|

तद्यथा- बाह्लीकसौराष्ट्रिकसैन्धवसौवीरकाः; ते हि पयसाऽपि सह लवणमश्नन्ति|

येऽपीह भूमेरत्यूषरा देशास्तेष्वोषधिवीरुद्वनस्पतिवानस्पत्या न जायन्तेऽल्पतेजसो वा भवन्ति, लवणोपहतत्वात्|

तस्माल्लवणं नात्युपयुञ्जीत|

ये ह्यतिलवणसात्म्याः पुरुषास्तेषामपि खालित्यपालित्यानि वलयश्चाकाले भवन्ति||१८||

Properties of salt:

lavaṇampunarauṣṇyataikṣṇyopapannam – Salt is associated with hot and sharp properties.

anatiguru, anatisnigdham – It is neither very heavy nor very unctuous.

upakledi, visraṃsanasamartham – It is deliquescent and is capable of producing laxative effect.

Annadravyarucikaram – It makes food delicious.

āpātabhadraṃprayogasamasādguṇyāt – When properly used, it produces good results.

tadrocanapācanopakledanavisraṃsanārthamupayujyate – It is however it is used as an appetizer, digestive, deliquescent and laxative.

tadatyarthamupayujyamānaṃglāniśaithilyadaurbalyābhinirvṛttikaraṃśarīrasyabhavati – When excessively used, it produces fatigueless, lassitude and weakness in the body.

ye hyenadgrāma nagara nigamajanapadāḥsatatamupayuñjatetebhūyiṣṭhaṃglāsnavaḥśithilamāṃsaśoṇitāaparikleśasahāścabhavanti – People of villages, towns, cities and countries, where it is continuously used in large quantity, are mostly languid and of loose flesh and blood, and they are unable to stand hardships.

bāhlīkasaurāṣṭrikasaindhavasauvīrakāḥ; – People of Bahilka (balkh), Saurastra, Sindh and Sauvira (people inhabiting at a district in the neighbourhood of Indus), belong to his category.

te hi payasā'pisahalavaṇamaśnanti – They take salt even with milk.

ye'pīhabhūmeratyūṣarādeśāsteṣvoṣadhivīrudvanaspativānaspatyānajāyante'lpatejasovābhavanti – Even in the localities having saline soil, herbs, creepers, Vanaspatis (trees having fruits without flowers) and Vanaspatyas (trees having fruits from flowers) do not grow at all or grow sluggishly because of the inhibiting effect of the salt in the soil.

lavaṇopahatatvāt – Therefore, salt is used in excess.

ye hyatilavaṇasātmyāḥpuruṣāsteṣāmapikhālityapālityānivalayaścākālebhavanti – People who are accustomed to the excessive use of salt, suffer from premature baldness, grey hair and wrinkles in the skin. [18]

Withdrawing from habits gradually:

तस्मातेषां तत्सात्म्यतः क्रमेणापगमनं श्रेयः|

सात्म्यमपि हि क्रमेणोपनिवर्त्यमानमदोषमल्पदोषं वा भवति||१९||

Therefore, people habituated with the intake of alkali and salt continuously in large quantities should give up this habit slowly (following the principle laid down in Sutra 7: 36-37). Even if the body is accustomed to these habits, the slow discontinuance of these habits does not have any harmful effect or even if it has, the harm caused is too insignificant. [19]

Satmya:

सात्म्यं नाम तद् यदात्मन्युपशेते; सात्म्यार्थो ह्युपशयार्थः|

तत्त्रिविधं प्रवरावरमध्यविभागेन; सप्तविधं तु रसैकैकत्वेन सर्वरसोपयोगाच्च|
तत्र सर्वरसं प्रवरम्, अवरमेकरसं, मध्यं तु प्रवरावरमध्यस्थम्|

Substance conducive to an individual is called "Satmya" and the use of such substances results in the well- being of that individual.

This is of 3 types, viz.

Pravara – Superior

Avara – inferior and

Madhyama – mediocre.

तत्रावरमध्याभ्यां सात्म्याभ्यां क्रमेणैव प्रवरमुपपादयेत् सात्म्यम्|
सर्वरसमपि च सात्म्यमुपपन्नः प्रकृत्याद्युपयोक्तृष्टमानि सर्वाण्याहारविधिविशेषायतनान्यभिसमीक्ष्य हितमेवानुरुध्येत||२०||

According to another mode of classification, it is of 7 types, depending upon the administration of individual Rasas or tastes (six types) and the use of Rasas or Tastes jointly (seventh type).

Use of all the Rasas is of the superior type of Satmya. Use of only one Rasa is of an inferior type and in between the superior and the inferior types is the mediocre type of Satmya.

The inferior and mediocre types are slowly changed over to the superior type of Satmya. If he is used to the superior type of Satmya, i.e. the habitual intake of substances having all the 6 tastes, the individual should adopt only the wholesome diet, considering the eight factors beginning with Prakrti (the nature of the food) and ending with Upayokta (the wholesomeness to the individual who takes it) which determine the utility or otherwise of a particular type of food. [20]

Ashta Ahara Vidhi VisheshaAyatana – Eight factors determining the utility of food:
तत्र खल्विमान्यष्टावाहारविधिविशेषायतनानि भवन्ति; तद्यथा- प्रकृतिकरणसंयोगराशिदेशकालोपयोगसंस्थोपयोक्तृष्टमानि (भवन्ति) ||२१||

The 8 factors determine the utility or otherwise of various types of food are:

Prakruti (nature of the food articles)

Karana (method of their processing)

Samyoga (combination)

Rashi (quantity)

Desha (habit)

Kala (time i.e., stage of the disease or the state of the individual)

Upayoga Samstha (rules governing the intake of food) and

Upayokta (wholesomeness to the individual who takes it [21]

Prakruti:

1. Prakruti – Nature of the substance:
तत्र प्रकृतिरुच्यते स्वभावो यः, स पुनराहारौषधद्रव्याणां स्वाभाविको गुर्वादिगुणयोगः; तद्यथा माषमुद्गयोः, शूकरैणयोश्च |२२|

Prakrti indicates the nature of the substance, i.e inherent attributes (heaviness etc) of diets and drugs e.g., Masha (Vigna mungo) is heavy and mudga (Phaseolus radiatus L) is light and meat of Sukara (boar) is heavy and that of Ena (deer) is light. [22-1]

Karana :

2. Karana – Processing of the substances:

करणं पुनः स्वाभाविकानां द्रव्याणामभिसंस्कारः|
संस्कारो हि गुणान्तराधानमुच्यते|
ते गुणास्तोयाग्निसन्निकर्षशौचमन्थनदेशकालवासनभावनादिभिः कालप्रकर्षभाजनादिभिश्चाधीयन्ते |२२|

Karna means the processing of the (inherent attributes of) substances. Processing results in the transformation of the inherent attributes of substances. Transformation of the attributes is affected by dilution, application of heat, cleansing, churning, storing, maturing, flavouring, impregnation, preservation, container etc. [22-II]

Samyoga :
3. Samyoga – Combination of substances:

संयोगः पुनर्द्वयोर्बहूनां वा द्रव्याणां संहतीभावः, स विशेषमारभते, यं पुनर्नैकैकशो द्रव्याण्यारभन्ते; तद्यथा- मधुसर्पिषोः, मधुमत्स्यपयसां च संयोगः |२२|

Samyoga is the combination of two or more substances. This results in the manifestation of specific attributes which cannot be manifested by individual substances e.g., combination of honey and ghee or honey, fish and milk. [22- III]

Rashi :
4. Rashi – Quantum of substance:

राशिस्तु सर्वग्रहपरिग्रहौ मात्रामात्रफलविनिश्चयार्थः|
तत्र सर्वस्याहारस्य प्रमाणग्रहणमेकपिण्डेन सर्वग्रहः, परिग्रहः पुनः प्रमाणग्रहणमेकैकश्येनाहारद्रव्याणाम्|
सर्वस्य हि ग्रहः सर्वग्रहः, सर्वतश्च ग्रहः परिग्रह उच्यते |२२|

Rashi is the quantum of total (Sarvagraha) or individual (parigraha) substances which determines the results of their administration in proper and improper dosage.

The quantity of food taken in its entirety is "Sarvagraha "and the quantity of each of its ingredients is "Parigraha". Quantity of all things involved is Sarvagraha and that of each and everything individually is Parigraha [22]

Desha :
5. Desha – Habitat of Substance:

देशः पुनः स्थानं; स द्रव्याणामुत्पत्तिप्रचारौ देशसात्म्यं चाचष्टे |२२|

Desha relates to the habitat. It determines attributes due to procreation (growth) or movement of substance in a particular locality or their acclimatization to that region. [22]

Kala :
6. Kala – Time:

कालो हि नित्यगश्चावस्थिकश्च; तत्रावस्थिको विकारमपेक्षते, नित्यगस्तु ऋतुसात्म्यापेक्षः |२२|

Kala stands for both the time in the form of day and night and the states of the individual, (viz. Condition of health and age). The latter is relevant to the disease (e.g. manifestation of diseases due to Kapha during childhood and fever etc). Due to dietetic errors) whereas the former for the determination of the wholesomeness to different types of seasons. [22]

Upayogasamstha :
7. UpayogaSamstha – Dietetic rules:

उपयोगसंस्था तूपयोगनियमः; स जीर्णलक्षणापेक्षः |२२|

Upayogasamstha stands for the dietetic rules. They are for the most part dependent on the symptoms of digestion.

[22]

Upayokta :
8. Upayokta – Habit of the individual:

उपयोक्ता पुनर्यस्तमाहारमुपयुङ्क्ते, यदायत्तमोकसात्म्यम्|
इत्यष्टावाहारविधिविशेषायतनानि व्याख्यातानि भवन्ति||२२||

Upayokta is he who takes food. He is, in the main, responsible for the wholesomeness by the habitual intake of things (Okasatmya). Thus the 8 factors which determine the utility or otherwise of various types of food are explained. [22]

एषां विशेषाः शुभाशुभफलाः परस्परोपकारका भवन्ति; तान् बुभुत्सेत, बुद्ध्वा च हितेप्सुरेव स्यात्; नच मोहात् प्रमादाद्वा प्रियमहितमसुखोदर्कमुपसेव्यमाहारजातमन्यद्वा किञ्चित्||२३||

These 8 factors (Ashta Vidhi AharaVisheshaAyatana) are associated especially with useful and harmful effects and they are conditioned by one another. One should try to understand them and after understanding, he should resort to useful things alone.

Neither due to ignorance nor intentionally, one should resort to such food articles or other things (drugs, regimens etc) as are instantaneously pleasing but harmful in the long run leading to unhappy consequences. [23]

Healthy Rules for taking food :
तत्रेदमाहारविधिविधानमरोगाणामातुराणां चापि केषाञ्चित् काले प्रकृत्यैव हिततमं भुञ्जानानां भवति- उष्णं, स्निग्धं, मात्रावत्, जीर्णे वीर्याविरुद्धम्, इष्टे देशे, इष्टसर्वोपकरणं, नातिद्रुतं, नातिविलम्बितम्, अजल्पन्, अहसन्, तन्मना भुञ्जीत, आत्मानमभिसमीक्ष्य सम्यक्||२४||

Healthy individuals as well as (some of the) patients should observe the following, even while using such of the food articles as are most wholesome by nature. One should eat only that food in proper quantity which is hot, unctuous and not contradictory in potency and that too, after the digestion of the previous meal. Food is taken in proper place equipped with all the accessories, without talking and laughing, with concentration of mind and paying due regard to oneself. [24]

Warm food benefits :
तस्य साद्गुण्यमुपदेक्ष्यामः- उष्णमश्नीयात्; उष्णं हि भुज्यमानं स्वदते, भुक्तं चाग्निमौदर्यमुदीरयति, क्षिप्रं जरां गच्छति, वातमनुलोमयति, श्लेष्माणं च परिह्राससयति ; तस्मादुष्णमश्नीयात् |२५|

Now we shall explain the utility of food articles. One should take warm food. When taken warm, it is delicious; after intake, it provokes the factors (enzymes) in the abdomen responsible for digestion; it provokes digestion factors; it gets digested quickly and helps in the downward passage of vata (wind) and detachment of Kapha. Therefore, one should take warm food. [25]

Unctuous (oily) food :
स्निग्धमश्नीयात्; स्निग्धं हि भुज्यमानं स्वदते, भुक्तं चानुदीर्णमग्निमुदीरयति क्षिप्रं जरां गच्छति, वातमनुलोमयति, शरीरमुपचिनोति, दृढीकरोतीन्द्रियाणि, बलाभिवृद्धिमुपजनयति, वर्णप्रसादं चाभिनिर्वर्तयति; तस्मात् स्निग्धमश्नीयात् |२५|

One should take unctuous food; unctuous food is delicious, after intake, it provokes the subdued power of digestion; it gets digested quickly; it helps in the downward movement of Vata (wind), it increases the plumpness of the body, strengthens complexion. Hence one should take unctuous food. [25]

Food in proper quantity :
मात्रावदश्नीयात्; मात्रावद्धि भुक्तं वातपित्तकफानपीडयदायुरेव विवर्धयति केवलं, सुखं गुदमनुपर्येति, न चोष्माणमुपहन्ति, अव्यथं च

परिपाकमेति; तस्मान्मात्रावदश्नीयात् |२५|

One should take food in the proper quantity. When taken in proper quantity, it promotes longevity in its entirety without afflicting vata, Pitta and Kapha; it easily passes down to the rectum; it does not impair the power of digestion and it gets digested without any difficulty. [25]

Intake after digestion of previous meal :

जीर्णेऽश्नीयात्; अजीर्णे हि भुञ्जानस्याभ्यवहृतमाहारजातं पूर्वस्याहारस्य रसमपरिणतमुत्तरेणाहाररसेनोपसृजत् सर्वान् दोषान् प्रकोपयत्याशु, जीर्णे तु भुञ्जानस्य स्वस्थानस्थेषु दोषेष्वग्नौ चोदीर्णे जातायां च बुभुक्षायां विवृतेषु च स्रोतसां मुखेषु विशुद्धे चोद्गारे हृदये विशुद्धे वातानुलोम्ये विसृष्टेषु च वातमूत्रपुरीषवेगेष्वभ्यवहृतमाहारजातं सर्वशरीरधातूनप्रदूषयदायुरेवाभिवर्धयति केवलं; तस्माज्जीर्णेऽश्नीयात् |२५|

One should take food only when the previous meal is digested. If one takes food before the digestion of the previous meal, the digestive product of the previous food, i.e. immature Rasa gets mixed up with the product of food taken afterwards, resulting in the provocation of all the Doshas instantaneously.

Signs of proper food digestion :

If food is taken after the digestion of the previous food while the Doshas are in their proper places and Agni (digestive enzymes) is provoked,

There is appetite

The entrances of the channels of circulation are open,

Eructation is purified

There is unimpaired cardiac function

Downward passage of the wind and

Proper manifestation of the urges for voiding flatus urine and stool,

Then the product of food does not vitiate the Dhatus of the body, but on the other hand it promotes longevity in its entirety. So one should take food only after digestion of the previous meal [25]

Intake of food having no contradictory potencies:

वीर्याविरुद्धमश्नीयात्; अविरुद्धवीर्यमश्नन् हि विरुद्धवीर्याहारजैर्विकारैर्नोपसृज्यते; तस्माद्वीर्याविरुद्धमश्नीयात् |२५|

One should take food having no contradictory potencies. By taking such food one does not get afflicted with such diseases as may arise from the intake of food having mutually contradictory potencies. Therefore, one should take food having no contradictory potencies. [25]

Intake in proper place and with all accessories:

इष्टे देशे इष्टसर्वोपकरणं चाश्नीयात्; इष्टे हि देशे भुञ्जानो नानिष्टदेशजैर्मनोविघातकरैर्भावैर्मनोविघातं प्राप्नोति, तथैवेष्टैः सर्वोपकरणैः; तस्मादिष्टे देशे तथेष्टसर्वोपकरणं चाश्नीयात् |२५|

One should take food properly equipped with all the accessories. By doing so he does not get afflicted with such factors as would result in emotional strain which (normally) occurs when one takes his food in improper places without the required accessories. Therefore, one should take food in a proper place equipped with all accessories. [25]

Intake not in hurry:

नातिद्रुतमश्नीयात्; अतिद्रुतं हि भुञ्जानस्योत्स्नेहनमवसादनं भोजनस्याप्रतिष्ठानं च, भोज्यदोषसाद्गुण्योपलब्धिश्च न नियता; तस्मान्नातिद्रुतमश्नीयात् |२५|

One should not take food too hurriedly. If food is taken too hurriedly it enters into a wrong passage; it does not enter into the stomach properly. In this situation one can never determine the taste of food articles and detect foreign bodies, mixed with them. [25]

Intake not too slow:

नातिविलम्बितमश्नीयात्; अतिविलम्बितं हि भुञ्जानो न तृप्तिमधिगच्छति, बहु भुङ्क्ते, शीतीभवत्याहारजातं, विषमं च पच्यते; तस्मान्नातिविलम्बितमश्नीयात् |२५|

One should not take food very slowly because this will not give satisfaction to the individual. In this situation he would take more than what is required; the food would become cold and there will be irregularity in digestion. Therefore, one should not take food very slowly. [25]

Intake with concentration:

अजल्पन्नहसन् तन्मना भुञ्जीत; जल्पतो हसतोऽन्यमनसो वा भुञ्जानस्य त एव हि दोषा भवन्ति, य एवातिद्रुतमश्नतः; तस्मादजल्पन्नहसंस्तन्मना भुञ्जीत |२५|

One should not talk or laugh or be unmindful while taking food. One taking food while talking, laughing or with detracted mind subjects to the same trouble as the one eating too hurriedly. So, one should not talk, laugh or be unmindful while taking food. [25]

Intake with self-confidence:

आत्मानमभिसमीक्ष्य भुञ्जीत सम्यक्; इदं ममोपशेते इदं नोपशेत इत्येवं विदितं ह्यस्यात्मन आत्मसात्म्यं भवति; तस्मादात्मानमभिसमीक्ष्य भुञ्जीत सम्यगिति||२५||

One should take food in a prescribed manner; with due regard to his own self. The knowledge of the usefulness or otherwise of food articles is the Sine Qua non for self- preservation. So, one should take food in a prescribed manner with due regard to his own self. [25]

Thus, it is said:

भवति चात्र-

रसान् द्रव्याणि दोषांश्च विकारांश्च प्रभावतः|

वेद यो देशकालौ च शरीरं च स नो भिषक्||२६||

He also is a good physician who knows specific nature of Rasas (tastes), drugs, Doshas and diseases as well as habitat time and physical constitution. [26]

To sum up:

तत्र श्लोकौ-

विमानार्थो रसद्रव्यदोषरोगाः प्रभावतः|

द्रव्याणि नातिसेव्यानि त्रिविधं सात्म्यमेव च||२७||

आहारायतनान्यष्टौ भोज्यसाद्गुण्यमेव च|

विमाने रससङ्ख्याते सर्वमेतत् प्रकाशितम्||२८||

The following topics are discussed in this chapter on the "Knowledge of Specific Attributes of Rasas (Rasa vimana): Scope of Vimana, Specific nature of Rasas (tastes), drugs, Doshas and diseases, substances which are not to be used continuously in excess, 3 types of wholesomeness, 8 factors which determines which food articles are useful. [27-28]

इत्यग्निवेशकृते तन्त्रे चरकप्रतिसंस्कृते विमानस्थाने रसविमानं नाम प्रथमोऽध्यायः|

Thus ends the first chapter on the "knowledge of specific Attributes of Rasa (taste)" of the Vimana section of Agniveshas' work as redacted by Charaka.

10

Vimanasthana Chapter 2
Trividhakukshiya Vimanam

Food Quantity, Ama :

The 2nd chapter of Charaka Vimana sthana is called Trividhakukshiya Vimana. It deals with the determination of specific characteristics of the stomach capacity together with its 3 parts.

Specific Characteristics of Stomach Capacity:

अथातस्त्रिविधकुक्षीयं विमानं व्याख्यास्यामः||१||

इति ह स्माह भगवानात्रेयः||२||

We shall now explore the chapter on the "Determination of the Specific Characteristics of the stomach capacity together with its 3 parts". Thus said Lord Atreya [1-2]

Division of stomach :

Division of stomach capacity into 3 parts:

त्रिविधं कुक्षौ स्थापयेदवकाशांशमाहारस्याहारमुपयुञ्जानः; तद्यथा- एकमवकाशांशं मूर्तानामाहारविकाराणाम्, एकं द्रवाणाम्, एकं पुनर्वातपित्तश्लेष्मणाम्; एतावतीं ह्याहारमात्रामुपयुञ्जानो नामात्राहारजं किञ्चिदशुभं प्राप्नोति||३||

For the purpose of taking food, the stomach capacity is divided into 3 parts:

One part of it is filled up with solid food,

The second part with liquids and

The third part is left for Vata, Pitta and Kapha.

One who takes food with due regard to this principle, does not fall victim to food with harmful effects which arise out of food taken in improper quantities. [3]

न च केवलं मात्रावत्त्वादेवाहारस्य कृत्स्नमाहारफलसौष्ठवमवाप्तुं शक्यं, प्रकृत्यादीनामष्टानामाहारविधिविशेषायतनानां प्रविभक्तफलत्वात्||४||

It is not possible to derive the entire benefit out of food, simply on the basis of the quantity of intake. For all the 8 factors like Prakrti, Karana etc (Ashta Vidha Ahara Vishesha Ayatana explained in Charak Vimana 1st chapter) etc. which determines the utility of food are jointly responsible for bringing about the requisite benefits. [4]

Signs of intake of food in proper quantity:

तत्रायं तावदाहारराशिमधिकृत्य मात्रामात्राफलविनिश्चयार्थः प्रकृतः|

एतावानेव ह्याहारराशिविधिविकल्पो यावन्मात्रावत्त्वममात्रावत्त्वं च||५||

In this chapter, Rashi (quantity of food) will be described with a view of determining the effect of the intake of food in proper and improper quantities. This is the only consideration to decide so as to how much is the proper and improper quantity of food.

तत्र मात्रावत्वं पूर्वमुद्दिष्टं कुक्ष्यंशविभागेन, तद्भूयो विस्तरेणानुव्याख्यास्यामः|

तद्यथा- कुक्षेरप्रणीडनमाहारेण, हृदयस्यानवरोधः, पार्श्वयोरविपाटनम्, अनतिगौरवमुदरस्य, प्रीणनमिन्द्रियाणां, क्षुत्पिपासोपरमः, स्थानासनशयनगमनोच्छ्वासप्रश्वासहास्यसङ्कथासु सुखानुवृत्तिः, सायं प्रातश्च सुखेन परिणमनं , बलवर्णोपचयकरत्वं च; इति मात्रावतो लक्षणमाहारस्य भवति||६||

How to determine whether the quantity of food is appropriate or not? – The quantity of food consumed is appropriate or inappropriate is determined on the basis of the stomach capacity and its division into three parts. This shall be described again in detail here.

Signs of intake of food in proper quantity:

kukṣerapraṇīḍanamāhāreṇa – There is no undue pressure on the stomach due to the food taken

hṛdayasyānavarodhaḥ – There is no obstruction to the proper functioning of the heat

pārśvayoravipāṭanam – There should not be any pressure in the sides of the chest

anatigauravamudarasya – There should not be excessive heaviness in the abdomen

prīṇanamindriyāṇām – There is proper nourishment of the senses

kṣutpipāsoparamaḥ – There is relief from hunger and thirst

sthānāsanaśayanagamanocchvāsapraśvāsahāsyasaṅkathāsusukhānuvṛttiḥ – There is the feeling of comfort in standing, sitting, sleeping, walking, exhaling, inhaling, laughing and talking

sāyamprātaścasukhenapariṇamanam – Food taken in the morning should get digested by the evening and the food taken during the evening should get digested by the next morning and

balavarṇopacayakaratvaṃ ca – There is promotion of strength, complexion and plumpness. [5-6]

Signs of intake of food in improper quantity :

अमात्रावत्वं पुनर्द्विविधमाचक्षते- हीनम्, अधिकं च|

Improper quantity of food is again of 2 types-deficient in quantity and excessive in quantity.

तत्र हीनमात्रमाहारराशिं बलवर्णोपचयक्षयकरमतृप्तिकरमुदावर्तकरमनायुष्यवृष्यमनौजस्यं शरीरमनोबुद्धीन्द्रियोपघातकरं सारविधमनमलक्ष्म्यावहमशीतेश्च वातविकाराणामायतनमाचक्षते

Food deficient in quantity will produce the following symptoms:

balavarṇopacayakṣayakaramatṛptikaram – Impairment of the strength, complexion and plumpness

udāvartakaram – Distension and absence of downward movement of food in stomach and intestines

anāyuṣyavṛṣyamanaujasyam – Impairment of longevity, virility and Ojas

śarīra mano buddhīndriyopaghātakaram – Affliction of body, mind, intellect and senses

sāravidhamanamalakṣmyāvahamaśīteśca – Impairment of excellence of Dhatus

vātavikārāṇāmāyatanamācakṣate – Causation of eighty varieties of Vatika diseases.

अतिमात्रं पुनः सर्वदोषप्रकोपणमिच्छन्ति कुशलाः|

यो हि मूर्तानामाहारजातानां सौहित्यं गत्वा द्रवैस्तृप्तिमापद्यते भूयस्तस्यामाशयगता वातपित्तश्लेष्माणोऽभ्यवहारेणातिमात्रेणातिप्रपीड्यमानाः सर्वे युगपत् प्रकोपमापद्यन्ते, ते प्रकुपितास्तमेवाहारराशिमपरिणतमविश्य कुक्ष्येकदेशमन्नाश्रिता विष्टम्भयन्तः सहसा वाऽप्युत्तराधराभ्यां मार्गाभ्यां प्रच्यावयन्तः पृथक् पृथगिमान् विकारानभिनिर्वर्तयन्त्यतिमात्रभोक्तुः|

Food taken in excessive quantities aggravates all the 3 Doshas. One who fills up his stomach with solid food and then takes liquid food in excessive quantity, all the 3 Doshas, viz. Vata (Samana Vayu), Pitta and Kapha residing in the stomach get too much compressed and simultaneously aggravated.The aggravated Doshas affect the undigested food and get mixed up with it. Then they obstruct a part of the stomach and instantaneously move through upward and downward and downward tracts separately to produce the following diseases in the individual, taking food in excess.

Effect of Doshas on ingested food :

तत्र वातः शूलानाहाङ्गमर्दमुखशोषमूर्च्छाभ्रमाग्निवैषम्य- पार्श्वपृष्ठकटिग्रहसिराकुञ्चनस्तम्भनानि करोति, पित्तं पुनर्ज्वरातीसारान्तर्दाहतृष्णामदभ्रमप्रलपनानि, श्लेष्मा तु छर्द्यरोचकाविपाकशीतज्वरालस्यगात्रगौरवाणि||७||

Vata produces

Shula-colic pain

Aanaha -constipation

Angamarda – malaise

Mukhaśoṣa – dryness of mouth

Bhrama –fainting

āgnivaiṣamya -irregularity in the power of digestion,

pārśvapṛṣṭhakaṭigraha – rigidity of sides, back and waist, and

sirākuñcanastambhanānikaroti – contraction and hardening of vessels.

Pitta produces

Jwara – fever

Atisara – diarrhea

Antardaha – burning sensation inside the body / viscera

Trshna – thirst

Mada – intoxication

Bhrama – giddiness

Pralapa – delirium

Kapha causes

Chardi – vomiting

Arochaka –anorexia

Avipaka – indigestion

Shitajvara – cold fever

Aalasya – laziness and

Gatragaurava – heaviness in the body. [7]

Ama vitiation factors :

Factors responsible for vitiation of Ama:

न च खलु केवलमतिमात्रमेवाहारराशिमामप्रदोषकरमिच्छन्ति , अपि तु खलु गुरुरूक्षशीतशुष्कद्विष्टविष्टम्भिविदाह्यशुचिविरुद्धानामकाले चान्नपानानामुपसेवनं, कामक्रोधलोभमोहेर्ष्याह्रीशोकमानोद्वेगभयोपतप्तमनसा वा यदन्नपानमुपयुज्यते, तदप्याममेव प्रदूषयति||८||

In addition to the intake of food in excess, the following factors also affect the body vitiating the undigested food products:

guru rūkṣaśītaśuṣkadviṣṭaviṣṭambhividāhyaśuciviruddhānāmakālecānnapānānāmupasevanaṃ – Untimely intake of food and drinks which are heavy, dry, cold, dry, despicable, constipative, irritant, unclean and mutually contradictory.

kāmakrodhalobhamoherṣyāhrīśokamānodvegabhayopataptamanasāvāyadannapānamupayujyate – Intake of food and drinks when the individual is afflicted with passion, anger, greed, confusion, envy, bashfulness, grief, indigestion, anxiety and fear.

भवति चात्र-

मात्रयाऽप्यभ्यवहृतं पथ्यं चान्नं न जीर्यति|

चिन्ताशोकभयक्रोधदुःखशय्याप्रजागरैः॥९॥

Thus, it is said: Wholesome food taken even in proper quantity do not get properly digested when the individual is afflicted with grief, fear, anger, sorrow, excessive sleep and excessive vigil [8-9]

Two types of Amapradosha :

तं द्विविधमामप्रदोषमाचक्षते भिषजः- विसूचिकाम्, अलसकं च॥१०॥

तत्र विसूचिकामूर्ध्वं चाधश्च प्रवृत्तामदोषां यथोक्तरूपां विद्यात्॥११॥

Amadosha (vitiation of undigested food) is known to physicians as of 2 types, viz.

Vishuchika (choleric diarrhea) and Alasaka (intestinal topper – kindly check for this).

In Vishuchika, undigested food gets expelled through the upper and lower tracks and it is accompanied with the symptoms already described (in para- 7 of this chapter). [10-11]

Alasaka

अलसकमुपदेक्ष्यामः- दुर्बलस्याल्पाग्नेर्बहुश्लेष्मणो वातमूत्रपुरीषवेगविधारिणः स्थिरगुरुबहुरूक्षशीतशुष्कान्नसेविनस्तदन्नपानमनिलप्रपीडितं श्लेष्मणा च विबद्धमार्गमतिमात्रप्रलीनमलसत्वान्न बहिर्मुखीभवति, ततश्छर्द्यतीसारवर्ज्यान्यामप्रदोषलिङ्गान्यभिदर्शयत्यतिमात्राणि।

Alasaka (intestinal toper):

If weak individual, having low power of digestion and excessive Kapha in his body, suppresses the urge for voiding flatus, urine and stool, and takes compact, heavy, dry, cold and dried food in excessive quantity, food and drinks get affected with Vata, simultaneously the passage gets obstructed by Kapha due to excessive adhesiveness of the food product. Because of which the undigested food product comes out of the stomach. Therefore, all the symptoms of Amadosha (described in Para- 7) except vomiting and diarrhoea are manifested in Alasaka.

अतिमात्रप्रदुष्टाश्च दोषाः प्रदुष्टामबद्धमार्गास्तिर्यग्गच्छन्तः कदाचिदेव केवलमस्य शरीरं दण्डवत् स्तम्भयन्ति, ततस्तं दण्डालसकमसाध्यं ब्रुवते।

The extremely vitiated Dosha moves side-ward due to the obstruction of the passage by undigested food or immature food product, and at times, makes the body of the patient rigid like a staff. This condition is known as Dandalasaka and it is incurable.

विरुद्धाध्यशनाजीर्णाशनशीलिनः पुनरामदोषमामविषमित्याचक्षते भिषजः, विषसदृशलिङ्गत्वात्; तत् परमसाध्यम्, आशुकारित्वाद्विरुद्धोपक्रमत्वाच्चेति॥१२॥

Ama visha :

Amadosha of an individual given to habitual intake of incompatible food, or food before the digestion of the previous meal or uncooked food is known as Amavisha (a condition characterized by the manifestation of toxic symptoms due to indigestion), because the manifestations of this condition resemble those of the poisoning. This is absolutely incurable because of the acuteness and also because of the contradiction involved in the line of treatment of this condition and tends to take away life in quick time. [12]

Management of Amapradosha :

तत्र साध्यमामं प्रदुष्टमलसीभूतमुल्लेखयेदादौ पाययित्वा सलवणमुष्णं वारि, ततः स्वेदनवर्तिप्रणिधानाभ्यामुपाचरेदुपवासयेच्चैनम्। विसूचिकायां तु लङ्घनमेवाग्रे विरिक्तवच्चानुपूर्वी।

The curable type of this disease having vitiated Ama (undigested food product) which has become stagnant is treated with emesis in the beginning, by administering hot salt water. Thereafter, fomentation and suppositories are employed and the patient is made to fast.

Visuchika treatment :

In case of Vishuchika (choleric diarrhea), the patient is kept on fasting in the beginning, and thereafter, he is given thin gruel etc. as is done after the administration of purgation etc.

आमप्रदोषेषु त्वन्नकाले जीर्णाहारं पुनर्दोषावलिप्तामाशयं स्तिमितगुरुकोष्ठमनन्नाभिलाषिणमभिसमीक्ष्य पाययेद्दोषशेषपाचनार्थमौषधमग्निसन्धुक्षणार्थं च, नत्वेवाजीर्णाशनम्; आमप्रदोषदुर्बलो ह्यग्निर्न युगपद्दोषमौषधमाहारजातं च शक्तः पक्तुम्।
अपि चामप्रदोषाहारौषधविभ्रमोऽतिबलत्वादुपरतकायाग्निं सहसैवातुरमबलमतिपातयेत्।

Even after the digestion of the food which was responsible for the causation of Amadosha (Vishuchika and Alasak), Doshas remain adhered to the stomach and during the meal-time also, the patient feels Stimita (timidity), Guru Kostha (heaviness of the abdomen) and Annanabhilasham (disinclination for food).

Treatment for Ama Pradosha :
At this stage, the patient is advised to take medicines in order to bring about the maturity of the remaining Doshas and also to stimulate the power of digestion. Food is never given when there is indigestion because the Agni (digestive fire) which is already weak due to the vitiation by Ama will not be able to digest the Doshas, drugs and food simultaneously.

The patient who is weak and whose Kayagni (enzymes responsible for the digestive and metabolic events in the body) is also weak will be seriously affected by the dominance of the untoward effects produced by Amapradosha, food and drugs simultaneously.

आमप्रदोषजानां पुनर्विकाराणामपतर्पणेनैवोपरमो भवति, सति त्वनुबन्धे कृतापतर्पणानां व्याधीनां निग्रहे निमित्तविपरीतमपास्यौषधमातङ्कविपरीतमेवावचारयेद्यथास्वम्।
सर्वविकाराणामपि च निग्रहे हेतुव्याधिविपरीतमौषधमिच्छन्ति कुशलाः, तदर्थकारि वा।

The diseases caused by Ama Dosha can be subsided / cured only by administration of Apatarpana. If the disease continues even after fasting, then the physician need not administer therapies as would be contrary (directly or indirectly) to the causative factors of the disease but administer therapies / medicines which are contrary to the respective diseases. They should be compatible and favourable to the prakriti, dosha etc of the patient. An expert physician should always administer such medicines which are opposite to the diseases or their causative factors so as to help cure all types of diseases. Or should prefer prescribing medicines which are similar to causative factors and diseases (and yet help in treating the diseases).

विमुक्तामप्रदोषस्य पुनः परिपक्वदोषस्य दीप्ते चाग्नावभ्यङ्गास्थापनानुवासनं विधिवत् स्नेहपानं च युक्त्या प्रयोज्यं प्रसमीक्ष्य दोषभेषजदेशकालबलशरीराहारसात्म्यसत्वप्रकृतिवयसामवस्थान्तराणि विकारांश्च सम्यगिति॥१३॥
Treatment after Ama Pachana :
When the patient is free from Amadosha, when Doshas are fully matured (digested) and when the powder of digestion is stimulated, the physician/ should employ massage, Asthapana and Anuvasana types of enema and Snehana, appropriately by following the prescribed procedure, after examining properly the different stages of doshas, therapies, Habitat, season, strength, physique, food, congeniality, mind, nature and age. [13]

Thus, it is said:
भवति चात्र-
आहारविध्यायतनानि चाष्टौ सम्यक् परीक्ष्यात्महितं विदध्यात्।
अन्यश्च यः कश्चिदिहास्ति मार्गो हितोपयोगेषु भजेत तं च॥१४॥
After properly examining the eight factors which determine the utility or otherwise of various types of food, one should take food which is wholesome for him. Other useful therapy which though not described here (but described in the chapter on the treatment of Grahani or sprue, and Atisara or diarrhea etc., for the cure of Amadosha) is

adopted. [14]

Amashaya and its functions :

अशितं खादितं पीतं लीढं च क्व विपच्यते|
एतत्त्वां धीर! पृच्छामस्तन्न आचक्ष्व बुद्धिमन्||१५||
इत्यग्निवेशप्रमुखैः शिष्यैः पृष्टः पुनर्वसुः|
आचचक्षे ततस्तेभ्यो यत्राहारो विपच्यते||१६||
नाभिस्तनान्तरं जन्तोरामाशय इति स्मृतः|
अशितं खादितं पीतं लीढं चात्र विपच्यते||१७||
आमाशयगतः पाकमाहारः प्राप्य केवलम्|
पक्वः सर्वाशयं पश्चाद्धमनीभिः प्रपद्यते||१८||

Amashaya and its functions:

O! Enlightened one; please tell us where (in which place, seat) the different types of food, viz

Aashitam – eatables

Khaditam – chewable

Pitam – drinkables and

Lidham- lickable gets digested.

Having heard this question of the disciples, viz Agnivesha etc. Lord Punarvasu replied, "It is in Amashaya (stomach) existing between umbilicus and nipples, that the eatables, chewable, drinkables and likables – all kinds of food get digested. When the foods reaching the amashaya get properly and totally digested the nutritive juices derived from the same reaches every part of the body circulating through the dhamanis (vessels). [15-18]

To sum up: -

तत्रश्लोकः:-

तस्यमात्रावतोलिङ्गंफलंचोक्तंयथायथम्|
अमात्रस्यतथालिङ्गंफलंचोक्तंविभागशः||१९||

Symptoms and the final outcome of the food taken in proper as well as improper quantities are appropriately described here separately. [19]

इत्यग्निवेशकृते तन्त्रेचरकप्रतिसंस्कृते विमानस्थाने त्रिविधकुक्षीयविमानं नाम द्वितीयोऽध्यायः||२||

Thus ends the 2nd chapter TrividhaKuksheeya Vimana, of the Vimana sthana of Agnivesha work as redacted by Charaka [2]

11
Vimanasthana Chapter 3
Janapadoddhvamsaniyam Vimanam

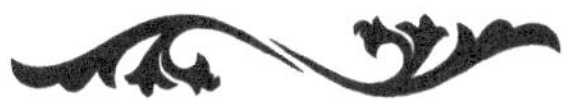

The 3rd chapter of CharakaSamhitha Vimana sthana is Janapadoddhvamsaneeya Vimanam. Janapada means a community. Udhwamsa means destruction. This deals with the determination of the specific characteristics of epidemics.

अथातो जनपदोद्ध्वंसनीयं विमानं व्याख्यास्यामः||१||

इति ह स्माह भगवानात्रेयः||२||

We shall now explore the chapter on the "Epidemic Diseases". Thus said Lord Atreya [1-2]

जनपदमण्डले पञ्चालक्षेत्रे द्विजातिवराध्युषिते काम्पिल्यराजधान्यां भगवान् पुनर्वसुरात्रेयोऽन्तेवासिगणपरिवृतः पश्चिमे घर्ममासे गङ्गातीरे वनविचारमनुविचरञ्छिष्यमग्निवेशमब्रवीत्||३||

In Kampilya (modern Kampil of Farokhabad District in Uttar Pradesh), the capital city of the country called Panchala, which was inhabited by the high-class people, Atreya was residing with his disciples. He was taking a stroll in the woods near the bank of the Ganga during the month of Jyestha (approximately May – June). He then, started speaking to his disciple Agnivesha. [3]

Collection, administration of herbs :

दृश्यन्ते हि खलु सौम्य! नक्षत्रग्रहगणचन्द्रसूर्यानिलानलानां दिशां चाप्रकृतिभूतानामृतुवैकारिका भावाः, अचिरादितो भूरपि च न यथावद्रसवीर्यविपाकप्रभावमोषधीनां प्रतिविधास्यति, तद्विवयोगाच्चातङ्कप्रायता नियता|

तस्मात् प्रागुद्ध्वंसात् प्राक् च भूर्मेविरसीभावादुद्धरध्वं सौम्य! भैषज्यानि यावन्नोपहतरसवीर्यविपाकप्रभावाणि भवन्ति|

वयं चैषां रसवीर्यविपाकप्रभावानुपयोक्ष्यामहे ये चास्माननुकाङ्क्षन्ति, यांश्च वयमनुकाङ्क्षामः|

न हि सम्यगुद्धृतेषु सौम्य! भैषज्येषु सम्यग्विहितेषु सम्यक् चावचरितेषु जनपदोद्ध्वंसकराणां विकाराणां किञ्चित् प्रतीकारगौरवं भवति||४||

Collection of herbs before the onset of epidemics:

O! Agnivesha, some abnormalities are now appearing in the stars, planets, moon, sun, air, fire and Disha (directions). This forecasts abnormality in the coming seasons. Very soon, the earth will cease to manifest proper tastes, potency, Vipaka (after digestion taste conversion) and Prabhava (special effects). This is bound to result in the wide-spread manifestation of diseases."

Therefore, O! Agnivesha, all of you should collect herbs before the time of destruction and before the earth loses its fertility, leading to the impairments of taste, potency, Vipaka and special effects.

Administration of herbs during epidemic disease:

We shall administer these herbs with proper taste, potency, vipaka, and Prabhava to treat diseases. It is not difficult to treat epidemic diseases, provided the herbs are collected, preserved and administered properly. [4]

Agnivesha's query :

एवंवादिनं भगवन्तमात्रेयमग्निवेश उवाच- उद्धृतानि खलु भगवन्! भैषज्यानि, सम्यग्विहितानि, सम्यगवचारितानि च; अपि तु खलु जनपदोद्ध्वंसनमेकेनैव व्याधिना युगपदसमानप्रकृत्याहारदेहबलसात्म्यसत्त्ववयसां मनुष्याणां कस्मादभवतीति||५||

Query about onset of epidemic disease:

Agnivesha asked Lord Atreya, "O! Lord, herbs will soon be collected, preserved and administered properly. How is it that people having dissimilar nature, diet, physical strength, congeniality, mental faculties, and age, simultaneously get afflicted by the same epidemic disease? [5]

Janapadodhwamsakara Bhava :

तमुवाच भगवानात्रेयः- एवमसामान्यावतामप्येभिरग्निवेश! प्रकृत्यादिभिर्भावैर्मनुष्याणां येऽन्ये भावाः सामान्यास्तद्वैगुण्यात् समानकालाः समानलिङ्गाश्च व्याधयोऽभिनिर्वर्तमाना जनपदमुद्ध्वंसयन्ति|

ते तु खल्विमे भावाः सामान्या जनपदेषु भवन्ति; तद्यथा- वायुः, उदकं, देशः, काल इति||६||

Factors responsible for epidemics:

Lord Atreya replied, "Agnivesha! Though there is dissimilarity in the physical constitution of human beings, there are such factors that are common to all individuals. They are – air, water, location and seasons. (Vayu, Udaka, Desha and Kala). Vitiation of these factors leads to the simultaneous manifestations of diseases having the same set of symptoms leading to the destruction of a country. [6]

Characteristics of pollution of air, water, land and time:

तत्र वातमेवंविधमनारोग्यकरं विद्यात्; तद्यथा- यथर्तुविषममतिस्तिमितमतिचलमतिपरुषमतिशीतमत्युष्णमतिरूक्षमत्यभिष्यन्दिनमतिभैरवारावमतिप्रतिहत- परस्परगतिमतिकुण्डलिनमसात्म्यगन्धबाष्पसिकतापांशुधूमोपहतमिति (१);

उदकं तु खल्वत्यर्थविकृतगन्धवर्णरसस्पर्शं क्लेदबहुलमपक्रान्तजलचरविहङ्गमुपक्षीणजलेशयमप्रीतिकरमपगतगुणं विद्यात् (२);

देशं पुनः प्रकृतिविकृतवर्णगन्धरसस्पर्शं क्लेदबहुलमुपसृष्टं सरीसृपव्यालमशकशलभमक्षिकामूषकोलूकश्माशानिकशकुनिजम्बूकादिभिस्तृणोलूपोपवनवन्तं प्रतानादिबहुलमपूर्ववदवपतितशुष्कनष्टशस्यं धूमपवनं प्रध्मातपत्रिगणमुत्कृष्टश्वगणमुद्भ्रान्तव्यथितविविधमृगपक्षिसङ्घमुत्सृष्टनष्टधर्मसत्यलज्जाचारशीलगुणजनपदं शश्वत्क्षुभितोदीर्णसलिलाशयं प्रततोल्कापातनिर्घातभूमिकम्पमतिभयारावरूपं रूक्षताम्रारुणसिताभ्रजालसंवृताक्चन्द्रतारकमभीक्ष्णं ससम्भ्रमोद्वेगमिव सत्रासरुदितमिव सतमस्कमिव गुह्यकाचरितमिवाक्रन्दितशब्दबहुलं चाहितं विद्यात् (३);

कालं तु खलु यथर्तुलिङ्गादिविपरीतलिङ्गमतिलिङ्गं हीनलिङ्गं चाहितं व्यवस्येत् (४);

इमानेवन्दोषयुक्तांश्चतुरो भावाञ्जनपदोद्ध्वंसकरान् वदन्ति कुशलाः; अतोऽन्यथाभूतांस्तु हितानाचक्षते||७||

विगुणेष्वपि खल्वेतेषु जनपदोद्ध्वंसकरेषु भावेषु भेषजेनोपपाद्यमानानामभयं भवति रोगेभ्य इति||८||

Polluted air features :

Air with following characteristics is injurious to health:

Atistimitamatichalam – Excessive calmness or violent waves

Excessive dryness, cold, hot air, roughness, or humidity

Excessive clashes among each other (wind blowing from one direction clashing with the one from the other)

Parasparagatimatikualinam – excessive cyclones

Presence of unwholesome smell, gasses, sand, ashes and smoke

Polluted water features :

Water that can cause endemic diseases:
Water having the following characteristics is considered to be devoid of its normal attributes
Abnormal smell, colour, taste and touch
Kleda – excessive stickiness
Absence of aquatic birds
Reduction in the number of aquatic animals
Unpleasantness in taste and odour

Polluted land features :
Land having the following characteristics is considered harmful:
Abnormal colour, smell, taste, and touch
Kledabahulam – Excessive stickiness, moistness
Abundance of serpents, wild animals, mosquitoes, locusts, flies, rats, owls, vulture and jackal
Having excess of grass and weeds
Abundance of highly branched creepers
Having a novel look
withered, dried
Abundance of smoke in the wind;
Presence of wild cries of birds and dogs
Bewilderment and pain in animals and birds.

Pollution of time features :
Time having following characteristics is considered to be harmful:

- Perversion or absence of religion, truth, modesty, manners, conducts and other qualities of the inhabitants of the land.
- Constant agitation and over-flow of water reservoirs
- Frequent occurrence of meteorites, thunderbolts and earthquakes
- Fierce look and cries in the nature
- Appearances of roughness and coppery red and white coloured sun, moon and stars; their appearance as if they are covered with a net of clouds
- Confusion, excitement; apprehension, lamentation and darkness in the atmosphere
- Presence of excessive crying noise as if the country is seized by demons
- Manifestation of the characteristic features contrary to the normal conditions of the various seasons is considered to be harmful.

The above mentioned four factors along with their respective features of vitiation are considered by the wise as responsible for destruction by epidemic diseases. When these factors are having qualities opposite to above, they are congenial for human beings.

Importance of treatment:
During the impairment of these Janapadodhwamsakara Bhavas (factors), if proper medicine administration is done, one need not be afraid of diseases. [7-8]

Most dangerous factor – Janapadodhwamsa kara Bhava:
भवन्ति चात्र-
वैगुण्यमुपपन्नानां देशकालानिलाम्भसाम्‌।
गरीयस्त्वं विशेषेण हेतुमत् सम्प्रवक्ष्यते॥९॥

वाताज्जलं जलाद्देशं देशात् कालं स्वभावतः|
विद्याद्दुष्परिहार्यत्वाद्गरीयस्तरमर्थवित् ||१०||
वार्वादिषु यथोक्तानां दोषाणां तु विशेषवित्|
प्रतीकारस्य सौकर्ये विद्याल्लाघवलक्षणम्||११||

Thus, it is said: – We shall now explain the vitiation of land, season, air and water in the order of their importance. Impairment of air, water, place and time are more lethal in their increasing order. (Impairment of time is most dangerous). A specialist should know that, it is easier to correct the vitiation of air, water and land, than those of time (Kala). [9-11]

Line of treatment of epidemic diseases :

चतुर्ष्वपि तु दुष्टेषु कालान्तेषु यदा नराः|
भेषजेनोपपाद्यन्ते न भवन्त्यातुरास्तदा||१२||
येषां न मृत्युसामान्यं सामान्यं न च कर्मणाम्|
कर्म पञ्चविधं तेषां भेषजं परमुच्यते||१३||
रसायनानां विधिवच्चोपयोगः प्रशस्यते|
शस्यते देहवृत्तिश्च भेषजैः पूर्वमुद्धृतैः||१४||
सत्यं भूते दया दानं बलयो देवतार्चनम्|
सद्वृत्तस्यानुवृत्तिश्च प्रशमो गुप्तिरात्मनः||१५||
हितं जनपदानां च शिवानामुपसेवनम्|
सेवनं ब्रह्मचर्यस्य तथैव ब्रह्मचारिणाम्||१६||
सङ्कथा धर्मशास्त्राणां महर्षीणां जितात्मनाम्|
धार्मिकैः सात्त्विकैर्नित्यं सहास्या वृद्धसम्मतैः||१७||
इत्येतद्भेषजं प्रोक्तमायुषः परिपालनम्|
येषामनियतो मृत्युस्तस्मिन् काले सुदारुणे||१८||

One does not suffer from this disease even while all these 4 vitiated factors (vitiated air, water, place and time) are at work if he is administered with medicines and treatment.

Panchakarma, Rasayana :
Panchakarma:
For those who are afflicted with these 4 factors, Panchakarma detoxification therapy is the best treatment.

Rasayana Therapy:
Proper Rasayana therapy done with medicines that are collected before onset of epidemic disease restores physical health.
Truthfulness,
Bhoote Daya – compassion for living beings,
Dana – donation, charity,
Bali – sacrifice,
Devatarchana – prayer to the gods,
Sadvrutta – good deeds,
adoption of preventive measures, tranquility, protection of the self by Mantra etc are very effective.
Devotion towards God, residence in auspicious localities, observance of Brahmacharya, service to those observing Brahmacharya is told as a remedy. Discussion on religious scriptures, befriending great sages, who have self- control, who follow religion, who are Satvika and who are learned people.

These therapies, which when adopted during epidemic disorders, can easily save lives of individuals provided the epidemics can easily save the lives of individuals provided the death of a particular individual is not predetermined (by destiny) [12-18]

इति श्रुत्वा जनपदोद्ध्वंसने कारणानि पुनरपि भगवन्तमात्रेयमग्निवेश उवाच- अथ खलु भगवन्! कुतोमूलमेषां वार्त्वादीनां वैगुण्यमुत्पद्यते? येनोपपन्ना जनपदमुद्ध्वंसयन्तीति||१९||

तमुवाच भगवानात्रेयः- सर्वेषामप्यग्निवेश! वार्त्वादीनां यद्वैगुण्यमुत्पद्यते तस्य मूलमधर्मः, तन्मूलं वाऽसत्कर्म पूर्वकृतं; तयोर्योनिः प्रज्ञापराध एव|

तद्यथा- यदा वै देशनगरनिगमजनपदप्रधाना धर्ममुत्क्रम्याधर्मेण प्रजां वर्तयन्ति, तदाश्रितोपाश्रिताः पौरजनपदा व्यवहारोपजीविनश्च तमधर्ममभिवर्धयन्ति, ततः सोऽधर्मः प्रसभं धर्ममन्तर्धत्ते, ततस्तेऽन्तर्हितधर्माणो देवताभिरपि त्यज्यन्ते; तेषां तथाऽन्तर्हितधर्माणामधर्मप्रधानानामपक्रान्तदेवतानामृतवो व्यापद्यन्ते; तेन नापो यथाकालं देवो वर्षति न वा वर्षति विकृतं वा वर्षति, वाता न सम्यगभिवान्ति, क्षितिर्व्यापद्यते, सलिलान्युपशुष्यन्ति, ओषधयः स्वभावं परिहायापद्यन्ते विकृतिं; तत उद्ध्वंसन्ते जनपदाः स्पृश्याभ्यवहार्यदोषात् ||२०||

Factors underlying vitiation of air :

Reasons for pollution of water etc leading to epidemics:

Having heard the causes of epidemics leading to the destruction of countries, Agnivesha again inquired from Lord Atreya, Sir! What is the factor underlying the vitiation of air etc., which destroys the entire country?

Lord Atreya replied "Sins of the present life or the misdeeds of the past life are at the root of the vitiation of all these factors. Intellectual blasphemy (Prajnaparadha) constitutes the origin of both the types of sins.

Causes – Sins :

For example, when the rulers of states, towns, cities and countries do not follow the righteous path and take up sins, then their subordinates and common people of villages and cities, and merchants add further to this sinful situation. Sinful acts make the righteous acts disappear. Because of the disappearance of Dharma, the gods desert the people living in these places. Such are the places where seasons get impaired. Consequently, there will not be rainfall, wind does not blow properly; there is abnormality in the earth, water dries up, drugs lose their qualities and get impaired. Then there is impairment of the country because of the impairment of food and drinks. [19-20]

तथा शस्त्रप्रभवस्यापि जनपदोद्ध्वंसस्याधर्म एव हेतुर्भवति येऽतिप्रवृद्धलोभक्रोधमोहमानास्ते दुर्बलानवमत्यात्मस्वजनपरोपघाताय शस्त्रेण परस्परमभिक्रामन्ति, परान् वाऽभिक्रामन्ति, परैर्वाऽभिक्राम्यन्ते||२१||

Sinful act leading to war:

Similarly a sinful act is at the root of destruction of a country by armaments. Because of increased greed, anger, and ego, some people may start fighting among themselves with killer intention or the enemy looking down- upon them as weak persons. They may attack the enemy or may get attacked by them. [21]

Sinful act leading to affliction by Rakshasas:

रक्षोगणादिभिर्वा विविधैर्भूतसङ्घैस्तमधर्ममन्यद्वाऽप्यपचारान्तरमुपलभ्याभिहन्यन्ते||२२||

People also get destroyed by Rakshasas (demons, germs, viruses) and varieties of other creatures due to sins. [22]

Sinful act leading to curse:

तथाऽभिशापप्रभवस्याप्यधर्म एव हेतुर्भवति|

ये लुप्तधर्माणो धर्मादपेतास्ते गुरुवृद्धसिद्धर्षिपूज्यानवमत्याहितान्याचरन्ति; ततस्ताः प्रजा गुर्वादिभिरभिशप्ता भस्मतामुपयान्ति प्रागेवानेकपुरुषकुलविनाशाय, नियतप्रत्ययोपलम्भादनियताश्चापरे ||२३||

Similarly the sinful act causes destruction of the population by curse. Those who get on without religious duties, they wrongly behave by showing disrespect to respectable ones. Many such families get immediately destroyed by curse. Even if they do not stay together, they get simultaneously destroyed because of the predetermined effect of the curse on them. [23]

Attributes in different Yugas :

प्रागपि चाधर्मादृते नाशुभोत्पत्तिरन्यतोऽभूत्|

आदिकाले ह्यदितिसुतसमौजसोऽतिविमलविपुलप्रभावाः प्रत्यक्षदेवदेवर्षिधर्मयज्ञविधिविधानाः शैलसारसंहतस्थिरशरीराः प्रसन्नवर्णेन्द्रियाः पवनसमबलजवपराक्रमाश्चारुस्फिचोऽभिरूपप्रमाणाकृतिप्रसादोपचयवन्तः   सत्यार्जवानृशंस्यदानदमनियमतपोपवासब्रह्मचर्यव्रतपरा व्यपगतभयरागद्वेषमोहलोभक्रोधशोकमानरोगनिद्रातन्द्राश्रमक्लमालस्यपरिग्रहाश्च पुरुषा बभूवुरमितायुषः|

तेषामुदारसत्त्वगुणकर्मणामचिन्त्यरसवीर्यविपाकप्रभावगुणसमुदितानि   प्रादुर्बभूवुः   शस्यानि   सर्वगुणसमुदितत्वात्   पृथिव्यादीनां कृतयुगस्यादौ|

भ्रश्यति तु कृतयुगे केषाञ्चिदत्यादानात् साम्पन्निकानां सत्त्वानां शरीरगौरवमासीत्, शरीरगौरवाच्छ्रमः, श्रमादालस्यम्, आलस्यात् सञ्चयः, सञ्चयात् परिग्रहः, परिग्रहाल्लोभः प्रादुरासीत् कृते|

ततस्त्रेतायां लोभादभिद्रोहः, अभिद्रोहानृतवचनम्, अनृतवचनात् कामक्रोधमानद्वेषपारुष्याभिघातभयतापशोकचिन्तोद्वेगादयः प्रवृत्ताः|

ततस्त्रेतायां धर्मपादोऽन्तर्धानमगमत्|

तस्यान्तर्धानात् युगवर्षप्रमाणस्य पादह्रासः, पृथिव्यादेश्च गुणपादप्रणाशोऽभूत्|

तत्प्रणाशकृतश्च शस्यानां स्नेहवैमल्यरसवीर्यविपाकप्रभावगुणपादभ्रंशः|

ततस्तानि प्रजाशरीराणि हीयमानगुणपादैराहारविहारैरयथापूर्वमुपष्टभ्यमानान्यग्निमारुतपरीतानि प्राग्व्याधिभिर्ज्वरादिभिराक्रान्तानि|

अतः प्राणिनो ह्रासमवापुरायुषः क्रमश इति||२४||

From the beginning of creation, manifestation of inauspiciousness has been preceded by sinful acts.

During Satyuga / Krutayuga:

During Satyuga, people were energetic like the sun; They were gods, divine saints, following Dharma, Yajna as per rules, Their bodies were firm like mountains; compact and stable; they had clear complexion and senses; they had strength, motion and valour like those of the wind.

They were endowed with the good shaped organs, features, proper body measurements, happiness and nourishment.

They were endowed with truthfulness, simplicity, non-violence, charity, self-control, observance of rules, meditation, fasting, Brahmacharya and religious rites, and they were devoid of fear, attachment, envy, delicious, greed, anger, grief, mental diseases, abnormal sleep, drowsiness, fatigue, exhaustion, laziness and tendency to collect things.

Because of these factors they were endowed with an unlimited span of life in the beginning of the Satyuga.
Because of the noble mind, qualities and actions of the people, the earth etc., got endowed with all the good qualities as a result of which excellent tastes, potencies, Vipaka and specific actions were manifested in food grains.

At the end of Satyuga / Krutayuga:

At the end of the Satyayuga, some rich people got heavy in their bodies due to over- indulgence. They suffered from fatigue because of the heaviness of the body. Fatigue gave rise to laziness; laziness made them accumulate things; accumulation led to the attachment for these things and attachment resulted in greed.

During Tretayuga greed gave rise to malice; malice gave rise to false statements, arose passion, anger, vanity, hatred, cruelty, infliction of injury, fear, sorrow, grief, worry, anxiety etc. therefore, during Tretayuga, a quarter of Dharma (religious duties) disappeared.

Because of this, the lifespan of human beings is reduced by a quarter. Similarly, there was a reduction in the attributes of earth etc, by one quarter. Because of the reduction of these attributes there was diminution by one quarter of the unctuousness, purity, tastes, potency, Vipakas, specific actions and qualities of grains.

Because of the reduction by a quarter of the attributes of diets and regimens there was an unusual change in the maintenance of equilibrium of Dhatus and there was vitiation of Agni (pitta) and Maruta (vata) by which, first of all, bodies of living being got afflicted with diseases like fever. Therefore, the lifespan of living beings underwent gradual diminution. [24]

Gradual decrease in lifespan:
युगे युगे धर्मपादः क्रमेणानेन हीयते|
गुणपादश्च भूतानामेवं लोकः प्रलीयते||२५||
संवत्सरशते पूर्णे याति संवत्सरः क्षयम्|
देहिनामायुषः काले यत्र यन्मानमिष्यते||२६||
इति विकाराणां प्रागुत्पत्तिहेतुरुक्तो भवति||२७||
Thus, it is said: – Religious duties and qualities of living beings got reduced in quarters gradually by the passage of each Yuga. This is how the entire universe must face dissolution. After the passage of 1/ 100th of the Yuga, the life span of living beings was reduced by one year, the actual span of life specific to that age. Thus, the origin of diseases in ancient times is described. [25-27]

एवंवादिनं भगवन्तमग्निवेश उवाच- किन्नु खलु भगवन्! नियतकालप्रमाणमायुः सर्वं न वेति||२८||
तं भगवानुवाच-
इहाग्निवेश! भूतानामायुर्युक्तिमपेक्षते|
दैवे पुरुषकारे च स्थितं ह्यस्य बलाबलम्||२९||
दैवमात्मकृतं विद्यात् कर्म यत् पौर्वदैहिकम्|
स्मृतः पुरुषकारस्तु क्रियते यदिहापरम्||३०||
बलाबलविशेषोऽस्ति तयोरपि च कर्मणोः|
दृष्टं हि त्रिविधं कर्म हीनं मध्यममुत्तमम्||३१||
तयोरुदारयोर्युक्तिर्दीर्घस्य च सुखस्य च|
नियतस्यायुषो हेतुर्विपरीतस्य चेतरा||३२||

Query about span of life:
Agnivesha inquired from lord Atreya, "O! Lord, is the span of life of all individuals predetermined or not?[28]

Daiva and purusakara :
Lord Atreya replied, O! Agnivesha, the lifespan of individuals depends upon the strength or weakness of both the Daiva (pre-determined) and Purusha (human effort).

Daiva and Purusha Kaara:
What is done during the past life is known as Daiva where the effect is predetermined and what is done during the existing life is known as Purusakaara- where the effect is based upon human effort.

Depending upon the strength or weakness, both the types of actions described above are classified into three categories, viz, mild, moderate and strong.

Association with the effects of both these types of actions belonging to the strong category results in a long and happy life with a predetermined span.

In the case of their mildness, the result is opposite and in the case of their mediocrity, the result is moderate. Hear the other cause of the predetermination or otherwise of the life-span [29-32]

मध्यमा मध्यमस्येष्टा कारणं शृणु चापरम्|३३|
दैवं पुरुषकारेण दुर्बलं ह्युपहन्यते||३३||
दैवेन चेतरत् कर्म विशिष्टेनोपहन्यते|
दृष्ट्वा यदेके मन्यन्ते नियतं मानमायुषः||३४||
कर्म किञ्चित् क्वचित् काले विपाके नियतं महत्|
किञ्चित्त्वकालनियतं प्रत्ययैः प्रतिबोध्यते||३५||

Daiva and Purusakaara dominance of one over the other:
A weak Daiva (actions during the past life) gets subdued by a strong Puruhsakara (action during the present life). Similarly, a strong Daiva subdues Purushakaara and because of this, some scholars hold the view that the span of life is invariably pre-determined. Effects of a strong Daiva (actions of the previous life) are invariably manifested. The time of this manifestation is conditioned by the availability of a congenial atmosphere. [33-35]

तस्मादुभयदृष्टत्वादेकान्तग्रहणमसाधु|
निदर्शनमपि चात्रोदाहरिष्यमः- यदि हि नियतकालप्रमाणमायुः सर्वं स्यात्, तदाऽऽयुष्कामाणां न मन्त्रौषधिमणिमङ्गलबल्युपहारहोमनियमप्रायश्चितोपवासस्वस्त्ययनप्रणिपातगमनाद्याः क्रिया इष्टयश्च प्रयोज्येरन्; नोद्भ्रान्तचण्डचपलगोजोष्ट्रखरतुरगमहिषादयः पवनादयश्च दुष्टाः परिहार्याः स्युः, न प्रपातगिरिविषमदुर्गाम्बुवेगाः, तथा न प्रमत्तोन्मत्तोद्भ्रान्तचण्डचपलमोहलोभाकुलमतयः, नारयः, न प्रवृद्धोऽग्निः, च विविधविषाश्रयाः सरीसृपोरगादयः, न साहसं, नादेशकालचर्या, न नरेन्द्रप्रकोप इति; एवमादयो हि भावा नाभावकराः स्युः, आयुषः सर्वस्य नियतकालप्रमाणत्वात्|
न चानभ्यस्ताकालमरणभयनिवारकाणामकालमरणभयमागच्छेत् प्राणिनां, व्यर्थाश्चारम्भकथाप्रयोगबुद्धयः स्युर्महर्षीणां रसायनाधिकारे, नापीन्द्रो नियतायुषं शत्रुं वज्रेणाभिहन्यात्, नाश्विनावार्तं भेषजेनोपपादयेतां, न महर्षयो यथेष्टमायुस्तपसा प्राप्नुयुः, न च विदितवेदितव्या महर्षयः ससुरेशाः सम्यक् पश्येयुरुपदिशेयुराचरेयुर्वा|
अपि च सर्वचक्षुषामेतत् परं यदैन्द्रं चक्षुः, इदं चाप्यस्माकं तेन प्रत्यक्षं; यथा- पुरुषसहस्राणामुत्थायोत्थायाहवं कुर्वतामकुर्वतां चातुल्यायुष्ट्वं, तथा जातमात्राणामप्रतीकारात् प्रतीकाराच्च, अविषविषप्राशिनां चाप्यतुल्यायुष्ट्वमेव, न च तुल्यो योगक्षेम उदपानघटानां चित्रघटानां चोत्सीदतां; तस्माद्धितोपचारमूलं जीवितम्, अतो विपर्ययान्मृत्युः|
अपि च देशकालात्मगुणविपरीतानां कर्मणामाहारविकाराणां च क्रमोपयोगः सम्यक्, त्यागः सर्वस्य चातियोगायोगमिथ्यायोगानां, सर्वातियोगसन्धारणम्, असन्धारणमुदीर्णानां च गतिमतां, साहसानां च वर्जनम्, आरोग्यानुवृत्तौ हेतुमुपलभामहे सम्यगुपदिशामः सम्यक् पश्यामश्चेति||३६||

Actions of past lives (Daiva) and present lives (purusakara) – their role in the determination of span of life:
Since the actions of past and present lives – both play their roles in the determination of the span of life, it is not correct to hold one sided view that one or the other is responsible for this.

If the lifespan is totally predetermined, then why there is need to do mantras, Aushadi (auspicious substances), Mani (wearing gems), Mangala Bali – auspicious rites, Upahara -offering, oblations, observance of religious rules (niyama), reconciliation, fasting, benedictory rites, paying obeisance, pilgrimage etc

If the lifespan is totally predetermined, one may not be afraid of fierce and excited bulls, elephants, camels, donkeys, horses, buffaloes, harmful winds, waterfalls, rivers passing through mountains and having dangerous currents which are difficult to cross; rough fierce people and whose minds are afflicted with confusion and greed, enemies, highly inflamed fire, various poisonous animals like reptiles, over straining, regimens which are not conducive to the locality and seasons and such deeds as would enrage the king of the land.

If lifespan is totally predetermined, then those who have not taken steps to prevent untimely death, is not be afraid of it. The instructions for initiation and discussions about the administration of Rasayana therapies would all be meaningless.

If lifespan is totally predetermined, even Lord Indra cannot kill his enemy by his Vajra (thunderbolt), even great sages cannot live as long as they like to live by means of meditation.

Why is predetermined lifespan theory a hoax?
The futility of the theory of predetermined lifespan can be observed even with the naked eyes. For example, thousands of people who go in for a battle and those who do not, have dissimilar spans of life.

Similarly, people whose diseases are treated immediately after their manifestation and those whose diseases are not treated in time or those who take poison and those who do not, have dissimilar spans of life. Earthen jars used as ornamental vases differ in respect of their durability.

Therefore, wholesome regimens lead to longevity, unwholesome ones to death. One should gradually resort to such actions and diets that are having qualities opposite to those of the locality, seasons and one's own body.

He should avoid the over utilization, non- utilization and wrong- utilization of all regimens (Heena, Mithya and Atiyoga). One should give up all types of over indulgences; the manifested urges and he should avoid over straining. We know, we properly advise and we properly observe the above-mentioned factors for the maintenance of health. [36]

Time of death:
अतः परमग्निवेश उवाच- एवं सत्यनियतकालप्रमाणायुषां भगवन्! कथं कालमृत्युरकालमृत्युर्वाभवतीति||३७||
Agnivesha's query about time of death :
Agnivesha enquired, "O! Lord, if the span of living beings is not predetermined then how is it said that some people die in the predetermined time and the rest otherwise?" [37]

तमुवाच भगवानात्रेयः- श्रूयतामग्निवेश! यथा यानसमायुक्तोऽक्षः प्रकृत्यैवाक्षगुणैरुपेतः स च सर्वगुणोपपन्नो वाह्यमानो यथाकालं स्वप्रमाणक्षयादेवावसानं गच्छेत्, तथाऽऽयुः शरीरोपगतं बलवत्प्रकृत्या यथावदुपचर्यमाणं स्वप्रमाणक्षयादेवावसानं गच्छति; स मृत्युः काले| यथा च स एवाक्षोऽतिभाराधिष्ठितत्वादिविषमपथादपथादक्षचक्रभङ्गाद्वाह्यवाहकदोषादणिमोक्षादनुपाङ्गात् पर्यसनाच्चान्तराऽवसानमापद्यते, तथाऽऽयुरप्ययथाबलमारम्भादयथाग्न्यभ्यवहरणादिविषमाभ्यावहरणादिविषमशरीरन्यासादतिमैथुनादसत्संश्रयादुदीर्ण-वेगविनिग्रहादिविधार्यवेगाविधारणाद्भूतविषवाय्वग्न्युपतापादभिघातादाहारप्रतीकारविवर्जनाच्चान्तराऽवसानमापद्यते, स मृत्युरकाले; तथा ज्वरादीनप्यातङ्कान्मिथ्योपचारेतानकालमृत्यून् पश्याम इति||३८||
Atreya's reply:
Lord Atreya replied, "O! Agnivesha, as a vehicle with an axle endowed with all good qualities and driven on a good road gets destroyed only after the expiry of its normal life, similarly the life inside the body of an individual endowed with strong physique and wholesome regimen will come to an end only at the end of its normal span (according to the Yuga).

This is called "timely death", the same vehicle along with its axle may subject itself to premature destruction in the event of a heavy load, uneven road, driving in places where there is no road, breakage of the wheel, defects in the vehicle or the driver, separation of the locking hook, lack of grease or an accident.

Similarly, in the event of excess strain, eating in excess, irregular meals, irregular body postures, excessive sex, association of urges which should be suppressed, affliction with evil spirits (germs), poison, wind and fire, exposure to injury and the avoidance of food and medicines, the life of an individual may soon come to an end. This is called "premature death"; when diseases like fever etc are not properly treated, they also lead to premature death. [38]

अथाग्निवेशः पप्रच्छ- किन्नु खलु भगवन्! ज्वरितेभ्यः पानीयमुष्णं प्रयच्छन्ति भिषजो भूयिष्ठं न तथा शीतम्, अस्ति च शीतसाध्योऽपि धातुर्ज्वरकर इति||३९||

Hot water in fever :

Query about prescription of hot water to patients suffering from fever:

Agnivesha enquired, O! Lord, why do physicians advise patients suffering from fever to take hot water in preference to cold water when the Dosha involved in the pathogenesis of this disease is ideal for cooling therapies? [39]

तमुवाच भगवानात्रेयः- ज्वरितस्य कायसमुत्थानदेशकालानभिसमीक्ष्य पाचनार्थं पानीयमुष्णं प्रयच्छन्ति भिषजः|

ज्वरो ह्यामाशयसमुत्थः, प्रायो भेषजानि चामाशयसमुत्थानां विकाराणां पाचनवमनापतर्पणसमर्थानि भवन्ति; पाचनार्थं च पानीयमुष्णं, तस्मादेतज्ज्वरितेभ्यः प्रयच्छन्ति भिषजो भूयिष्ठम्|

तद्धि तेषां पीतं वातमनुलोमयति, अग्निं चोदर्यमुदीरयति, क्षिप्रं जरां गच्छति, श्लेष्माणं परिशोषयति, स्वल्पमपि च पीतं तृष्णाप्रशमनायोपकल्पते; तथायुक्तमपि चैतन्नात्यर्थोत्सन्नपित्ते ज्वरे सदाहभ्रमप्रलापातिसारे वा प्रदेयम्, उष्णेन हि दाहभ्रमप्रलापातिसारा भूयोऽभिवर्धन्ते, शीतेन चोपशाम्यन्तीति||४०||

Rationale behind administering hot water:

Lord Atreya replied, "Keeping in view physician advises the patient suffering from fever to take hot water so that the immaturely formed Doshas which are responsible for the disease may get matured. The origin of fever is Amashaya (stomach).

For the treatment of disease originating from the stomach, usually Pachaka (digestive), as well as emetic (Vamana) and Apatarpana (depleting) drugs are administered. It is because of this that the physician advises the patient suffering from fever to take hot water.

If hot water is taken, this results in a downward movement of Vata (flatus), stimulation of Agni (digestive enzymes), easy digestion (the hot water itself gets easily digested) and drying up of Kapha. Even then, hot water is not given to those patients with excessive vitiation of Pitta or if there is burning sensation, dizziness, delirium and diarrhoea. Hot things lead to the burning sensation, giddiness, delirium and diarrhoea. Only cold food and drinks are helpful in this situation. [40]

भवति चात्र-

शीतेनोष्णकृतान् रोगाञ्छमयन्ति भिषग्विदः|
ये तु शीतकृता रोगास्तेषामुष्णं भिषग्जितम्||४१||

Thus, it is said: - enlightened physicians administer cold things to cure diseases caused by hot things. For diseases caused by cold things, hot drugs are useful. [41]

Santarpana and Apatarpana:

एवमितरेषामपि व्याधीनां निदानविपरीतं भेषजं भवति; यथा- अपतर्पणनिमित्तानां व्याधीनां नान्तरेण पूरणमस्ति शान्तिः, तथा पूरणनिमित्तानां व्याधीनां नान्तरेणापतर्पणम्||४२||

अपतर्पणमपि च त्रिविधं- लङ्घनं, लङ्घनपाचनं, दोषावसेचनं चेति||४३||

तत्र लङ्घनमल्पबलदोषाणां, लङ्घनेन ह्यग्निमारुतवृद्ध्या वातातपपरीतमिवाल्पमुदकमल्पो दोषः प्रशोषमापद्यते; लङ्घनपाचने तु मध्यबलदोषाणां, लङ्घनपाचनाभ्यां हि सूर्यसन्तापमारुताभ्यां पांशुभस्मावकिरणैरिव चानतिबहूदकं मध्यबलो दोषः प्रशोषमापद्यते; बहुदोषाणां पुनर्दोषावसेचनमेव कार्यं, न ह्यभिन्ने केदारसेतौ पल्वलाप्रसेकोऽस्ति, तद्वद्दोषावसेचनम्||४४||

Nourishing and depleting therapies: Santarpana and Apatarpana:

Similarly, the treatment of other diseases involve the administration of therapies that are antagonistic to their causes. For example, diseases caused by the depletion of Dhatus cannot get cured without nourishing therapy; similarly, diseases caused by over-nourishment cannot be cured without depletion therapy.

Apatarpana – Depletion therapy is of three types, viz,

Langhana (fasting),

Langhana-pachana (fasting and administration of such medicaments as would help in burning out the maturity of doshas) and

Doshavasecahna (elimination of Doshas).

Langhana (fasting) is suitable when the vitiation of Doshas is mild. By fasting, there is aggravation of Agni (power of digestion) and Vata, as a small quantity of water gets absorbed by heat and wind similarly Doshas get subsided by the aggravation of Agni and Vata due to fasting.

Langhana Pachana (fasting and administration of such medications as would help in bringing out the maturity (paka) of Doshas) is suitable when the vitiation of Doshas is moderate. As exposure to sun rays, wind and sprinkling of ashes and dust dry up moderately vitiated (accumulated) water. If the aggravation of Doshas is very strong, then it is necessary to eliminate them. Without breaking the boundary wall, it will not be eliminated to dry up a pond. Similar is the case when the doshas are exceedingly vitiated. [42-44]

Patients unsuitable for treatment:

दोषावसेचनमन्यद्वा भेषजं प्राप्तकालमप्यातुरस्य नैवंविधस्य कुर्यात् ।

तद्यथा - अनपवादप्रतीकारस्याधनस्यापरिचारकस्य वैद्यमानिनश्चण्डस्यासूयकस्य तीव्राधर्मारुचेरतिक्षीणबलमांसशोणितस्यासाध्यरोगोपहतस्य मुमूर्षुलिङ्गान्वितस्य चेति ।

एवंविधं ह्यातुरमुपचरन् भिषक् पापीयसाऽयशसा योगमृच्छतीति ॥४५॥

Even though required, as per state of the disease, elimination therapies, other forms of depletion therapies and nourishing therapy is not be administered to such patients who are:

Anapavada Pratikara – have not been absolved of the allegations against them, those who are incapable of meeting their expenditure, those who pose themselves as physicians, those who are given to violent behaviour and envy, those who draw pleasure from vicious acts, those whose strength, flesh and blood have undergone excessive diminution, these who are suffering from incurable diseases and those who are having symptoms of imminent death. If the physician takes such patients under his treatment, then he is defamed because of sinful acts. [45]

भवति चात्र-

तदात्वे चानुबन्धे वा यस्य स्यादशुभं फलम्|

कर्मणस्तन्न कर्तव्यमेतद्बुद्धिमतां मतम्||४६||

(अल्पोदकद्रुमो यस्तु प्रवातः प्रचुरातपः|

ज्ञेयः स जाङ्गलो देशः स्वल्परोगतमोऽपि च||४७||

प्रचुरोदकवृक्षो यो निवातो दुर्लभातपः|

अनूपो बहुदोषश्च, समः साधारणो मतः)||४८||

Thus, it is said: -

If an action produces inauspicious results immediately or in the long run, then according to wise persons, one should not resort to such type of work.

Different kinds of places:

Jangala or arid type of country is characterized by scarcity of water and trees, and plentiful air and sunshine. It causes minimum number of diseases.

Anupa or marshy land is characterized by abundance of water and trees and scarcity of air and sunshine. It causes many diseases.

Sama or moderate type of country is characterized by moderation in the above-mentioned factors. [46-48]

तत्र श्लोकाः-
पूर्वरूपाणि सामान्या हेतवः सस्वलक्षणाः|
देशोद्ध्वंसस्य भैषज्यं हेतूनां मूलमेव च||४९||
प्राग्विकारसमुत्पत्तिरायुषश्च क्षयक्रमः|
मरणं प्रति भूतानां कालाकालविनिश्चयः||५०||
यथा चाकालमरणं यथायुक्तं च भेषजम्|
सिद्धिं यात्यौषधं येषां न कुर्याद्येन हेतुना||५१||
तदात्रेयोऽग्निवेशाय निखिलं सर्वमुक्तवान्|
देशोद्ध्वंसनिमित्तीये विमाने मुनिसत्तमः||५२||
To sum up:-
Premonitory signs, causative factors in general, characteristic features and management of epidemics which destroy countries, source of the causative factors, origin of diseases in ancient times, process of the reduction in the span on life, determination of the timely and premature death of living beings, cause of premature death, appropriate medicine, selection of therapy for success, reasons for which a particular patient is not be treated- all these topics are described by lord Atreya to Agnivesha in this chapter on " Janapadodhwamsa." [49-52]

इत्यग्निवेशकृते तन्त्रे चरकप्रतिसंस्कृते विमानस्थाने जनपदोद्ध्वंसनीयविमानं नाम तृतीयोऽध्यायः||३||
Thus ends the third chapter on the Determination of the Specific Characteristics of epidemics of the Vimana section of Agnivesha's work as redacted by Charaka. [3]

12

Vimanasthana Chapter 4 Trividha Roga Vishesha Vijnaniya Vimanam

अथातस्त्रिविधरोगविशेषविज्ञानीयं विमानं व्याख्यास्यामः||१||

इति ह स्माह भगवानात्रेयः||२||

The 4th chapter of Charaka Samhitha Vimana Sthana is TrividhaRogaVisheshaVijaniniya Vimana. It deals with usage of Aptopadesha (scriptural knowledge), Pratyaksha (patient examination) and inference in patient and disease examination.

We shall now explore Trivodha Roga Vishesha Vijnaneeyaadhyaya. This chapter deals with the determination of three Factors for understanding the disease characteristics". Thus said Lord Atreya [1-2]

Three sources of knowledge :

त्रिविधं खलु रोगविशेषविज्ञानं भवति; तद्यथा आप्तोपदेशः, प्रत्यक्षम्, अनुमानं चेति||३||

There are three means to know about disease features:

Aaptopadesha – authoritative instruction, preaching of saints

Pratyaksham – direct observation and

Anumana – inference. [3]

Aptopadesha :

तत्राप्तोपदेशो नामाप्तवचनम्|

आप्ता ह्यवितर्कस्मृतिविभागविदो निष्प्रीत्युपतापदर्शिनश्च|

तेषामेवङ्गुणयोगाद्यद्वचनं तत् प्रमाणम्|

अप्रमाणं पुनर्मत्तोन्मत्तमूर्खरक्तदुष्टादुष्टवचनमिति; प्रत्यक्षं तु खलु तद्यत् स्वयमिन्द्रियैर्मनसा [२] चोपलभ्यते|

अनुमानं खलु तर्को युक्त्यपेक्षः||४||

Aptopadesha – preaching of saints / authoritative instructions are the teachings of Aptas (persons who are reliable and truthful).

AptaLakshana: features of truthful reliable person:

Aptas are free from doubts and their memory is unimpaired (AvitarkaSmruti), i.e., they know things in their entirety by determinate experience. They see things without any attachment or affliction.

Because of these qualities, their teaching is authentic. The statements made by intoxicated, mad, illiterate and attached persons are not to be considered as authoritative.

Pratyaksha and Anumana Pramana :
Pratyaksha or direct observation is that which is comprehensive by an individual through his own sense organs and mind. Anumana or inference is the indirect knowledge acquired by reasoning. [4]

Patient examination :

Patient examination with 3 Pramanas:
त्रिविधेन खल्वनेन ज्ञानसमुदायेन पूर्वं परीक्ष्य रोगं सर्वथा सर्वमथोत्तरकालमध्यवसानमदोषं भवति, न हि ज्ञानावयवेन कृत्स्ने ज्ञेये ज्ञानमुत्पद्यते।
त्रिविधे त्वस्मिन् ज्ञानसमुदये पूर्वमाप्तोपदेशाज्ज्ञानं, ततः प्रत्यक्षानुमानाभ्यां परीक्षोपपद्यते।
किं ह्यनुपदिष्टं पूर्वं यत्तत् प्रत्यक्षानुमानाभ्यां परीक्षमाणो विद्यात्।
तस्मादि्द्विविधा परीक्षा ज्ञानवतां प्रत्यक्षम्, अनुमानं च; त्रिविधा वा सहोपदेशेन।।५।।
First, one should examine various aspects of diseases with the help of the above 3 Pramanas (sources of knowledge). This helps to get accurate disease knowledge. First knowledge is gained by Aptopadesha (by reading text books and getting to know theoretical aspects of disease). After that, disease knowledge is gained by Pratyaksha – direct observation and then by Anumana – inference.

What is to be examined by direct observation, and inference unless something is Prima Facie stated? Therefore, a thing can be examined in two ways, viz, "Direct observation" and inference or in three ways which include Aptopadesha in addition. [5]

Different aspects of the examination of diseases:
तत्रेदमुपदिशन्ति बुद्धिमन्तः- रोगमेकैकमेवम्प्रकोपणमेवंयोनिमेवमुत्थानमेवमात्मानमेवमधिष्ठानमेवंवेदनमेव संस्थानमेवंशब्दस्पर्शरूपरसगन्धमेवमुपद्रवमेवंवृद्धिस्थानक्षयसमन्वितमेवमुदर्क मेवन्नामानमेवंयोगं विद्यात्; तस्मिन्निर्यं प्रतीकारार्था प्रवृत्तिरथवा निवृत्तिरित्युपदेशाज्ज्ञायते।।६।।
Learned physicians described the following features) of each and every disease:
Prakopana – Provoking factors, viz, dry food intake etc.
Yoni – Source of Doshas involved
Utthana – Mode of manifestation.
Atma – nature and seriousness of disease
Adhishtana – site of disease manifestation
Vedana – Pain
Samsthana – Symptoms
Association with specific touch, colours, tastes and smell
Complications
Association with symptoms of aggravations, maintenance and abatement
Prognosis
Names
Concomitants and
Prescriptions and prohibitions in the treatment, e.g. prescription of fasting and use of digestive drugs, and prohibition of day sleep and bath in fever.
One can understand the above mentioned characteristic features of diseases from authorities' testimony. [6]

Factors examined by Pratyaksha :
प्रत्यक्षतस्तु खलु रोगतत्त्वं बुभुत्सुः सर्वैरिन्द्रियैः सर्वानिन्द्रियार्थानातुरशरीरगतान् परीक्षेत, अन्यत्र रसज्ञानात्; तद्यथा- अन्त्रकूजनं, सन्धिस्फुटनमङ्गुलीपर्वणां च, स्वरविशेषांश्च, ये चान्येऽपि केचिच्छरीरोपगताः शब्दाः स्युस्ताञ्छ्रोत्रेण परीक्षेत; वर्णसंस्थानप्रमाणच्छायाः,

शरीरप्रकृतिविकारौ, चक्षुर्वैषयिकाणि यानि चान्यान्यनुक्तानि तानि चक्षुषा परीक्षेत; रसं तु खल्वातुरशरीरगतमिन्द्रियवैषयिकमप्यनुमानादवगच्छेत्, न ह्यस्य प्रत्यक्षेण ग्रहणमुपपद्यते, तस्मादातुरपरिप्रश्नेनैवातुरमुखरसं विद्यात्, यूकापसर्पणेन त्वस्य शरीरवैरस्यं, मक्षिकोपसर्पणेन शरीरमाधुर्यं, लोहितपित्तसन्देहे तु किं धारिलोहितं लोहितपित्तं वेति श्वकाकभक्षणाद्धारिलोहितमभक्षणाल्लोहितपित्तमित्यनुमातव्यम्, एवमन्यानप्यातुरशरीरगतान् रसाननुमिमीत; गन्धांस्तु खलु सर्वशरीरगतानातुरस्य प्रकृतिवैकारिकान् घ्राणेन परीक्षेत; स्पर्शं च पाणिना प्रकृतिविकृतियुक्तम्|
इति प्रत्यक्षतोऽनुमानादुपदेशतश्च परीक्षणमुक्तम्||७||

Factors to be examined by Pratyaksha – direct observation:
The doctor should examine the patient with all his senses organs except tongue.

The following is examined by auscultation / ears :
antrakujana – Gurgling sound in the intestine
sandhisphutanama – Cracking sound in the joints including those in the fingers
Voice of the patient and
Such other sounds in the body of the patient like the sounds of coughing and hiccup.

Factors examined by eyes – ChakshuIndriya:
The following is examined visually:-
Colour, shape, measurement and complexion
Natural and unnatural states of the body and
Others which can be examined visually like signs of the diseases and luster.

Examination of taste :
Tastes of the various factors in the body of the patient are however ascertained by Anumana and not by direct observation (Pratyaksha). Therefore, the taste in the mouth of the patient is ascertained by interrogation. Impairment of the taste of the body is inferred when lice etc., go away from the body.

Use of animals to examine body fluids:
Sweet taste of the body can be inferred when flies are attracted towards the body. In the case of bleeding from the body, if there is a doubt about the nature of the blood, it is resolved by giving the blood to dogs and crows to eat. Intake of the blood by these animals indicates that patient's blood is vitiated by Pitta Dosha (Raktapitta)

Patient examination by smell and touch:
Normal and abnormal smell of the entire body of the patient is examined by nose. Similarly, the normal and abnormal touch of the patient is examined by hand. Thus, the examination of a patient by direct observation, inference and Aptopadesh is described. [7]

Factors observed by Anumana:
इमे तु खल्वन्येऽप्येवमेव भूयोऽनुमानजेया भवन्ति भावाः|
तद्यथा- अग्निं जरणशक्त्या परीक्षेत, बलं व्यायामशक्त्या, श्रोत्रादीनि शब्दाद्यर्थग्रहणेन, मनोऽर्थव्यभिचरणेन, विज्ञानं व्यवसायेन, रजःसङ्गेन, मोहमविज्ञानेन, क्रोधमभिद्रोहेण, शोकं दैन्येन, हर्षमामोदेन, प्रीतिं तोषेण, भयं विषादेन, धैर्यमविषादेन, वीर्यमुत्थानेन, अवस्थानमविभ्रमेण, श्रद्धामभिप्रायेण, मेधां ग्रहणेन, सञ्ज्ञां नामग्रहणेन, स्मृतिं स्मरणेन, ह्रियमपत्रपणेन, शीलमनुशीलनेन, द्वेषं प्रतिषेधेन, उपधिमनुबन्धेन, धृतिमलौल्येन, वश्यतां विधेयतया, वयोभक्तिसात्म्यव्याधिसमुत्थानानि कालदेशोपशयवेदनाविशेषेण, गूढलिङ्गं व्याधिमुपशयानुपशयाभ्यां, दोषप्रमाणविशेषमपचारविशेषेण, आयुषः क्षयमरिष्टैः, उपस्थितश्रेयस्त्वं कल्याणाभिनिवेशेन, अमलं सत्त्वमविकारेण, ग्रहणास्तु मृदुदारुणत्वं स्वप्नदर्शनमभिप्रायं दिवष्टेष्टसुखदुःखानि चातुरपरिप्रश्नेनैव विद्यादिति||८||

Factors to be observed by Inference – Anumana:

The following among others are the factors to be observed by inference:

Agni (digestive fire) from the power of digestion

Strength from the capacity for exercise

Condition of the senses, viz. auditory facility faculty etc. from their capacity to perceive the respective objects, viz sound etc.

The mind perceptions are observed by its activities,

Knowledge of a thing from proper reaction to it,

Rajoguna from attachment to woman etc;

Moha (unconsciousness) from lack of understanding

Anger from the revengeful intentions

Grief from the sorrow feelings

Joy from happiness, viz, indulgence in dancing, singing, playing musical instruments and remaining in a festive mood.

Priti (Pleasure) form satisfaction which is reflected by happiness of face, eyes etc.

Fear from apprehension

Dhairyamavidena – Courage from strength of mind even in dangerous situations.

Energy from his initiative in difficult situations

stability of the mind from the avoidance of any mistake

desire from request

intelligence from the power of comprehension of scriptures etc

Recognition from the recollection of the name

Memory from the recollection of the name

Modesty from bashfulness

Liking from habitual intake of things

Dislike from disinclination

Upadhimanubandhena – Deception from subsequent manifestations

Courage from firmness

Obedience from compliance with orders

Age, liking, homologation (Satmya) and cause of the disease from the stage of the life, habit, conduction and characteristic features of pain respectively.

Age of the patient can be determined by the stage of his life.

Desha is determined by habits

Disease curability is guessed by symptoms

The curability of disease is inferred by hidden symptoms.

Quantity of Dosha vitiation is inferred by amount of apathya – unsuitable diet and lifestyle

Arishtalakshanas give a hint toward life expectancy

Promotion of Sattvika qualities of the mind from the absence of its impairments, viz, attachment, envy etc

Softness or chronic symptoms of Grahani, dreams, desires for food etc., likes and dislikes, happiness and unhappiness etc, are known by Prashna – interrogating the patient. [8]

भवन्ति चात्र-

आप्ततश्चोपदेशेन प्रत्यक्षकरणेन च|

अनुमानेन च व्याधीन् सम्यग्विद्यादिवचक्षणः||९||

सर्वथा सर्वमालोच्य यथासम्भवमर्थवित्|

अथाध्यवस्येतत्त्वे च कार्ये च तदनन्तरम्||१०||

कार्यतत्त्वविशेषज्ञः प्रतिपत्तौ न मुह्यति|

अमूढः फलमाप्नोति यदमोहनिमित्तजम्||११||

ज्ञानबुद्धिप्रदीपेन यो नाविशति तत्त्ववित्|

आतुरस्यान्तरात्मानं न स रोगांश्चिकित्सति||१२||

Thus, it is said: – The wise should properly understand a disease by the Aptopadesh, Pratyaksha and Anumana – inference.

As far as possible all factors are discussed in their entirety. After examining the disease by Aptopadesha etc., the physician should obtain knowledge regarding the nature of disease and the therapies required thereafter.

One who is well versed in the specific nature of disease and therapies, therefore, seldom fails to act properly. It is only he who acts properly reaps the results of proper action (success).

When a physician who even if well versed in the knowledge of the disease and its treatment does not try to enter into the heart of the patient by virtue of the light of his knowledge, he will not be able to treat the diseases. [9-12]

तत्र श्लोकौ-
सर्वरोगविशेषाणां त्रिविधं ज्ञानसङ्ग्रहम्|
यथा चोपदिशन्त्याप्ताः प्रत्यक्षं गृह्यते यथा||१३||
ये यथा चानुमानेन ज्ञेयास्तांश्चाप्युदारधीः|
भावांस्त्रिरोगविज्ञाने विमाने मुनिरुक्तवान्||१४||

To sum up: -
The methods for the determination of disease, factors to be understood by the instruction of Aptas (sages), by Pratyaksha and Anumana are explained in detail in this chapter. [13-14]

इत्यग्निवेशकृते तन्त्रे चरकप्रतिसंस्कृते विमानस्थाने त्रिविधरोगविशेषविज्ञानीयं विमानं नाम चतुर्थोऽध्याय: |४|
Thus ends the 4th chapter Trividha Roga Vishesha Vijnaniya of Vimana Section of Agnivesha's work as redacted by Charaka. [4]

13

Vimanasthana Chapter 5 Srotasam Vimanam

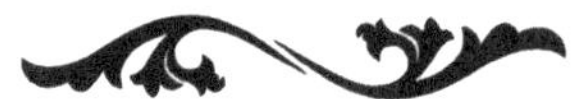

अथातः स्रोतसां विमानं व्याख्यास्यामः||१|| इति ह स्माह भगवानात्रेयः||२||

The 5th chapter of CharakaSamhitha Vimana Sthana is Srotasam Vimana or Sroto Vimana. It explains in detail about different body channels of the body, called Srotas.

We shall now explore the chapter on "Srotasam Vimana Adhyaya." Thus said Lord Atreya [1-2]

यावन्तः पुरुषे मूर्तिमन्तो भावविशेषास्तावन्त एवास्मिन् स्रोतसां प्रकारविशेषाः|

सर्वे हि भावा पुरुषे नान्तरेण स्रोतांस्यभिनिर्वर्तन्ते, क्षयं वाऽप्यभिगच्छन्ति|

स्रोतांसि खलु परिणाममापद्यमानानां धातूनामभिवाहीनि भवन्त्ययनार्थेन||३||

Srotas, varieties :

Srotas: Channels of circulation and their varieties:

The specific varieties of channels of circulation in the human body are the same in number as the organs. All the organs in the body have their own channels. The flow of all mobile things between these structures happens through Srotas – channels. The Kshaya or depletion or disease of organs is reflected in srotas as well. The channels of circulation carry the Dhatus (tissue elements or their constituents) undergoing transformation to their destination. [3]

Srotas and Purusha :

अपि चैके स्रोतसामेव समुदयं पुरुषमिच्छन्ति, सर्वगतत्वात् सर्वसरत्वाच्च दोषप्रकोपणप्रशमनानाम्|

न त्वेतदेवं, यस्य हि स्रोतांसि, यच्च वहन्ति, यच्चावहन्ति, यत्र चावस्थितानि, सर्वं तदन्येतेभ्यः||४||

अतिबहुत्वात् खलु केचिदपरिसङ्ख्येयान्याचक्षते स्रोतांसि, परिसङ्ख्येयानि पुनरन्ये||५||

Another view:

How Srotas is different from Purusha?

Because srotas is present all over the body, because all the movements inside the body happen in Srotas only, and because increase or decrease of Dosha happen in Srotas only, some authors say that Srotas itself is the whole body – Purusha. But it is not true.

The elements which compose them, the elements they carry, the elements to which they provide nourishment and their abodes (muscles etc) they are different from these channels. Some scholars hold them to be innumerable. [4-5]

Sites of organs and signs of vitiation of various channels of circulation:

तेषां तु खलु स्रोतसां यथास्थूलं कतिचित्प्रकारान्मूलतश्च प्रकोपविज्ञानतश्चानुव्याख्यास्यामः; ये भविष्यन्त्यलमनुक्तार्थज्ञानाय ज्ञानवतां,

विज्ञानाय चाज्ञानवताम्||६||

तद्यथा- प्राणोदकान्नरसरुधिरमांसमेदोस्थिमज्जशुक्रमूत्रपुरीषस्वेदवहानीति; वातपित्तश्लेष्मणां पुनः सर्वशरीरचराणां सर्वाणि स्रोतांस्ययनभूतानि, तद्वदतीन्द्रियाणां पुनः सत्त्वादीनां केवलं चेतनावच्छरीरमयनभूतमधिष्ठानभूतं च|

तदेतत् स्रोतसां प्रकृतिभूतत्वान्न विकारैरुपसृज्यते शरीरम्||७||

Important varieties of channels of circulation:

Of all these Srotas, important ones will be described here with reference to their controlling organs, symptoms manifested by their controlling organs and the symptoms manifested by their vitiation. This description will be sufficient for an ignorant man to understand the characteristic features of these channels, while for a wise man this description will provide enough material to understand the characteristic features of other channels which are not described here.

These channels are those carrying:

Prana (Vital breath)

Udaka (water)

Anna (food)

Rasa (Plasma, nutrition)

Rudhira (blood specifically the haemoglobin fraction of it)

Mamsa (muscle tissue)

Medas (fat or adipose tissue)

Asthi (bone or osseous tissue)

Majja (marrow)

Shukra (semen specifically the sperm)

Mutra (urine)

Purisha (faeces) and

Sveda (sweat)

Vata, Pitta and Kapha move in all the srotas of the body. Therefore, all srotas are pathways for circulation of doshas. Similarly for factors which are beyond sensory perception (trans- sensory) like mind etc the entire body (channels located in the entire body) are the pathways. When these srotas are healthy the body will not be afflicted from any diseases. [6]

PranavahaSrotas vitiation features :

तत्र प्राणवहानां स्रोतसां हृदयं मूलं महास्रोतश्च, प्रदुष्टानां तु खल्वेषामिदं विशेषविज्ञानं भवति; तद्यथा- अतिसृष्टमतिबद्धं कुपितमल्पाल्पमभीक्ष्णं वा सशब्दशूलमुच्छ्वसन्तं दृष्ट्वा प्राणवहान्यस्य स्रोतांसि प्रदुष्टानीति विद्यात्|

उदकवहानां स्रोतसां तालुमूलं क्लोम च, प्रदुष्टानां तु खल्वेषामिदं विशेषविज्ञानं भवति; तद्यथा- जिह्वातालुओष्ठकण्ठक्लोमशोषं पिपासां चातिप्रवृद्धां दृष्ट्वोदकवहान्यस्य स्रोतांसि प्रदुष्टानीति विद्यात्|

अन्नवहानां स्रोतसामामाशयो मूलं वामं च पार्श्व, प्रदुष्टानां तु खल्वेषामिदं विशेषविज्ञानं भवति; तद्यथा- अनन्नाभिलषणमरोचकविपाकौ छर्दि च दृष्ट्वाऽन्नवहान्यस्य स्रोतांसि प्रदुष्टानीति विद्यात्|

रसवहानां स्रोतसां हृदयं मूलं दश च धमन्यः|

शोणितवहानां स्रोतसां यकृन्मूलं प्लीहा च|

मांसवहानां च स्रोतसां स्नायुमूलं त्वक् च|

मेदोवहानां स्रोतसां वृक्कौ मूलं वपावहनं च|

अस्थिवहानां स्रोतसां मेदो मूलं जघनं च|

मज्जवहानां स्रोतसामस्थीनि मूलं सन्धयश्च|

शुक्रवहानां स्रोतसां वृषणौ मूलं शेफश्च|

प्रदुष्टानां तु खल्वेषां रसादिवहस्रोतसां विज्ञानान्युक्तानि विविधाशितपीतीये; यान्येव हि धातूनां प्रदोषविज्ञानानि तान्येव यथास्वं प्रदुष्टानां धातुस्रोतसाम्|

मूत्रवहानां स्रोतसां बस्तिर्मूलं वङ्क्षणौ च, प्रदुष्टानां तु खल्वेषामिदं विशेषविज्ञानं भवति; तद्यथा- अतिसृष्टमतिबद्धं प्रकुपितमल्पाल्पमभीक्ष्णं वा बहलं सशूलं मूत्रयन्तं दृष्ट्वा मूत्रवहान्यस्य स्रोतांसि प्रदुष्टानीति विद्यात्।

पुरीषवहानां स्रोतसां पक्वाशयो मूलं स्थूलगुदं च, प्रदुष्टानां तु खल्वेषामिदं विशेषविज्ञानं भवति; तद्यथा- कृच्छ्रेणाल्पाल्पं सशब्दशूलमतिद्रवमतिग्रथितमतिबहु चोपविशन्तं दृष्ट्वा पुरीषवहान्यस्य स्रोतांसि प्रदुष्टानीति विद्यात्।

स्वेदवहानां स्रोतसां मेदो मूलं लोमकूपाश्च, प्रदुष्टानां तु खल्वेषामिदं विशेषविज्ञानं भवति; तद्यथा- अस्वेदनमतिस्वेदनं पारुष्यमतिश्लक्ष्णतामङ्गस्य परिदाहं लोमहर्षं च दृष्ट्वा स्वेदवहान्यस्य स्रोतांसि प्रदुष्टानीति विद्यात्॥८॥

PranavahaSrotas – vital energy channels:

Root (sites of origin) are Heart and the Mahasrotas (alimentary tract). It carries Prana – vital energy.

The characteristic features of the vitiation of Pranavaha channel are

Atisrushtashwasa – too long breaths

Atibaddhashwasa – too restricted breathing

Kupita – aggravated breathing

AlpaAlpa – shallow or

Abhikshna – frequent breaths

Sashabda, Sashula are associated with sound and pain.

UdakavahaSrotas: channels of watery elements:

Talu (palate) and Kloma (pancreas) are the sites of origin / controlling organs of UdakavahaSrotas. Vitiation of these channels lead to

Jihva, Talu, Osha, Kanta, KlomaShosha – dryness of tongue, palate, lips, throat and Kloma and Pipasa – excessive thirst.

Annavahasrotas – channels that carry food elements:

Sites of origin: Amashaya – Stomach and Vamaparshva (left side) are the sites of origin of the channels carrying food and its products.

Vitiation characteristic features:

Anannaabhilasha – disinterest in food,

Arochaka – anorexia,

Vipaka – impaired digestion

Chardi – vomiting.

DhatuvahaSrotas:- carrying tissue elements:

Site of origin of RasavahaSrotas is Hrudaya (heart) and Dasha Dhamani (10 big arteries)

Raktavahasrotas moola – Yakrut – Liver and Pleeha – spleen

Mamsavahasrotas (muscle tissue) – Snayu – Ligaments and Twak – skin

Medovahasrotas Moola – (fat or adipose tissue) – Vrukka – Kidneys and Vapavahana – omentum

AsthivahaSrotomoola – (bone)- Meda (fat/Adipose tissue), Jaghana – buttock

Majjavahasrotomoola – (marrow) Asthi – bones and Sandhayaha – joints

Shukravahasrotomoola – (semen specially the sperms) – Vrushana – Testicles and Shepha – pudendum

Vitiations of Dhatuvaha srotas are already described in Charaka sutrasthana 28th chapter 9-19. Symptoms manifested by the vitiation of these Dhatus and their specific channels are the same.

MutravahaSrotas: Urinary system:

Moola – root of origin – Basti (bladder) and vankshanas (kidneys).

MutravahaSrotoDushtiLakshana:

The characteristic manifestations of the vitiation of these channels are
Atisrushta mutra – voiding of too much of urine
Vibaddha mutra – the complete suppression of urine,
impairment of the composition of urine and occasionally or frequently passing of thick urine Sashoola – urination associated with pain.

Purishavaha Srotas:
Pureeshavaha srotomoola :
Pakvashaya – pakvashaya (large intestine) and the sthulaguda (rectum)
Purisavahasroto dustilakshana:
The characteristic manifestations of their vitiation are the
Kruchrena – difficulty in passing stools
Alpalpla – low quantity of stools
Sashabda – noisy evacuation
Sashoola – painful evacuation
Atidrava – diarrhoea, liquid stools
Atigrathiata – granular
voiding of small quantity of feces with difficulty, voiding of large quantity of very watery and very scybalous stool associated with sound and pain.

Svedahavaha srotas:
Swedavahasrotomoola :
The site of origin of the channels carrying sweat are -
Meda – adipose tissue and
Lomakoopa – hair follicles.
The characteristic manifestations of their vitiation are absence of perspiration, excessive perspiration, roughness and excessive smoothness of the body, general burning sensation and horrification. [7-8]

Effect of vitiation of different srotas:
Srotas (channels), Sira (Vein), Dhamani (artery), Rasayani (Lymphatic channel), Rasavahini (capillary), Nadi (duct), Pantha (passage), Marga (track), Shariracchidra (spaces inside the body), Samvrtasamrta (duct closed at one end and open at the other), Sthana (residence), Ashaya (container) and Niketa (Abode)- these are the names attributed to various visible and invisible spaces inside the tissue elements of the body.

Affliction of these channels leads to the vitiation of the tissue elements residing there or passing through them- vitiation of one lead to the vitiation of the other. They vitiate channels and Dhatus respectively. Because of their vitiating nature, Doshas, viz, Vata, and Kapha are responsible for the vitiation of all them (channels and tissue elements). [9]

Causes of vitiations of different channels of circulation:
भवन्ति चात्र-
क्षयात् सन्धारणाद्रौक्ष्याद्व्यायामात् क्षुधितस्य च।
प्राणवाहीनि दुष्यन्ति स्रोतांस्यन्यैश्च दारुणैः॥१०॥
औष्ण्यादामादभयात् पानादतिशुष्कान्नसेवनात्।
अम्बुवाहीनि दुष्यन्ति तृष्णायाश्चातिपीडनात्॥११॥
अतिमात्रस्य चाकाले चाहितस्य च भोजनात्।
अन्नवाहीनि दुष्यन्ति वैगुण्यात् पावकस्य च॥१२॥

गुरुशीतमतिस्निग्धमतिमात्रं समश्नताम्‌|
रसवाहीनि दुष्यन्ति चिन्त्यानां चातिचिन्तनात्‌||१३||
विदाहीन्यन्नपानानि स्निग्धोष्णानि द्रवाणि च|
रक्तवाहीनि दुष्यन्ति भजतां चातपानलौ||१४||
अभिष्यन्दीनि भोज्यानि स्थूलानि च गुरूणि च|
मांसवाहीनि दुष्यन्ति भुक्त्वा च स्वपतां दिवा||१५||
अव्यायामादिदवास्वप्नान्मेद्यानां चातिभक्षणात्‌|
मेदोवाहीनि दुष्यन्ति वारुण्याश्चातिसेवनात्‌||१६||
व्यायामादतिसङ्क्षोभादस्थ्नामतिविघट्टनात्‌|
अस्थिवाहीनि दुष्यन्ति वातलानां च सेवनात्‌||१७||
उत्पेषादत्यभिष्यन्दादभिघातात् प्रपीडनात्‌|
मज्जवाहीनि दुष्यन्ति विरुद्धानां च सेवनात्‌||१८||
अकालयोनिगमनान्निग्रहादतिमैथुनात्‌|
शुक्रवाहीनि दुष्यन्ति शस्त्रक्षाराग्निभिस्तथा||१९||
मूत्रितोदकभक्ष्यस्त्रीसेवनान्मूत्रनिग्रहात्‌|
मूत्रवाहीनि दुष्यन्ति क्षीणस्याभिक्षतस्य च||२०||
सन्धारणादत्यशनादजीर्णाध्यशनात्तथा|
वर्चोवाहीनि दुष्यन्ति दुर्बलाग्नेः कृशस्य च||२१||
व्यायामादतिसन्तापाच्छीतोष्णाक्रमसेवनात् |
स्वेदवाहीनि दुष्यन्ति क्रोधशोकभयैस्तथा||२२||

Pranavahasrotodusti – vitiation occurs due to
Kshaya – depletion of body tissues, tuberculosis
Sandharana – suppressing natural urges
Raukshyat – excessive dryness
VyayamaKshudhita – excessive exercise by a hungry person.

Ambuvaha Srotodushti Karana :
Ambuvahasrotas (channels carrying water) get vitiated,
Aushnyat – by exposure to heat, indigestion, alcoholic drinks, intake of excessively dry food and excessive thirst.

Annavaha srotodushti karana :
Annavahasrotamsi (channels carrying Rasa or Plasma) get vitiated due to the excessive intake of heavy, cold and excessively unctuous food, and over worry.

Rasavaha srotodushti Karana :
Excessive intake of heavy, cold, excess unctuous foods, excess quantity of food, tension, stress and worries.

Raktavaha srotodushtikarana:
Channels carrying blood get vitiated due to the intake of food and drinks which are irritant, unctuous, hot and liquid, and exposure to sun and fire.

Mamsavahasrotodushti Karana :
Mamsavahasrotamsi (channels carrying muscle tissue) get vitiated by intake of
Abhishyandhibhojana – semisold, semi-cooked foods
food with bulkiness and heavy qualities and sleeping soon after taking food.

Medovaha srotodushti Karana:
Fat channels are vitiated due to lack of exercise, sleeping during day time, excess consumption of Varuni (fermented drink prepared by palm dates and date fruits).

Asthivaha srotodushti Karana:
Bone tissue channels get vitiated by excessive exercise, not consuming food, excessive friction and intake of Vata increasing food and drinks.

Majjavaha srotodushti Karana:
Crushing of bones (due to accident, fall etc), intake of abhishyandi food, injury, and intake of bad food combinations (ViruddhaAhara).

Shukravaha srotodushtikarana:
Causes for vitiation of reproductive channels – untimely sexual intercourse, withholding ejaculation during orgasm, excess use of kshara, surgical procedure and agnikarma.

Mutravaha srotodushtikarana:
Causes for vitiation of urinary system are :
consuming liquids during an urge to urinate,
excess sexual intercourse,
suppressing urge to urinate,
Kshaya – depletion of body tissues and due to external injury to it.

Varchovaha srotodushtikarana:
Channels carrying faeces get vitiated by the suppression of the urge for defecation, intake of food in large quantities, intake of food before the digestion of the previous meal especially in those who are emaciated and having weak power of digestion.

Svedovaha srotodushtikarana:
Channels carrying sweat get vitiated due to excess exercise, exposure to excess of heat, indulgence, in cold and hot things without following the prescribed order, anger, grief and fear. [10-22]

Causative factors for vitiation of channels of circulation:
आहारश्च विहारश्च यः स्याद्दोषगुणैः समः|
धातुभिर्विगुणश्चापि स्रोतसां स प्रदूषकः||२३||
Food and regimens that promote the morbidity of (aggravate) Doshas and go contrary to the well- being of Dhatus (tissue elements) vitiate the channels. [23]

Signs of the vitiation of channels of circulation:
अतिप्रवृत्तिः सङ्गो वा सिराणां ग्रन्थयोऽपि वा|
विमार्गगमनं चापि स्रोतसां दुष्टिलक्षणम्||२४||
Increase or obstruction of the flow of the contents of the channels, appearance of nodules in the channels and diversion of the flow of the contents to improper channels- these are, in general, the signs (results) of the vitiation of the channels [24]

Characteristic features of channels of circulation:

स्वधातुसमवर्णानि वृत्तस्थूलान्यणूनि च|
स्रोतांसि दीर्घाण्याकृत्या प्रतानसदृशानि च||२५||

These channels have the colour like that of the Dhatu they carry; they are tubular, either large or small in size and either straight or reticulated in shape. [25]

Line of treatment :

प्राणोदकान्नवाहानां दुष्टानां श्वासिकी क्रिया|
कार्या तृष्णोपशमनी तथैवामप्रदोषिकी||२६||
विविधाशितपीतीये रसादीनां यदौषधम्|
रसादिस्रोतसां कुर्यात्तद्यथास्वमुपक्रमम्||२७||
मूत्रविट्स्वेदवाहानां चिकित्सा मौत्रकृच्छ्रिकी|
तथाऽतिसारिकी कार्या तथा ज्वरचिकित्सिकी||२८||

Therapies for the treatment of the vitiation of Prana, Udaka and Annavaha Srotamsi (channels carrying vital breath, water and food) are the same as those described for the treatment of respiratory disorders (viz, bronchial asthma), morbid thirst and Amasosha (vitiation of the undigested food product) respectively.

Therapies prescribed in **CharakaSutrasthana 28/25- 30**for the treatment of condition caused by the vitiation of tissue elements viz, Rasa etc. is adopted here for the treatment of the condition caused by vitiation of the respective channels. Therapies prescribed for difficulty in passing urine, diarrhoea and fever are adopted for the treatment of the diseases caused by the vitiation of Mutra, Purisha and SvedaVahasrotamsi (channels carrying urine, feces and sweet) respectively. [26-28]

Summary:
तत्र श्लोकाः-
त्रयोदशानां मूलानि स्रोतसां दुष्टिलक्षणम्|
सामान्यं नामपर्यायाः कोपनानि परस्परम्||२९||
दोषहेतुः पृथक्त्वेन भेषजोद्देश एव च|
स्रोतोविमाने निर्दिष्टस्तथा चादौ विनिश्चयः||३०||
केवलं विदितं यस्य शरीरं सर्वभावतः|
शारीराः सर्वरोगाश्च स कर्मसु न मुह्यति||३१||

Determination of the characteristic features of channels, sites of origin and the general symptoms manifested by the vitiation of the 13 channels of circulation in the body, names and symptoms of these channels, vitiation of one by the other, causes of vitiation of each channel separately and the treatment in brief all these topics are described in this chapter of Srotovimanaadhyaya".

A physician who is well acquainted with all aspects of the entire body and all the diseases manifested there seldom commits mistakes in treatment. [29-31]

इत्यग्निवेशकृते तन्त्रे चरकप्रतिसंस्कृते विमानस्थाने स्रोतोविमानं नाम पञ्चमोऽध्यायः |5|
Thus ends the 5th chapter on "Srotovimana", of Vimana section of Agnivesha's work as redacted by Charaka. [5]

14

Vimanasthana Chapter 6
Roganikam Vimanam

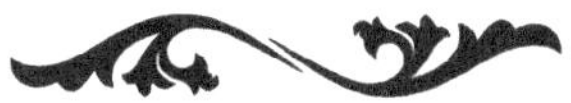

The 6th chapter of Charaka Samhitha Vimana Sthana is RoganikamVimanam. It deals with management of diseases affecting persons with different body types and determination of the specific characteristics of diseases, etc.

अथातो रोगानीकं विमानं व्याख्यास्यामः||१||

इति ह स्माह भगवानात्रेयः||२||

"Let us explore Roganika Vimana Adhyaya – the chapter on the determination of the specific characteristics of diseases" thus said Lord Atreya [1-2]

Disease Classification :

द्वे रोगानीके भवतः प्रभावभेदेन- साध्यम्, असाध्यं च; द्वे रोगानीके बलभेदेन- मृदु, दारुणं च; द्वे रोगानीके अधिष्ठानभेदेन- मनोऽधिष्ठानं, शरीराधिष्ठानं च; द्वे रोगानीके निमित्तभेदेन- स्वधातुवैषम्यनिमित्तम्, आगन्तुनिमित्तं च; द्वे रोगानीके आशयभेदेन- आमाशयसमुत्थं, पक्वाशयसमुत्थं चेति|

एवमेतत् प्रभावबलाधिष्ठाननिमित्ताशयभेदाद्द्वैधं सद्भेदप्रकृत्यन्तरेण भिद्यमानमथवाऽपि सन्धीयमानं स्यादेकत्वं बहुत्वं वा|

एकत्वं तावदेकमेव रोगानीकं, दुःखसामान्यात्; बहुत्वं तु दश रोगानीकानि प्रभावभेदादिना भवन्ति; बहुत्वमपि सङ्ख्येयं स्यादसङ्ख्येयं वा|

तत्र सङ्ख्येयं तावद्यथोक्तमष्टोदरीये, अपरिसङ्ख्येयं पुनर्यथा- महारोगाध्याये रुग्वर्णसमुत्थानादीनामसङ्ख्येयत्वात्||३||

Various types of classification of diseases:
Diseases are classified into two groups on the basis of the five different criteria, as follows:
Types of diseases as per Ayurveda:
PrabhavaBheda – Based on Prognosis – Curable, Incurable (Sadhya, Asadhya)
BalaBheda – Based on intensity – mild, severe (Mrudu, Daruna)
AdhishtanaBheda – based on location – Mental, Physical (Mano Adhishtana, ShariraAdhishtana)
NimittaBheda – based on nature of the causative factors – Endogenous, Exogenous (sva dhatu vaishamyanimitta, agantunimitta)
Ashayabheda – based on site of origin – Having origin from Amashaya (stomach), Having origin from Pakvashaya (colon) (Amashayasamutta, Pakvasaysamuttha)
Even though diseases are of two groups based on prognosis, intensity, location, nature of the causative factors and site of origin, still by different permutations and combinations they can be classified as one or in many ways.

Diseases as single classification:
All diseases may be of one group because manifestation of pain is common for all- Dukha Samanyaat. They may be of many groups on the basis of their tenfold classification according to prognosis etc., described above.

Multiplicity of the classification of diseases :

Diseases can be numerable or innumerable. Their innumerability has been described in the 19th chapter of Sutra sthana – MaharogaAdhyaya and their innumerability on the basis variations in pain, colour. [3]

न च सङ्ख्येयाग्रेषु भेदप्रकृत्यन्तरीयेषु विगीतिरित्यतो दोषवती स्यादत्र काचित् प्रतिज्ञा, न चाविगीतिरित्यतः स्याददोषवती|

भेत्ता हि भेद्यमन्यथाभिनत्ति, अन्यथा पुरस्ताद्भिन्नं भेदप्रकृत्यन्तरेण भिन्दन् भेदसङ्ख्याविशेषमापादयत्यनेकधा, न च पूर्वं भेदाग्रमुपहन्ति|

समानायामपि खलु भेदप्रकृतौ प्रकृतानुप्रयोगान्तरमपेक्ष्यम्|

सन्ति ह्यर्थान्तराणि समानशब्दाभिहितानि, सन्ति चानर्थान्तराणि पर्यायशब्दाभिहितानि|

समानो हि रोगशब्दो दोषेषु च व्याधिषु च; दोषा ह्यपि रोगशब्दमातङ्कशब्दं यक्ष्मशब्दं दोषप्रकृतिशब्दं विकारशब्दं च लभन्ते, व्याधयश्च रोगशब्दमातङ्कशब्दं यक्ष्मशब्दं दोषप्रकृतिशब्दं विकारशब्दं च लभन्ते|

तत्र दोषेषु चैव व्याधिषु च रोगशब्दः समानः, शेषेषु तु विशेषवान्||४||

Justification for different types of classification:

If the diseases are classified in different bases does not take away the validity of those classifications.

An individual has the liberty to classify things as he likes. If something is already classified into some groups in a particular manner, he may reclassify it on the basis of different criterion which may result in changes in the number of groups in different ways.

This does not invalidate the number of groups according to some other mode of classification. In some cases, the criterion of classification may appear to be the same as the previous one but the specific features of each of these criterions is observed based on the validity of this classification.

The same term may carry different meanings; e.g., the word "Roga" denotes both the Doshas as well as diseases. similarly various terms which are synonymous may denote only one thing, e.g., Roga, Atanka, Yakshman, Doshaprakrti (having polluting nature) and Vikara (morbidity)- these terms carry the meaning of or are synonymous with both Dosha and Vyadhi (diseases). For the rest like Hetu (aetiology) etc., this term, viz Roga carries a different meaning. [4]

Doshas and vitiation :

तत्र व्याधयोऽपरिसङ्ख्येया भवन्ति, अतिबहुत्वात्|

दोषास्तु खलु परिसङ्ख्येया भवन्ति, अनतिबहुत्वात्|

तस्माद्यथाचित्रं विकारानुदाहरणार्थम्, अनवशेषेण च दोषान् व्याख्यास्यामः|

रजस्तमश्च मानसौ दोषौ|

तयोर्विकाराः कामक्रोधलोभमोहेर्ष्यामानमदशोकचितो(न्तो)द्वेगभयहर्षादयः|

वातपित्तश्लेष्माणस्तु खलु शारीरा दोषाः|

तेषामपि च विकारा ज्वरातीसारशोफशोषश्वासमेहकुष्ठादयः|

इति दोषाः केवला व्याख्याता विकारैकदेशश्च||५||

तत्र खल्वेषां द्वयानामपि दोषाणां त्रिविधं प्रकोपणं; तद्यथा- असात्म्येन्द्रियार्थसंयोगः, प्रज्ञापराधः, परिणामश्चेति||६||

Physical and mental Doshas and their vitiations:

Because of their highly multitudinous nature, diseases are innumerable. On the other hand, Doshas are numerable because of their limitation in number. So only some of the diseases will be explained by way of illustrations whereas Doshas will be explained in their entirety.

Mano Doshas:

Rajas and Tamas are the Doshas pertaining to the mind and the type of morbidity caused by them are Kama (lust), Krodha – anger, Lobha – greed, Moha – attachment, Irshya – envy, Mana – ego, Mada – pride, Shoka – depression, Chinta – worry, Udvega – anxiety, Bhaya – fear, Harsha – excitement etc. Vata, Pitta and Kapha- these three are the Doshas pertaining to the body.

Sharirika Dosha :

Diseases caused by them are fever, diarrhoea, oedema, emaciation, dyspnoea, Meha – diabetes, urinary tract disorders, skin diseases. Thus, Doshas and diseases are explained.

Causes for vitiation :
Causes for vitiation of mental and physical Doshas:

Both the types of Doshas have three types of etiological factors, viz .,

AsatmyaIndriyaArthaSamyoga – unwholesome contact with the object of senses,

Prajnaparadha – intellectual Blasphemy and

Parinama – seasonal changes. [5-6]

Factors responsible for manifestation of innumerable disease:

प्रकुपितास्तु खलु ते प्रकोपणविशेषाद्दूष्यविशेषाच्च

विकारविशेषानभिनिर्वर्तयन्त्यपरिसङ्ख्येयान्॥७॥

Depending upon the specific nature of the causative factors and also the specificity of the nature elements afflicted, Doshas when aggravated manifest innumerable types of diseases. [7]

Psycho-somatic disease:

ते च विकाराः परस्परमनुवर्तमानाः कदाचिदनुबध्नन्ति कामादयो ज्वरादयश्च॥८॥

When allowed to persist for long, these psychic diseases, Viz, Kama (lust) etc, and somatic diseases viz, fever etc., at times get combined with each other. [8]

Psychic Doshas- their eternal union:

नियतस्त्वनुबन्धो रजस्तमसोः परस्परं, न ह्यरजस्कं तमः प्रवर्तते ॥९॥

There is an eternal union between the two Mano Doshas – Rajas and tamas. Tamas cannot manifest its actions without Rajas. [9]

Combination of physical Doshas:

(प्रायः) शारीरदोषाणामेकाधिष्ठानीयानां सन्निपातः संसर्गो वा समानगुणत्वात्; दोषा हि दूषणैः समानाः॥१०॥

Vata, Pitta and Kapha located in the same place and having similar attributes mostly combine with one another (samsarga) or with all together (Sannipata) to form disease. Attributes of Doshas resemble those of the factors which vitiated them. [10]

Anubandhya, AnubandhaRoga:

तत्रानुबन्ध्यानुबन्धकृतो विशेषः- स्वतन्त्रो व्यक्तलिङ्गो यथोक्तसमुत्थानप्रशमो भवत्यनुबन्ध्यः, तद्विपरीतलक्षणस्त्वनुबन्धः।

अनुबन्ध्यलक्षणसमन्वितास्तत्र यदि दोषा भवन्ति तत्त्रिकं सन्निपातमाचक्षते, द्वयं वा संसर्गम्।

अनुबन्ध्यानुबन्धविशेषकृतस्तु बहुविधो दोषभेदः।

एवमेष सञ्ज्ञाप्रकृतो भिषजां दोषेषु व्याधिषु च नानाप्रकृतिविशेषव्यूहः ॥११॥

तत्रानुबन्ध्यानुबन्धकृतो विशेषः- स्वतन्त्रो व्यक्तलिङ्गो यथोक्तसमुत्थानप्रशमो भवत्यनुबन्ध्यः, तद्विपरीतलक्षणस्त्वनुबन्धः।

अनुबन्ध्यलक्षणसमन्वितास्तत्र यदि दोषा भवन्ति तत्त्रिकं सन्निपातमाचक्षते, द्वयं वा संसर्गम्।

अनुबन्ध्यानुबन्धविशेषकृतस्तु बहुविधो दोषभेदः।

एवमेष सञ्ज्ञाप्रकृतो भिषजां दोषेषु व्याधिषु च नानाप्रकृतिविशेषव्यूहः ||११||

Primary and secondary diseases: Anubandhya, AnubandhaRoga :
Characteristic features of primary and secondary (subordinate) diseases:

Anubandhya – primary disorder and

Anubandha – secondary disorder.

Anubandhya – primary disease will have its own specific characteristic features. It is caused due to specific etiological factors mentioned in textbooks. The other type of disease, without specific features or causes is called Anubandha – secondary.

Sannipata – Here, all the three Doshas are primarily vitiated at a time.

Samsarga – Here two Doshas get vitiated at a time to produce disease.

Based on permutation and combination of causative factors and symptoms, both the above two types of diseases can be classified in different ways. Considering such characteristic features, physician attribute various names (like Jvara – fever or fever) and Atisara – diarrhoea, dysentery or diarrhoea) to different conditions caused by Doshas and diseases. [11]

Four types of Agni :

अग्निषु तु शारीरेषु चतुर्विधो विशेषो बलभेदेन भवति| तद्यथा- तीक्ष्णो, मन्दः, समो, विषमश्चेति|

तत्र तीक्ष्णोऽग्निः सर्वोपचारसहः, तद्विपरीतलक्षणस्तु मन्दः, समस्तु खल्वपचारतो विकृतिमापद्यतेऽनपचारतस्तु प्रकृताववतिष्ठते, समलक्षणविपरीतलक्षणस्तु विषम इति| एते चतुर्विधा भवन्त्यग्नयश्चतुर्विधानामेव पुरुषाणाम्|

तत्र समवातपित्तश्लेष्मणां प्रकृतिस्थानां समा भवन्त्यग्नयः, वातलानां तु वाताभिभूतेऽग्न्यधिष्ठाने विषमा भवन्त्यग्नयः, पित्तलानां तु पित्ताभिभूते ह्यग्न्यधिष्ठाने तीक्ष्णा भवन्त्यग्नयः, श्लेष्मलानां तु श्लेष्माभिभूतेऽग्न्यधिष्ठाने मन्दा भवन्त्यग्नयः||१२||

Depending upon strength, Agni (factors responsible for digestion and metabolism) can be classified under four categories, viz

Teekshna – sharp, high intensity

Manda – mild, low intensity

Sama – regular, normal intensity

Vishama – irregular intensity

Teeksnagni – Capable of tolerating all types of diet irregularities

mandagni – minor food irregularity leads to diseases

Samagni – moderate food irregularity leads to disease, otherwise maintains health

Vishamagni – Sometimes it gets impaired and sometimes it does not get impaired by food irregularities (unpredictable variations).

Agni and Dosha body types :

Four types of Agni occur in 4 types of individuals.

In a person with balanced Tridoshas – Samagni.

Vata body type person will have Vishamagni

Pitta person will have Teekshnagni

Kapha person will have mandagni . [12]

Prakruti :

तत्र केचिदाहुः- न समवातपित्तश्लेष्माणो जन्तवः सन्ति, विषमाहारोपयोगित्वान्मनुष्याणां; तस्माच्च वातप्रकृतयः केचित्, केचित् पित्तप्रकृतयः, केचित् पुनः श्लेष्मप्रकृतयो भवन्तीति|

तच्चानुपपन्नं, कस्मात् कारणात्? समवातपित्तश्लेष्माणं ह्यरोगमिच्छन्ति भिषजः, यतः प्रकृतिश्चारोग्यम्, आरोग्यार्था च भेषजप्रवृत्तिः, सा चेष्टरूपा, तस्मात् सन्ति समवातपित्तश्लेष्माणः; न खलु सन्ति वातप्रकृतयः पित्तप्रकृतयः श्लेष्मप्रकृतयो वा|

तस्य तस्य किल दोषस्याधिक्यात् सा सा दोषप्रकृतिरुच्यते मनुष्याणां, न च विकृतेषु दोषेषु प्रकृतिस्थत्वमुपपद्यते, तस्मान्नैताः प्रकृतयः सन्ति; सन्ति तु खलु वातलाः पित्तलाः श्लेष्मलाश्च, अप्रकृतिस्थास्तु ते ज्ञेयाः||१३||

तत्र केचिदाहुः- न समवातपित्तश्लेष्माणो जन्तवः सन्ति, विषमाहारोपयोगित्वान्मनुष्याणां; तस्माच्च वातप्रकृतयः केचित्, केचित् पित्तप्रकृतयः, केचित् पुनः श्लेष्मप्रकृतयो भवन्तीति|

तच्चानुपपन्नं, कस्मात् कारणात्? समवातपित्तश्लेष्माणं ह्यरोगमिच्छन्ति भिषजः, यतः प्रकृतिश्चारोग्यम्, आरोग्यार्था च भेषजप्रवृत्तिः, सा चेष्टरूपा, तस्मात् सन्ति समवातपित्तश्लेष्माणः; न खलु सन्ति वातप्रकृतयः पित्तप्रकृतयः श्लेष्मप्रकृतयो वा|

तस्य तस्य किल दोषस्याधिक्यात् सा सा दोषप्रकृतिरुच्यते मनुष्याणां, न च विकृतेषु दोषेषु प्रकृतिस्थत्वमुपपद्यते, तस्मान्नैताः प्रकृतयः सन्ति; सन्ति तु खलु वातलाः पित्तलाः श्लेष्मलाश्च, अप्रकृतिस्थास्तु ते ज्ञेयाः||१३||

Prakruti – Physical constitution:

Some scholars opine that no person can have all the three doshas in equilibrium, because food always has one or the other dosha dominance in it. They only believe that there are three Prakrutis – Vata, Pitta and Kapha.

But this is not true because physicians consider an individual as healthy only when Vata, Pitta, and Kapha are in equilibrium and health represents the natural state of the body. It is with a view to maintaining good health that all types of treatments are prescribed.

Hence, there exists people with Tridosha equilibrium.

The Dosha body types are determined by aggressive, but healthily dominant Dosha in the body, not by vitiated Doshas.

The 4 types of body type (Sama, Vata, Pitta and Kapha) should follow 4 types of regimens. The person with Sama prakruti – all Doshas in equilibrium should adopt a normal and healthy diet and lifestyle. The Vata, Pitta and Kapha body type people should follow a diet and lifestyle with opposite characteristics to their Dosha.

Vata Prakruti treatment:
Treatment principles in Vata Prakriti:

The single Dosha prakruti persons are called Sadatura – they get afflicted by their respective Doshic disorders easily. In a Vata Prakruti person, Vata gets aggravated very easily with Vata vitiating causes. Here, Pitta and kapha do not vitiate easily. Vata aggravation leads to depletion of

Bala – strength

Varna – colour

Sukha – health

Ayusha – quality of life.

Such disorders are treated with

Sneha – oleation

Sweda – sweating treatment

MruduSamshodhana – mild Shodhana (elimination) therapies with medicines having

Sneha – unctuousness, hot, sweet, sour, salt properties.

Abhyanga – Massage, Upanaha – poultice, Udveshtana – bandage, Mardana – kneading, Parisheka – effusion, Avagaha- tub bath, Samvahana, (pressing and massaging by hand), Peedana – pressing, Vitrasana – terrorizing,

Vismapana – surprising and

Vismarana – re-memorizing.

Use of Sura and Asavas (fermented drinks)

usage of different fats with Deepana, Pachana, Vatahara, Virechanaeeyopaga properties, boiled hundred and thousand times and be administered in different ways viz, internal use, massage, enema with all proper rules and regulations of enema therapies etc

Pitta Prakruti treatment :

Characteristics of Pitta Parkriti and its management:

If a Pittala individual resorts to Pitta aggravating activities, he develops diseases immediately. In him, Vata and Kapha Doshas do not aggravate easily. The imbalanced Pitta afflicts the individual by the manifestation of diseases resulting in the impairment of strength, complexion, happiness and longevity.

The following therapies alleviates Pitta Dosha :

Intake of ghee

Oleation by ghee

Purgation – Virechana treatment

Use of medicines and diets having sweet, bitter and astringent tastes and cooling property

Use of scents which are mild, sweet, fragrant, cooling and cordial

Use in the chest of pearls, jewels and garlands which are kept in excessively cold water

Frequent sprinkling of cold water and cold air of Agrya Chandana (Santalum Album Linn), Priyangu (Callicarpa macrophylla), Kaliya (yellow variety of Chandana (Sandalwood – Santalum album) and Mrunala(Lotus stalk) mixed with Utpala (Nymphaea alba), Kumuda (a variety of Utpala), Sugandhikaand Padma – Lotus

Hearing of songs and music which are pleasing to ears, mild, sweet and agreeable

Hearing the information regarding prosperity

Keeping company of friends

Company of agreeable ladies wearing cooling garments and garlands

Residence in building which is cooled by the moon rays and exposed to the breezes from all sides

Residence in cold places in mountains and river banks , use of cold apparel and exposure to the cold winds of fans

Visiting beautiful gardens having pleasing, cold and the body is the most cherished one.[13]

Management of Persons having different types of physical constitution:

तेषां तु खलु चतुर्विधानां पुरुषाणां चत्वार्यनुप्रणिधानानि श्रेयस्कराणि भवन्ति|

तत्र समसर्वधातूनां सर्वाकारसमम्, अधिकदोषाणां तु त्रयाणां यथास्वं दोषाधिक्यमभिसमीक्ष्य दोषप्रतिकूलयोगीनि त्रीण्यनु(न्न)प्रणिधानानि श्रेयस्कराणि भवन्ति यावदग्नेः समीभावात्, समे तु सममेव कार्यम्; एवं चेष्टा भेषजप्रयोगाश्चापरे|

तान् विस्तरेणानुव्याख्यास्यामः||१४||

Four types of regimens are prescribed for the benefit of these four categories of individuals. For an individual having the balanced state of all Doshas, all the regimens to be adopted by balanced state of all Doshas, all the regimens to be adopted by him is of balanced type. When there is predominance of Doshas, depending upon the nature of the Doshas involved, it is useful to adopt such there regimens as would be in contradiction with these three predominating Doshas till there is normalcy of Agni. It is only after the normalcy of the Agni is attained, balanced regimens are adopted. Similarly, various therapies and other regimens are administered to these four categories of individuals. We shall now explain them in detail. [14]

त्रयस्तु पुरुषा भवन्त्यातुराः, ते त्वनातुरास्तन्त्रान्तरीयाणां भिषजाम्|

तद्यथा- वातलः, पित्तलः, श्लेष्मलश्चेति|

तेषामिदं विशेषविज्ञानं- वातलस्य वातनिमित्ताः, पित्तलस्य पित्तनिमित्ताः, श्लेष्मलस्य श्लेष्मनिमित्ता व्याधयः प्रायेण बलवन्तश्च भवन्ति||१५||

तत्र वातलस्य वातप्रकोपणान्यासेवमानस्य क्षिप्रं वातः प्रकोपमापद्यते, न तथेतरौ दोषौ; स तस्य प्रकोपमापन्नो यथोक्तैर्विकारैः शरीरमुपतपति बलवर्णसुखायुषामुपघाताय|

तस्यावजयनं- स्नेहस्वेदौ विधियुक्तौ, मृदूनि च संशोधनानि स्नेहोष्णमधुराम्ललवणयुक्तानि, तद्वदभ्यवहार्याणि, अभ्यङ्गोपनाहनोद्वेष्टनोन्मर्दनपरिषेकावगाहनसंवाहनावपीडनवित्रासनविस्मापनविस्मारणानि, सुरासवविधानं, स्नेहाश्चानेकयोनयो दीपनीयपाचनीयवातहरविरेचनीयोपहितास्तथा शतपाकाः सहस्रपाकाः सर्वशश्च प्रयोगार्थाः, बस्तयः, बस्तिनियमः सुखशीलता चेति||१६||

Characteristic of Vatala constitution and its management:

Vatala (dominance of Vata), Pittala (dominance of Pitta) and Sleshmala (dominance of Kapha) these three are the morbid states in individuals, even though, according to another school of thought they represent the natural states of the body. Their characteristic features are as given below:

Vatala, Pitala and Sleshmala types of individuals are more susceptible to Vatika, Paittika and Sleshmika diseases respectively and such diseases in the respective types of individuals become very severe.

If a Vatala type of individual resorts to such thing as are aggravators of Vata, Vata in his body gets aggravated immediately. This does not happen in the case of the remaining two Doshas. The aggravated Vata afflicts individuals by manifestation of diseases already described], resulting in the impairment of strength, complexion, happiness and longevity.

The following therapies alleviate this Doshas:

Proper administration of oleation and fomentation;

Mild purgative prepared by the addition of fat, hot things and substances having sweet, sour and saline tastes

Food having the ingredients of the above mentioned properties

Massage, poultices, bandage, kneading, effusion, bath, samvahana (pressing and by hand) pressing, terrorizing, surmising and rememorizing,

Use of wine and Asavas (fermented drinks)

Fats from different source mixed with drugs having digestive, stimulant, carminative, Vata- alleviating and purgative properties- they may be boiled hundred and thousand times and be used for being administered in different times ways, viz, internal use, massage, enemata etc and

Enemata and regimens to be adopted along with it, the number of enemata may be according to the description available in Siddhi section for Karmabasti, Kalabasti, Yogabasti etc., Siddhi 1:47 [15-16]

पित्तलस्यापि पित्तप्रकोपणान्यासेवमानस्य क्षिप्रं पित्तं प्रकोपमापद्यते, न तथेतरौ दोषौ; तदस्य प्रकोपमापन्नं यथोक्तैर्विकारैः शरीरमुपतपति बलवर्णसुखायुषामुपघाताय|

तस्यावजयनं- सर्पिष्पानं, सर्पिषा च स्नेहनम्, अधश्च दोषहरणं, मधुरतिक्तकषायशीतानां चौषधाभ्यवहार्याणामुपयोगः, मृदुमधुरसुरभिशीतहृद्यानां गन्धानां चोपसेवा, मुक्तामणिहारावलीनां च परमशिशिरवारिसंस्थितानां धारणमुरसा, क्षणे क्षणेऽग्र्यचन्दनप्रियङ्गुकालीयमृणालशीतवातवारिभिरुत्पलकुमुदकोकनदसौगन्धिकपद्मानुगतैश्च वारिभिरभिप्रोक्षणं, श्रुतिसुखमृदुमधुरमनोऽनुगाना च गीतवादित्राणां श्रवणं, श्रवणं चाभ्युदयानां, सुहृदिभः संयोगः, संयोगश्चेष्टाभिः स्त्रीभिः शीतोपहितांशुकस्रग्धारिणीभिः, निशाकरांशुशीतलप्रवातहर्म्यवासः, शैलान्तरपुलिनशिशिरसदनवसनव्यजनपवनसेवनं, रम्याणां चोपवनानां सुखशिशिरसुरभिमारुतोपहितानामुपसेवनं, सेवनं च पद्मोत्पलनलिनकुमुदसौगन्धिकपुण्डरीकशतपत्रहस्तानां, सौम्यानां च सर्वभावानामिति||१७||

Characteristics of Pittala constitution and its management:

If a Pittala individual resorts to such things as aggravators of Pitta, Pitta in his body gets aggravated immediately. This does not happen in the case of the remaining two Doshas. The aggravated Pitta afflicts the individual by the manifestation of diseases already described resulting in the impairment of strength, complexion, happiness and longevity.

The following therapies alleviate Pitta Dosha:

Intake of ghee

Oleation by ghee

Purgation

Use of drugs and diets having sweet, bitter and astringent tastes and cooling property

Use of scents which are mild, sweet, fragrant, cooling and cordial

Use in the chest of pearls, jewels and garlands which are kept in excessively cold water

Frequent sprinkling of cold water and cold air of Agrya Chandana (Santalum album Linn), Priyangu (Callicarpa macrophylla VahL), Kaliya (yellow variety of Chandana) and Mrnala (lotus stalk) mixed with Utpala, Kumuda (a variety of Uptpala) Kokanada , Sugandhika and Padma

Hearing of songs and music which are pleasuring to ears, mild, sweet and agreeable

Hearing the information regarding prosperity

Keeping company of friends

Company of agreeable ladies wearing cooling garments and garlands;

Residence in buildings which is cooled by the moon rays and exposed to the breezes from all sides;

Residence in cold places in mountains and river banks, use of cold apparel and exposure to the cold winds of fans.

Visiting beautiful gardens having pleasing, cold and fragrant wind

Use of the flower of Padma (Nelumbo nucifera Gaertn), Utpala (Nymphaea alba Linn), Nalina (a type of lotus), Kumuda (a variety of Utpla), Saugandhika (a variety of Utpala) pundarika (Nymphaea lotus Linn) and Satapatra (a variety of lotus) and

Adaptation of such other regimens as are of soothing nature. [17]

Kapha Prakruti treatment :

श्लेष्मलस्यापि श्लेष्मप्रकोपणान्यासेवमानस्य क्षिप्रं श्लेष्मा प्रकोपमापद्यते, न तथेतरौ दोषौ; स तस्य प्रकोपमापन्नो यथोक्तैर्विकारैः शरीरमुपतपति बलवर्णसुखायुषामुपघाताय।

तस्यावजयनं- विधियुक्तानि तीक्ष्णोष्णानि संशोधनानि, रूक्षप्रायाणि चाभ्यवहार्याणि कटुकतिक्तकषायोपहितानि, तथैव धावनलङ्घनप्लवनपरिसरणजागरणनियुद्धव्यवायव्यायामोन्मर्दनस्नानोत्सादनानि, विशेषतस्तीक्ष्णानां दीर्घकालस्थितानां च मद्यानामुपयोगः, सधूमपानः सर्वशश्चोपवासः, तथोष्णं वासः, सुखप्रतिषेधश्च सुखार्थमेवेति॥१८॥

Characteristics of KaphaPrakruti and management of aggravation:

If a Sleshmala type of individual resorts to Kapha increasing activities, Kapha easily gets aggravated. In him, Vata and Pitta do not aggravate easily.

The aggravated kapha afflicts the individual by the manifestation of diseases, leading to impairments of strength, complexion, happiness and longevity.

The following therapies alleviate Kapha Dosha:

Proper administration of strong and hot elimination therapies – Vamana

Intake of diet which is mostly un-unctuous and is composed of ingredients having pungent, bitter and astringent tastes

Running, jumping, swimming whirling, keeping awake during night, fighting, sexual intercourse, exercise, unction, bath and oil massage.

Intake of strong wines preserved for a long time

All lightening therapies (Langhana) along with Dhumapana – herbal smoking

Use of warm apparels and

Giving up comforts of life for enjoying happiness ultimately. [18]

भवति चात्र-

सर्वरोगविशेषज्ञः सर्वकार्यविशेषवित्।

सर्वभेषजतत्त्वज्ञो राज्ञः प्राणपतिर्भवेदिति॥१९॥

Thus, it is said:

A man well versed with the specific features of all diseases, principles of their treatment and properties of all medications, is entitled to be a royal physician. [19]

तत्र श्लोकाः
प्रकृत्यन्तरभेदेन रोगानीकविकल्पनम्|
परस्पराविरोधश्च सामान्यं रोगदोषयोः||२०||
दोषसङ्ख्या विकाराणामेकदेशः प्रकोपणम्|
जरणं प्रति चिन्ता च कायाग्नेर्धुक्षणानि च||२१||
नराणां वातलादीनां प्रकृतिस्थापनानि च|
रोगानीके विमानेऽस्मिन् व्याहृतानि महर्षिणा||२२||

To sum up:
Various categories of diseases classified on the basis of different criteria, absence of any contradiction in these statements, identical nature of Roga (disease) and Dosha, number of Doshas, partial description of diseases, factors responsible for the aggravation of Doshas, digestive powers of digestion, therapies for the maintenance of the health of various types of individuals, viz, Vatala etc, all these topics have been described in this Chapter on "Roganeeka Vimanam". [20-22]

इत्यग्निवेशकृते तन्त्रे चरकप्रतिसंस्कृते विमानस्थाने रोगानीकविमानं नाम षष्टोऽध्यायः |6|
Thus ends the Sixth Chapter – Roganeeka Vimana Adhyaya – Determination of Specific Characteristics of Diseases of the Vimana Section of Agnivesha's work, redacted by Charaka. [6]

15

Vimanasthana Chapter 7 Vyadhita Rupiya Vimanam

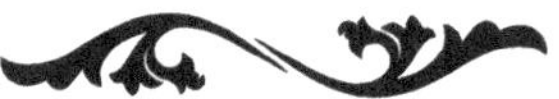

The 7th chapter of Charaka Samhitha Vimana Sthana is Vyadhita Rupiya Vimana. It deals with the determination of the specific types of patients, different types of parasites and their treatment through Panchakarma and oral medicines.

अथातो व्याधितरूपीयं विमानं व्याख्यास्यामः||१||
इति ह स्माह भगवानात्रेयः||२||

Let us explore the chapter on the "Vyadhita Rupeeya Viaman – Determination of the specific different types of Patients". Thus said Lord Atreya [1-2]

Two types of patients:
इहखलुद्वौपुरुषौव्याधितरूपौभवतः- गुरुव्याधितः, लघुव्याधितश्च|
तत्र- गुरुव्याधितएकःसत्त्वबलशरीरसम्पदुपेतत्वाल्लघुव्याधितइवदृश्यते,
लघुव्याधितोऽपरःसत्वादीनामधमत्वाद्गुरुव्याधितइवदृश्यते|
तयोरकुशलाःकेवलंचक्षुषैवरूपंदृष्ट्वाऽध्यवस्यन्तोव्याधिगुरुलाघवेविप्रतिपद्यन्ते||३||

Patients can be classified into two groups, viz,
Guru Vyadhita – those suffering from serious diseases and
Laghu Vyadhita – those suffering from mild diseases.

The patient suffering from a Guru Vyadhi (serious disease) may appear to be suffering from a mild disease due to :
Good Satva – good tolerance capacity
Bala – immunity of the patient
Shareera Sampath – physical strength.

Due to bad tolerance capacity, weak immunity and weak physical strength, a Laghu Vyadhi can look like a Guru Vyadhi in some patients.

Unskilled physicians, who try to diagnose just by seeing, commit mistakes in determining Laghu and Guru Vyadhis. [3]

Need for careful examination :
नहि ज्ञानावयवेन कृत्स्ने ज्ञेये विज्ञानमुत्पद्यते|

विप्रतिपन्नास्तु खलु रोगज्ञाने उपक्रमयुक्तिज्ञाने चापि विप्रतिपद्यन्ते।

ते यदा गुरुव्याधितं लघुव्याधितरूपमासादयन्ति, तदा तमल्पदोषं मत्वा संशोधनकालेऽस्मै मृदु संशोधनं प्रयच्छन्तो भूय एवास्य दोषानुदीरयन्ति।

यदा तु लघुव्याधितं गुरुव्याधितरूपमासादयन्ति, तदा तं महादोषं मत्वा संशोधनकालेऽस्मै तीक्ष्णं संशोधनं प्रयच्छन्तो दोषानतिनिर्हृत्य शरीरमस्य क्षिण्वन्ति।

एवमवयवेन ज्ञानस्य कृत्स्ने ज्ञेये ज्ञानमभिमन्यमानाः परिस्खलन्ति।

विदितवेदितव्यास्तु भिषजः सर्वं सर्वथा यथासम्भवं परीक्ष्यं परीक्ष्याध्यवस्यन्तो न क्वचिदपि विप्रतिपद्यन्ते, यथेष्टमर्थमभिनिर्वर्तयन्ति चेति||४||

One cannot perceive a thing in its entirety with partial knowledge. In the absence of the correct knowledge of the disease, one commits mistakes in deciding the rationale behind the line of treatment. When the doctor mistakes a patient suffering from a serious disease (Guru Vyadhita) for Laghu Vyadhita, he would administer Mrudu Samshodhana – soft treatment, leading to further aggravation of Doshas and diseases. (Dosha Udeerana).

Similarly, if the doctor mis-diagnoses a weak disease as Guru Vyadhita, then he may administer Teekshna Shodhana – very strong purification procedures, leading to depletion of body tissues and health – Shareera Kshaya.

Physicians, who diagnose diseases accurately, by comprehensive patient examination, seldom err in deciding about Guruvyadhita or Laghu Vyadhita and achieve cure for the diseases. [4]

भवन्तिचात्र-

सत्त्वादीनांविकल्पेनव्याधिरूपमथातुरे |

दृष्ट्वाविप्रतिपद्यन्तेबालाव्याधिबलाबले||५||

तेभेषजमयोगेनकुर्वन्त्यज्ञानमोहिताः|

व्याधितानांविनाशायक्लेशायमहतेऽपिवा||६||

प्राज्ञास्तुसर्वमाज्ञायपरीक्ष्यमिहसर्वथा|

नस्खलन्तिप्रयोगेषुभेषजानांकदाचन||७||

Thus, it is said:
Because of the variation in
Satva – patient's mental tolerance capacity toward treatment,
Bala – physical strength and immunity of the patient etc., an ignorant doctor may commit mistakes in deciding the seriousness or mildness of the disease, leading to selection of wrong therapies. This results in aggravation of the disease.

Physicians well versed in the science, ascertain all aspects of the disease and examine it by employing all the methods; they seldom err in administering correct therapies. [5-7]

Agnivesha's query about Parasites:

इति व्याधितरूपाधिकारे व्याधितरूपसङ्ख्याग्रसम्भवं व्याधितरूपहेतुविप्रतिपत्तौ कारणं सापवादं सम्प्रतिपत्तिकारणं चानपवादं निशम्य, भगवन्तमात्रेयमग्निवेशोऽतः परं सर्वक्रिमीणां पुरीषसंश्रयाणां समुत्थानस्थानसंस्थानवर्णनामप्रभावचिकित्सितविशेषान् पप्रच्छोपसङ्गृह्य पादौ||८||

Thus, the classification of patients, cause of incorrect diagnosis along with its bad consequences, factors responsible for correct diagnosis and good results born out of it- these topics are elaborately described.

Having listened to all this, Agnivesha fell at the feet of Lord Atreya and inquired about the specific cause, habit, from colour, name, effect and treatment of all parasites (Krumi) having human body. [8]

Four groups of Krumi:

अथास्मै प्रोवाच भगवानात्रेयः- इह खल्वग्निवेश! विंशतिविधाः क्रिमयः पूर्वमुद्दिष्टा नानाविधेन प्रविभागेनान्यत्र सहजेभ्यः; ते पुनः प्रकृतिभिर्विभज्यमानाश्चतुर्विधा भवन्ति; तद्यथा- पुरीषजाः, श्लेष्मजाः, शोणितजा, मलजाश्चेति॥९॥

Lord Atreya replied to Agnivesha,

"There are twenty types of Krumi, which can be grouped into four, on the basis of their source,

Malaja born of external excreta

Pureeshaja Krumi – born of faeces,

Sleshmaja – born of Phlegm

Shonitaja – born of blood [9]

Pureeshaja Krumi (Malaja Krimi) – Yuka, Pipeelika

Shonitaja Krumi – Keshada, Lomada, Lomadvipa, Saurasa, Audumbara, Jantumata

Shleshmaja Krumi – Antrada, Udarada, Hrudayachara, Churava, Darbhapushpa, Saugandhika, Mahaguda

Purishaja – Kakeruka, Makeruka, Leliha, Sashulaka, Sausurada

Malaja Krimi :

तत्र मलो बाह्यश्चाभ्यन्तरश्च।

तत्र बाह्यमलजातान् मलजान् सञ्चक्ष्महे।

तेषां समुत्थानं- मृजावर्जनं; स्थानं- केशश्मश्रुलोमपक्ष्मवासांसि; संस्थानम्- अणवस्तिलाकृतयो बहुपादाश्च; वर्णः- कृष्णः, शुक्लश्च; नामानि- यूकाः, पिपीलिकाश्च; प्रभावः- कण्डूजननं, कोठपिडकाभिनिर्वर्तनं च; चिकित्सितं तु खल्वेषामपकर्षणं, मलोपघातः, मलकराणां च भावानामनुपसेवनमिति॥१०॥

Waste products are of two types – external and internal. Malaja Krumi are considered to be born of external waste products.

Cause for Malaja Krimi – lack of cleanliness

Samutthana – Habitat: hair on the head, face and other parts of the body, eye lashes and dresses.

Shape and size – minute, Millipede and having the shape of sesame grains.

Color: Black and white

Effects: Itching, production of urticaria and pimples

Treatment:

Apakarshana – killing of these Krumis

Malopaghata – removal of waste products

such regimens which produce the excreta. [10]

Shonitaja Krumi :

शोणितजानां तु खलु कुष्ठैः समानं समुत्थानं; स्थानं- रक्तवाहिन्यो धमन्यः; संस्थानम्- अणवो वृत्ताश्चापादाश्च, सूक्ष्मत्वाच्चैके भवन्त्यदृश्याः; वर्णः- ताम्रः; नामानि- केशादा, लोमादा, लोमद्वीपाः, सौरसा, औडुम्बरा, जन्तुमातरश्चेति; प्रभावः- केशश्मश्रुनखलोमपक्ष्मापध्वंसः, व्रणगतानां च हर्षकण्डूतोदसंसर्पणानि, अतिवृद्धानां च त्वक्सिरास्नायुमांसतरुणास्थिभक्षणमिति; चिकित्सितमप्येषां कुष्ठैः समानं, तदुत्तरकालमुपदेक्ष्यामः॥११॥

Shonitaja Krumi – Parasites of blood:

Cause: the same as for Kushta – skin diseases

Samutthana – Raktavahi Dhamani – blood vessels

Samsthana – Form: minute, round and having no pedicle (Apada). Because of minuteness some of them are not visible to the naked eye.

Color: coppery

Names:

Keshada (which eat away hair of the head)

Lomada (which eat-away the small hair of the body), Lomadvikpa,

Saurasa, Audumbara and Jantumatara.

Prabhava of Shonitaja Krumi :

Destruction of the hair from the head, face, other parts of the body, eye-lashes and nails.

When a wound is affected, it causes

Harsha – hyperesthesia,

Kandu – itching,

Toda – pain and

Samsarpana – creeping sensation in the ulcerated area are caused;

When excessively grown they eat away the skin, vessels, ligaments, muscles tissue and cartilages;

Treatment: same as that of Kushta, which is described in 7th chapter of Chikitsa sthana of Charaka Samhita. [11]

Shleshmaja Krimi :

श्लेष्मजाः   क्षीरगुडतिलमत्स्यानूपमांसपिष्टान्नपरमान्नकुसुम्भस्नेहाजीर्णपूतिक्लिन्नसङ्कीर्णविरुद्धासात्म्यभोजनसमुत्थानाः; तेषामामाशयः स्थानं, ते प्रवर्धमानास्तूर्ध्वमधो वा विसर्पन्त्युभयतो वा; संस्थानवर्णविशेषास्तु- श्वेताः पृथुब्रध्नसंस्थानाः केचित्, केचिद्वृत्तपरिणाहा गण्डूपदाकृतयः श्वेतास्ताम्रावभासाश्च, केचिदणवो दीर्घास्तन्त्वाकृतयः श्वेताः; तेषां त्रिविधानां श्लेष्मनिमितानां क्रिमीणां नामानि- अन्त्रादाः, उदरादाः, हृदयचराः, चुरवः, दर्भपुष्पाः, सौगन्धिकाः, महागुदाश्चेति; प्रभावो- हल्लासः, आस्यसंस्रवणम्, अरोचकाविपाकौ, ज्वरः, मूर्च्छा, जृम्भा, क्षवथुः, आनाहः, अङ्गमर्दः, छर्दिः कार्श्यं, पारुष्यं, चेति॥१२॥

Causes for Sleshmaj Krumi:

Intake of milk, Sugar-candy, excess sesame seeds, fish, meat of animals inhabiting marshy land (Anupa Mamsa),

Pishtanna – Pastries,

Paramanna – milk preparations,

Kusumabha taila (Carthamus tinctorious Linn). Uncooked, putrefied and softened food, food mixed with despicable articles like faeces, food having mutually contradictory properties and unwholesome food.

Habitat: Amashaya; when excessively grown, they move upwards, or to both the sides.

Form and color: some are big and fat (tape like) in shape and white in colour; some are round in shape like earthworm and white in colour with a coppery tinge; some are minute and long in shape like a thread and white in colour.

Names of Shleshmaja Krumi:

Antrada (which eats away the intestine)

Udarada (which disturbs stomach)

Hrdayacara (lit. which moves in the heart), Guru, Darbhapuspa (which is like the flower of Darbha), Saugandhika, Mahagruda (Lit having a big anus).

Effects: Nausea, salivation, anorexia, indigestion, fever, fainting, yawning, sneezing, constipation, malaise, vomiting, emaciation and dryness of the body. [12]

Pureeshaja Krumi:

पुरीषजास्तुल्यसमुत्थानाः श्लेष्मजैः; तेषां स्थानं पक्वाशयः, ते प्रवर्धमानास्त्वधो विसर्पन्ति, यस्य पुनरामाशयाभिमुखाः स्युर्यदन्तरं तदन्तरं तस्योद्गारनिःश्वासाः पुरीषगन्धिनः स्युः; संस्थानवर्णविशेषास्तु- सूक्ष्मवृत्तपरिणाहाः श्वेता दीर्घा ऊर्णाशुसङ्काशाः केचित्, केचित् पुनः स्थूलवृत्तपरिणाहाः श्यावनीलहरितपीताः; तेषां नामानि ककेरुकाः, मकेरुकाः, लेलिहाः; सशूलकाः, सौसुरादाश्चेति; प्रभावः- पुरीषभेदः, कार्श्यं, पारुष्यं, लोमहर्षाभिनिर्वर्तनं च, त एव चास्य गुदमुखं परितुदन्तः कण्डूं चोपजनयन्तो गुदमुखं पर्यासते, त एव जातहर्षा गुदनिष्क्रमणमतिवेलं कुर्वन्ति; इत्येष श्लेष्मजानां पुरीषजानां च क्रिमीणां समुत्थानादिविशेषः॥१३॥

Pureeshaja Krumi: Parasites of faeces:

Causes of Pureeshaja Krumi: Same as Shleshmaja Krumi.

Habitat: Pakvashaya or colon; when excessively grown they move downwards; when they move towards Amasaya or stomach, then the eructation and breath of the patient produce faecal odour.

Form and colour:some of them are minute, cylindrical and long, they appear like the fibres of wool and they are white in colour; some others are thick, cylindrical and their colour are gray, blue, green or yellow.

Names of Purishaja Krumi: Kakeruka, Makeruka, Leliha, Sasulaka (which cause colic pain) and Sausurada.

Effects: diarrhoea, emaciation, dryness and horrification inhabit the oral region and cause irritation and itching there; when excited they frequently come out of the anus.

Thus the cause etc., of parasites born of phlegm and faeces as described. [13]

Krimi Chikitsa Sutra :

Krumi Chikitsa Suthra – Line of treatment:

तत्र सर्वक्रिमीणामपकर्षणमेवादितः कार्य, ततः प्रकृतिविघातः, अनन्तरं निदानोक्तानां भावानामनुपसेवनमिति॥१४॥

Line of treatment of Krumi in brief:

Apararshana – extraction of Krumi- by hand and by Shod hana

Prakruti Vighata – acting against the nature of the Krumi. Eg: Shleshmahara procedures in Shleshmaja Krumi.

Nidana Anupasevana – avoiding causative factors [14]

Krumi Apakarshana :

तत्रापकर्षणं- हस्तेनाभिगृह्य विमृश्योपकरणवताऽपनयनमनुपकरणेन वा; स्थानगतानां तु क्रिमीणां भेषजेनापकर्षणं न्यायतः, तच्चतुर्विधं; तद्यथा- शिरोविरेचनं, वमनं, विरेचनम्, आस्थापनं च; इत्यपकर्षणविधिः।

प्रकृतिविघातस्त्वेषां कटुतिक्तकषायक्षारोष्णानां द्रव्याणामुपयोगः, यच्चान्यदपि किञ्चिच्छ्लेष्मपुरीषप्रत्यनीकभूतं तत् स्यात्; हति प्रकृतिविघातः।

अनन्तरं निदानोक्तानां भावानामनुपसेवनं- यदुक्तं निदानविधौ तस्य विवर्जनं तथाप्रायाणां चापरेषां द्रव्याणाम्।

इति लक्षणतश्चिकित्सितमनुव्याख्यातम्।

एतदेव पुनर्विस्तरेणोपदेक्ष्यते॥१५॥

Krumi Apakarshana – Procedure to be followed for parasite extraction :

Apakarshana :

Parasites may be extracted by hand with or without the help of instruments (forceps etc). Parasites residing inside the body can be extracted by the Shodhana therapies.

Shirovirechana (errhines),

Vamana

Virechana and Asthapana Basti.

Prakruti Vighata

Prakruti Vighata treatment for Krumi :

Counteracting the factors responsible for the production of parasites. Drugs and diets which are pungent, bitter and astringent tastes, Kshara, Ushna medicines, in nature are given, along with other Kaphahara Pureesha hara medicines are administered.

Nidana Anupasevana :

Factors which produce these parasites and similar other substances are to be avoided. [15]

Preparatory treatment :

अथैनं क्रिमिकोष्ठमातुरमग्रे षड्रात्रं सप्तरात्रं वा स्नेहस्वेदाभ्यामुपपाद्य श्वोभूते एनं संशोधनं पाययिताऽस्मीति क्षीरगुडदधितिलमत्स्यानूपमांसपिष्टान्नपरमान्नकुसुम्भस्नेहसम्प्रयुक्तैर्भोज्यैः सायं प्रातश्चोपपादयेत् समुदीरणार्थं क्रिमीणां

कोष्ठाभिसरणार्थं च भिषक्|
अथ व्युष्टायां रात्र्यां सुखोषितं सुप्रजीर्णभक्तं च विज्ञायास्थापनवमनविरेचनैस्तदहरेवोपपादयेदुपपादनीयश्चेत् स्यात् सर्वान् परीक्ष्यविशेषान् परीक्ष्य सम्यक्||१६||

Preparatory treatment for Krimi treatment:
The patient afflicted is given Snehana, Swedana for 6 – 7 days,
Next day (a day before the administration of elimination therapy) during morning and evening meals he is given food consisting of milk, sugar candy, curd, sesame, fish, Anupa mamsa, Pishtanna, milk preparation and oil of Kusumbha (Carthamus tinctorius Linn) with a view to arousing the parasites and impelling them to migrate to the alimentary tract.

If the patient passes the night comfortably and the food taken by him in the previous day is fully digested, he is given Asthapana Basti, Vamana, Virechana – all on the same day, provided the patient is found fit for all these therapies. [16]

Asthapana Basti :
अथाहरेति ब्रूयात्- मूलकसर्षपलशुनकरञ्जशिग्रुमधुशिग्रुखरपुष्पाभूस्तृणसुमुखसुरसकुठेरकगण्डीरकालमालकपर्णासक्षवकफणिञ्झकानि सर्वाण्यथवा यथालाभं; तान्याहृतान्यभिसमीक्ष्य खण्डशश्छेदयित्वा प्रक्षाल्य पानीयेन सुप्रक्षालितायां स्थाल्यां समावाप्य गोमूत्रेणार्धोदकेनाभिषिच्य साधयेत् सततमवघट्टयन् दर्व्या, तमुपयुक्तभूयिष्ठेऽम्भसि गतरसेष्वौषधेषु स्थालीमवतार्य सुपरिपूतं कषायं सुखोष्णं मदनफलपिप्पलीविडङ्गकल्कतैलोपहितं स्वर्जिकालवणितमभ्यासिच्य बस्तौ विधिवदास्थापयेदेनं; तथाऽर्कालर्ककुटजाढकीकुष्ठकैदर्यकषायेण वा, तथा शिग्रुपीलुकुस्तुम्बुरुकटुकासर्षपकषायेण, तथाऽऽमलकशृङ्गवेरदारुहरिद्रापिचुमर्दकषायेण मदनफलादिसंयोगसम्पादितेन, त्रिवारं सप्तरात्रं वाऽऽस्थापयेत्||१७||
Radish, mustard, garlic, Karanja, Moringa leaves and seed, Kharapushpa, Bhutruna, Sumuka, Srasa, Kuteraka, Gandiraka, Alamala, Parnasa, Kshavaka, Phaninjaka – all these herbs or whichever are available, are taken, washed well, cut into small pieces, taken in a vessel, added with cow urine and half part of water, boiled till Gatarasa (herbs leave their taste), – filtered. While they are Sukhoshna – lukewarm, Madanaphala pippali, Vidanga Kalka, sesame oil, Swarjika Lavana are added as prakshepa and administered as Asthapana Basti.

Or, Basti prepared with Decoction of these – Arka, Alarka, Kutaja, Adhaki, Kushta, Kaidarya + madanaphala pippali etc. herbs or Basti with Decoction of Amalaki, ginger, Daruharidra, Pichumardha, Madanapippali etc Prakshepa are administered as Asthapana basti for 3 0r 7 days.

प्रत्यागते च पश्चिमे बस्तौ प्रत्याश्वस्तं तदहरेवोभयतोभागहरं संशोधनं पाययेद्युक्त्या; तस्य विधिरुपदेक्ष्यते- मदनफलपिप्पलीकषायस्यार्धाञ्जलिमात्रेण त्रिवृत्कल्काक्षमात्रमालोड्य पातुमस्मै प्रयच्छेत्, तदस्य दोषमुभयतो निर्हरति साधु; एवमेव कल्पोक्तानि वमनविरेचनानि प्रतिसंसृज्य पाययेदेनं बुद्ध्या सर्वविशेषानवेक्षमाणो भिषक्||१८||
अथैनं सम्यग्विरिक्तं विज्ञायापराह्णे शैखरिककषायेण सुखोष्णेन परिषेचयेत्|
तेनैव च कषायेण बाह्याभ्यन्तरान् सर्वोदकार्थान् कारयेच्छश्वत्; तद्भावे कटुतिक्तकषायाणामौषधानां क्वाथैर्मूत्रक्षारैर्वा परिषेचयेत्|
परिषिक्तं चैनं निवातमागारमनुप्रवेश्य पिप्पलीपिप्पलीमूलचव्यचित्रकशृङ्गवेरसिद्धेन यवाग्वादिना क्रमेणोपाचरेत्, विलेपीक्रमागतं चैनमनुवासयेद्विडङ्गतैलेनैकान्तरं द्विस्त्रिर्वा||१९||
After Basti treatment, Ubhayato Bhagahara Samshodana is adminsitered. (Vamana and Virechana)
For this, Madanapahala pippali Kashaya – half anjali, along with Trivrit Kalpa – 12 grams is mixed and administered. This will induce vomiting and purgation. After the patient is well-purged, in the afternoon, he is sponged with the lukewarm decoction of Vidanga (Embelia ribes).

He should use Vidanga Kashaya for washing and drinking in place of water. If this decoction is not available then the decoction of drugs having pungent, bitter and astringent tastes or Kshara or prepared urine may be used for sponging over the patient.

After getting sprinkled with the decoction etc, the patient should enter into a closed room (a room which is not windy) and gradually be given with Panchakola Yavagu.

When the patient comes to the stage of being given Vilepi (thin gruel) then he is administered two to three Anuvasana Basti with Vidanga taila on alternate days. [18-19]

Administration of nasya :

यदि पुनरस्यातिप्रवृद्धाञ्छीर्षादान् क्रिमीन् मन्येत शिरस्यैवाभिसर्पतः कदाचित्,
ततः स्नेहस्वेदाभ्यामस्य शिर उपपाद्य विरेचयेदपामार्गतण्डुलादिना शिरोविरेचनेन॥२०॥

If it is observed that these parasites have invaded the head because of their excessive growth, thereby causing injury to the head, the head of patient is oleated and fomented and Doshas from the head is purged by the administration of errhines prepared with the de-husked seeds of Apamarga (Achyranthes aspera) as described in the second chapter of Sutra section [20]

Antidotes :

यस्त्वभ्यवहार्यविधिः प्रकृतिविघातायोक्तः क्रिमीणामथ तमनुव्याख्यास्यामः- मूलकपर्णीं समूलाग्रप्रतानामाहृत्य खण्डशश्छेदयित्वोलू(द्)खले क्षोदयित्वा पाणिभ्यां पीडयित्वा रसं गृह्णीयात्, तेन रसेन लोहितशालितण्डुलपिष्टं समालोड्य पूपलिकां कृत्वा विधूमेष्वङ्गारेष्वपकुड्य विडङ्गतैललवणोपहितां क्रिमिकोष्ठाय भक्षयितुं प्रयच्छेत्, अनन्तरं चाम्लकाञ्जिकमुदश्विद्वा पिप्पल्यादिपञ्चवर्गसंसृष्टं सलवणमनुपाययेत्।
अनेन कल्पेन मार्कवार्कसहचरनीपनिर्गुण्डीसुमुखसुरसकुठेरकगण्डीरकालमालकपर्णासक्षवकफणिज्झक-बकुलकुटजसुवर्णक्षीरीस्वरसानामन्यतमस्मिन् कारयेत् पूपलिकाः; तथा किणिहीकिराततिक्तकसुवहामलकहरीतकीबिभीतकस्वरसेषु कारयेत् पूपलिकाः; स्वरसांश्चैतेषामेकैकशो द्वन्द्वशः सर्वशो वा मधुविलुलितान् प्रातरनन्नाय पातुं प्रयच्छेत्॥२१॥

Antidotes for production of parasites :

We shall now explore the measures to be adopted for counteracting the factors responsible for the production of parasites.

Recipe 1 :
Mulakaparni along with its roots and branches is collected, cut into pieces, crushed in a mortar and its juice is extracted by manual pressure. Juice and made of Pupalikas (a type of cake) which are again to be fried with smokeless fire- brands.

The patient suffering from parasitic infection is given this cake to take along with the salt and the oil of Vidanga Then, he is made to drink sour Kanji (sour gruel) or Udashvit (a mixture of water and buttermilk in equal quantity) along with salt and the powder of
Pippali – Long pepper fruit – Piper longum
Root of Pippali
Chavya (Piper chaba hunter),
Chitraka (Plumbago zeylanica Linn) and
Shringavera – Ginger.

On the same way, Pupalika type of cake may be prepared by the juice of any of the following plants;
Markava , Arka – Calotropis gigantea R. Br. Ex Ait), Sahacara (Barleria cristata)
Nipa, Nirgundi (Vitex negundo), various types of Basils, Viz, Sumukka, Surasa, Kutheraka, Gandira, Kalamalaka, Parnasa, ksavaka, and Phnijjhaka, Bakula (Mimusops elengi Linn), Kutaja Suvarnaksriri .Kinihi (Achyranthes aspera

Linn), Kriratatikta (Swertia chirata Buch_Ham), Suvaha– Operculina turpethum, Amalaka (Emblica officinalis Gaern), Haritaki (Terminalia chebula Linn) and Bibhitaka (Terminalia bellirica Roxb).

The patient may be given the juice of all these plants or one or two of them mixed with honey in the morning on an empty stomach. [21]

Recipe 2:
अथाश्वशकृदाहृत्य महति किलिञ्जके प्रस्तीर्यातपे शोषयित्वोदूखले क्षोदयित्वा दृषदि पुनः सूक्ष्मचूर्णानि कारयित्वा विडङ्गकषायेण त्रिफलाकषायेण वाऽष्टकृत्वो दशकृत्वो वाऽऽतपे सुपरिभावितानि भावयित्वा दृषदि पुनः सूक्ष्माणि चूर्णानि कारयित्वा नवे कलशे समावाप्यानुगुप्तं निधापयेत्|
तेषां तु खलु चूर्णानां पाणितलं यावद्वा साधु मन्येत तत् क्षौद्रेण संसृज्य क्रिमिकोष्ठिने लेढुं प्रयच्छेत्||२२||

Another recipe for counter action:
Another recipe for counteracting the factors responsible for the production of parasites is also follows: horse-dung is collected, spread over a tray and kept exposed to sun till it gets dried up. This should therefore be crushed in a mortor and again pounded on a stone slab so as to make it into a fine powder.

The powder is well impregnated in the sun, with the decoction of Vidanga or Triphala – eight or ten times. This again is made to a fine powder over a stone slab and stored in an air tight new earthen jar carefully so as to avoid any infection.

This powder, in the dose of one Panitala (12 g) or in another suitable dose mixed with honey and in the form of linctus is given to the patient suffering from the parasitic infection. [22]

Recipe 3:
तथा भल्लातकास्थीन्याहृत्य कलशप्रमाणेन चापोथ्य स्नेहभाविते दृढे कलशे सूक्ष्मानेकच्छिद्रबद्ध्ने शरीरमुपवेष्ट्य मृदावलिप्ते समावाप्योडुपेन पिधाय भूमावाकण्ठं निखातस्य स्नेहभावितस्यैवान्यस्य दृढस्य कुम्भस्योपरि समारोप्य समन्ताद्गोमयैरुपचित्य दाहयेत्, स यदा जानीयात् साधु दग्धानि गोमयानि विगतस्नेहानि च भल्लातकास्थीनीति ततस्तं कुम्भमुद्धरेत्|
अथ तस्मादि्द्वतीयात् कुम्भात् स्नेहमादाय विडङ्गतण्डुलचूर्णैः स्नेहार्धमात्रैः प्रतिसंसृज्यातपे सर्वमहः स्थापयित्वा ततोऽस्मै मात्रां प्रयच्छेत् पानाय; तेन साधु विरिच्यते, विरिक्तस्य चानुपूर्वी यथोक्ता|
एवमेव भद्रदारुसरलकाष्ठस्नेहानुपकल्प्य पातुं प्रयच्छेत्||२३||
अनुवासयेच्चैनमनुवासनकाले ||२४||
Third recipe for Counter-action:
Another recipe for counteracting the factors responsible for the production of parasites is as below:
One Kalasa 912. 288 Kg) of the stones / seeds of Bhallataka (Semecarpus anacardium Linn.) is collected, crushed and kept in an earthen jar. The interior of this jar should be made unctuous by anointing it with oil many times. The outer surface of the jar is wrapped with 4-5 layers of cloth coated with clay and dried. It is not wrapped on the bottom of the jar and the neck and opening. Many small orifices are made at the bottom of the jar. The opening is closed with an earthen lid and sealed with clay coated cloth.

This jar is placed over another jar which is strong, smeared inside with oil and buried under ground up to its neck. Cow-dung cakes are piled "all around the jar and ignited.

When the cow dung cakes are well burnt and the stones / seeds of Bhallataka (Semecarpus anacardium Linn.) have been drained of their oil contents, then the upper jar is removed and the oil from the lower jar is collected. This oil mixed with a halt of its quantity of the de-husked seeds of Vidanga is kept in the sun for the whole day.

This is given to the patient in a proper dose will cause purgation. Follow- up measures to be adopted after purgation have already been described. Similarly, the oil extracted from the wood of Bhadradaru (Cedrus deodara Loud) and Sarala (Pinus roxburghii) may be administered.

Thereafter, in appropriate time, the patient is given Anuvasana (oleation) type of enema [23-24]

Recipe 4:

अथाहरेति ब्रूयात्- शारदान्नवांस्तिलान् सम्पदुपेतान्; तानाहृत्य सुनिष्पूतान्निष्पूय, सुशुद्धान् शोधयित्वा, विडङ्गकषाये सुखोष्णे प्रक्षिप्य निर्वापयेदादोषगमनात्, गतदोषानभिसमीक्ष्य, सुप्रलूनान् प्रलुञ्च्य, पुनरेव सुनिष्पूतान् निष्पूय, सुशुद्धान् शोधयित्वा, विडङ्गकषायेण त्रिःसप्तकृत्वः सुपरिभावितान् भावयित्वा, आतपे शोषयित्वा, उलू(द्)खले सङ्क्षुद्य, दृषदि पुनः श्लक्ष्णपिष्टान् कारयित्वा, द्रोण्यामभ्यवधाय, विडङ्गकषायेण मुहुर्मुहुरवसिञ्चन् पाणिमर्दमेव मर्दयेत्; तस्मिंस्तु खलु प्रपीड्यमाने यत्तैलमुदियात्तत् पाणिभ्यां पर्यादाय, शुचौ दृढे कलशे न्यस्यानुगुप्तं निधापयेत्||२५||

Fourth recipe for counter action:

Another recipe for counteracting the factors responsible for the production of parasites is as follows: -
Fresh sesame seeds of good quantity harvested in the autumn are collected, separated from dirt particles, washed well and kept in the lukewarm decoction of Vidanga (Embelia ribes Burm f) till all the dirt particles are removed.

Then the decoction is drained out. When the Taila is free from impurities, it is de-husked, cleaned well again, washed well, impregnated well for twenty-one times in the decoction of Vidanga, dried in sun, crushed in a mortar and made to a fine powder over a stone slab, keeping this fine powder in a container, it is rubbed well with hands again and again, sprinkling frequently the decoction of Vidanga. The oil which comes out of it by the application of presence is collected by hand and kept in a safe place in a clean and strong earthen jar. [25]

Recipe 5 :

अथाहरेति ब्रूयात्- तिल्वकोद्दालकयोर्द्वौ बिल्वमात्रौ पिण्डौ श्लक्ष्णपिष्टौ विडङ्गकषायेण, तदर्धमात्रौ श्यामात्रिवृत्योः, अतोऽर्धमात्रौ दन्तीद्रवन्त्योः, अतोऽर्धमात्रौ च चव्यचित्रकयोरिति|

एतं सम्भारं विडङ्गकषायस्यार्धाढकमात्रेण प्रतिसंसृज्य, तत्तैलप्रस्थं समावाप्य, सर्वमालोड्य, महति पर्योगे समासिच्याग्नावधिश्रित्यासने सुखोपविष्टः सर्वतः स्नेहमवलोकयन्नजस्रं मृद्वग्निना साधयेद्दर्व्या सततमवघट्टयन्|

स यदा जानीयादिवरमति शब्दः, प्रशाम्यति च फेनः, प्रसादमापद्यते स्नेहः, यथास्वं च गन्धवर्णरसोत्पत्तिः, संवर्तते च भैषज्यमङ्गुलिभ्यां मृद्यमानमनतिमृद्वनतिदारुणमनङ्गुलिग्राहि चेति, स कालस्तस्यावतारणाय|

ततस्तमवतार्य शीतीभूतमहतेन वाससा परिपूय, शुचौ दृढे कलशे समासिच्य, पिधानेन पिधाय, शुक्लेन वस्त्रपट्टेनावच्छाद्य, सूत्रेण सुबद्धं सुनिगुप्तं निधापयेत्|

ततोऽस्मै मात्रां प्रयच्छेत् पानाय, तेन साधु विरिच्यते; सम्यगपहृतदोषस्य चानुपूर्वी यथोक्ता|

ततश्चैनमनुवासयेदनुवासनकाले|

एतेनैव च पाकविधिना सर्षपातसीकरञ्जकोषातकीस्नेहानुपकल्प्य पाययेत् सर्वविशेषानवेक्षमाणः|

तेनागदो भवति||२६||

Fifth recipe for counter action:

Another therapy for counteracting the factors responsible for the production of parasites is as follows:
Tilvaka (Symplocos racemosa Roxb) and Uddalaka – one Bilva (48 g) of each is collected, Made to a fine paste by the addition of the decoction of Vidanga (Embelia ribes Burm. f) and kept in bolus form.

Similarly half Bilva (24g) each of Syama (black variety of Operculina turpethum R.B), one fourth Bilva (12 g) each of Danti (Baliospermum montanum Muell-Arg) and Dravanti and one eight Bilva (6g) each of Chavya (Piper chaba Hunter) and Citraka (Plumbago zeylanica Linn) is collected. The above-mentioned ingredients are mixed with half Adhaka – 3.072 kg (1.53 liter) of the decoction of Vidanga and one Prastha – 768 ml (0.768 liter) of oil. All of them are mixed well in a sufficiently big vessel and kept over fire.

This oil is constantly stirred through a ladle over very mild fire by a person comfortably sitting near the hearth and carefully watching the oil from all sides. the time of removing the oil- pan out of fire is determined by the following criteria: -
Stoppage of the budding sound
Subsidence of the foam
Appearance of clarity in the oil
Manifestation of the desired smell; colour and taste.

When a portion of the pasted drugs mixed with the oil is rubbed with the fingers then it takes the shape of a wick, it does not adhere to the finger and it is neither very hard nor very soft to touch.

When it cools after having been taken out of fire, it is filtered with a new cloth and kept in a clean and strong earthen jar. This jar is closed with a lid and covered with a piece of white cloth, tied well with rope and kept in a safe place. This oil, given to the patient in the proper dose to drink, will cause Virechana. When all the impurities are removed from the body, follow up measures as already described (in para- 19 of this chapter) is adopted. In proper time he is given Anuvasana (oil enema) also.

Following the same method, oil is prepared with drugs like Sarsapa (Brassica nigra Koch), Atasi (Linum usitatissimum Linn), Karanja (Pongamia pinnata Merr) and Kosataki (Luffa acutangula) and after having examined all aspects, the patient is administered this therapy. This cures the patient of his disease. [26]

एवं द्वयानां श्लेष्मपुरीषसम्भवानां क्रिमीणां समुत्थानसंस्थानवर्णनामप्रभावचिकित्सितविशेषा व्याख्याताः सामान्यतः|
विशेषतस्तु स्वल्पमात्रमास्थापनानुवासनानुलोमहरणभूयिष्ठं तेष्वेवौषधेषु पुरीषजानां क्रिमीणां चिकित्सितं कर्तव्यं, मात्राधिकं पुनः शिरोविरेचनवमनोपशमनभूयिष्ठं तेष्वेवौषधेषु श्लेष्मजानां क्रिमीणां चिकित्सितं कार्यम्; इत्येष क्रिमिघ्नो भेषजविधिरनुव्याख्यातो भवति|
तमनुतिष्ठता यथास्वं हेतुवर्जने प्रयतितव्यम्|
यथोद्देशमेवमिदं क्रिमिकोष्ठचिकित्सितं यथावदनुव्याख्यातं भवति||२७||
Thus, the specific cause, shape, colour, names, effects and treatment of parasites with origin both from phlegm and faeces are generally explained. Difference in the treatment of these two types of parasites is as follows: - for the faeces- born parasites, the treatment involves the administration of the above-mentioned drugs in small quantity, mostly in the form of Asthapana (corrective) and Anuvasana (oleation) types of enema and purgative.

For phlegm- born parasites, however, the drug is in large quantities and mostly having the property of eliminating Doshas from the head (errhines), emesis and sedation. Thus, the anti-parasitic therapies are explained. While administering these therapies, efforts are made to avoid such of the causative factors which are responsible for the production of these parasites. Thus, the treatment of parasites of the alimentary tract as was suggested in paragraph 14 is explained. [27]

भवन्ति चात्र-
अपकर्षणमेवादौ क्रिमीणां भेषजं स्मृतम्|
ततो विघातः प्रकृतेर्निदानस्य च वर्जनम्||२८||
अयमेव [१] विकाराणां सर्वेषामपि निग्रहे|
विधिर्दृष्टस्त्रिधा योऽयं क्रिमीनुद्दिश्य कीर्तितः||२९||
संशोधनं संशमनं निदानस्य च वर्जनम्|
एतावद्भिषजा कार्यं रोगे रोगे यथाविधि||३०||
Thus, it is said:
The treatment of Krumis involves

Apakarshana – removal in the beginning.

Prakruti Vighanta – Then the causative factors for their production of parasites is countered and

Nidana Tyaga – avoiding causes.

These three principles of treatment described for curing the parasitic infestation are also applicable for the cure of all diseases in general. Elimination therapy, alleviation therapy and avoidance of causative factors- these three principles along with their proper procedure is adopted for treatment of each and every disease by the physician. [28-30]

तत्र श्लोकौ-
व्याधितौ पुरुषौ ज्ञाज्ञौ भिषजौ सप्रयोजनौ|
विंशतिः क्रिमयस्तेषां हेत्वादिः सप्तको गणः||३१||
उक्तो व्याधितरूपीये विमाने परमर्षिणा|
शिष्यसम्बोधनार्थाय व्याधिप्रशमनाय च||३२||

To sum up:

Two types of patients, ignorant and wise physicians, need for correct determination, twenty types of parasites, seven aspects, viz., aetiology etc., of these parasites- all these topics are described by Lord Atreya in this chapter – Vyadhita Rupiya with a view to proper understanding of the disciples and curing the disease. [31- 32]

इत्यग्निवेशकृते तन्त्रे चरकप्रतिसंस्कृते विमानस्थाने व्याधितरूपीयविमानं नाम सप्तमोऽध्यायः||७||

Thus ends the seventh chapter on the "Determination of the specific characteristics of Different Types of Patients" of the Vimana section of Agnivesha's work as redacted by Master Charaka. [7]

16

Vimanasthana Chapter 8 Roga Bhishagjiteeya Vimanam

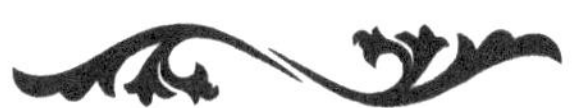

Specific Requirements for Treatment

अथातो रोगभिषग्जितीयं विमानं व्याख्यास्यामः||१||

इति ह स्माह भगवानात्रेयः||२||

athāto rogabhiṣagjitīyaṃ vimānaṃ vyākhyāsyāmaḥ||1||

iti ha smāha bhagavānātreyaḥ||2||

We shall now explore the chapter on the "Determination of the specific Requirements for the Treatment of Diseases". Thus said Lord Atreya [1-2]

Selection of a suitable medical text :

बुद्धिमानात्मनः कार्यगुरुलाघवं कर्मफलमनुबन्धं देशकालौ च विदित्वा युक्तिदर्शनादिभिषग्बुभूषुः शास्त्रमेवादितः परीक्षेत|

विविधानि हि शास्त्राणि भिषजां प्रचरन्ति लोके; तत्र यन्मन्येत सुमहद्यशस्विधीरपुरुषासेवितमर्थबहुलमाप्तजनपूजितं त्रिविधशिष्यबुद्धिहितमपगतपुनरुक्तदोषमार्षं सुप्रणीतसूत्रभाष्यसङ्ग्रहक्रमं स्वाधारमनवपतितशब्दमकष्टशब्दं पुष्कलाभिधानं क्रमागतार्थमर्थतत्त्वविनिश्चयप्रधानं सङ्गतार्थमसङ्कुलप्रकरणमाशुप्रबोधकं लक्षणवच्चोदाहरणवच्च, तदभिप्रपद्येत शास्त्रम्|

शास्त्रं ह्येवंविधममल इवादित्यस्तमो विधूय प्रकाशयति सर्वम्||३||

A wise man, desirous of adopting the medical profession should, first of all, carefully select a suitable text on medicine, depending upon his competence to undertake light or serious type of work, his willingness for short term or long-term results, his habit and age. There are several such texts available for physicians. Only the texts having the following:-

Which are followed by great, illustrious and wise physicians (for those texts which are great and popular and are followed by wise persons)

which are pregnant with ideas and respected by reputed experts

Which are conducive to the intellectual growth of disciples of all the three categories (viz highly intelligent and less intelligent)

Which are free from defects of repetition, transmitted by seers and have well knit aphorisms together with commentaries thereon in proper order

Which have elegant ideas to convey

Which are free from vulgar and difficult expressions and have clear and unambiguous expressions

Which convey ideas in an orderly manner

Which primarily deal with the determination of real objects

Which are free from contradictions

Where there is no confusion relating to contexts

Which convey ideas quickly and

Which are equipped with definitions (of etiology, symptomatology and therapeutics) and illustrations. a text of this type may be compared to the sun which removes darkness and illuminates all. [3]

Selection of a suitable preceptor:

ततोऽनन्तरमाचार्यं परीक्षेत; तद्यथा- पर्यवदातश्रुतं परिदृष्टकर्माणं दक्षं दक्षिणं शुचिं जितहस्तमुपकरणवन्तं सर्वेन्द्रियोपपन्नं प्रकृतिज्ञं प्रतिपत्तिज्ञमनुपस्कृतविद्यमनहङ्कृतमनसूयकमकोपनं क्लेशक्षमं शिष्यवत्सलमध्यापकं ज्ञापनसमर्थं चेति|

एवङ्गुणो ह्याचार्यः सुक्षेत्रमार्तवो मेघ इव शस्यगुणैः सुशिष्यमाशु वैद्यगुणैः सम्पादयति||४||

Thereafter one should assess the qualities of the preceptor. an ideal preceptor is he who is well grounded in scriptures; equipped with practical knowledge, wise, skilful, whose, prescriptions are infallible, who is pious, who has all the necessary equipments for treatment, who is not deficient in respect of any of the sense organs, who is acquainted with human nature, and the rationale of treatment, whose knowledge of other scriptures), who is free from vanity, envy and anger, who is hard working, who is affectionately disposed towards his disciples and is capable of expressing his views with clarity. A preceptor posed of such qualities infuses medical knowledge to a good disciple as the seasonal cloud helps bring about good crop in a fertile land. [4]

तमुपसृत्यारिराधयिषुरुपचरेदग्निवच्च देववच्च राजवच्च पितृवच्च भर्तृवच्चाप्रमत्तः|

ततस्तत्प्रसादात् कृत्स्नं शास्त्रमधिगम्य शास्त्रस्य दृढतायामभिधानस्य सौष्ठवेऽर्थस्य विज्ञाने वचन शक्तौ च भूयो भूयः प्रयतेत सम्यक्||५||

One should approach such a preceptor and respect him like fire, God, king, father with all cares. After having obtained the knowledge of the entire scripture, through his blessing one should strive again and again for achieving depth in scriptures, clarity of expressions, comprehension of the various concepts and power of oration. [5]

Three methods of obtaining knowledge:

तत्रोपायाननुव्याख्यास्यामः- अध्ययनम्, अध्यापनं, तद्विद्यसम्भाषा चेत्युपायाः||६||

तत्रायमध्ययनविधिः- कल्यः कृतक्षणः प्रातरुत्थायोपव्यूषं वा कृत्वाऽऽवश्यकमुपस्पृश्योदकं देवर्षिगोब्राह्मणगुरुवृद्धसिद्धाचार्येभ्यो नमस्कृत्य समे शुचौ देशे सुखोपविष्टो मनःपुरःसराभिर्वाग्भिःसूत्रमनुक्रामन् पुनः पुनरावर्तयेद् बुद्ध्वा सम्यगनुप्रविश्यार्थतत्त्वं स्वदोषपरिहारार्थं परदोषप्रमाणार्थं च; एवं मध्यन्दिनेऽपराह्णे रात्रौ च शश्वदपरिहापयन्नध्ययनमभ्यस्येत्|

इत्यध्ययनविधिः||७||

We shall now explain the ways and means for attaining objectives. They are:

1. Study
2. Teaching
3. Participations in debates.

Procedure for study:

The disciple is healthy and solely devoted to study. He should get up early in the morning or in the last quarter of the night. He should then perform ablution and offer enlightened persons and preceptors and should then sit comfortable in an even and clean place. Thereafter, he should recite the Sutras orally with due concentration.

Benefits after proper understanding, he should repeat his recitation with a view to removing his own deficiencies and testifying to the deficiencies of others. He should continue with his practice in the noon, in the afternoon and at night without any break. This is the procedure for study. [7]

Procedure for teaching:

अथाध्यापनविधिः- अध्यापने कृतबुद्धिराचार्यः शिष्यमेवादितः परीक्षेत; तद्यथा- प्रशान्तमार्यप्रकृतिकमक्षुद्रकर्माणमृजुचक्षुर्मुखनासावंशं तनुरक्तविशदजिह्वमविकृतदन्तौष्ठमिन्निमनं धृतिमन्तमनहङ्कृतं मेधाविनं वितर्कस्मृतिसम्पन्नमुदारसत्त्वं तद्विद्यकुलजमथवा तद्विद्यवृत्तं तत्त्वाभिनिवेशिनमव्यङ्गमव्यापन्नेन्द्रियं निभृतमनुद्धतमर्थतत्त्वभावकमकोपनमव्यसनिनं शीलशौचाचारानुरागदाक्ष्यप्रादक्षिण्योपपन्नमध्ययनाभिकाममर्थविज्ञाने कर्मदर्शने चानन्यकार्यमलुब्धमनलसं

सर्वभूतहितैषिणमाचार्यसर्वानुशिष्टिप्रतिकरमनुरक्तं च, एवङ्गुणसमुदितमध्याप्यमाहुः॥८॥

The preceptor planning to undertake teaching should, first of all, examine the disciple himself. Qualities of a good disciple are as follows:

tranquility

generosity

aversion to mean acts

normal condition of eyes, face and nasal ridge

thin, red and clear tongue

absence of any morbidity in teeth, lips and voice

perseverance

freedom from vanity

presence of intellect, power of reasoning and memory

liberal mindedness

birth in the family of a physician or the one having the description of truth

physical perfection

unimpaired senses

modesty and absence of ego

ability to understand the real meaning of things

absence of irritability

absence of addictions

good character, purity, conduct, love for study, enthusiasm and sympathetic disposition

devotion to study

uninterrupted taste for the theory and practice of the science

absence of greed and laziness

good- will for living beings

obedience to all the instructions of the preceptor and

Devotion to the preceptor. [8]

एवंविधमध्ययनार्थिनमुपस्थितमारिराधयिषुमाचार्योऽनुभाषेत - उदगयने शुक्लपक्षे प्रशस्तेऽहनि तिष्यहस्तश्रवणाश्वयुजामन्यतमेन नक्षत्रेण योगमुपगते भगवति शशिनि कल्याणे कल्याणे च करणे मैत्रे मुहूर्ते मुण्डः कृतोपवासः स्नातः काषायवस्त्रसंवीतः सगन्धहस्तः समिधोऽग्निमाज्यमुपलेपनमुदकुम्भान् माल्यदागदीगतिरिण्याहेमरजतमणिमुक्ताविद्रुमक्षौमपरिधीन् कुशलाजसर्षपाक्षतांश्च शुक्लानि सुमनांसि ग्रथिताग्रथितानि मेध्यान् भक्ष्यान् गन्धांश्च घृष्टानादायोपतिष्ठस्वेति॥९॥

स तथा कुर्यात्॥१०॥

When the disciple having the above mentioned (in para- 8) qualities approaches the preceptor with reverence for study, he is advised as follows:

During a favorable Muhurta (a unit of time consisting of 48 minutes and named as Shiva, Bhujaga etc.,) and auspicious Ksana (a division of the day used in astrological science), when the moon is auspicious by virtue of its conjunction with either of Pushya, Hasta, Shravana or Asvayuk constellations, in an auspicious day of the light fort- night of Uttarayana (summer solstice) the disciple should come with his hair saved, observing fast, after bath, wearing a saffron colored cloth and with fragrant material in hand. he should also bring with him Samidha (dry twigs used for offering oblation), fire, ghee, sandalwood paste, earthen jar filled with water, garlands, lamp, gold, ornaments of gold, silver, jewels, pearl, coral, silken garments, Paridhi (sticks of Palasha (Butea monosperma kuntze) of one cubic in length for being placed in the four sides of Homakunda i.e a rectangularly dug fire place for offering oblations), Kusa (Desmostachya bipinnata Stapf) , fried paddy, Sarsapa (Brassica nigra Koch), Aksata (unbroken dehusked rice), white loose flowers and garlands, prepared out of them, food articles which promote intellect and sweet scented pastes. The disciple should do accordingly. [9-10]

तमुपस्थितमाज्ञाय समे शुचौ देशे प्राक्प्रवणे उदक्प्रवणे वा चतुष्किष्कुमात्रं चतुरस्रं स्थण्डिलं गोमयोदकेनोपलिप्तं कुशास्तीर्णं सुपरिहितं परिधिभिश्चतुर्दिशं यथोक्तचन्दनोदकुम्भक्षौमहेमहिरण्यरजतमणिमुक्ताविद्रुमालङ्कृतं मेध्यभक्ष्यगन्धशुक्लपुष्पलाजसर्षपाक्षतोपशोभितं कृत्वा, तत्र पालाशीभिरैङ्गुदीभिरौदुम्बरीभिर्माधुकीभिर्वा समिद्भिरग्निमुपसमाधाय प्राङ्मुखः शुचिरध्ययनविधिमनुविधाय मधुसर्पिभ्र्यां त्रिस्त्रिर्जुहुयादग्निमाशीःसम्प्रयुक्तैर्मन्त्रैर्ब्रह्माणमग्निं धन्वन्तरिं प्रजापतिमश्विनाविन्द्रमृषींश्च सूत्रकारानभिमन्त्रयमाणः पूर्वं स्वाहेति||११||

शिष्यश्चैनमन्वालभेत|

हुत्वा च प्रदक्षिणमग्निमनुपरिक्रामेत्|

परिक्रम्य ब्राह्मणान् स्वस्ति वाचयेत्; भिषजश्चाभिपूजयेत्||१२||

When the disciple comes with the preparations mentioned above, the physician should get constructed a Sthanila (an elevated place of the shape of a square and of four cubits in size) in an even and pure place having slope towards the east or the north.

The place is smeared with cow dung, spread with Kusha grass (Desmostachya bipinnata Stapf) and provided with good brooder on all the four sides. This place is then decorated with sandal paste, earthen jar, water, silken garments, gold, ornaments of gold, silver, jewels, pearls, corals, food articles which promote intellect, fragrant things, white flowers, fried paddy, mustard seeds, and broken dehusked rice which have already been described above (in para 9). Then fire is ignited in that place with the help of dried twig of Palasa (Butea monosperma), Ingudi, Udumbara (Ficus racemosa Linn) or Madhuka Glycyrrhiza glabra

The physician facing towards the east with purity of mind and reciting the benedictory Mantras ending with Svaha for Brahma, Agni, Dhanvatari, Prajapati, the Asvins, Indra, Rises and Authors of Hymns- three times each.

The disciple should follow the preceptor. After offering oblations he should take a round of the fire keeping it to the right side. After taking the round, Brahmanas may be made to recite propitiatory hymns. He should then offer prayers to the physicians. [11-12]

Instruction about general behavior of the student:

अथैनमग्निसकाशे ब्राह्मणसकाशे भिषक्सकाशे चानुशिष्यात्- ब्रह्मचारिणा श्मश्रुधारिणा सत्यवादिनाऽमांसादेन मेध्यसेविना निर्मत्सरेणाशस्त्रधारिणा च भवितव्यं, न च ते मद्वचनात् किञ्चिदकार्यं स्यादन्यत्र राजद्विष्टात् प्राणहरादिवपुलादधर्म्यादनर्थसम्प्रयुक्तादवाऽप्यर्थात्; मदर्पणेन मत्प्रधानेन मदधीनेन मत्प्रियहितानुवर्तिना च शश्वद्भवितव्यं, पुत्रवद्दासवदर्थिवच्चोपचरताऽनुवस्तव्योऽहम्, अनुत्सेकेनावहितेनानन्यमनसा विनीतेनावेक्ष्यावेक्ष्यकारिणाऽनसूयकेन चाभ्यनुज्ञातेन प्रविचरितव्यम्, अनुज्ञातेन (चाननुज्ञातेन च) प्रविचरता पूर्वं गुर्वर्थोपाहरणे यथाशक्ति प्रयतितव्यं, कर्मसिद्धिमर्थसिद्धं यशोलाभं प्रेत्य च स्वर्गमिच्छता भिषजा त्वया गोब्राह्मणमादौ कृत्वा सर्वप्राणभृतां शर्माशासितव्यमहरहरुत्तिष्ठता चोपविशता च, सर्वात्मना चातुराणामारोग्याय प्रयतितव्यं, जीवितहेतोरपि चातुरेभ्यो नाभिद्रोग्धव्यं, मनसाऽपि च परस्त्रियो नाभिगमनीयास्तथा सर्वमेव परस्वं, निभृतवेशपरिच्छदेन भवितव्यम्, अशौण्डेनापापेनापापसहायेन च, श्लक्ष्णशुक्लधर्म्यशर्म्यधन्यसत्यहितमितवचसा देशकालविचारिणा स्मृतिमता ज्ञानोत्थानोपकरणसम्पत्सु नित्यं यत्नवता च; न च कदाचिद्राजद्विष्टानां राजद्वेषिणां वा महाजनद्विष्टानां महाजनद्वेषिणां वाऽप्यौषधमनुविधातव्यं, तथा सर्वेषामत्यर्थविकृतदुष्टदुःखशीलाचारोपचाराणामनपवादप्रतिकारणां मुमूर्षूणां च, तथैवासन्निहितेश्वराणां स्त्रीणामनध्यक्षाणां वा; न च कदाचित् स्त्रीदत्तमामिषमादातव्यमननुज्ञातं भर्त्राऽथवाऽध्यक्षेण, आतुरकुलं चानुप्रविशता विदितेनानुमतप्रवेशिना सार्धं पुरुषेण सुसंवीतेनावाक्शिरसा स्मृतिमता स्तिमितेनावेक्ष्यावेक्ष्य मनसा सर्वमाचरता सम्यगनुप्रवेष्टव्यम्, अनुप्रविश्य च वाङ्मनोबुद्धीन्द्रियाणि न क्वचित् प्रणिधातव्यान्यन्यत्रातुरादातुरोपकारार्थादातुरगतेष्वन्येषु वा भावेषु, न चातुरकुलप्रवृत्तयो बहिर्निश्चारयितव्याः, ह्रसितं चायुषः प्रमाणमातुरस्य जानताऽपि त्वया न वर्णयितव्यं तत्र यत्रोच्यमानमातुरस्यान्यस्य वाऽप्युपघाताय सम्पद्यते; ज्ञानवताऽपि च नात्यर्थमात्मनो ज्ञाने विकत्थितव्यम्, आप्तादपि हि विकत्थमानादत्यर्थमुद्विजन्त्यनेके||१३||

In front of the fire, Brahmanas and physicians, the preceptor should instruct his disciples as below:

You should observe Brahmacharya, maintain your beard, speak the truth, take vegetarian food, resort to such food and regimens as are conducive to the promotion of intellect, refrain from envy and carry no weapon with you.

You should always obey my instruction except when they go against the ruler of the land, or they are directed towards your death or they involve sinful commitments considerably or bring about calamity.

You should always be devoted to me, surrender yourself to my superiority, be subordinate to me and behave in a manner which will be pleasant and useful to me.

You should due regards to me as if you are my son, servant or supplicant.

You should act without ego, with cares and affection, with undisturbed mind, with modesty, with proper vigilance, without jealousy and with obedience for my instructions.

Acting either at my instance or otherwise, you should first of all try to collect to the best of your ability the things desired by your preceptor.

If you want to achieve success in your medical perfection, earn wealth as well as fame and attain heaven the well-being of cows, Brahmanas and all other living beings.

We should make efforts to cure the patient.

You must never give any ill will towards your patients even at the cost of your life.

You should not even think of committing adultery and should not aspire for any property belonging to others.

Your appearance and apparel should make you look modest.

You should not take wine, commit sins or have association with those committing sinful acts.

Your speech is pleasant, pure, righteous, blissful, excellent, truthful, useful and moderate.

Your behavior is in conformity with the time and place, based on the recollections of the past experience.

You should always make efforts for the upliftment of your knowledge and adoption of such methods as would give you good health.

You should not prescribe medicines for those who are despaired by the king or noble persons and those who despised the king or noble persons and those who despise the King or noble persons.

You should not treat all those who are excessively artificial in their behavior, are wicked or of miserable conduct and behavior or who have not been absolved of the allegations against them or who are going to succumb to death.

Women in the absence of their husbands and guardians should not be treated by you.

You should not do any joyful thing given by a woman without the permission of her husband or guardian.

You should enter the residence of the patient accompanied by a person who knows the place and who, on his part, has obtained permission to enter there. While doing so you are well clad, with your head bowed down, having a good memory, having concentration of mind and acting with proper thinking. After having entered three your speech, mind, intellect and senses is entirely devoted to nothing except the welfare of the patient and allied matters.

Family customs (secrets) should not be disclosed by you to outsiders.

Even having known that the patient's span of life has come to a close, you should not disclose this to the patient because it may cause shock to the patient or to his relatives.

Even though you are actually possessed of wisdom, you should not exhibit it to others. Many people get very irritated with others. Many people get very much irritated to hear such self- praise even from a saint. [13]

न चैव ह्यस्ति सुतरमायुर्वेदस्य पारं, तस्मादप्रमत्तः शश्वदभियोगमस्मिन् गच्छेत्, एतच्च कार्यम्, एवम्भूयश्च वृत्तसौष्ठवमनसूयता परेभ्योऽप्यागमयितव्यं, कृत्स्नो हि लोको बुद्धिमतामाचार्यः शत्रुश्चाबुद्धिमताम्, अतश्चाभिसमीक्ष्य बुद्धिमताऽमित्रस्यापि धन्यं यशस्यमायुष्यं पौष्टिकं लौक्यमभ्युपदिशतो वचः श्रोतव्यमनुविधातव्यं चेति|

अतः परमिदं ब्रूयात्- देवताग्निद्विजगुरुवृद्धसिद्धाचार्येषु ते नित्यं सम्यग्वर्तितव्यं, तेषु ते सम्यग्वर्तमानस्यायमग्निः सर्वगन्धरसरत्नबीजानि यथेरिताश्च देवताः शिवाय स्युः, अतोऽन्यथा वर्तमानस्याशिवायेति|

एवं ब्रुवति चाचार्ये शिष्यः 'तथा' इति ब्रूयात्|

यथोपदेशं च कुर्वन्नध्याप्यः, अतोऽन्यथा त्वनध्याप्यः|

अध्याप्यमध्यापयन् ह्याचार्यो यथोक्तैश्चाध्यापनफलैर्योगमाप्नोत्यन्यैश्चानुक्तैः श्रेयस्करैर्गुणैः शिष्यमात्मानं च युनक्ति|

इत्यध्यापनविधिरुक्तः||१४||

It is not easy to acquire comprehensive knowledge of the "Science of life". Therefore, one should make honest efforts to be in constant touch with this science. One should strive to acquire quantities (described in para- 13), one should learn similar noble qualities even from his enemies without having any sense of jealousy.

The wise consider the entire unversed as their preceptor; it is only the unwise who consider it to be their enemy. One should, therefore, have the proper advice which brings fame, which promotes longevity and nourishment and which is acceptable to the people. Such advice can be had even from an enemy and be adopted in practice.

Thereafter, the preceptor should say, always behave well with the gods, fire Brahmanas, preceptors, elders, persons who have attained perfection and teachers. If you do so, fire, all types of smell, tastes, jewels, seeds and the gods will bless you. Otherwise, they will be unfavorably disposed towards you."

To the preceptor advising as above, the disciple should say, "tatha". I.e., I shall act accordingly. It is only when the disciple acts accordingly; he can be considered eligible for studies. a teacher gets all the auspicious fruits of teaching those described in scriptures and those that are not described- and gets himself and the disciple endowed with the virtuous qualities only when the disciple is worthy of teaching. Thus, the procedure of teaching has been described. [14]

Procedure for debates:

सम्भाषाविधिमत ऊर्ध्वं व्याख्यास्यामः- भिषक् भिषजा सह सम्भाषेत|

तद्विद्यसम्भाषा हि ज्ञानाभियोगसंहर्षकरी भवति, वैशारद्यमपि चाभिनिर्वर्तयति, वचनशक्तिमपि चाधत्ते, यशश्चाभिदीपयति, पूर्वश्रुते च सन्देहवतः पुनः श्रवणाच्छुतसंशयमपकर्षति, श्रुते चासन्देहवतो भूयोऽध्यवसायमभिनिर्वर्तयति, अश्रुतमपि च कञ्चिदर्थं श्रोत्रविषयमापादयति, यच्चाचार्यः शिष्याय शुश्रूषवे प्रसन्नः क्रमेणोपदिशति गुह्याभिमतमर्थजातं तत् परस्परेण सह जल्पन् पिण्डेन विजिगीषुराह संहर्षात्, तस्मात्तद्विद्यसम्भाषामभिप्रशंसन्ति कुशलाः||१५||

द्विविधा तु खलु तद्विद्यसम्भाषा भवति- सन्धायसम्भाषा, विगृह्यसम्भाषा च||१६||

Hereafter we shall explore the procedure for debates. A physician should participate in a discussion with another physician. Professional discussion indeed promotes the power of application of knowledge and competition leading to enlightenment. It manifests the clarity of knowledge, promoters the power of speech, spreads fame, eliminates doubts reminiscent of the previous study by repeated hearing and brings about confirmation of what is undoubtedly understood before.

During the course of discussion, one comes to know of many new things which were not heard by him previously. Being pleased over the devoted disciple, the preceptor during the course of teaching elaborates some secret meanings.

The participants during the course of mutual discussion enthusiastically disclose these secret meanings in brief with a view to achieving a victory over the competitor. Therefore, participation in professional debates is always applauded by the wise.

Professional discussions are of the types, viz (i) friendly discussions and (ii) hostile discussions. [15-16]

Procedure for friendly discussion:

तत्र ज्ञानविज्ञानवचनप्रतिवचनशक्तिसम्पन्नेनाकोपनेनानुपस्कृतविद्येनानसूयकेनानुनयेनानुनयकोविदेन क्लेशक्षमेण प्रियसम्भाषणेन च सह सन्धायसम्भाषा विधीयते|

तथाविधेन सह कथयन् विस्रब्धः कथयेत्, पृच्छेदपि च विस्रब्धः, पृच्छते चास्मै विस्रब्धाय विशदमर्थं ब्रूयात्, न च निग्रहभयादुद्विजेत्, निगृह्य चैनं न हृष्येत्, न च परेषु विकत्थेत, न च मोहादेकान्तग्राही स्यात्, न चाविदितमर्थमनुवर्णयेत्, सम्यक् चानुनयेनानुनयेत्, तत्र चावहितः स्यात्|

इत्यनुलोमसम्भाषाविधिः||१७||

One should have friendly discussions with persons of learning possessed of scientific knowledge, powder of argument and counter argument, who do not get irritated, who are endowed with correct knowledge, who are not jealous, who can be made to understand, who are competent in convincing others, who are capable of facing difficult situations and who can address in a sweet tone.

One should confidently discuss with such persons and ask them questions. When he asks anything, it is elaborately; described with confidence. One should not get worried under the apprehension of getting defecated, one should not rejoice by defeating such opponents. One should not hold extreme views under delusion. One should try to bring round the other party with politeness and not by deception. One is very careful to behave politely with his opponents.

This is the procedure for "Friendly discussions". [17]

Procedure to be adopted in a discussion:
अत ऊर्ध्वमितरेण सह विगृह्य सम्भाषायां जल्पेच्छ्रेयसा योगमात्मनः पश्यन्|
प्रागेव च जल्पाज्जल्पान्तरं परावरान्तरं परिषदि्वशेषांश्च सम्यक् परीक्षेत|
सम्यक्परीक्षा हि बुद्धिमतां कार्यप्रवृत्तिनिवृत्तिकालौ शंसति, तस्मात् परीक्षामभिप्रशंसन्ति कुशलाः|
परीक्षमाणस्तु खलु परावरान्तरमिमान् जल्पकगुणाञ् श्रेयस्करान्दोषवतश्च परीक्षेत सम्यक्; तद्यथा- श्रुतं विज्ञानं धारणं प्रतिभानं वचनशक्तिरिति, एतान् गुणान् श्रेयस्करानाहुः; इमान् पुनर्दोषवतः, तद्यथा- कोपनत्वमवैशारद्यं भीरुत्वमधारणत्वमनवहितत्वमिति|
एतान् गुणान् गुरुलाघवतः परस्य चैवात्मनश्च तुलयेत्||१८||
With persons other than preceptor and Brahmacarins (class-mates), one should go in for a "hostile discussion", provided he is confident of his superiority. Before entering into the discussion, the procedure proposed to be adopted by the opponent and the disposition of the members of the assembly is carefully examined. A wise person determines the time of entering into or giving up the discussion only through proper examination. Hence proper examination is always advisable.

There are some good and bad qualities of the participants in a discussion. With a view to determining the superiority or inferiority of onself in respect of his or his opponent, one should carefully examine these good and bad qualities.

Good qualities of participants are the knowledge of the text, practical experience, and power of retention, presence of mind and eloquence.

Bad qualities of the participants are irritation, lack of skill, cowardice, lack of the powder of retention and carelessness. One should compare the strength or weakness of himself and of his opponent in respcct of these qualities. [18]

Three types of opponents:
तत्र त्रिविधः परः सम्पद्यते- प्रवरः, प्रत्यवरः, समो वा, गुणविनिक्षेपतः; नत्वेव कात्स्न्र्येन||१९||
Depending upon the presence of the above-mentioned qualities, the opponent may belong to the three categories, viz., (i) superior (ii) inferior or, (iii) equal.
However, other factors like family status, conduct, religious etc., should not be taken into account in this connection. [19]

Two types of Assembly:
परिषत् खलु दि्विविधा- ज्ञानवती, मूढपरिषच्च|
सैव दि्विविधा सती त्रिविधा पुनरनेन कारणविभागेन- सुहृत्परिषत्, उदासीनपरिषत्, प्रतिनिविष्टपरिषच्चेति [१]|
तत्र प्रतिनिविष्टायां परिषदि ज्ञानविज्ञानवचनप्रतिवचनशक्तिसम्पन्नायां मूढायां वा न कथं चित् केनचित् सह जल्पो विधीयते; मूढायां तु सुहृत्परिषदुदासीनायां वा ज्ञानविज्ञानवचनप्रतिवचनशक्तीरन्तरेणाप्यीदीप्तयशसा महाजनविदि्वष्टेनापि सह जल्पो विधीयते|

तद्विधेन च सह कथयता आविद्धदीर्घसूत्रसङ्कुलैर्वाक्यदण्डकैः कथयितव्यम्, अतिहृष्टं मुहुर्मुहुरुपहसता परं निरूपयता च पर्षदमाकारैर्ब्रुवतश्चास्य वाक्यावकाशो न देयः; कष्टशब्दं च ब्रुवता वक्तव्यो नोच्यते, अथवा पुनर्हीना ते प्रतिज्ञा, इति|

पुनश्चाहू(ह्व)यमानः प्रतिवक्तव्यः- परिसंवत्सरो भवान् शिक्षस्व तावत्; न त्वया गुरुरुपासितो नूनम्, अथवा पर्याप्तमेतावत्; सकृदपि हि परिक्षेपिकं निहतं निहतमाहुरिति नास्य योगः कर्तव्यः कथञ्चित्|

अप्येवं श्रेयसा सह विगृह्य वक्तव्यमित्याहुरेके; नत्वेवं ज्यायसा सह विग्रहं प्रशंसन्ति कुशलाः||२०||

An assembly is of two types viz, (i) enlightened and (ii) dull on the basis of different criteria; both these types of an assembly may be classified into three types viz. (i) friendly, (ii) netural and (iii) prejudicial.

Members of an assembly may be enlightened (endowed with knowledge, experience, power of speech and contradiction) or dull but if they are prejudicial, then one should never enter into a discussion with anybody, not even with the most wetched on, in such an assembly.

If the members of the assembly are dull but friendly or neutral, then the individual should enter into discussion with an opponent who is not very famous and is even despised by great people even without theoreticaland practical knowledge or power.

While discussing with such an opponent, one should use such long sentences as difficult to understand or are composed of long and complicated aphorisms. An over excited opponent is ridiculed and the individual should continue his speech acting as if addressing the assembly, without giving an opportunity for the opponent to speak.

One should speak using such terms as are difficult to understand and the opponent is told that he was incapable of advancing any argument in the matter and his proposition had failed. If the opponent challenges again, he is told, "You should study for at least one more year to have some more experience in debates. Probably you have not observed the guidance of your preceptor well. "Or else, he is told, "this is sufficient for you." Once the opponent is defeated, he remains defeated forever; hence his further challenge for discussion should not be accepted.

Some people advise that the same procedure is followed even while discussing with a superior opponent. But the wise do not approve of such a proposition to enter into hostile discussion with a superior opponent.

While discussing with the opponent in a debate, methods of which are not enlightened, one should use complicated sentences so that members of the assembly will find it very difficult to understand. By implication, the user of such words and sentences will be credited with success. [20]

Procedure for debate with an opponent of inferior or equal type:

प्रत्यवरेण तु सह समानाभिमतेन वा विगृह्य जल्पता सुहृत्परिषदि कथयितव्यम्, अथवाऽप्युदासीनपरिषद्यवधानश्रवणज्ञानविज्ञानोपधारणवचनप्रतिवचनशक्तिसम्पन्नायां कथयता चावहितेन परस्य साद्गुण्यदोषबलमवेक्षितव्यं, समवेक्ष्य च यत्रैनं श्रेष्ठं मन्येत नास्य तत्र जल्पं योजयेदनाविष्कृतमयोगं कुर्वन्; यत्र त्वेनमवरं मन्येत तत्रैवैनमाशु निगृह्णीयात्|

तत्र खल्विमे प्रत्यवराणामाशु निग्रहे भवन्त्युपायाः; तद्यथा- श्रुतिहीनं महता सूत्रपाठेनाभिभवेत्, विज्ञानहीनं पुनः कष्टशब्देन वाक्येन, वाक्यधारणाहीनमाविद्धदीर्घसूत्रसङ्कुलैर्वाक्यदण्डकैः, प्रतिभाहीनं पुनर्वचनेनैकविधेनानेकार्थवाचिना, वचनशक्तिहीनमर्धोक्तस्य वाक्यस्याक्षेपेण, अविशारदमपत्रपणेन, कोपनमायासनेन, भीरुं वित्रासनेन, अनवहितं नियमनेनेति|

एवमेतैरुपायैः परमवरमभिभवेच्छीघ्रम्||२१||

With an opponent of inferior or equal type, one should enter into hostile discussion if the members of the assembly are favorably disposed towards him. In an assembly where members are natural and are attentive, inclined to hear, learned, experienced, having the power of retention, speech and contradistinction; one should carefully observe the good and bad qualities of the opponent as a participant in the discussion.

On the basis of these observations, if the opponent is found to belong to a superior category, then one should not enter into discussion on the same topic. Without letting the assembly know, he should change the topic of discussion to a favorable one. If the opponent is found to be of inferior category, then efforts are made to defeat him immediately in a hostile discussion.

The following procedure is adopted for immediately defeating an opponent of inferior category. If the opponent is not a learned person, then he is defeated by citing long aphorisms; if he is not experienced then by such words and sentences as are difficult to understand; if he is unable to retain sentences by memory then by sentences composed of complicated and long aphorisms; if he is dull then by statements of the same type (composed of the same words) but carrying different meaning with half of a sentence (the opponent in that case is required to fill up the other half); if he has no experience of participating in seminars then by putting him to a disgraceful situation; if he is irritable, then by creating difficult situations for him; if he is cowardice then by creating fearful situations and if he is not careful by adhering to the discipline of discussion.

These are the procedures to be followed for immediately defeating the opponent of an inferior category. [21]

तत्र श्लोकौ-
विगृह्य कथयेद्युक्त्या युक्तं च न निवारयेत्।
विगृह्यभाषा तीव्रं हि केषाञ्चिद्द्रोहमावहेत्||२२||
नाकार्यमस्ति क्रुद्धस्य नावाच्यमपि विद्यते।
कुशला नाभिनन्दन्ति कलहं समितौ सताम्||२३||
एवं प्रवृत्ते वादे कुर्यात्||२४||
Thus, it is said: In fighting discussion one should make careful statements and should not overrule the statements (of opponents) which are well authenticated. Some people get excessively irritated during hostile discussions and there is nothing which cannot be done or said by the enraged one. Therefore, in an assembly of learned people, the wise never appreciate a quarrel. This is how one should participate in a debate. [22-24]

प्रागेव तावदिदं कर्तुं यतेत- सन्धाय पर्षदाऽयनभूतमात्मनः प्रकरणमादेशयितव्यं, यद्वा परस्य भृशदुर्गं स्यात्, पक्षमथवा परस्य भृशं विमुखमानयेत्; परिषदि चोपसंहितायामशक्यमस्माभिर्वक्तुम्, एषैव ते परिषद्यथेष्टं यथायोगं यथाभिप्रायं वादं वादमर्यादां च स्थापयिष्यतीत्युक्त्वा तूष्णीमासीत्||२५||

The prevail upon should proceed like this: one should prevail upon the assembly to select such a topic as is favorable to himself and is exceedingly difficult for the opponent to discuss.

Or the opponent is made to take such a side in the discussion which will be disliked by the members of the assembly. When the assembly supports the stand taken by him, he should say, "I have nothing more to say. The assembly, according to the choice, may sufficiently and appropriately decide upon the validity of the debate and its limitations, "he should observe silence, thereafter. [25]

तत्रेदं वादमर्यादालक्षणं भवति- इदं वाच्यम्, इदमवाच्यम्, एवं पराजितो भवतीति||२६||
The following factors bear importance in deterring the limits of a fighting debate:
Things which is said
Things which should not be said
The point of defeat [26]

Logical terms to be acquainted with by debaters:

इमानि तु खलु पदानि भिषग्वादमार्गज्ञानार्थमधिगम्यानि भवन्ति; तद्यथा- वादः, द्रव्यं, गुणाः, कर्म, सामान्यं, विशेषः, समवायः, प्रतिज्ञा, स्थापना, प्रतिष्ठापना, हेतुः, दृष्टान्तः, उपनयः, निगमनम्, उत्तरं, सिद्धान्तः, शब्दः, प्रत्यक्षम्, अनुमानम्, ऐतिह्यम्, औपम्यं, संशयः, प्रयोजनं, सव्यभिचारं, जिज्ञासा, व्यवसायः, अर्थप्राप्तिः, सम्भवः, अनुयोज्यम्, अननुयोज्यम्, अनुयोगः, प्रत्यनुयोगः, वाक्यदोषः, वाक्यप्रशंसा, छलम्, अहेतुः, अतीतकालम्, उपालम्भः, परिहारः, प्रतिज्ञाहानिः, अभ्यनुज्ञा, हेत्वन्तरम्, अर्थान्तरं, निग्रहस्थानमिति||२७||

Acquaintances with the following term help in the determination of the course of debate among physicians:

Vada (debate)

Dravya (Substance)

Guna (attributes)

Karman(action)

Samanya (generic concomitance)

Vishesha (variant factor)

Samavaya (inseparable concomittance)

Pratijna(proposition)

Sthapana(justification)

Pratisthapana (counter argument)

Hetu (cause)

Drstanta (example)

Upanaya (subsumptive correlation)

Nigamana (final conclusion

Uttara(rejoinder)

Siddhanta (conclusion truth)

Sabda(words)

Pratyaksa (direct observation)

Anumana (Inference)

Aitihya (words of divine origin)

Aupamya (analogy)

Samsaya(doubt)

Prayojana(object)

Savyabhicara (statements with exceptions)

Jijnasa (enquiry)

Vyavasaya (determination)

Arthaprapti (defective statement)

Sambhava (source)

Ananuyoja (defective statement)

Anuyoja (infallible statement)

Anuyoga (scriptural equity)

Pratyanuyoga (scriptural counter enquiry)

Vakyadosha (syntactical defects)

Vakyaprasamsa (syntactical excellence)

Chala (causuistry)

Ahetu (casual fallacy)

Atitakala (defiance of temporal order)

Upalambha (pointing out defects in casuistry)

Parihara (correction)

Pratijnahani (shift from the original proposition)

Abhyanujna (confessional retort)

Hetvantara (fallacy of reason)

Arthantara (irrelevant statement)

Nigrahasthana (clinchers) [27]

Vada (debate):
तत्र वादो नाम स यत् परेण सह शास्त्रपूर्वकं विगृह्य कथयति|
स च द्विविधः सङ्ग्रहेण- जल्पः, वितण्डा च|
तत्र पक्षाश्रितयोर्वचनं जल्पः, जल्पविपर्ययो वितण्डा|
यथा- एकस्य पक्षः पुनर्भवोऽस्तीति, नास्तीत्यपरस्य; तौ च स्वस्वपक्षहेतुभिः स्वस्वपक्षं स्थापयतः, परपक्षमुद्भावयतः, एष जल्पः|
जल्पविपर्ययो वितण्डा|
वितण्डा नाम परपक्षे दोषवचनमात्रमेव||२८||
A debate may be defined as a hostile discussion with an opponent based on scriptures. This is of two types, viz (i) Jalpa (disputation) and Vitanda (Wrangling). Advancement of one's own view while contradicting the opponent is Jalpa (disputation); otherwise, the discussion is Vitanda (Wrangling).

For example, if one of the participants debated in favor of the existence of Punarjanma (rebirth) and the other against it, and both of them advance arguments in support of their own views contradicting the other's viewpoint, this is known as Jalpa (disputation).

In Vitanda (Wrangling) type of debate, only the opponents' views are contradicted without advancing arguments in support of the individual's own views. [28]

द्रव्य-गुण-कर्म-सामान्य-विशेष-समवायाः स्वलक्षणैः श्लोकस्थाने पूर्वमुक्ताः||२९||
Dravya (matter), Guna (attributes), Karman (action), Samanya (generic concomitance), Vishesha (variant factor) and Samanya (inseparable concomitance) all these along with their definitions are already described in the first chapter of Sutra section. [29]

Pratijna (Proposition):
अथ प्रतिज्ञा- प्रतिज्ञा नाम साध्यवचनं; यथा- नित्यः पुरुष इति||३०||
Pratijna may be defined as an assertion about the object to be proved (major terms); e.g the purusha (soul) is eternal. [30]

Sthapana (justification):
अथ स्थापना स्थापना नाम तस्या एव प्रतिज्ञाया हेतुदृष्टान्तोपनयनिगमनैः स्थापना|
पूर्वं हि प्रतिज्ञा, पश्चात् स्थापना, किं ह्यप्रतिज्ञातं स्थापयिष्यति; यथा- नित्यः पुरुष इति प्रतिज्ञा; हेतुः- अकृतकत्वादिति; दृष्टान्तः - यथाऽऽकाशमिति; उपनयः- यथा चाकृतकमाकाशं, तच्च नित्यं, तथा पुरुष इति; निगमनं- तस्मान्नित्य इति||३१||
अथ हेतुः- हेतुर्नामोपलब्धिकारणं; तत् प्रत्यक्षम्, अनुमानम्, ऐतिह्यम्, औपम्यमिति; एभिर्हेतुभिर्यदुपलभ्यते तत् तत्त्वम्||३३||
Sthapana may be defined as the justification of the proposition by dint of the Hetu (statement of probans), Drstanta (corroborative instance), Upanaya (subsumptive correlation), a Nigamana (final conclusion) the proposition comes first and then its justification.

How can one justify anything, unless it is proposed? For example, one can propose that the "soul is eternal "Therefore, he would make a statement that it is so because it is not produced by anyone. Then he would cite Akasha as the corroborative instance elucidating (subsumptive correlation) further that as Akasha is not produced by anybody and is, therefore, eternal so is the soul, he would finally conclude (final conclusion) that the soul is eternal. [31]

Pratisthapana (counter argument):
अथ प्रतिष्ठापना- प्रतिष्ठापना नाम या तस्या एव परप्रतिज्ञाया विपरीतार्थस्थापना|

यथा- अनित्यः पुरुष इति प्रतिज्ञा ; हेतुः- ऐन्द्रियकत्वादिति; दृष्टान्तः- यथा घट इति, उपनयो- यथा घट ऐन्द्रियकः स चानित्यः, तथा चायमिति; निगमनं- तस्मादनित्य इति||३२||

Pratisthapana stands for a counter- argument against the proposition set forth by an opponent. E. G, if the opponent argues in favor of the eternity of the soul, the corresponding counter argument would be "the soul is ephemeral" because it is perceived by a sense organ like a pitcher; that is to say, as a picture is perceived by sense organs and it is ephemeral, so also the soul is perceivable by sense organs and it is ephemeral, the conclusion is that the soul is ephemeral. [32]

Hetu (cause):

अथ हेतुः- हेतुर्नामोपलब्धिकारणं; तत् प्रत्यक्षम्, अनुमानम्, ऐतिह्यम्, औपम्यमिति; एभिर्हेतुभिर्यदुपलभ्यते तत् तत्त्वम्||३३||

Means for obtaining the knowledge (observing the object) constitute the Hetu or cause. They are of four types, viz, (1) direct observation, (2) inference, (3) tradition and, (4) analogy the knowledge obtained through these factors is valid. [33]

Drstanta (example):

अथ दृष्टान्तः- दृष्टान्तो नाम यत्र मूर्खविदुषां बुद्धिसाम्यं, यो वर्ण्य वर्णयति |
यथा- अग्निरुष्णः, द्रवमुदकं, स्थिरा पृथिवी, आदित्यः प्रकाशक इति; यथा आदित्यः प्रकाशकस्तथा साङ्ख्य ज्ञानं प्रकाशकमिति||३४||

Description of universal truths comprehensible by the wise and ignorant alike is known as Drstanta or it illustrates the object. For example, fire is hot, water is liquid, earth is stable and the sun is illuminating. As the sun is illuminating so also the knowledge obtained from the Samkhya system of philosophy is illuminating. [34]

उपनयो निगमनं चोक्तं स्थापनाप्रतिष्ठापनाव्याख्यायाम्||३५||

While explaining Sthapana (proposition) and Pratisthapana (counter proposition) in verses 31-32 above, Upanaya (subsumptive correlation) and Nigamana (final conclusion) have already been explained. [35]

Uttara (rejoinder):

अथोतरम्- उतरं नाम साधर्म्योपदिष्टे हेतौ वैधर्म्यवचनं, वैधर्म्योपदिष्टे वा हेतौ साधर्म्यवचनम्|
यथा- 'हेतुसधर्माणो विकाराः, शीतकस्य हि व्याधेर्हेतुभिः साधर्म्य हिमशिशिरवातसंस्पर्शाः', इति ब्रुवतः परो ब्रूयात्- हेतुविधर्माणो विकाराः, यथा शरीरावयवानां दाहौष्ण्यकोथप्रपचने हेतुवैधर्म्य हिमशिशिरवातसंस्पर्शा इति|
एतत् सविपर्ययमुत्तरम्||३६||

Uttara (rejoinder) stands for refutation of the argument showing correlation of homologous and heterogonous substances by citing examples of homologous and heterogeneous casual relationships respectively.

E.g, if somebody says, "Diseases are similar to their causative factors because cold fever is caused by factors having identical properties, viz, exposure to snow and cold wind" the Uttara (rejoinder) would be, "diseases are dissimilar to their causative factors because burning and heating sensations, suppuration and Flammation of organs of the body are caused by the exposure to snow and cold wind."

Thus, the Rejoinder along with the counter-rejoinder is described. [36]

Siddhanta (Demonstrated Truth):

अथ सिद्धान्तः- सिद्धान्तो नाम स यः परीक्षकैर्बहुविधं परीक्ष्य हेतुभिश्च साधयित्वा स्थाप्यते निर्णयः|
स चतुर्विधः- सर्वतन्त्रसिद्धान्तः, प्रतितन्त्रसिद्धान्तः, अधिकरणसिद्धान्तः, अभ्युपगमसिद्धान्तश्चेति|
तत्र सर्वतन्त्रसिद्धान्तो नाम तस्मिंस्तस्मिन् सर्वस्मिंस्तन्त्रे ततत् प्रसिद्धं; यथा सन्ति निदानानि, सन्ति व्याधयः, सन्ति सिद्ध्युपायाः साध्यानामिति|
प्रतितन्त्रसिद्धान्तो नाम तस्मिंस्तस्मिन्नेकैकस्मिंस्तन्त्रे ततत् प्रसिद्धं; यथा- अन्यत्राष्टौ रसाः षडत्र, पञ्चेन्द्रियाण्यत्र षडिन्द्रियाण्यन्यत्र

तन्त्रे, वातादिकृताः सर्वे विकारा यथाऽन्यत्र, अत्र वातादिकृता भूतकृताश्च प्रसिद्धाः|
अधिकरणसिद्धान्तो नाम स यस्मिन्नधिकरणे प्रस्तूयमाने सिद्धान्यन्यान्यप्यधिकरणानि भवन्ति, यथा- 'न मुक्तः कर्मानुबन्धिकं कुरुते,
निस्पृहत्वात् इति प्रस्तुते सिद्धाः कर्मफल-मोक्ष-पुरुष-प्रत्यभावा भवन्ति|
अभ्युपगमसिद्धान्तो नाम स यमर्थमसिद्धमपरीक्षितमनुपदिष्टमहेतुकं वा वादकालेऽभ्युपगच्छन्ति भिषजः; तद्यथा- द्रव्यं प्रधानमिति
कृत्वा वक्ष्यामः, गुणाः प्रधानमिति कृत्वा वक्ष्यामः, वीर्यं प्रधानमिति कृत्वा वक्ष्यामः, इत्येवमादिः|
इति चतुर्विधः सिद्धान्तः||३७||

A demonstrated truth established after several examinations and reasoning is known as Siddhanta. It is of four types
as follows:

- Sarvatantra Siddhanta or truth common to all scriptures. e.g., existence of causative factors of diseases and
  existence of curatives for curable diseases.
- Pratitantra Siddhanta or truth specific to a given scripture, e.g., in other scriptures Rasas (tastes) are described
  to be of eight types but in this text, they are of six types only; here Indriyas (senses) are described to be five in
  number but in other scriptures they are six; in other scriptures all diseases are described to be caused by Doshas
  viz, vata etc, but here diseases are caused by Doshas Viz, Vata etc., as well as evil spirits) (germs).
- Adhikarna Siddhanta or truth implied from a given context. E.G no liberated soul indulges in action leading
  to bondage for he is free from all desires; his proposition implies truths like action, liberation of the soul and
  existence of life after death.
- Abhyupagama Siddhanta or truth taken for granted i.e a hypothesis (postulation). E.G things are explained
  sometimes on the basis of the pre-dominance of matter, sometimes that of the qualities and sometimes that of the
  potentiality.

So, the four-fold "Demonstrated Truth" is described. [37]

Shabda (words):

अथ शब्दः:- शब्दो नाम वर्णसमाम्नायः; स चतुर्विधः- दृष्टार्थश्च, अदृष्टार्थश्च, सत्यश्च, अनृतश्चेति|
तत्र दृष्टार्थो नाम- त्रिभिर्हेतुभिर्दोषाः प्रकुप्यन्ति, षड्भिरुपक्रमैश्च प्रशाम्यन्ति, सति श्रोत्रादिसद्भावे शब्दादिग्रहणमिति|
अदृष्टार्थः पुनः- अस्ति प्रेत्यभावः, अस्ति मोक्ष इति|
सत्यो नाम- यथार्थभूतः; सन्त्यायुर्वेदोपदेशाः, सन्ति सिद्ध्युपायाः साध्यानां व्याधीनां, सन्त्यारम्भफलानीति|
सत्यविपर्ययश्चानृतः||३८||

Words are made of sound. They are of four types viz:

- Drstartha or those based on observations, e.g Doshas get aggravated by their groups of factors, viz intellectual
  blasphemy sures, viz fasting etc. sounds etc., can be perceived only in the presence of auditory or other sense
  organs.
- Adstrartha or those based on unobservable phenomena, e.g there is life after death and there is salvation.
- Satya or factual, E.G there are the prescriptions of the science of medicine, there are the therapeutic measures
  meant for the alleviation of curable diseases and therapeutic measures produce their effects.
- Anrta or false: - words contrary to facts are false, E.g., there are no prescriptions of the science of medicine. [38]

Pratyaksha (direct observation):

अथ प्रत्यक्षं- प्रत्यक्षं नाम तद्यदात्मना चेन्द्रियैश्च स्वयमुपलभ्यते; तत्रात्मप्रत्यक्षाः सुखदुःखेच्छाद्वेषादयः,
शब्दादयस्त्विन्द्रियप्रत्यक्षाः||३९||

Things perceived by one self or with the help of sense organs come under the category of direct observation, e.g
happiness, misery, desire, and hatred etc., are perceived by the "Self he; sound etc are perceived with the help of
sense organs. [39]

Anumana (Inference):

अथानुमानम्- अनुमानं नाम तर्को युक्त्यपेक्षः; यथा- अग्निं जरणशक्त्या, बलं व्यायामशक्त्या, श्रोत्रादीनि शब्दादिग्रहणेनेत्येवमादि||४०||

Inference is based on argument accompanied with reasoning: - E.g one can infer Agni (digestive fire) from the power of digestion, strength from capacity to perform exercise and auditory sense organs etc., from the perception of sound etc. [40]

Aitihya (words of the divine origin):

अथैतिह्यम्- ऐतिह्यं नामाप्तोपदेशो वेदादिः||४१||

Words of the divine origin are those uttered by the gods who are enlightened par excellence e.g the Vedas transmitted by Lord Brahma {41}

Aupamya (Analogy):

अथौपम्यम्- औपम्यं नाम यदन्येनान्यस्य सादृश्यमधिकृत्य प्रकाशनं; यथा- दण्डेन दण्डकस्य, धनुषा धनुःस्तम्भस्य, इष्वासेनाऽऽरोग्यदस्येति||४२||

Exposition based on the similarly of the one with the other is Anupamya or analogy, E.g the disease Dandaka (a disease characterized by the rigidity of the muscles of the body) is explained as similar to Danda (Staff), the disease Dhanustambha (tetanus) to Dhanus (bow) and a good physician to a successful archer. [42]

Samshaya (doubt):

अथ संशयः- संशयो नाम सन्देहलक्षणानुसन्दिग्धेष्वर्थेष्वनिश्चयः; यथा- दृष्टा ह्यायुष्मल्लक्षणैरुपेताश्चानुपेताश्च तथा सक्रियाश्चाक्रियाश्च पुरुषाः शीघ्रभङ्गाश्चिरजीविनश्च, एतदुभयदृष्टत्वात् संशयः- किमस्ति खल्वकालमृत्युरुत नास्तीति||४३||

Want of decision in relation to the various doubtful objects of similar implications is Samshaya or doubt E.g., there are persons who are endowed with the signs of long life, some are not there are persons who resort to therapeutics, some are not; there are persons who resort to therapeutics, some do not, of all these people some are seen to die early and some live long. This creates a doubt whether there is a possibility of premature death or not? [43]

Prayojana (object):

अथ प्रयोजनं- प्रयोजनं नाम यदर्थमारभ्यन्त आरम्भाः; यथा- यद्यकालमृत्युरस्ति ततोऽहमात्मानमायुष्यैरुपचरिष्याम्यनायुष्याणि च परिहरिष्यामि, कथं मामकालमृत्युः प्रसहेतेति||४४||

The object is the one to accomplish which various measures are adopted. E.G "Granting that there is a possibility of premature death, I would get myself treated with drugs which promote longevity and avoid taking recourse to unwholesome regimens. How would then premature death can attack me?[44]

Savyabhicara (Statements with exception):

अथ सव्यभिचारं- सव्यभिचारं नाम यद्व्यभिचरणं; यथा- भवेदिदमौषधमस्मिन् व्याधौ यौगिकमथवा नेति||४५||

A statement with exceptions is known as Savyabhicara. E.g such statements might create doubts as to whether a given medicine would be appropriate for a particular disease or not? [45]

Jijnasa (Enquiry):

अथ जिज्ञासा- जिज्ञासा नाम परीक्षा; यथा भेषजपरीक्षोत्तरकालमुपदेक्ष्यते||४६||

An inquiry with a view to examining a thing is known as Jijnasa. E.G the examination relating to drugs which will be subsequently explained. [46]

Vyavasaya (determination):

अथ व्यवसायः- व्यवसायो नाम निश्चयः; यथा- वातिक एवायं व्याधिः, इदमेवास्य भेषजं चेति||४७||

Determination of a given object is Vyavasaya E.g there is Verily a Vatika type of disease and a given medicine is the best suited for its cure. [47]

Arthaprapti (Implied meaning):

अथार्थप्राप्तिः- अर्थप्राप्तिर्नाम यत्रैकेनार्थेनोक्तेनापरस्यार्थस्यानुक्तस्यापि सिद्धिः; यथा- नायं सन्तर्पणसाध्यो व्याधिरित्युक्ते भवत्यर्थप्राप्तिः- अपतर्पणसाध्योऽयमिति, नानेन दिवा भोक्तव्यमित्युक्ते भवत्यर्थप्राप्तिः- निशि भोक्तव्यमिति||४८||

When from something explicitly stated some other thing which is not stated is understood I this known as Arthaprapti (understanding by implication). E.g, if it is said that a given disease cannot be cured by nourishing therapy, it evidently follows that the disease is curable by emaciating therapy. Again, if it is said that a patient should not eat during time implies that he is given food at night. [48]

Sambhava (Source):

अथ सम्भवः- यो यतः सम्भवति स तस्य सम्भवः; यथा- षड्धातवो गर्भस्य, व्याधेरहितं, हितमारोग्यस्येति||४९||

Something from which another thing originates is regarded as Sambhava or source. E.g the six Dhatus are the source of embryo, unwholesome regimens of a disease and wholesome regimens of good health. [49]

Anuyojya (defective statement):

अथानुयोज्यम्- अनुयोज्यं नाम यद्वाक्यं वाक्यदोषयुक्तं तत्|
सामान्यतो व्याहृतेष्वर्थेषु वा विशेषग्रहणार्थं यद्वाक्यं तदप्यनुयोज्यं;

A statement which is not lucid is Anuyoja or a defective statement. In the event of general statements having been made, making statements to specify the object is also called Anuyoja. E.g if somebody says that a given disease is curable by elimination therapy, it is enquired, "whether it is curable by emetic or purgation therapy. [50]

Ananuyoja (infallible statement):

यथा- 'संशोधनसाध्योऽयं व्याधिः' इत्युक्ते 'किं वमनसाध्योऽयं, किंवा विरेचनसाध्यः' इत्यनुयुज्यते||५०||

Where there is no room for any query, lie statements so made is known as Ananuyojya or infallible statement. E.g a given disease is incurable. [51]

Anuyoga (Scriptural Enquiry):

अथानुयोगः- अनुयोगो नाम स यत् तद्विद्यानां तद्विद्यैरेव सार्धं तन्त्रे तन्त्रैकदेशे वा प्रश्नःप्रश्नैकदेशो वा ज्ञानविज्ञानवचनप्रतिवचनपरीक्षार्थमादिश्यते|
यथा- 'नित्यः पुरुषः' इति प्रतिज्ञाते यत् परः 'को हेतुः' इत्याह, सोऽनुयोगः||५२||

When scholars proficient in scriptures enquire from similar scholars something relating to a scripture or a part of the scripture or a question or a part of the question with a view to testing the knowledge, power of comprehension and expression and capacity to reply to the latter, this is known as scriptural enquired" why is it so? This is Anuyoga or scriptural enquiry. [52]

Pratyanuyoga (Scriptural counter Enquiry):

अथ प्रत्यनुयोगः- प्रत्यनुयोगो नामानुयोगस्यानुयोगः; यथा- अस्यानुयोगस्य पुनः को हेतुरिति||५३||

To put another enquiry in respect of an enquiry is known as Pratyanuyoga or scriptural counter- enquiry. e.g., in respect of the enquiry presented above, it might further be asked, "what is the justification for this enquiry relating to the eternity of the soul [53]

Vakyadosha (syntactical defects):

अथ वाक्यदोषः- वाक्यदोषो नाम यथा खल्वस्मिन्नर्थे न्यूनम्, अधिकम्, अनर्थकम्, अपार्थकं, विरुद्धं चेति; एतानि ह्यन्तरेण न प्रकृतोऽर्थः प्रणशयेत्|
तत्र न्यूनं- प्रतिज्ञाहेतूदाहरणोपनयनिगमनानामन्यतमेनापि न्यूनं न्यूनं भवति; यद्वा बहूपदिष्टहेतुकमेकेन हेतुना साध्यते तच्च न्यूनम्|
अथाधिकम्- अधिकं नाम यन्न्यूनविपरीतं, यद्वाऽऽयुर्वेदे भाष्यमाणे बार्हस्पत्यमौशनसमन्यद्वा यत्किञ्चिदप्रतिसम्बद्धार्थमुच्यते, यद्वा

सम्बद्धार्थमपि द्विरभिधीयते तत् पुनरुक्तदोषत्वादधिकं; तच्च पुनरुक्तं द्विविधम्- अर्थपुनरुक्तं, शब्दपुनरुक्तं च; तत्रार्थपुनरुक्तं यथा-
भेषजमौषधं साधनमिति, शब्दपुनरुक्तं पुनर्भेषजं भेषजमिति|

अथानर्थकम्- अनर्थकं नाम यद्वचनमक्षरग्राममात्रमेव स्यात् पञ्चवर्गवन्न चार्थतो गृह्यते|

अथापार्थकम्- अपार्थकं नाम यदर्थवच्च परस्परेणासंयुज्यमानार्थकं; यथा- चक्र-न(त)क्र-वंश-वज्र-निशाकरा इति|

अथ विरुद्धं- विरुद्धं नाम यद्दृष्टान्तसिद्धान्तसमयैर्विरुद्धं; तत्र पूर्वं दृष्टान्तसिद्धान्तावुक्तौः समयः पुनस्त्रिधा भवति; यथा-
आयुर्वैदिकसमयः, याज्ञिकसमयः, मोक्षशास्त्रिकसमयश्चेति; तत्रायुर्वैदिकसमयः- चतुष्पादं भेषजमिति, याज्ञिकसमयः- आलभ्या यजमानैः
पशव इति, मोक्षशास्त्रिकसमयः- सर्वभूतेष्वहिंसेति; तत्र स्वसमयविपरीतमुच्यमानं विरुद्धं भवति|

इति वाक्यदोषाः||५४||

Syntactical defects are; semantic deficiency, superfluity, nonsensical statement, semantic incongruity and contradictory statement. It is only when a sentence is free from these defects, its semantic potentiality remains intact.

When a statement is deficient in any one of the five constituents of a statement, viz proposition, statement of probans, corroborating instance, subsumptive correlation and final conclusion then it suffers from semantic deficiency. Or, where from out of several statements of profanes only one is presented, the sentence is again considered to be deficient semantically. (e.g., the statements of probans in respect of the eternity of the soul are the state of having no beginning, state of not having been created and the state of freedom from any transformation; if instead of presenting all these statements of probans, one presents only one of them the statement would suffer from the defect of semantic deviancy)

Superfluity is just opposite to semantic deficiency. Or if in the core of a discussion relating to the science of medicine, somebody starts talking about Barhaspatya or Shukranti and such other irrelevant things, this is also considered to be superfluous. Or even if relevant, when things are unnecessarily respected that is again superfluous. Repetitions are of two kinds: -
Semantic repetition i.e to give more than one synonym for expressing one and the same concept e.g Bhesaja Ausadha, Sadhana etc.
Verbal repetition i.e repeating the same words again and again e.g Bhesaja, Bhesaja etc

Nonsensical statements are those which are made of unmeaningful letters e.g unrelated five groups of stops like Ka, Kha, GamGha and na.

If a sentence consists of unconnected words- those meaningful, in isolation but with no meanings whatsoever in the combination from e.g Vakra, Nakra, Vamsa, Vamsa and Nisakara etc. this is known as anrthaka (meaningless).

When a statement is not in keeping with illustrations, basic doctrines and traditions, it is known as Viruddha or contradictory statement. The illustrations statements contradictory to Drstanta (illustration) and siddhanta (fundamental doctrines) have already been cited above.
(1) contradictory to illustration; e.g a statement that fever produces heat as cold water produces heat
(2) contradictory to the fundamental principles; e.g the statement of a physician to the effect that a medicine does nor cure a disease.

Tradition is of three types as follows:

- Transition relating to the science of medicine e.g a therapy has four constitutions
- Ritualistic transition e.g animals are to be sacrificed by the worshippers
- Spiritual tradition e.g non-violent attitude towards all creatures.

Thus, a statement contradicting the traditions of a given scripture is known as a contradictory statement. Thus are the defects in statements [54]

Vakyaprasamsa (syntactical excellence):

अथ वाक्यप्रशंसा- वाक्यप्रशंसा नाम यथा खल्वस्मिन्नर्थे त्वन्यूनम्, अनधिकम्, अर्थवत्, अनपार्थकम्, अविरुद्धम्, अधिगतपदार्थं चेति यतद्वाक्यमननुयोज्यमिति प्रशस्यते||५५||

Syntactical excellence is attained when the statement is free from syntactical deficiency, superfluity, incongruity, contradiction and breach of tradition. That is to say where there is no room for further enquiry, the statement is considered to be of excellent type. [55]

Chala (casuistry):

अथ च्छलं- छलं नाम परिशठमर्थाभासमनर्थकं वाग्वस्तुमात्रमेव|

तद्दिद्विविधं- वाक्छलं, सामान्यच्छलं च|

Chala (casuistry) stands for confusion created by play on words not relevant to the question, nonsensical in nature, and only apparently having some meanings. This is of two kinds, viz, Vakcchala (verbal casuistry) and Samanyacchala (casuistry in general).

तत्र वाक्छलं नाम यथा- कश्चिद्ब्रूयात्- नवतन्त्रोऽयं भिषगिति, अथ भिषग् ब्रूयात्- नाहं नवतन्त्र एकतन्त्रोऽहमिति; परो ब्रूयात्- नाहं ब्रवीमि नव तन्त्राणि तवेति, अपि तु नवाभ्यस्तं ते तन्त्रमिति; भिषक् ब्रूयात्- न मया नवाभ्यस्तं तन्त्रम्, अनेकधाऽभ्यस्तं मया तन्त्रमिति; एतद्वाक्छलम्|

Verbal Casuistry: - if somebody says that the physician is "Navatantra "meaning therapy that he has learnt the science of medicine but too recently, the opponent replies, "I am not "Navatantra" (meaning thereby that he has not studied nine scripture) but has studied only one scripture. Then again, the questioner replies, "I did not mean that the physician has studied nine scriptures but I meant that your experience in the field of medicine is quite new (Navabhyasta). Then again, the opponent replies. "I have not studied the scriptures nine times (Navabhayasta) but have studies it several times. "This illustrates verbal casuistry.

सामान्यच्छलं नाम यथा- व्याधिप्रशमनायौषधमित्युक्ते, परो ब्रूयात्- सत् सत्प्रशमनायेति किं नु भवानाह; सन् हि रोगः, सदौषधं; यदि च सत् सत्प्रशमनाय भवति, तत्र सत् कासः, सत् क्षयः, सत्सामान्यात् कासस्ते क्षयप्रशमनाय भविष्यतीति|

एतत् सामान्यच्छलम्||५६||

Casuistry in General: - if somebody makes a statement that the medicine is meant for alleviating a disease, the opponent asks, did you mean to say that something existent alleviates some other existent. If something existent and so is the medicine existent. If something existent could alleviate some other existent. If something existent could alleviate another thing in existence, then Kasa (cough) is also existent and so is Ksaya (consumption). Therefore, according to this general principal cough in existence could also cure consumption. This illustrates "casuistry in general". [56]

Ahetu (causal fallacy):

अथाहेतुः- अहेतुर्नामप्रकरणसमः, संशयसमः, वर्ण्यसमश्चेति|

Casual fallacy is of three kinds as given below:

तत्र प्रकरणसमो नामाहेतुर्यथा- अन्यः शरीरादात्मा नित्य इति; परो ब्रूयात्- यस्मादन्यः शरीरादात्मा, तस्मान्नित्यः; शरीरं ह्यनित्यमतो विधर्मिणा चात्मना भवितव्यमित्येष चाहेतुः; नहि य एव पक्षः स एव हेतुरिति|

Prakaranasama or stultified fallacy: If somebody says, The soul is eternal because it is different from the body, then the opponent will point out the fallacy underlying the statement, if the soul is eternal simply because it is different from the body then the statement does not add to any reasoning for the proposition relating to the eternity of the soul because the body being ephemeral and soul being different from the body, it (the soul) would naturally have opposite qualities and so the minor and major terms of the proposition would almost be the same". this illustrates the fallacy of stultified reasoning.

संशयसमो नामाहेतुर्य एव संशयहेतुः स एव संशयच्छेदहेतुः; यथा- अयमायुर्वेदैकदेशमाह, किन्न्वयं चिकित्सकः स्यान्न वेति संशये परो ब्रूयात्- यस्मादयमायुर्वेदैकदेशमाह तस्माच्चिकित्सकोऽयमिति, न च संशयच्छेदहेतुं विशेषयति, एष चाहेतुः; न हि य एव संशयहेतुः, स एव संशयच्छेदहेतुर्भवति|

Samsayasama or Doubtful fallacy: Fallacy of doubtful reasoning is the one where a doubt reasoning in itself is intended to remove doubts. If somebody puts a query about a physician, "Can a person who knows only a part of the science of medicine be considered as a physician?". The opponent replies, because he knows only a part of Ayurveda so he is a physician. "Thus, the very point of doubt is taken to remove the doubt. This is the fallacy of doubtful reasoning.

वर्ण्यसमो नामाहेतुः- यो हेतुर्वर्ण्याविशिष्टः; यथा- कश्चिद्ब्रूयात्- अस्पर्शत्वाद्बुद्धिरनित्या शब्दवदिति; अत्र वर्ण्यः शब्दो बुद्धिरपि वर्ण्या, तदुभयवर्ण्याविशिष्टत्वाद्वर्ण्यसमोऽप्यहेतुः||५७||

Varnyasama or fallacy of insignificant causality: Somebody says, Intellect is ephemeral because of its intractability, as sound," here intractability does not help in establishing the ephemerality of intellect as of the sound as both these items are equally unproven, and sound whose ephemerality is yes to be proven cannot be cited as an illusion. This is the fallacy of insignificant reasoning. [57]

Atitakala (defiance of Temporal order):

अथातीतकालम्- अतीतकालं नाम यत् पूर्वं वाच्यं तत् पश्चादुच्यते, तत् कालातीतत्वादग्राह्यं भवतीति; पूर्वं वा निग्रहप्राप्तमनिगृह्य परिगृह्य पक्षान्तरितं पश्चान्निगृहीते, ततस्यातीतकालत्वान्निग्रहवचनमसमर्थं भवतीति||५८||

If something which is to be stated first in the order of priority is stated later, this constitutes Atitakala or defiance of temporal order. Being devoid of temporal prosperity this is also not acceptable in the debate. E.G the proposition is to come first and then the final conclusion. But if somebody gives the final conclusion first and then he states the proposition. This should constitute the refinance of temporal order. Or where there is an occasion for clinchers, if one keeps quiet at that time and after sometime he applies clinchers on some other point, this also constitutes the defiance of temporal order and it is equally unacceptable and irrelevant in the debate. [58]

Upalambha (defective causality):

अथोपालम्भः- उपालम्भो नाम हेतोर्दोषवचनं; यथा- पूर्वमहेतवो हेत्वाभासा व्याख्याताः||५९||

Upalambha stands for pointing out defects in causality as explained in Para – 57 above. [59]

Parihara (correction):

अथ परिहारः- परिहारो नाम तस्यैव दोषवचनस्य परिहरणं; यथा- नित्यमात्मनि शरीरस्थे जीवलिङ्गान्युपलभ्यन्ते, तस्य चापगमान्नोपलभ्यन्ते, तस्मादन्यः शरीरादात्मा नित्यश्चेति||६०||

Parihara stands for correcting the defects pointed out in respect of the proposition. E.g., in Para – 57 above, it is shown that being different from the body does not constitute a valid reasoning for the eternity of the soul. The opponents'view point may however, be marks of life that are visible in the body and not otherwise. So, the soul is different from the body and is also eternal. [60]

Pratijnahani (Shift from the original stand):

अथ प्रतिज्ञाहानिः- प्रतिज्ञाहानिर्नाम सा पूर्वपरिगृहीतां प्रतिज्ञां पर्यनुयुक्तो यत् परित्यजति, यथा प्राक् प्रतिज्ञां कृत्वा नित्यः पुरुष इति, पर्यनुयुक्तस्त्वाह- अनित्य इति||६१||

If one makes a statement and then being attacked by his opponents contradicts his own statement, this is known as Pratijnahani or shift from the original stand.If somebody makes a statement that the soul is eternal and then attacked by his opponent subsequently changes his view and says, "The soul is ephemeral", this would amount to a shift in the stand. [61]

Abhyanujna (confessional retort):

अथाभ्यनुज्ञा- अभ्यनुज्ञा नाम सा य इष्टानिष्टाभ्युपगमः||६२||

Where the allegations made by the opponent are accepted and the opponent is also charged with the same allegation this is known as Abhyanujna or confessional retort. E.g if an opponent says, "You are also a thief". [62]

Hetvantara (fallacy of reason):

अथ हेत्वन्तरं- हेत्वन्तरं नाम प्रकृतहेतौ वाच्ये यदि्विकृतहेतुमाह||६३||

When instead of relevant rezoning an irrelevant reasoning is given, it is known as Hetvantara or fallacy of reason. [63]

Arthantara (Irrelevant statement):

अथार्थान्तरम्- अर्थान्तरं नामैकस्मिन् वक्तव्येऽपरं यदाह|

यथा- ज्वरलक्षणे वाच्ये प्रमेहलक्षणमाह||६४||

If somebody starts defining Prameha (obstinate urinary disorders including Diabetes mellitus), when he ought to define fever, this would constitute irrelevant statements. [64]

Nigrahasthana (Clincher):

अथ निग्रहस्थानं- निग्रहस्थानं नाम पराजयप्राप्तिः; तच्च त्रिरभिहितस्य वाक्यस्यापरिज्ञानं परिषदि विज्ञानवत्यां, यद्वा अननुयोज्यस्यानुयोगोऽनुयोज्यस्य चाननुयोगः|

Clinchers stand for defeat. When an enlightened scholarly assemblage, a statement is repeated three times but the opponent is unable to understand it or if he enquires about something which ought not to be enquired or he enquired about such situations constitute clinchers

प्रतिज्ञाहानिः, अभ्यनुज्ञा, कालातीतवचनम्, अहेतुः, न्यूनम्, अधिकं, व्यर्थम्, अनर्थकं, पुनरुक्तं, विरुद्धं, हेत्वन्तरम्, अर्थान्तरं च निग्रहस्थानम्||६५||

इति वादमार्गपदानि यथोद्देशमभिनिर्दिष्टानि भवन्ति||६६||

Besides Pratijnahani (shift from the original stand), Abhyanujna (confessional retort), Kalatitavabcana (definance of the temporal order), Ahetu (Superfluity), Vyartha (semantic incongruity), Anarthaka (nonsensical statement), Punarrukta (repetition), Viruddha (contradictory statement), Hetvantara (fallacy of reason) and Arthantara (irrelevant statement) also constitute clinchers.

Thus, the various aspects of debate have been duly explained. [65-66]

Guidelines for a debate:

वादस्तु खलु भिषजां प्रवर्तमानो प्रवर्तेतायुर्वेद एव, नान्यत्र|

अत्र हि वाक्यप्रतिवाक्यविस्तराः केवलाश्चोपपत्तयः सर्वाधिकरणेषु|

ताः सर्वाः समवेक्ष्यावेक्ष्य सर्वं वाक्यं ब्रूयात्, नाप्रकृतकमशास्त्रमपरीक्षितमसाधकमाकुलमव्यापकं वा|

सर्वं च हेतुमद्ब्रूयात्|

हेतुमन्तो ह्यकलुषाः सर्व एव वादविग्रहाश्चिकित्सिते कारणभूताः, प्रशस्तबुद्धिवर्धकत्वात्; सर्वारम्भसिद्धिं ह्यावहत्यनुपहता बुद्धिः||६७||

The debate among physicians relates to nothing else but the science of medicine. The various details about statements and rejoinders as well as fundamental principles (of the debates) mentioned above of course relate to all the scriptures. A physician should make statements with due regard to the principles of debates. He should not make statements out of the context or country to scriptural prescriptions or without due examination or o irrelevant, confused or too sketchy statements. Whatever he states is based on arguments. All debates equipped with arguments and flawlessness the enlightening powers of mental faculty. The mental faculty undisturbed well accomplishes all the objects in view.[67]

Important topics to be known by physicians:

इमानि खलु तावदिह कानिचित् प्रकरणानि भिषजां ज्ञानार्थमुपदेक्ष्यामः|

ज्ञानपूर्वकं हि कर्मणां समारम्भं प्रशंसन्ति कुशलाः|

ज्ञात्वा हि कारण-करण-कार्ययोनि-कार्य-कार्यफलानुबन्ध-देश-काल-प्रवृत्त्युपायान् सम्यगभिनिर्वर्तमानः कार्याभिनिर्वृतताविष्टफलानुबन्धं कार्यमभिनिर्वर्तयत्यनतिमहता यत्नेन कर्ता||६८||

There are some of the important topics which we shall explain for the sake of knowledge of the physicians. The wise admire action initiated with the due knowledge. A physician can accomplish the desire object without any special effort, provided he duly initiates action after having full knowledge of Karana (cause), Karana (instrument), Karyayoni (source of action), Karya (action itself), Karyaphala (fruits of action), Anubandha (subsequent manifestation), do (habit), Kala (season), Pravrtti(initiation) and Upaya (means of action). [68]

Karana:

तत्र कारणं नाम तद् यत् [१] करोति, स एव हेतुः, स कर्ता||६९|||

The cause here is the one who initiates action independently, that is to say, the doer or the agent constitutes the cause of action. [69]

Karana:

करणं पुनस्तद् यदुपकरणायोपकल्पते कर्तुः कार्याभिनिर्वृतौ प्रयतमानस्य||७०||

Karana stands for an instrument which helps an agent in the performance of his action. [70]

Karyayoni:

कार्ययोनिस्तु सा या विक्रियमाणा कार्यत्वमापद्यते||७१||

The Karyayoni (source of an action) is the one which becomes an action by the process of transformation. [71]

Karya:

कार्यं तु तद्यस्याभिनिर्वृतिमभिसन्धाय कर्ता प्रवर्तते||७२||

Action is the one whose accomplishment is kept in view before an agent proceeds to act. [72]

Karyaphala:

कार्यफलं पुनस्तद् यत्प्रयोजना कार्याभिनिर्वृतिरिष्यते||७३||

The object of action stands for the object for which the action is imitated. [73]

Anubandha:

अनुबन्धः खलु स यः कर्तारमवश्यमनुबध्नाति कार्यादुतरकालं कार्यनिमितः शुभो वाऽप्यशुभो भावः||७४||

An after effect- good or bad-is the one which is bound to leave its impact on the agent after he has performed his action.[74]

Desha:

देशस्त्वधिष्ठानम्||७५|||

Desha (location) represents the site favorable or unfavorable to an action

Kala:

कालः पुनः परिणामः||७६||

Time is nothing but a recess of transformation into seasons, solstices etc., [76]

Pravriti:

प्रवृत्तिस्तु खलु चेष्टा कार्यार्था; सैव

Pravrtti (Endeavour) represents the initiation of action as a means to the accomplishment of an object. This is action; this is an object and this is an effort as well as the beginning of action. [77]

Upaya:

उपायः पुनस्त्रयाणां कारणादीनां सौष्ठवमभिविधानं च सम्यक् कार्यकार्यफलानुबन्धवर्ज्यानां, कार्याणामभिनिर्वर्तक इत्यतस्तूपायः; कृते नोपायार्थोऽस्ति, न च विद्यते तदात्वे, कृताच्चोतरकालं फलं, फलाच्चानुबन्ध इति||७८||

Upaya (device) stands for bringing about excellence in the agent, the instrument and the origin of action and their proper setting. That is to say, a device is the one which accomplishes the object. Device has no meaning after an action has been performed. The action itself does not exist before it is performed. (So, the action cannot in itself be a device). After an action has been performed, the object is revealed and it (the object) leads to an after effect. So, the stage of a proper device comes long before an action is initiated. [78]

Thorough examination prior to initiating action:

एतद्दशविधमग्रे परीक्ष्यं, ततोऽनन्तरं कार्यार्था प्रवृत्तिरिष्टा|

तस्मादिभषक् कार्य चिकीर्षुः प्राक् कार्यसमारम्भात् परीक्षया केवलं परीक्ष्यं परीक्ष्य कर्म समारभेत कर्तुम्||७९||

These ten factors are examined first. One should try to initiate action thereafter. So, a physician desirous of initiating an action should examine all that are required to be examined before initiating his action. [79]

Queries about Panchakarma:

तत्र चेदिभषगभिषग्वा भिषजं कश्चिदेवं खलु पृच्छेद्- वमन विरेचनास्थापनानुवासन शिरोविरेचनानि प्रयोक्तुकामेन भिषजा कतिविधया परीक्षया कतिविधमेव परीक्ष्यं, कश्चात्र परीक्ष्यविशेषः, कथं च परीक्षितव्यः, किम्प्रयोजना च परीक्षा, क्व च वमनादीनां प्रवृत्तिः, क्व च निवृत्तिः, प्रवृति निवृति लक्षण संयोगे च किं नैष्ठिकं, कानि च वमनादीनां भेषजद्रव्याण्युपयोगं गच्छन्तीति||८०||

So, if another physician or a layman asks the physician, "what are the types of examinations and what are the types of objects to be examined by a physician desirous of administering Vamana (emesis), Virecana (purgation), Asthapana type of enema, Anuvasana type of enema and Sirovirecana (errhines) what is it that is to be specifically examined? How is it to be examined? What is the object of examination? When should emesis etc. be administered? What is done to determine the administrability or otherwise of these therapies? What are the drugs which are used for Vamana (emesis) etc? The physician may reply as follows [80]

A bewildering reply:

स एवं पृष्टो यदि मोहयितुमिच्छेत्, ब्रूयादेनं- बहुविधा हि परीक्षा तथा परीक्ष्य विधि भेदः, कतमेन विधिभेदप्रकृत्यन्तरेण भिन्नया परीक्षया केन वा विधिभेदप्रकृत्यन्तरेण परीक्ष्यस्य भिन्नस्य भेदाग्रं भवान् पृच्छत्याख्यायमानं; नेदानीं भवतोऽन्येन विधिभेदप्रकृत्यन्तरेण भिन्नया परीक्षयाऽन्येन वा विधिभेदप्रकृत्यन्तरेण परीक्ष्यस्य भिन्नस्याभिलषितमर्थं श्रोतुमहमन्येन परीक्षाविधिभेदेनान्येन वा विधिभेदप्रकृत्यन्तरेण परीक्ष्यं भित्वाऽन्यथाऽऽचक्षाण इच्छां पूरयेयमिति||८१||

If he wants to bewilder his opponent, he should say, "Diverse are the types of examinations and methods of examining the various objects of examinations. What particular method of examination or what particular type to satisfy your query by describing the method of examination or the type of the object of examination different from what you wish to know". [81]

Situations for giving correct answer:

स यदुतरं ब्रूयातत् समीक्ष्योतरं वाच्यं स्याद्यथोक्तं च प्रतिवचनविधिमवेक्ष्य; सम्यक् यदि तु ब्रूयान्न चैनं मोहयितुमिच्छेत्, प्राप्तं तु वचनकालं मन्येत, काममस्मै ब्रूयादाप्तमेव निखिलेन||८२||

In case the opponent answers these queries, he should duly explain the required method and other aspects of the examination. If, on the other hand, somebody asks a question in good faith and at the appropriate time and the physician does not want to bewilder the questioner, he should explain everything in detail according as it has been explained in the scriptures [82]

Three methods of examination:

द्विविधातु खलु परीक्षा ज्ञानवतां- प्रत्यक्षम्, अनुमानं च|
एतद्दि द्वयमुपदेशश्च परीक्षा स्यात्|
एवमेषा द्विविधा परीक्षा, त्रिविधा वा सहोपदेशेन||८३||

The wise take recourse to two types of examinations-perceptual and inferential. These two combined with instructions constitute the methods of examination. So, the examination is of two types or of three types if "instruction" is included in it. [83]

Ten important topics for examination:

दशविधं तु परीक्ष्यं कारणादि यदुक्तमग्रे, तदिह भिषगादिषु संसार्य सन्दर्शयिष्यामः- इह कार्यप्राप्तौ कारणं भिषक्, करणं पुनर्भैषजं, कार्य योनि धातुवैषम्यं, कार्य धातुसाम्यं, कार्यफलं सुखावाप्तिः, अनुबन्धः खल्वायुः, देशो भूमिरातुरश्च, कालः पुनः संवत्सरश्चातुरावस्था च, प्रवृतिः प्रतिकर्मसमारम्भः, उपायस्तु भिषगादीनां सौष्ठवमभिविधानं च सम्यक्|
इहाप्यस्योपायस्य विषयः पूर्वेणैवोपाय sविशेषेण व्याख्यातः|
इति कारणादीनि दश दशसु भिषगादिषु संसार्य सन्दर्शितानि, तथैवानुपूर्व्यैतद्दशविधं परीक्ष्यमुक्तं च||८४||

In Para 68 cause etc. are mentioned as the ten factors that are to be examined. Each of them is described below with relevant illustrations:

Karana (cause): the physician serves as the causative factors for the achievement of the object i.e the maintenance of the equilibrium of Dhatus.

Karana (instrument): Medicaments

Karyayoni (source of action): - Disturbance of the equilibrium of Dhatus

Karya (action itself): - maintenance of the equilibrium of Dhatus

Karyaphala (fruits of action): - Attainment of happiness, i.e the star of freedom from a disease.

Anubandha (subsequent manifestation): - Longevity.

Desha (Habiat): - both the land as well as the patient constitute Desha or habitat.

Kala (Time): - the year consisting of seasons and the state of the disease constitute Kala or time.

Pravrti(institution): - therapeutic action

Upaya (means of action): - excellence of the physician and the correctness of the therapy constitute Upaya or means of action. Factors which are described as the objects of Upaya in Para 78 are also implied here.

Thus, the ten factors, viz, cause etc, are described along with ten illustrations, viz physician etc, these are the ten factors to be examined in succession [84]

Examination of physician:

तस्य यो यो विशेषो यथा यथा च परीक्षितव्यः, स तथा तथा व्याख्यास्यते||८५||
कारणं भिषगित्युक्तमग्रे, तस्य परीक्षा- भिषङ्नाम यो भिषज्यति, यः सूत्रार्थप्रयोग कुशलः, यस्य चायुः सर्वथा विदितं यथावत्|
स च सर्वधातुसाम्यं चिकीर्षन्नात्मानमेवादितः परीक्षेत गुणिषु गुणतः कार्याभिनिर्वृत्तिं पश्यन्, कच्चिदहमस्य कार्यस्याभिनिर्वर्तने समर्थो न वेति; तत्रेमे भिषग्गुणा यैरुपपन्नो भिषग्धातुसाम्याभिनिर्वर्तने समर्थो भवति; तद्यथा- पर्यवदातश्रुतता, परिदृष्टकर्मता, दाक्ष्यं, शौचं, जितहस्तता, उपकरणवत्ता, सर्वेन्द्रियोपपन्नता, प्रकृतिज्ञता, प्रतिपत्तिज्ञाता चेति||८६||

Specific of each of these ten items and the manner in which they are required to be examined are now being explained. It is stated in the beginning that the physician is the Sine Qua non for the successful administration of therapies. A physician is he who treats patients, who are well versed in the applied aspects of the meaning contained in tense aphorisms and who are well acquainted with all aspects of life.

Four factors, viz. The physician, the drug, the attendant and the patient should possess something specific in order to be effective for curing a disease. Of them, the physician desirous of bringing about the state of equilibrium of Dhatus should, first of all. Examine him with a view to ascertaining if he is competent or otherwise to handle the case.

A physician possessed of the following qualities is capable of bringing about the equilibrium of Dhatus:
Knowledge of medical texts in their entirety
Practical experience
Skill
Purity
Infallibility of prescriptions
Possession of normal sense faculties and all the requisite equipments
Knowledge of the various natural manifestations
Presence of mind [85-86]

Examination of drug:

करणं पुनर्भेषजम्|
भेषजं नाम तद्यदुपकरणायोपकल्पते भिषजो धातु साम्याभिनिर्वृत्तौ प्रयतमानस्य विशेषतश्चोपायान्तेभ्यः|
तद्दिद्विविधं व्यपाश्रयभेदात्- दैव व्यपाश्रयं, युक्तिव्यपाश्रयं चेति|

Medicaments constitute the instruments for achieving the object i.e the cure of the disease. Medicaments are those which are employed by physicians with a view to bringing about the equilibrium of Dhatus. They are used by the subject as instruments and include factors other than Karyayoni (source of action), Pravritti (Initiation), Desha (Habitat), Kala (time) and Upaya (means of action).

Depending upon their nature, they are of two types, viz,
Spiritual
Rational.

तत्र दैवव्यपाश्रयं- मन्त्रौषधि मणि मङ्गल बल्युपहारहोम नियम प्रायश्चित्तोपवासस्वस्त्ययनप्रणिपातगमनादि, युक्तिव्यपाश्रयं- संशोधनोपशमने चेष्टाश्च दृष्टफलाः|
एतच्चैव भेषजमङ्गभेदादपि द्विविधं- द्रव्यभूतमः, अद्रव्यभूतं च|
तत्र यदद्रव्यभूतं तदुपायाभिप्लुतम्|

Spiritual therapy comprises incantation, Talisman, Jewels, auspicious rites, religious sacrifices, oblations, religious rites, vow, atonement, fasting, chanting of auspicious hymns, paying obeisance, pilgrimage etc. elimination as well as alleviation therapies and such other regimens effects of which can be directly perceived belong to the category of rational therapy.

उपायो नाम भय दर्शन विस्मापन विस्मारण क्षोभण हर्षणभर्त्सनवधबन्धस्वप्नसंवाहनादिरमूर्तो भावविशेषो यथोक्ताः सिद्ध्युपायाश्चोपायाभिप्लुता इति|
यत्तु द्रव्यभूतं तद्वमनादिषु योगमुपैति|
तस्यापीयं परीक्षा- इदमेवम्प्रकृत्यैवङ्गुणमेवम्प्रभावमस्मिन् देशे जातमस्मिन्नृतावेवं गृहीतमेवं निहितमेवमुपस्कृतमनया च मात्रया युक्तमस्मिन् व्याधावेवंविधस्य पुरुषस्यैवतावन्तं दोषमपकर्षत्युपशमयति वा, यदन्यदपि चैवंविधं भेषजं भवेत्तच्चानेन विशेषेण युक्तमिति||८७||

Depending upon the nature of their composition, they also are of two types, viz. those having material substrata and those without having any material substrata. The later category of therapy has indirect action on the disease. It is not an inseparable con-commit ant cause for the cure of diseases

Terracing, surprising, rememorizing, shocking, exiting, chiding, threatening for murder, binding, inducing sleep, massage etc, are the means employed in the Adravyabhuta therapy (therapy without involving any material substrata). Therapies having material base are used for emesis etc. they are examined with reference to their characteristics as follows:

Nature

Qualities

Specific actions

Place of growth

Season of collection mode of collection

Method of preservation

Method of processing

Dosage in which employed

Quantum of Doshas elevated or alleviated from various types of patients suffering from particular types of diseases. Other drugs having similar characteristics may also be used. [87]

Examination of disease:

कार्ययोनिर्धातुवैषम्यं, तस्य लक्षणं विकारागमः|

परीक्षा त्वस्य विकार प्रकृतेश्चैवोनातिरिक्तलिङ्गविशेषावेक्षणं विकारस्य च

साध्यासाध्य मृदु दारुण लिङ्ग विशेषावेक्षणमिति||८८||

The disturbance of the equilibrium of Dhatus is the source of action. The disturbance of the equilibrium of Dhatus is invariably indicated by the cosset of the disease. This state of health can be ascertained from the appearance "Of specific symptoms in smaller or greater digress due to the Doshas responsible for the causation of the disease and also from the "Specific characteristics of the disease e.g curability, incurability, mildness, seriousness etc. [88]

Examination to ascertain if the disease is cured:

कार्य धातुसाम्यं, तस्य लक्षणं विकारोपशमः|

परीक्षा त्वस्य- रुग्उपशमनं, स्वरवर्णयोगः, शरीरोपचयः, बल वृद्धिः, अभ्यवहार्याभिलाषः, रुचिराहारकाले, अभ्यवहृतस्य चाहारस्य काले सम्यग्जरणं, निद्रालाभो यथाकालं, वैकारिणां च स्वप्नानामदर्शनं, सुखेन च प्रतिबोधनं, वातमूत्रपुरीषरेतसां मुक्तिः, सर्वाकारैर्मनोबुद्धीन्द्रियाणां चाव्यापत्तिरिति||८९||

Equilibrium of Dhatus represents the "Action itself". It is insatiably associated with the alleviation or absence of the disease. This state of health can be ascertained from the following:

Alleviation of pain

Appearance of normal voice and complexion

Nourishment of the body

Increase in strength

Desire for taking food

Appetite for food during meal- time

Proper digestion of the food taken during meal- time

Getting sleep at the appropriate time

Absence of dreams indicating morbidity

Happy awakening

Proper elimination of wind, urine, stool and semen

Unimpairement of mind, intellect and senses and association of all healthy symptoms there with [89]

Signs of normalcy:

कार्यफलं सुखावाप्तिः, तस्य लक्षणं- मनो बुद्धीन्द्रिय शरीर तुष्टिः||९०||

Attainment of spiritual happiness is the result of therapeutic action/ it is characterised by the pleasure or satisfaction of the mind, intellect, senses and the body. [90]

Signs of Ayus:

अनुबन्धस्तु खल्वायुः, तस्य लक्षणं- प्राणैः सह संयोगः||९१||

Anubandha or subsequent manifestation is the maintenance of life (longivity). It is characterized by its union with prana type of Vayu. [91]

Examination of the land to ascertain particulars about the patient:

देशस्तु भूमिरातुरश्च||९२||

तत्र भूमिपरीक्षा आतुर परिज्ञान हेतोर्वा स्यादौषधपरिज्ञानहेतोर्वा|

तत्र तावदियमातुरपरिज्ञानहेतोः|

तद्यथा- अयं कस्मिन् भूमिदेशे जातः संवृद्धो व्याधितो वा; तस्मिंश्च भूमिदेश मनुष्याणामिदमाहारजातम्, इदं विहारजातम्, इदमाचारजातम्, एतावच्च बलम्, एवंविधं सत्त्वम्, एवंविधं सात्म्यम्, एवंविधो दोषः, भक्तिरियम्, इमे व्याधयः, हितमिदम्, अहितमिदमिति प्रायोग्रहणेन |

औषधपरिज्ञानहेतोस्तु कल्पेषु भूमिपरीक्षा वक्ष्यते||९३||

Both the land as well as the patient constitutes Desha or habitat. Nature of the land is examined with a view to ascertaining the specific features of individual patients as well as the medical plants in different localities. The following points are to be examined with reference to the patient:

Place of birth, growth and affliction with the disease.

Specific features concerning food, exercise, customs, strength, mental condition, homologation by habit, dominance of one or the other of the Doshas liking, manifestation of diseases and things which are useful and harmful.

Above information is generally obtained by the examination of the land.

The characteristic features of different types of land leading to the determination of specific features of medical plants will be described in Kalpa 1:8 [92-93]

Examination of Patient:

आतुरस्तु खलु कार्यदेशः|

तस्य परीक्षा आयुषः प्रमाण ज्ञान हेतोर्वा स्याद्, बल दोष प्रमाण ज्ञान हेतोर्वा|

तत्र तावदियं बल दोष प्रमाण ज्ञान हेतोः; दोष प्रमाणानुरूपो हि भेषज प्रमाण विकल्पो बल प्रमाण विशेषापेक्षो भवति|

A patient constitutes the KaryaDesha or the site for the administration of therapies with a view to bringing about equilibrium of Dhatus. He is examined so as to obtain knowledge relating to the to the strength of the individual and the intensity of morbidity, because, it is on the basis of the intensity of morbidity that the dosage of the therapy is determined and the latter is dependant upon the strength or the power of resistance of the individual.

सहसा ह्यतिबलमौषधमपरीक्षकप्रयुक्तमल्पबलमातुरमतिपातयेत्; न ह्यतिबलान्याग्नेयवायवीयान्यौषधान्यग्नि क्षार शस्त्र कर्माणि वा शक्यन्तेऽल्पबलैः सोढुम्; असह्याति तीक्ष्ण वेगत्वादि्धतानि सद्यःप्राणहराणि स्युः|

एतच्चैव कारणमपेक्षमाणा हीन बलमातुरमविषादकरैर्मृदु सुकुमार प्रायैरुत्तरोत्तर गुरुभिरविभ्रमैरनात्ययिकैश्चोपचरन्त्यौषधैः; विशेषतश्च नारीः, ता ह्यनवस्थित मृदु विवृत विक्लवहृदयाः प्रायः सुकुमार्योऽबलाः परसंस्तभ्याश्च|

If strong things are immediately administered without proper examination, to a weak patient, this might result in his death. Weak patients are incapable of resisting strong therapies like medicaments dominating in Agni and Vayu Mahabhutas, application of alkalies and heat (cauterization) and surgical operations. These therapies cause immediate death of the patient because of their very sharp actions which are too strong for the individual. Thus, a weak patient is given such mild and tender therapies as are not injurious to the body and the mind.

तथा बलवति बलवद्व्याधिपरिगते स्वल्पबलमौषधमपरीक्षकप्रयुक्तमसाधकमेव भवति|

तस्मादातुरं परीक्षेत प्रकृतितश्च, विकृतितश्च, सारतश्च, संहननतश्च, प्रमाणतश्च, सात्म्यतश्च, सत्त्वतश्च, आहारशक्तितश्च, व्यायामशक्तितश्च, वयस्तश्चेति, बल प्रमाण विशेष ग्रहण हेतोः||९४||

Stronger therapies are not injurious to the body and the mind. Stronger therapies which are neither distressing during their digestion nor associated with serious complications may be administered slowly and gradually. Such therapies are specially needed for ladies because they are by nature unsteady, light (not deep) and of sensitive or weak temperament and also because they are mostly thunder and subordinate to others, similarly, if weak therapies are administered to a strong individual having a serious disease without proper examination, the disease does not get cured.

Therefore, the patient is examined with reference to his Prakrti (Physical constitution), Vikrti (Morbidity), Sara (excellence of Dhatus, or tissue elements), Samhanana (compactness of organs), Pramana (measurement of the organs of the body), Satmya (Homogation), Sattva (psychic conditions), Aharasakti (power of intake and digestion of food), Vyayamashakti (power of performing exercise) and Vayas (age) in order to ascertain his strength and the intensity of the malady. [94]

Prakriti:

तत्र प्रकृत्यादीन् |

तद्यथा- शुक्रशोणितप्रकृतिं, कालगर्भाशयप्रकृतिं, आतुराहारविहारप्रकृतिं, महाभूत विकार प्रकृतिं च गर्भशरीरमपेक्षते|

एतानि हि येन येन दोषेणाधिकेनैकेनानेकेन वा समनुबध्यन्ते, तेन तेन दोषेण गर्भोऽनुबध्यते; ततः सा सा दोषप्रकृतिरुच्यते मनुष्याणां गर्भादिप्रवृत्ता|

तस्माच्छ्लेष्मलाः प्रकृत्या केचित्, पित्तलाः केचित्, वातलाः केचित्, संसृष्टाः केचित्, समधातवः केचिद्भवन्ति|

तेषां हि लक्षणानि व्याख्यास्यामः||९५||

Now we shall explain the characteristic feature of Prakrti (physical constitution etc) Prakrti or physical constitution of the fetus is determined by the following factors:

Sperms and ovum

Season and condition of the uterus

Food and regimens of the mother

Nature of the Mahabhutas comprising the fetus

The fetus gets afflicted with one or more of the Doshas which are dominantly associated with the above-mentioned factors. The physical constitution of an individual is a determining factor when they initially unite in the form of a fetus. Therefore, the physical constitution of some is dominated by Kapha (Sleshmala), of some others by Pitta (Pittala), of others by Vata (vatala) and of some others by the combination of two Doshas (Samsrsata). In some other cases, however, the equilibrium of Doshas (Samaprakrti) is well maintained. We shall now expound their characteristics one after the other. [95]

Characteristics of Sleshmala individual:

श्लेष्मा हि स्निग्ध श्लक्ष्ण मृदु मधुर सार सान्द्र मन्द स्तिमित गुरु शीत विज्जलाच्छः|

तस्य स्नेहाच्छ्लेष्मलाः स्निग्धाङ्गाः, श्लक्ष्णत्वाच्छ्लक्ष्णाङ्गाः, मृदुत्वाद्दृष्टि सुख सुकुमारावदातगात्राः, माधुर्यात् प्रभूत शुक्र व्यवायापत्याः, सारत्वात् सार संहत स्थिर शरीराः, सान्द्रत्वादुपचितपरिपूर्णसर्वाङ्गाः, मन्दत्वान्मन्द चेष्टाहारव्याहाराः, स्तैमित्याद शीघ्रारम्भक्षोभ विकाराः, गुरुत्वात् साराधिष्ठितावस्थितगतयः, शैत्यादल्पक्षुत्तृष्णासन्तापस्वेददोषाः, विज्जलत्वात् सुश्लिष्टसारसन्धिबन्धनाः, तथाऽच्छत्वात् प्रसन्नदर्शनाननाः प्रसन्नस्निग्धवर्णस्वराश्च भवन्ति|

त एवङ्गुणयोगाच्छ्लेष्मला बलवन्तो वसुमन्तो विद्यावन्त ओजस्विनः शान्ता आयुष्मन्तश्च भवन्ति||९६||

Kapha is unctuous, smooth, soft, sweet, firm, dense, slow, stable, heavy, cold, viscous and clear.

The various manifestations in the human body having Sleshmala type of constitution are given below:

1. Unctuous - Unctuousness of organs
2. Smooth - Smoothness of organs
3. Soft - Pleasing appearance, tenderness and clarity of complexion
4. Sweet - Increase in the quantity of semen, desire for sex-act and number of procreations
5. Firm - Firmness, compactness and stability of the body

6. Dense - Plumpness and roundness of all organs
7. Slow - Slow in action, intake of food and movement
8. Stable - Slowness in initiating actions, getting irritated and morbid manifestations
9. Heavy - Non-slippery and stable gait with the entire sole of the feet pressing against the earth
10. Cold - Lack of intensity in hunger, thirst, heat and perspiration
11. Viscous - Firmness and compactness in joints
12. Clear - Happiness in the look and face; happiness and softness of complexion and voice

Characteristics of Pittala individual:

पित्तमुष्णं तीक्ष्णं द्रवं विस्रमम्लं कटुकञ्च|

तस्यौष्ण्यात् पित्तला भवन्त्युष्णासहा, उष्णमुखाः, सुकुमारावदातगात्राः , प्रभूत विप्लुव्यङ्ग तिल पिडकाः, क्षुत्पिपासावन्तः, क्षिप्र वली पलित खालित्य दोषाः, प्रायोमृद्वल्पक पिल श्मश्रु लोम केशाश्च; तैक्ष्ण्यातीक्ष्णपराक्रमाः, तीक्ष्णाग्नयः, प्रभूताशनपानाः, क्लेशासहिष्णवो, दन्दशूकाः; द्रवत्वाच्छिथिलमृदु सन्धि मांसाः, प्रभूत सृष्ट स्वेद मूत्र पुरीषाश्च; विस्रत्वात् प्रभूत पूतिकक्षास्यशिरःशरीरगन्धाः; कट्वम्लत्वादल्पशुक्रव्यवायापत्याः; त एवङ्गुणयोगात् पित्तला मध्यबला मध्यायुषो मध्यज्ञानविज्ञानवित्तोपकरणवन्तश्च भवन्ति||९७||

Pitta is hot, sharp, liquid, of fleshy smell, sour and Pungnet, Various manifestations due to these attributes in the human body having pittala type of constitution are given below:

- Hot - Intolerance for hot things, having hot face, tender and clear body, of Port- wine stain, freckles, black moles, excessive hunger and thirst; quick development of bodywrinkles, graying of hair and baldness; presence of lesser body hair and scalp hair with mustache that are soft in nature.
- Sharp - Sharp (demonstration of) physical strength, strong digestive power, intake of food and drink in large quantity, inability to face difficult situations and glutton habits
- Liquor - Looseness and softness of joints and muscles; voiding of sweet, urine and feces in large quantity.
- Fleshy smell - Excessive putrid smell of axilla, mouth, head and body
- Pungent and sour tastes - Insufficiency of semen, sexual desire and procreation.

By virtue of the above-mentioned qualities, a man having Pittala type of constitution is endowed with moderate strength, moderate life, moderate spiritual and materialistic knowledge, wealth and the accessories of life. [97]

Characteristics of Vatala individual:

वातस्तु रूक्ष लघु चल बहु शीघ्र शीत परुष विशदः|

तस्य रौक्ष्याद्वातला रूक्षापचिताल्पशरीराः प्रतत रूक्ष क्षामसन्नसक्तजर्जरस्वरा जागरूकाश्च भवन्ति, लघुत्वाल्लघु चपल गति चेष्टाहार व्याहाराः, चलत्वादनवस्थित सन्ध्यक्षिभूहन्वोष्ठ जिह्वा शिरःस्कन्ध पाणि पादाः, बहुत्वाद्बहु प्रलाप कण्डरासिरा प्रतानाः, शीघ्रत्वाच्छीघ्रसमारम्भक्षोभविकाराः शीघ्र त्रास राग विरागाः श्रुत ग्राहिणोऽल्पस्मृतयश्च, शैत्याच्छीतासहिष्णवः प्रतत शीतकोद्वेपक स्तम्भाः, पारुष्यात् परुष केश श्मश्रु रोम नख दशन वदन पाणि पादाः, वैशद्यात् स्फुटिताङ्गावयवाः सतत सन्धि शब्द गामिनश्च भवन्ति; त एवङ्गुणयोगाद्वातलाः प्रायेणाल्पबलाश्चाल्पायुष्श्चाल्पापत्याश्चाल्पसाधनाश्चाल्पधनाश्च भवन्ति||९८||

संसर्गात् संसृष्टलक्षणाः||९९||

Vata is un, unctuous, light, mobile, and abundant in quantity, swift, cold, rough and non-slime. B various manifestations due to these attributes of Vata in human body having Vatala type of constitution are given below:

1. Ununctous - Ununctuousness emaciation and dwarfness of the body, long drawn, dry low, broken, obstructed and hoarse voice, always keeping awake
2. Light - Light and inconsistent gait, action, food and movement
3. Mobile - Unstable joints- eyes, eye brows, jaw, lips, tongue, head, shoulder, hands and legs
4. Abundance - Talkativeness, abundance in tendons and veins

5. Swift - Quick in initiating actions, getting irritated and the onset of morbid manifestation; quick in affliction with fear, quick in likes and dislikes; quick in understanding and forgetting things

6. Cold - Intolerance for cold things; often getting afflicted with cold, shivering and stiffness

7. Rough - Roughness in the hair of the head, face and other parts of the body, nails, teeth, face, hands and feet

8. Non-slime - Cracking of the limbs and organs, production of cracking sound in joints when they move.

Because of the above-mentioned qualities, individuals having Vatala type of constitution are mostly processed of strength, span of life, procreation, accessories of life and wealth in lesser quantity. Individuals having constitution dominated by the combination of two Doshas are characterized of respective Doshas. [98-99]

सर्वगुणसमुदितास्तु समधातवः|
इत्येवं प्रकृतितः परीक्षेत||१००||

A Samadhatu type of individual who has all the Doshas in the state of equilibrium is endowed with the good qualities of all the three types of individuals described in para 96-98. Thus, an individual is examined for his constitution. [100]

Factors required to be examined to ascertain the nature of disease:

विकृतितश्चेति विकृतिरुच्यते विकारः|
तत्र विकारं हेतु-दोष-दूष्य-प्रकृति-देश-काल-बल विशेषैर्लिङ्गतश्च परीक्षेत, न ह्यन्तरेण हेत्वादीनां बल विशेषं व्याधि बल विशेषोपलब्धिः|
यस्य हि व्याधेर्दोष-दूष्य-प्रकृति-देश-काल-बलसाम्यं भवति, महच्च हेतु लिङ्ग बलं, स व्याधिर्बलवान् भवति; तद्विपर्ययाच्चाल्पबलः;
मध्यबलस्तु दोषदूष्यादीनामन्यतमसामान्याद्धेतुलिङ्ग मध्य बलत्वाच्चोपलभ्यते||१०१||

According to para 94, a patient is to be examined for the Vikrti or morbid manifestations. These morbid manifestations are to be examined with reference to the specific causative factors, Dosha and Dhatus involved in the pathogenesis, constitution of the individual, habitat, season and strength and also the symptoms of the diseases. Without determining the strength of the causative factors etc., it is not possible to obtain the knowledge regarding the intensity of the disease.

If the afflicted Doshas and Dhatus, physical constitution of the patient, habit, season and strength of the individual resemble that of the disease in quality and the causative factors and symptoms are too strong and numerous, the disease so manifested is acute; otherwise, it is mild. If either of the Doshas, Dhatus etc, resembles that of threat of the disease in quality and the causative factors and symptoms of the disease are of moderate nature, the disease so manifested is also moderate. [101]

Examination of Sara:

सारतश्चेति साराण्यष्टौ पुरुषाणां बल मान विशेष ज्ञानार्थमुपदिश्यन्ते; तद्यथा- त्वग्रक्त मांस मेदोऽस्थि मज्ज शुक्र सत्त्वानीति||१०२||

According to para 94, patients are to be examined with reference to Sara or the excellence of their Dhatus. When a view to determining the specific measure of strength they are classified into eight categories, depending upon the Sara or excellence of their Dhatus, viz, Tvak (Lit, meaning skin but contextual meaning Rasadhatu), Rakta (blood), Mamsa (muscle tissue), Medas (adipose tissue), Asthi (bone tissue), Majja(marrow) Shukra (semen) and Sattva (mental faculties). [102]

Tvak-sara:

तत्र स्निग्ध श्लक्ष्ण मृदु प्रसन्न सूक्ष्माल्प गम्भीर सुकुमार लोमा सप्रभेव च त्वक् त्वक्साराणाम्|
सा सारता सुख सौभाग्यैश्वर्योपभोग बुद्धि विद्यारोग्य प्रहर्षणान्यायुष्यत्वं चाचष्टे||१०३||

Individuals having the excellence of Tvak or skin are characterized by unctuous, smooth, soft, clear, fine, less numerous, deep rooted and tender hair and lustrous skin. Such individuals are endowed with happiness, good fortunes, power, enjoyment, intellect knowledge, health, excitement and longevity [103]

Rakta-Sara:

कर्णाक्षि मुख जिह्वा नासौष्ठ पाणिपाद तल नख ललाट मेहनं स्निग्ध रक्त वर्ण श्रीमद्भ्राजिष्णु रक्त साराणाम्|
सा सारता सुखमुद्धतां मेधां मनस्वित्वं सौकुमार्यमनतिबलमक्लेश सहिष्णुत्वमुष्णासहिष्णुत्वं चाचष्टे||१०४||

Individuals having the excellence of Rakta or blood are characterized by unctousness, red color, beautiful dazzling appearance of the ears, eyes, face, tongue, nose, lips, sole of the hands and feet, nails, forehead and genital organs, such individuals are endowed with happiness, great genius, enthusiasm, tenderness, moderate strength and inability to face difficulties their body remains hot. [104]

Mamsa –Sara:

शङ्ख ललाट कृकाटिकाक्षिगण्ड हनु ग्रीवास्कन्धोदर कक्ष वक्षःपाणिपाद सन्धयः स्थिर गुरु शुभ मांसोपचिता मांससाराणाम्|
सा सारता क्षमां धृतिमलौल्यं वित्तं विद्यां सुखमार्जवमारोग्यं बलमायुश्च दीर्घमाचष्टे||१०५||

Individual having the excellence of the Mamsa or muscle tissue are characterized by stability, heaviness, beautiful appearance and plumpness of temples, forehead, nape, eyes, cheeks, jaws, neck, shoulder, abdomen maxillae, chest and joints of upper and lower limbs being covered with flesh. Such individuals are endowed with forgiven, patience, noun greediness, wealth, knowledge, happiness, simplicity, health, strength and longevity. [105]

Medah –Sara:

वर्ण स्वर नेत्र केश लोम नख दन्तौष्ठ मूत्र पुरीषेषु विशेषतः स्नेहो मेदःसाराणाम्|
सा सारता वित्तैश्वर्य सुखोपभोगप्रदानान्यार्जवं सुकुमारोपचारतां चा चष्टे||१०६||

Individuals having the excellence of Medas or adipose tissue are characterized by the abundance of unctuousness in completion, voice, eyes, hair of the head and other parts of the body, nail, teeth, lips, urine and feces. Such individuals are endowed with health, power, happiness, enjoyment, charity, simplicity and delicate habits. [106]

Asthi-Sara:

पार्ष्णि गुल्फ जान्वरत्नि जत्र चिबुक शिरःपर्वस्थूलाः स्थूलास्थि नख दन्ताश्चास्थिसाराः|
ते महोत्साहाः क्रियावन्तः क्लेश सहाः सारस्थिर शरीरा भवन्त्यायुष्मन्तश्च||१०७||

Individuals having the excellence of Asthi or bone tissue are characterized by robust heels, ankles, keeps, fore-arms, collar bones, chin, head, joints, bones, nails and teeth. Such individuals are very enthusiastic and active, and are endowed with strong and firm bodies as well as longevity. [107]

Majja- Sara:

मृद्वङ्गा बलवन्तः स्निग्ध वर्ण स्वराः स्थूल दीर्घ वृत्तसन्धयश्च मज्जसाराः|
ते दीर्घायुषो बलवन्तः श्रुत वित्त विज्ञानापत्यसम्मानभाजश्च भवन्ति||१०८||

Individuals having the excellence of Majja or narrow are characterized by softness of organs, strength, unctuous complexion and voice and robust long and rounded joints. Such individuals are endowed with longevity, strength, learning, wealth, knowledge, progeny and honor. [108]

Shukra- Sara:

सौम्याः सौम्यप्रेक्षिणः क्षीरपूर्ण लोचना इव प्रहर्षबहुलाः स्निग्धवृत सार समसंहत शिखर दशनाः प्रसन्न स्निग्ध वर्ण स्वरा भ्राजिष्णवो महास्फिचश्च शुक्रसाराः|
ते स्त्रीप्रियोपभोगा बलवन्तः सुखैश्वर्यारोग्यवित्तसम्मानापत्यभाजश्च भवन्ति||१०९||

Individuals having the excellence of Shukradhatu or semen are characterized by gentleness, gentle look, having eyes as if filled with milk, cheerfulness, having teeth which are unctuous, round, strong, even and beautiful, clean and unctuous complexion and voice, dazzling appearance and large buttocks. Such individuals are loved by women; they are strong and endowed with happiness, power, health, wealth, honors and children. [109]

Sattva-sara:

स्मृतिमन्तो भक्तिमन्तः कृतज्ञाः प्राज्ञाः शुचयो महोत्साहा दक्षा धीराः समर विक्रान्तयोधिनस्त्यक्तविषादाः सुव्यवस्थित गति गम्भीर बुद्धि चेष्टाः कल्याणाभिनिवेशिनश्च सत्त्वसाराः|

तेषां स्वलक्षणैरेव गुणा व्याख्याताः||११०||

Individuals having the excellence of mental faculties are characterized by good memory, devotion, gratefulness, wisdom, purity, excessive enthusiasm, and skill, and courage, valour in fighting, absence and virtuous acts. (These characteristic features represent the qualities of such individuals) [110]

Individuals having all saras:

तत्र सर्वैः सारैरुपेता पुरुषा भवन्त्यतिबलाः परम सुख युक्ताः क्लेशसहाः सर्वारम्भेष्वात्मनि जातप्रत्ययाः कल्याणाभिनिवेशिनः स्थिर समाहित शरीराः सुसमाहितगतयः सानुनाद स्निग्ध गम्भीर महास्वराः सुखैश्वर्य वित्तोप भोग सम्मानभाजो मन्दजरसो मन्दविकाराः प्रायस्तुल्यगुणविस्तीर्णापत्याश्चिरजीविनश्च||१११||

Individuals possessed of the excellence of all the above mentioned Dhatus including mental faculties (as described in para Nos. 103-110) are endowed with great strength and happiness, resistance to difficulties, self-confidence in all enterprises, virtuous acts, firm and well built body, correct gait; resonant, melodies and high pitched voice, happiness, power, wealth, enjoyments, honor, slowness of aging process, resistance for diseases, large number of children with similar qualities and longevity. [111]

अतो विपरीतास्त्वसाराः||११२||

मध्यानां मध्यैःसार विशेषैर्गुण विशेषा व्याख्याता भवन्ति||११३||

Qualities opposite to what are described in paragraphs 103-111 are indicative of the absence of the excellence of respective Dhatus in the individual. Individuals having excellence of these Dhatus of moderate nature are possessed of respective qualities in moderate intensity. [112-113]

इति साराण्यष्टौ पुरुषाणां बल प्रमाण विशेष ज्ञानार्थमुपदिष्टानि भवन्ति||११४||

Thus the eight categories of individuals expanding upon the Sara or excellence of Dhatus are described in brief strength. [114]

Need for examination of Sara:

कथं नु शरीरमात्रदर्शनादेव भिषङ्मृह्येदयमुपचितत्वाद्बलवान्, अयमल्पबलः कृशत्वात्, महाबलोऽयं महाशरीरत्वात्, अयमल्पशरीरत्वादल्पबल इति; दृश्यन्ते ह्यल्पशरीराः कृशाश्चैके बलवन्तः; तत्र पिपीलिकाभारहरणवत् सिद्धिः|

अतश्च सारतः परीक्षेतेत्युक्तम्||११५||

It is fallacious to consider an individual to be strong or weak either from his plump or emaciated body or from the large one small size of his body. Some people having a small sized and emaciated body are seen to be strong. They are like ants that have a small body and look emaciated but can carry too heavy a load. Thus, one should examine the individual with reference to the excellence of his Dhatus. [115]

Samhanana:

संहननश्चेति संहननं, संहतिः, संयोजनमित्येकोऽर्थः|

तत्र समसुविभक्तास्थि, सुबद्धसन्धि, सुनिविष्टमांसशोणितं, सुसंहतं शरीरमित्युच्यते|

तत्र सुसंहत शरीराः पुरुषा बलवन्तः, विपर्ययेणाल्पबलाः, मध्यत्वात् संहननस्य मध्यबला भवन्ति||११६||

According to Para- 94, a patient is to be examined with reference to his samhanana or compactness of the body. Samhanana, Samhati and Samyojana – these three terms are synonymous. A compact body is characterized by the symmetrial and well divided bones, well-knit joints and well bound muscles and blood. An individual having a compact body is very strong; otherwise, he is weak. When the body is moderately compact, the individual is passed of moderate strength. [116]

Pramana:

प्रमाणतश्चेति शरीर प्रमाणं पुनर्यथास्वेनाङ्गुलि प्रमाणेनोपदेक्ष्यते उत्सेध विस्तारायामैर्यथाक्रमम्‌|

तत्र पादौ चत्वारि षट् चतुर्दशाङ्गुलानि, जङ्घे त्वष्टादशाङ्गुले षोडशाङ्गुलपरिक्षेपे च, जानुनी चतुरङ्गुले षोडशाङ्गुल परिक्षेपे, त्रिंशदङ्गुल परिक्षेपावष्टादशाङ्गुलावूरू, षडङ्गुल दीर्घौ वृषणावष्टाङ्गुलपरिणाहौ, शेफः षडङ्गुलदीर्घं पञ्चाङ्गुलपरिणाहं, द्वादशाङ्गुलिपरिणाहो भगः, षोडशाङ्गुलविस्तारा कटी, दशाङ्गुलं बस्तिशिरः, दशाङ्गुलविस्तारं द्वादशाङ्गुलमुदरं, दशाङ्गुलविस्तीर्ण द्वादशाङ्गुलायामे पार्श्वे, द्वादशाङ्गुलं स्तनान्तरं, द्व्यङ्गुलं स्तनपर्यन्तं, चतुर्विंशत्यङ्गुलविशालं द्वादशाङ्गुलोत्सेधमुरः, द्व्यङ्गुलंहृदयम्, अष्टाङ्गुलौ स्कन्धौ, षडङ्गुलावंसौ, षोडशाङ्गुलौ प्रबाहू, पञ्चदशाङ्गुलौ प्रपाणी, हस्तौ द्वादशाङ्गुलौ, कक्षावष्टाङ्गुलौ, त्रिकं द्वादशाङ्गुलोत्सेधम्‌, अष्टादशाङ्गुलोत्सेधं पृष्ठं, चतुरङ्गुलोत्सेधा द्वाविंशत्यङ्गुलपरिणाहा शिरोधरा, द्वादशाङ्गुलोत्सेधं चतुर्विंशत्यङ्गुलपरिणाहमाननं, पञ्चाङ्गुलमास्यं, चिबुकौष्ठकर्णाक्षिमध्यनासिकाललाटं चतुरङ्गुलं, षोडशाङ्गुलोत्सेधं द्वात्रिंशदङ्गुलपरिणाहं शिरः; इति पृथक्त्वेनाङ्गावयवानां मानमुक्तम्‌|

केवलं पुनःशरीरमङ्गुलिपर्वाणि चतुरशीतिः|

तदायामविस्तारसमं समुच्यते|

तत्रायुर्बलमोजः सुखमैश्वर्य वित्तमिष्टाश्चापरे भावा भवन्त्यायताः प्रमाणवति शरीरे; विपर्ययस्त्वतो हीनेऽधिके वा||११७||

According to Para- 94, the patient is also to be examined with reference to Pramana or the measurement of his bodily organs. This is determined by measuring the height, length and breadth of the organs by taking the finger breadth of the individual as the unit of measurement. (One finger breadth of a medium sized adult is approximately 1.95 cm)

Measurement of organs as are endowed with all good qualities is given below. Measurement with finger breadth of the individual as a unit:

Measurement with finger breadth of the individual as a unit:

abbreviations – ht = Height, ln = length, br = breadth, cn – Circumference, Ot = Others (not specified), Unit – Angula

1. Feet: ht – 4, ln - 14, br – 6
2. Jangha (calf region): ln - 18, cn – 16
3. Knees: ln – 4, cn – 16
4. Thighs - ln - 18, cn – 30
5. Testicles: ln - 6, cn – 8
6. Phallus: ln - 6, cn – 5
7. Vagina: cn – 12
8. Waist: br – 16
9. Bastisira (top of pelvis): Ot – 10
10. Abdomen: ln - 12, br – 10
11. Parsva (sides of chest): ln - 12, br – 10
12. Distance between the nipples: ht – 12 Ot – 12
13. Nipples: cn – 2
14. Chest: cn – 2
15. Hrdaya (Heart): br – 24
16. Shoulders: Ot – 18
17. Shoulder blades: Ot – 6
18. Prabahu(arms): Ot – 16
19. Fore-arms: Ot – 15
20. Hands: Ot – 20
21. Axillae: Ot – 8
22. Trika (sac-12 rum incuding coceyx): -
23. Back: ht – 18
24. Neck: ht – 4, cn – 22
25. Face: ht – 12, cn – 24

26. Mouth: br – 5,

27. Chin: Ot – 4

28. Lips: Ot – 4

29. Ears: Ot – 4

30. Distance between the eyes (external angles of the eyes): Ot – 4

31. Nose - Ot – 4

32. Fore-head: Ot – 4

33. Head: ht – 16, cn – 32

34. Entire body: ht – 84, br - 84

(When hands are fully out-spread)

Thus, the measurement of individual organs of the body is described. A body consisting of organs having proper measurement is involved with longevity, strength, Ojas (energy), happiness, power, wealth and virtues. If the measurement is either on the high or low side, the individual possesses qualities contrary to what are mentioned above, [117]

Satmya:

सात्म्यतश्चेति सात्म्यं नाम तद्यत् सातत्येनोपसेव्यमानमुपशेते|

तत्र ये घृत क्षीर तैल मांस रस सात्म्याः सर्वरससात्म्याश्च ते बलवन्तः क्लेशसहाश्चिरजीविनश्च भवन्ति,

रूक्षसात्म्याः पुनरेकरससात्म्याश्च ये ते प्रायेणाल्पबला अल्पक्लेशसहा अल्पायुषोऽल्पसाधनाश्च भवन्ति,

व्यामिश्रसात्म्यास्तु ये ते मध्यबलाः सात्म्य निमित्ततो भवन्ति||११८||

According to para-34 again, a patient is to be examined with reference to his Satmya or homogation. Satmya stands for such factors as wholesome to the individual even when continually used. Individuals for whom ghee, milk, oil and meat soup as well as the drugs and diets having all the six tastes are wholesome are endowed with strength, the power of facing difficult situations and longevity. Those who are accustomed to ununctuous things, and drugs and diets having only one particular taste, are mostly possessed of less strength, less power (or resistance) to face difficult situations, are of smaller life-span and of meager accessories like drugs for the treatment of his diseases. If there is combination of both these types of homologations, individuals are posed of moderate strength. [118]

Sattva:

सत्त्वतश्चेति सत्त्वमुच्यते मनः|

तच्छरीरस्य तन्त्रकमात्मसंयोगात्|

तत् त्रिविधं बलभेदेन- प्रवरं, मध्यम्, अवरं चेति; अतश्च प्रवर मध्यावर सत्त्वाः पुरुषा भवन्ति|

तत्र प्रवरसत्त्वाः सत्त्वसारास्ते सारेष्पदिष्टाः, स्वल्पशरीरा ह्यपि ते निजागन्तुनिमित्तासु महतीष्वपि पीडास्वव्यथा दृश्यन्ते सत्त्वगुणवैशेष्यात्; मध्यसत्त्वास्त्वपरानात्मन्युपनिधाय संस्तम्भयन्त्यात्मनाऽऽत्मानं परैर्वाऽपि संस्तभ्यन्ते; हीनसत्त्वास्तु नात्मना नापि परैः सत्त्वबलं प्रति शक्यन्ते उपस्तम्भयितुं, महाशरीरा ह्यपि ते स्वल्पानामपि वेदनानामसहा दृश्यन्ते, सन्निहितभयशोकलोभमोहमाना रौद्रभैरवद्विष्टबीभत्सविकृतसङ्कथास्वपि च पशु पुरुष मांस शोणितानि चावेक्ष्य विषाद वैवर्ण्य मूर्च्छोन्माद भ्रम प्रपतनानामन्यतममाप्नुवन्त्यथवा मरणमिति||११९||

The patient is again to be examined with reference to his Sattva or mental faculties. Sattva is the mind and it regulates the body because of its association with the soul. Depending upon its strength, it is of three types, viz, superior, mediocre and inferior mental faculties. Individuals having mental faculties of their mental faculties Individuals are described in para- 110 above. Even if possessed of weak physique, such individuals, because of the specific manifestations of Sattva qualities in them, tolerate serious exogenous and endogenous diseases without much difficulty.

Individuals having mediocrity of mental faculties tolerate the pain themselves when they realize that others can also tolerate the pain themselves when they realize that others can also tolerate it, then they of mental faculties, neither by themselves nor through others can sustain their mental strength and even mild pain. They are susceptible to fear, grief, greed, delusion and ego. When they hear even stones describing wrathful, fearful, hateful, terrifying and ugly situation or come across vision of flesh or blood of an animal or man, they fall victims to depression, pallor, fainting, madness, giddiness of falling on the ground, or such aviates may even lead them to death. [119]

Capacity for food:

आहारशक्तितश्चेति आहारशक्तिरभ्यवहरण शक्त्या जरण शक्तया च परीक्ष्या; बलायुषी ह्याहारायते||१२०||

A patient is further to be examined with reference to his Aharasakti or the capacity for intake of food. One's capacity for food can be examined from two angles, viz, the power of ingestion as well as the power of digestion; both the strength and life-span are determined by the diet of the individual. [120]

Capacity for exercise:

व्यायामशक्तितश्चेति व्यायाम शक्तिरपि कर्मशक्त्या परीक्ष्या|

कर्मशक्त्या ह्यनुमीयते बलत्रैविध्यम् ||१२१||

The patient is examined with reference to his capacity for exercise which is determined by one's ability to perform work like lifting weight etc. strength of individuals is classified into three categories, depending upon their ability to perform work. [121]

Span of life:

वयस्तश्चेति काल प्रमाण विशेषापेक्षिणी हि शरीरावस्था वयोऽभिधीयते|

तद्वयो यथा स्थूल भेदेन त्रिविधं- बालं, मध्यं, जीर्णमिति|

The patient is examined with reference to his age which represents the state of his body depending upon the length of the time that has passed since birth. Age is broadly of three types, viz, young age, middle age and old age.

तत्र बालमपरिपक्वधातुमजातव्यञ्जनं सुकुमारमक्लेशसहमसम्पूर्णबलं श्लेष्मधातुप्रायमाषोडशवर्षं, विवर्धमानधातुगुणं पुनः प्रायेणानवस्थितसत्त्वमात्रिंशद्वर्षमुपदिष्टं; मध्यं पुनः समत्वागत बल वीर्य पौरुष पराक्रम ग्रहण धारण स्मरण वचन विज्ञान सर्वधातुगुणं बलस्थितमवस्थित सत्त्वमविशीर्यमाण धातु गुणं पित्त धातु प्रायमाषष्टिवर्षमुपदिष्टम्; अतः परं हीयमानधात्विन्द्रिय बल वीर्य पौरुष पराक्रम ग्रहण धारण स्मरण वचन विज्ञानं भ्रश्यमान धातुगुणं वायु धातु प्रायं क्रमेण जीर्णमुच्यते आयर्षशताग्| वर्षशतं खल्वायुषः प्रमाणमस्मिन् काले; सन्ति च पुनरधिकोनवर्षशतजीविनोऽपि मनुष्याः; तेषां विकृतिवर्जैः प्रकृत्यादिबलविशेषैरायुषो लक्षणतश्च प्रमाणमुपलभ्य वयसस्त्रित्वं विभजेत्||१२२||

Young age is again of two types, viz (i) immature stage lasting upon 16th year of age and (ii) maturing stage lasting upon the 30th year of age. During the immature stage various organs of the body are not well developed, there is tenderness, the individual cannot tolerate difficulties, and there is incomplete strength and the dominance of Kapha Dosha in the body. During the second stage i.e the stage of maturing lasting up to 30th year of age, the mental faculties are not properly developed.

During the middle age lasting up to the 60th year of age, there is diminution of the Dhatus (tissue elements), strength of sense organs, energy, manliness and velour, power of understanding, retention, memorizing, speech and analyzing facts and the qualities of all Dhatus; there is the dominance of Pittadosha.

Thereafter during old age lasting upto the 100th year of age, there is diminution of the Dhatus (tissue elements), strength of sense organs, energy, manliness, valor, power of understanding, retention, memorizing, speech and analyzing facts. There is gradual diminution in the qualities of Dhatus and dominance of Vata during this age.

During this Kali age, the span of life is 100 years. Of course. There are people who live for a longer or shorter period than this. Their age is classified in para 94, viz. Prakrti (physical constitution) etc. excluding morbidity and also with the help of characteristic features of individuals having various categories of life-span. [122]

Strength of the body, Doshas and drugs:

एवं प्रकृत्यादीनां विकृतिवर्ज्यानां भावानां प्रवर मध्यावर विभागेन बल विशेषं विभजेत्|

विकृतिबलैविविध्येन तु दोषबलं त्रिविधमनुमीयते|

ततो भैषज्यस्य तीक्ष्ण मृदु मध्य विभागेन त्रैविध्यं विभज्य यथादोष भैषज्यमवचारयेदिति||१२३||

The strength of individuals can be classified, depending upon the superiority, mediocrity and inferiority of the above-mentioned factors, viz, Prakrti (physical constitution) etc., except Vikrti or morbidity. Three types of the strength of the Doshas are inferred from the three types of the intensity of morbidity. Thereafter, depending upon the nature of the Doshas involved, three types of medicaments, viz strong, mild and moderate, are administered. [123]

आयुषः प्रमाण ज्ञान हेतोः पुनरिन्द्रियेषु जातिसूत्रीये च लक्षणान्युपदेक्ष्यन्ते||१२४||

With a view to ascertaining the life-span of an individual, symptoms will be described in the Indriya section and also in the 8th chapter of Sharira section. [124]

Division of year:

कालः पुनः संवत्सरश्चातुरावस्था च|

तत्र संवत्सरो द्विधा त्रिधा षोढा द्वादशधा भूयश्चाप्यतः प्रविभज्यते तत्तत्कार्यमभिसमीक्ष्य|

अत्र खलु तावत् षोढा प्रविभज्य कार्यमुपदेक्ष्यते- हेमन्तो ग्रीष्मो वर्षाश्चेति शीतोष्णवर्षलक्षणास्त्रय ऋतवो भवन्ति, तेषामन्तरेष्वितरे साधारण लक्षणास्त्रय ऋतवः- प्रावृट्शरद्वसन्ता इति|

प्रावृडिति प्रथमः प्रवृष्टः कालः, तस्यानुबन्धो हि वर्षाः|

एवमेते संशोधनमधिकृत्य षट् विभज्यन्ते ऋतवः||१२५||

Kala or time connotes two meanings, viz, the year and the state of the disease in the patient. Depending upon the necessity, year is variously divided into two, three, six, twelve and even, ore. In the present context, six divisions of the year are envisaged Hemanta (winter) Grishma (summer) and Varsha (rainy) weather. Flanked by them are three other seasons, viz, ate nature. Pravrt season is characterized by the beginning of rains of elimination therapies in view, seasons are thus divided into six. [125]

Suitable season for administration of Elimination Therapy:

तत्र साधारणलक्षणेष्वृतुषु वमनादीनां प्रवृत्तिर्विधीयते, निवृत्तिरितरेषु|

साधारणलक्षणा हि मन्दशीतोष्णवर्षत्वात् सुखतमाश्च भवन्त्यविकल्पकाश्च शरीरौषधानाम्,

इतरे पुनरत्यर्थशीतोष्णवर्षत्वाद्दुःखतमाश्च भवन्ति विकल्पकाश्च शरीरौषधानाम्||१२६||

A year can be classified in different ways depending upon the different purposes in view. On the basis of Ayana or solstitial movement of the sun to north or south., year is divided into two; on the basis of the intensity of cold, heat or rain, it is divided into three; on the basis of seasons, it is divided into six; on the basis of months, it is divided into twelve and on the basis of fortnights, it is divided into twenty-four. Similarly, it can have many divisions on the basis of Prahara (a unit of three hoarse) etc

Asadha (June- july) and Shravana (July –August) – these months constitute the Pravrt season. In their season, viz Varsha (rainy season) etc. are also composed of two months each. Division of the year into six seasons each comprising two months is detailedand given below:

1. Pravrt :

Months according to Hindu calendar - Asadha, Shravana

Months according to Greek calendar (appropriately) - June-July, July - August

2. Varsha :

Months according to Hindu calendar - Bhadrapada, Ashvina
Months according to Greek calendar (appropriately) - August- September, September- October
3. Sarat :
Months according to Hindu calendar - Kartika, Mrugashira
Months according to Greek calendar (appropriately) - October- November, November - December
4. Hemanta :
Months according to Hindu calendar - Pausa, Magha
Months according to Greek calendar (appropriately) - December-January, January- February
5. Vasanta :
Months according to Hindu calendar - Phalguna, Chaitra
Months according to Greek calendar (appropriately) - February- March, March-April
6. Grishma :
Months according to Hindu calendar - Vaisakha, Jyestha
Months according to Greek calendar (appropriately) - April-May, May-June

Suitable season for administration of elimination therapy:
Elimination therapies, viz, Vamana (emesis) etc.., are administered only in seasons of moderate nature. In other seasons having extreme cold, heat or rain, such therapies should not be administered.

Moderate seasons are characterized by moderation in cold heat and rain. They are very enjoyable and they do not adversely affect the conditions of the body and drugs. Remaining seasons are characterized by extreme cold, heat or rain. They are very unpleasant and the body as well as medicines are adversely affected by them. [126]

Unsuitable seasons for Elimination Therapy:
तत्र हेमन्ते ह्यतिमात्रशीतोपहतत्वाच्छरीरमसुखोपपन्नं भवत्यतिशीतवाताध्मातमतिदारुणीभूतमवबद्धदोषं च, भेषजं पुनः संशोधनार्थमुष्णस्वभावमतिशीतोपहतत्वान्मन्दवीर्यत्वमापद्यते, तस्मात्तयोः संयोगे संशोधनमयोगायोपपद्यते शरीरमपि च वातोपद्रवाय|
During the Hemanta or winter season, the body is exposed to great discomfort because of affliction by excessive cold. The Doshas do not get detached and remain adhered to the channels in the body due to their excessive firmness caused by the contact with the terrific cold- wind. Medicaments used for elimination therapy are by nature hot but because of affliction with excessive cold their therapeutic effectiveness is diminished. When these therapeutically less potent drugs are administered to an individual whose body is unsuitable for the therapy it does not produce the desired effect and the body gets afflicted with Vata.

ग्रीष्मे पुनर्भृशोष्णोपहतत्वाच्छरीरमसुखोपपन्नं भवत्युष्णवातातपाध्मातमतिशिथिलमत्यर्थप्रविलीनदोषं, भेषजं पुनः संशोधनार्थमुष्णस्वभावमुष्णानुगमनात्तीक्ष्णतरत्वमापद्यते, तस्मात्तयोः संयोगे संशोधनमतियोगायोपपद्यते शरीरमपि पिपासोपद्रवाय|
During the Grishma or summer season there is great discomfort in the body because of the affliction with excessive heat. Doshas remain excessively detached due to their excessive looseness caused by the contact with excessively hot wind as well as hot sun. Medicaments used for elimination therapy are by nature hot and because of the afflicted with excessive heat, their therapeutic effect becomes all the sharper. When these drugs having sharp effect are administered to an individual having an impaired body, there is excessive elimination of Doshas and the body gets afflicted with complications including excessive thirst.

वर्षासु तु मेघजलावतते गूढार्कचन्द्रतारे धाराकुले वियति भूमौ पङ्कजलपटलसंवृतायामत्यर्थापक्लिन्नशरीरेषु भूतेषु विहतस्वभावेषु च केवलेष्वौषधग्रामेषु तोयतोयदानुगतमारुतसंसर्गाद् गुरुप्रवृतीनि वमनादीनि भवन्ति, गुरुसमुत्थानानि च शरीराणि|
During the Varsha or Rainy season, bodies of animals become excessively deliquescent because of their exposure to rain water, invisibility of the sun, moon and stars, over- casting of the sky by clouds and the presence of mud and water all over the earth. There is impairment of all medications because of their contact with water and the moist

wind associated with clouds. Thus, there is improper manifestation of drugs of emesis etc. and it takes a long time for the body to recover from the effects of these elimination therapies.

तस्मादवमनादीनां निवृत्तिर्विधीयते वर्षान्तेष्वृतुषु, न चेदात्ययिकं कर्म|
आत्ययिके पुनः कर्मणि काममृतुं विकल्प्य कृत्रिमगुणोपधानेन यथर्तुगुणविपरीतेन भेषजं संयोगसंस्कारप्रमाणविकल्पेनोपपाद्य प्रमाणवीर्यसमं कृत्वा ततः प्रयोजयेदुत्तमेन यत्नेनावहितः||१२७||

Therefore, in the above mentioned three seasons ending with rainy season elimination therapy, viz emesis etc. should not be administered unless there is an emergency. In such emergencies, natural manifestations of seasons, viz, excessive cold, heat and rains are counter-acted by artificial means (air conditioning). Similarly, the quantities of medicines are rendered opposite to those of the respective seasons by suitable combination, processing and determination of proper dosage. Thus, bringing the dosage and potency of medicaments to the required level, elimination therapies are administered with utmost care. [127]

Another connotation of kala:

आतुरावस्थास्वपि तु कार्याकार्य प्रति कालाकालसञ्ज्ञा; तद्यथा- अस्यामवस्थायामस्य भेषजस्याकालः, कालः पुनरन्यस्येति; एतदपि हि भवत्यवस्थाविशेषेण; तस्मादातुरावस्थास्वपि हि कालाकालसञ्ज्ञा|
तस्य परीक्षा- मुहुर्मुहुरातुरस्य सर्वावस्थाविशेषावेक्षणं यथावद्भेषजप्रयोगार्थम्|
न ह्यतिपतितकालमप्राप्तकालं वा भेषजमुपयुज्यमानं यौगिकं भवति; कालो हि भैषज्यप्रयोगपर्याप्तिमभिनिर्वर्तयति||१२८||

Another connotation of the term Kala or time is the state of the patient which determines the initiation of timely actions and prohibitions of untimely ones. For example, in a particular condition or the state of the patient one medicine may not be useful. Administration of this medicine will be termed untimely whereas administration of another medicine may be useful which will be termed as timely.

Thus, the determination of the utility or otherwise of a particular medicine depends upon the state of the patient and this in other words is known as "timely" or "untimely" to ascertain tis with a view to administering the therapy, the specific characteristics of all the states of the patient is frequently observed. The therapy does not produce its desired effect, if administered after the passage or before the arrival of the correct time. It is the time which determines the manifestation of the desired efffects of a drug administered. [128]

Pravrtti:

प्रवृत्तिस्तु प्रतिकर्म समारम्भः|
तस्य लक्षणं भिषगौषधधातुरपरिचारकाणां क्रियासमायोगः||१२९||

Pravrati or endeavour is the initiation of the therapeutic action. It represents the combined action of the physician, medicaments, patient and the attendant. [129]

Upaya:

उपायः पुनर्भिषगादीनां सौष्ठवमभिविधानं च सम्यक्|
तस्य लक्षणं- भिषगादीनां यथोक्तगुणसम्पत् देश काल प्रमाण सात्म्य क्रियादिभिश्च सिद्धिकारणैः सम्यगुपपादितस्यौषधस्यावचारणमिति||१३०||

Upaya or means comprises the excellence of the physician etc., and the correct therapy. This is characterised by the existence of the desired qualities in the physician and the administration of the correctly processed drugs, depending upon the locality, time, dosage and homologation. [130]

एवमेते दश परीक्ष्यविशेषाः पृथक् पृथक् परीक्षितव्या भवन्ति||१३१||
Thus, these are the ten factors to be examined separately [131]

Objects of examination:

परीक्षायास्तु खलु प्रयोजनं प्रतिपत्तिज्ञानम्|

प्रतिपत्तिर्नाम यो विकारो यथा प्रतिपत्तव्यस्तस्य तथाऽनुष्ठानज्ञानम्||१३२||

Purpose of this examination is so obtained knowledge regarding the line of treatment that is adopted with a view to correcting the morbidity. [132]

यत्र तु खलु वमनादीनां प्रवृत्तिः, यत्र च निवृत्तिः, तद्व्यासतः सिद्धिषूत्तरमुपदेक्ष्यामः||१३३||

Indications and contra-indications of elimination therapies viz, emesis etc., will be described later in detail in the Siddhi section. [133]

प्रवृत्ति निवृत्ति लक्षण संयोगे तु गुरु लाघवं सम्प्रधार्य सम्यगध्यवस्येदन्यतरनिष्ठायाम्|

सन्ति हि व्याधयः शास्त्रेषूत्सर्गापवादैरुपक्रमं प्रति निर्दिष्टाः|

तस्माद्गुरुलाघवं सम्प्रधार्य सम्यगध्यवस्येदित्युक्तम्||१३४||

If there are symptoms which are simultaneously responsive as well as unresponsive to a given therapy. The physician should decide for or against the administration of that therapy, on asertaining the seriousness orlightness of the therapy, on ascertaining the seriousness or lightness of the (mutually contadictory) symptoms. Generally, rules together with the exceptional ones for the treatment of diseases are described in the text. The physician should accordingly initiate action (treatment) with the care and on ascertaining the seriousness or lightness of the symptoms concerned. [134]

Drugs used in emesis:

यानि तु खलु वमनादिषु भेषज द्रव्याण्युपयोगं गच्छन्ति तान्यनुव्याख्यास्यामः|

तद्यथा- फल जीमूतकेक्ष्वाकु धामार्गव कुटज कृतवेधन फलानि, फल जीमूतकेक्ष्वाकु धामार्गव पत्र पुष्पाणि आरग्वध वृक्षक मदन स्वादु कण्टक पाठा पाटला शाङ्र्गेष्टा मूर्वा सप्तपर्ण नक्तमाल पिचुमर्द पटोल सुषवी गुडूची- चित्रक सोमवल्क शतावरी द्वीपीशिग्रु मूल कषायैः, मधुक मधूक कोविदार कर्वुदारनीप विदुल बिम्बी शणपुष्पी सदापुष्पा प्रत्यक्पुष्पा कषायैश्च, एला हरेणु प्रियङ्गु पृथ्वीका कुस्तुम्बुरु तगर नलद ह्रीवे रतालीशोशीर कषायैश्च, इक्षुकाण्डेक्षिवक्षुवालिका दर्भ पोटगलकालङ्कृ(इक)तकषायैश्च, सुमनासौमनस्यायनी हरिद्रा दारुहरिद्रा वृश्चीर पुनर्नवा महा सहाक्षुद्र सहाकषायैश्च, शाल्मलि शाल्मलिकभद्रपर्ण्येलापण्र्युपोदिकोद्दालक धन्वनराजादनोपचित्रागोपी शृङ्गाटिका कषायैश्च, पिप्पली पिप्पलीमूल चव्य चित्रक शृङ्गवेर सर्षप फाणित क्षीर क्षार लवणोदकैश्च, यथालाभं यथेष्टं वाऽप्युपसंस्कृत्य वर्तिक्रियाचूर्णावलेह स्नेह कषाय मांस रस यवागू यूष काम्बलिक क्षीरोपधेयान्मोदकानन्यांश्च भक्ष्य प्रकारान् विविधाननुविधाय यथार्हं वमनार्हाय दद्यादिवधिवद्वमनम्|

इति कल्पसङ्ग्रहो वमनद्रव्याणाम्| कल्पमेषां विस्तारेणोत्तरकालमुपदेक्ष्यामः||१३५||

We shall now expound the drugs which enter into the composition of emetic therapics. They are:

The fruits of

Phala (Randia dumetorum Lam)

Jimutaka (Luffa echinata Roxb)

Iksvaki (Lagenaria vulgaris)

Dhamargava (Luffa cylindrica)

Kutaja (Holarrhena antidysenterica)

Krtavedhana (Luffa acutangula Roxb)

Leaves and flowers of

Phala (Randia dumetorum Lam)

Jimutaka (Luffa echinata Roxb)

Iksvaka (Lagenaria vulgaris Standl) and

Dhamargava (Luffa cylindrica M. Roem)

Decoction of the roots of:
Aragvadha (Cassia fistula Linn)
Vrksaka (Holarrhena antidysenterica)
Mandana (Randia dumetrorum Lam)
Svadukantaka (Tribulus terrestris Linn)
Patha (Cissampelos pareiraLinn)
Patala (Stereospermum suaveolens DG)
Sarngestha (Abrus precatorius Linn)
Murva (Clematis triloba Heyene ex Roth)
Saptaparna (Alstonia scholaris)
Naktamala (Pongamia pinnata merr)
Pichumarda (Azadirachta indica A. juss)
Patola (Trichosanthes cucumerina Linn)
Susavi (Momordica charantia Linn)
Guduchi (Tinospora cordifolia Miers)
Chitraka (Plumbago zeylanica Linn)
Somavalka (Acacia catechu Willd)
Shatavari (Asparagus racemosus Wild)
Dvipi (Solanum xanthocarpum Schrad and wendl)
Shigru (Moringa oleifera Lam)

Decoctions of
Madhuka (Glycyrrhiza glabra Linn)
Madhuka (Madhuca indica J.F Gmel)
Kovidara (red variety of Bauhinia variegata Linn)
Karvaudara (red vareity of Bauhinia variegata Linn)
Nipa (Anthocephalus indicus A: Rich)
Vidula
Bimbi (Coccinia indica W & A)
Sanapuspi (Crotalaria verrucosa Linn)
Sadapuspa (Calotropis gigantea R. Br Ex Ait)
Pratyakpuspa (Achyranthes aspera Linn)

Decoctions of
Ela (Elettaria cardamomum Maton)
Harenu (Pisum sativum Linn)
Priyangu (Callicarpa macrophylla Vahi)
Prthvika (Nigella sativa Linn)
Kustumburu (Coriandrum sativum Linn)
Tagara (Valeriana wallichii Dc)
Nalada (Nardostachys jatamansi DG)
Hrivera (Pavonia odorata willd)
Talisa (Abies webbiana Lindl)
Usira (Vetiveria zizanioides Nash)

Decoctions of
Iksu (Saccharum officinarum Linn)
Kandeksu (Saccharum spontaneum Linn)

Iksuvalika (Asteracantha longifolia Nees)
Darbha (Desmostachya bipinnata Stapf)
Potagala (Arundo donax linn)
Kalankrta (Cassia occidentalis Linn)

Decoctions of
Sumana (Jasminum officinale)
Saumanasyayani (Myristica fragrans Hovtt)
Haridra (Curcuma longa Linn)
Daruharidra (Berberis aristata DC)
Vrscira (white variety of Boerhaavia diffusa Linn)
Punarnava (red Variety of Boerhavia diffusa Linn)
Mahasaha (Teramnus labialis Spreng)
Ksudrasaha (Phaseolus trilobus Ait)

Decoctions of
Salmali (Salmalia malabarica Schott and Endl)
Salmalika (Tecomella undulata Seem)
Bhadraparni (Paederia foetida linn)
Elaparni (Alpinia galanga Swartz)
Upodika
Uddalaka
Dhanvana
Rajadana (Mimusops hexandra)
Upacitra (Gopi - Hemidesmus indicus R.B)
Srngatika (Trapa bispinosa Roxb)

Powder of
Pippali (Piper longum Linn)
Root of Pippali
Chavya (Pipper chaba Hunter)
Chitraka (Plumbago zeylanica Linn)
Srngavera (Zingiber officinale Rose)

Water mixed with
Penidium
Milk
Alkali preparations
Salt

The above-mentioned drugs in sufficient quantity or as much as available is processed in the forms Vartiables in an elongated from like a suppository), powder, linctus, medicated oil, decoction, meat-soup, gruel, yusa (soap), Linctus, medicated oil, decoction, meat- soup, gruel, Yusha (soup), Kambabalika (a preparation of sour milk mixed with whey and vinegar M. W) milk preparation, sweet-meats and the like. These preparations are properly administered for emesis to a patient after ascertaining his suitability for this therapy. This in brief, is the description of various preparations for emetic therapy. A detailed description of these preparations will be furnished in the Kalpa section later. [135]

Drugs used for purgation:

विरेचन द्रव्याणि तु श्यामात्रिवृच्चतुरङ्गुल तिल्वक महावृक्ष सप्तला शङ्खिनी दन्ती द्रवन्तीनां क्षीर मूलत्वक्पत्रपुष्पफलानि यथायोगं तैस्तैः क्षीरमूल त्वक्पत्र पुष्प फलै विक्लिप्ता विक्लिप्तैः , अजगन्धाश्वगन्धाजशृङ्गी क्षीरिणी नीलिनी क्लीतक कषायैश्च, प्रकीर्योदकीर्या मसूर विदला कम्पिल्लक विडङ्गगवाक्षीकषायैश्च, पीलु प्रियाल मृद्वीका काश्मर्य परूषक बदर दाडिमामलक हरीतकी बिभीतक वृश्चीर पुनर्नवा विदारिगन्धादिकषायैश्च, सीधु सुरा सौवीरक तुषोदक मैरेय मेदक मदिरा मधु मधूलक धान्याम्लकुवल बदर खर्जूर कर्कन्धुभिश्च, दधि दधिमण्डोदश्विद्भिश्च, गोमहिष्यजावीनां च क्षीरमूत्रैर्यथालाभं यथेष्टं वाऽप्युपसंस्कृत्य वर्तिक्रियाचूर्णासवलेह स्नेह कषाय मांस रस यूष काम्बलिक यवागू क्षीरोपधेयान् मोदकानन्यांश्च भक्ष्यप्र(वि)कारान् विविधांश्च योगाननुविधाय यथार्हं विरेचनार्हाय दद्यादिवरेचनम्| इति कल्पसङ्ग्रहो विरेचनद्रव्याणाम्|

कल्पमेषां विस्तरेण यथावदुत्तरकालमुपदेक्ष्यामः||१३६||

Drugs which can be included under the composition of purgation therapy are the latex, roots, barks, leaves, flowers and fruitys of:

Syama (black variety of Operculina turpethum R. B)

Trivrt (white variety of O. turpethum R., B)

Chaturangula (Cassia fistula Linn)

Tilvaka (Symplocos racemosa Roxb)

Mahavrksa (Euphorbia neriifolia Linn)

Saptala (Acacia concinna DC)

Sankhini (Canscora decussata Roem et. sch)

Danti (Baliospermum montanum muell Arg)

Dravanti (Jatropha glandulifera Roxb)

According to the requirements, the latex, roots, barks, leaves, flowers and fruits and fruits may be combined or used individually. These drugs may be mixed with the following group of drugs.

Decoctions of

Ajagandha (Gynandropsis gynandra Briquet)

Asvagandha (Withania somnifera Dunal)

Ajasrngi (Rhus succedanea Linn)

Ksirini (Mimusops hexandra Roxb)

Nilini (Indigofera tinctoria)

Klitaka (Glycyrrhiza glabra Linn)

Decoctions of

Prakirya (Caesalpinia crista Linn)

Udakriya (Pongamia pinnata Merr)

Masuravidala (Ichnocarpus frutescens R. Br)

Kampillaka (Mallotus philippinensis Muell Arg)

Vidanga (Embelia ribes Burm F)

Gavaksi (Citrullus colocynthis Schard)

Decoctions of

Pilu (Salvadora persica Linn)

Priyala (Buchanania lanzan spreng)

Mrdvika (Vitis vinifera Linn)

Kasmarya (Gmelina arborea Linn)

Parusaka (Grewia asiatica Linn)

Badara (Ziziphus jujuba Lam)

Dadima (Punica granatum Linn)

Amalaka (Emblica officinalis Gaertn)

Haritaki (Terminalia chebula linn)

Bibhitaka (Terminalia belerica Roxb)

Viscira (white variety of Boerhavia diffusa Linn)

Punarnava (red variety of Boerhavia diffusa Linn)

Vidarignddha

Sidhu (fermented liquor from mixture of thickened cane juice and dark brown crude sugar-CSSS)

Sura (fermented liquor from barley etc- CSSS)

Sauviraka (a type of wine)

tusodaka (sour gruel prepared by fermenting barley along with its husk)

maireya 9 a type of wine)

medaka (a type of wine)

madira (distilled wine of high alcoholic content)

madhu (a type of wine)

Dhanyamla (sour fermented liquor from rice gruel)

Kuvala (Ziziphus ativa Gaertn)

Badara (Ziziphus jujuba Lam)

Kharjura (Phoenix sylvestris Roxb)

Karkandhu

Curd

Dadhimanda (whey)

Udasvi (a mixture of water and butter milk in equal quantity MW)

Milk and urine of cow, buffalo, goat and sheep

The above-mentioned drugs in sufficient quantity or as much as available is processed in the forms of Vartikriya (eatables in an elongated form like a suppository), powder, Alcholic preparation, linctus, medicated oil, decoction, meat-soup, Yusa (soup), Kambalika (a preparation of sour milk- preparation, sweet meats like. these preparations is properly administered for this therapy. this in brief, is the description of these preparations will be furnished in the Kalpa section later. [136]

आस्थापनेषु तु भूयिष्ठकल्पानि द्रव्याणि यानि योगमुपयान्ति तेषु तेष्ववस्थान्तरेष्वातुराणां, तानि द्रव्याणि नामतो विस्तरेणोपदिश्यमानान्यपरिसङ्ख्येयानि स्युरतिबहुत्वात्; इष्टश्चानतिसङ्क्षेपविस्तरोपदेशस्तन्त्रे, इष्टं च केवलं ज्ञानं, तस्माद्रसत एव तान्यत्र व्याख्यास्यामः| रससंसर्गविकल्पविस्तरो ह्येषामपरिसङ्ख्येयः, समवेतानां रसानामंशांशबलविकल्पातिबहुत्वात्| तस्माद्द्रव्याणां चैकदेशमुदाहरणार्थं रसेष्वनुविभज्य रसैकैकश्येन च नामलक्षणार्थं षडास्थापनस्कन्धा रसतोऽनुविभज्य व्याख्यास्तन्ते||१३७||

There are many drugs which are used in Asthapana (corrective enema) for patients suffering from different ailments. The details are too exhaustive to be enumerated. It is desirable that the description of the science should neither be too lengthy nor too brief. At the same time the text should contain the entire scientific knowledge. Hence (some important ones of) these drugs grouped according to their tastes will be described here. [137]

Rarity of drugs having single taste:

यत् षड्विधमास्थापनमेकरसमित्याचक्षते भिषजः, तद्दुर्लभतमं संसृष्ट रस भूयिष्ठत्वाद्द्रव्याणाम्|
तस्मान्मधुराणि मधुरप्रायाणि मधुरविपाकानि मधुरप्रभावाणि च मधुरस्कन्धे मधुराण्येव कृत्वोपदेक्ष्यन्ते, तथेतराणि द्रव्याण्यपि||१३८||

Substances are mostly composed of many tastes. Drugs having only one taste so as to be unquestionably included under one of the six groups are very rare. Therefore, drugs that are sweet or are predominantly sweet or are sweet in Vipaka (taste conversion after digestion) or that produce the effects similar to those of the drugs having sweet taste, are included under the Madhuraskandha (group of drugs having sweet taste). Drugs belonging to other five groups are also selected on the basis of similar criteria. [138]

Drugs having sweet taste:

तद्यथा- जीवकर्षभकौ जीवन्ती वीरा तामलकी काकोली क्षीरकाकोली मुद्गपर्णी माषपर्णी शालपर्णी पृश्निपर्ण्यसनपर्णी मधुपर्णी मेदा महामेदा कर्कटशृङ्गी शृङ्गाटिका छिन्नरुहा च्छत्राऽतिच्छत्रा श्रावणी महाश्रावणी सहदेवा विश्वदेवा शुक्ला क्षीरशुक्ला बलाऽतिबला विदारी क्षीरविदारी क्षुद्रसहा महासहा ऋष्यगन्धाऽश्वगन्धा वृश्चीरः पुनर्नवा बृहती कण्टकारिकोरुबूको मोरटः श्वदंष्ट्रा संहर्षा शतावरी शतपुष्पा मधूकपुष्पी यष्टीमधु मधूलिका मृद्वीका खर्जूरं परूषकमात्मगुप्ता पुष्करबीजं कशेरुकं राजकशेरुकं राजादनं कतकं काश्मर्य शीतपाक्योदनपाकी ताल खर्जूर मस्तकमिक्षुरिक्षुवालिका दर्भः कुशः काशः शालिगुन्द्रेत्कटकः शरमूलं राजक्षवकः ऋष्यप्रोक्ता द्वारदा भारद्वाजी वनत्रपुष्प्यभीरुपत्री हंसपादी काकनासिका कुलिङ्गाक्षी क्षीरवल्ली कपोलवल्ली कपोतवल्ली सोमवल्ली गोपवल्ली मधुवल्ली चेति; एषामेवंविधानामन्येषां च मधुरवर्गपरिसङ्ख्यातानामौषधद्रव्याणां छेद्यानि खण्डशश्छेदयित्वा भेद्यानि चाणुशो भेदयित्वा प्रक्षाल्य पानीयेन सुप्रक्षालितायां स्थाल्यां समावाप्य पयसाऽर्धोदकेनाभ्यासिच्य साधयेद्द्रव्या सततमवघट्टयन्; तदुपयुक्तभूयिष्ठेऽम्भसि गतरसेष्वौषधेषु पयसि चानुपदग्धे स्थालीमुपहृत्य सुपरिपूतं पयः सुखोष्णं घृत तैल वसा मज्ज लवण फाणितोपहितं बस्तिं वातविकारिणे विधिज्ञो विधिवद्दद्यात्; शीतं तु मधुसर्पिर्भ्यामुपसंसृज्य पित्तविकारिणे विधिवद्दद्यात्| इति मधुरस्कन्धः||१३९||

The following belong to the group of sweet drugs:

Jivaka

Rsabhaka

Jivanti (Leptadenia reticulatae)

Vira (Asparagus racemosus Willd)

Tamalaki (Phyllanthus niruri Linn)

Kakoli

Ksirakakoli

Mudgaparni (Phaseolus trilobus Ait)

Masaparni (Teramnus labialis Spreng)

Salaparni (Desmodium gangeticum Dc)

Prsniparni (Uraria picta Desv)

Asanaparni (Clitoria ternatea Linn)

Madhuparni (Tinospora cordifolia Miers)

Meda

Mahameda

Karkatasrngi (Rhus succedanea Linn)

Srngatika (Trapa bispinosa Roxb)

Chinnaruha (Tinospora cordifolia Miers)

Chatra (Asteracantha longifolia Nees)

Aticchatra (red variety of Asteracantha longifolia Nees)

Sravani (Sphaeranthus indicus Linn)

Mahasrvani (a variety of Sravani)

Sahadeva (Sida rhombifolia Linn)

Visadeva

Sukla (Sugar)

Ksirasukla

Bala (Sida cordifolia linn)

Atibala

Vidari (Ipomoea paniculata R. Br)

Ksiravidari (Ipomoea paniculata R. Br)

Kusdrasaha

Mahasaha (Teramnus labialis Spreng)

Rsyagandha

Asvagandha (Withania somnifera Dunal)

Vrscira (white variety of Boerhavia diffusa Linn)

Punarnava (red variety of Boerhavia diffusa Linn)

Brhati (Solanum indicum Linn)

Kantakarika (Solanum xanthocarpum Schrad & Wendl)

Urubuka (a type of Ricinus communis Linn)

Morata (Clematis triloba Heyne ex Roth)

Svadamstra (Tribulus terrestris Linn)

Samharsa

Satavari (Asparagus racemosa Willd)

Satapuspa

Madhukapuspi

Yastimadhu

Madhulika (Madhuca longifolia)

Mrdvika (Tribulus terrestris)

Kharjura (Phoenix sylvestris Roxb)

Paruska (Grewia asiatica linn)

Atmagupta

Seeds puskara

Kaseruka

Rajakaseruka

Rajadana

Kataka (Strychnos potatorum)

Kasmarya (Gmelina arborea linn)

Sitapaki

Odanapaki

Tala

Upper Portion of Kharjura (Phoenix sylvestris Roxb)

Iksu (Saccharum officinarum Linn)

Iksuvalika (Asteracantha longifolia Nees)

Darbha (a variety of Desmostachya bipinnata Stapf)

Kusa (Desmostachya bipinnata Stapf)

Kasa (Saccharum spontaneum Linn)

Sali (Oryza sativa Linn)

Gundra

Itkataka

Root of Sara (Saccharum munja Roxb)

Rajaksavaka

Rsyaprokta (a variety of Sida cordifolia Linn)

Dvarada

Bharadvaja

Vanatrapusi

Abhirupatri (a variety of Asparagus racemosus willd)

Hamsapadi - Adiantum lunulatum

Kakanasik

Ksiravavalli

Kapotavalli (Plectranthus amboinicus)

Kapotavalli

Ela (Elettaria cardamomum Maton)

Somavalli

Gopaballi (Hemidesmus indicus R. B)

Madhuvalli (a variety of Glycyrrhiza glabra Linn)

The above-mentioned ones and such others belonging to the group of sweet drugs are cut or pierced into small pieces, washed well in water, kept in a vessel added with milk diluted with fifty percent water and boiled.

During the process of boiling, they are constantly stirred with a label. When the water comes to the desired level, and drugs given up their active principles and before milk gets charred, the vessel is removed from the heath and milk is filtered well.

An expert physician should administer this luke-warm milk mixed with ghee, oil muscle fat, marrrow, salt and penidium as enema to a patient sufering from diseases due to vitiation of Vata, following the proper procedure. To a patient suffering from diseases due to the vitiation of Piia) this milk is administered as enema after it is cooled down and mixed with honey and ghee, following the proper procedure.

Thus ends the description of the froup of sweet drugs [139]

Drugs having sour taste:
आम्राम्रातक लकुच करमर्द वृक्षाम्लाम्लवेतस कुवल बदर दाडिम मातुलुङ्ग गण्डीरामलक नन्दीतक शीतक- तिन्तिण्डीक दन्तशठैरावतक कोशाम्र धन्वनानां फलानि, पत्राणि चाम्रातकाश्मन्तकचाङ्गेरीणां चतुर्विधानां चाम्लिकानां द्वयोश्च कोलयोश्चामशुष्कयोर्द्वयोश्चैव शुष्काम्लिकयोर्ग्राम्यारण्ययोः, आसवद्रव्याणि च सुरा सौवीरक तुषोदक मैरेय मेदक मदिरा मधुशुक्तशीधु दधि दधिमण्डोदश्विद्धान्याम्लादीनि च, एषामेवंविधानामन्येषां चाम्लवर्ग परिसङ्ख्यातानामौषध द्रव्याणां छेद्यानि खण्डशश्छेदयित्वा भेद्यानि चाणुशो भेदयित्वा द्रवैः स्थाल्यामभ्यासिच्य साधयित्वोपसंस्कृत्य यथावतैलवसामज्जलवणफाणितोपहितं सुखोष्णं बस्तिं वातविकारिणे विधिज्ञो विधिवद्दद्यात्।
इत्यम्लस्कन्धः॥१४०॥

The following belong to the group of sour drugs:
Fruits of
Amra (Mangifera indica Linn)

Amrataka (Spondias pinnata Kurz)

Lakuca (Artocarpus lakoocha Roxb)

Karamarda (Carissa carandas Linn)

Vrksamla (Garcinia indica chois)

Amlavetasa (Garcinia pedunculata wall)

Kuvala (Ziziphus sativa Gaertn)

Badara (Ziziphus jujuba Lam)

Dadima (Punica granatum Linn)

Matulunga (Citrus medica Linn)

Gandira (Typha angustata Linn)

Amalaka (Emblica officinalis)

Nanditaka

Sitaka

Tintidika

Dantasatha

Airavata

Kosamra

Dhanvana

Leaves of

Amrataka

Asmantaka

Cangeri (Oxalis corniculata Linn)

Four varieties of

Amlika (Tamarindus indica Linn)

Dry and wet Kola (Ziziphus jujuba Lam)

Wild and cultivated varieties of dried Amlika (Tamarindus indica Linn)

Alcoholic preparations viz

Sura (fermented liquor from barely etc)

Sauviraka (a type of wine)

Tusodaka (sour gruel prepared by fermenting barley along with its husk)

Maireya (a type of wine)

Medaka (a type of wine)

Madira (distilled wine of high alcoholic content)

Madhu (a type of wine)

Sukta (fermented drink)

Sidhu (fermented liquor from mixture of thickened cane juice and dark brown crude sugar)

Curd

Dadhimanda (whey)

Udasvit (a mixture of water butter- milk in equal quantity)

Dhanyamla (sour fermented liquor from rice gruel)

The above-mentioned ones and such others belonging to the group of sour drugs are cut or pierced into small pieces, added with liquids and are boiled. They are added with oil, muscle fat, marrow, salt and pendium as per early administered as enema by an expert physician to a patient suffering disease caused by the vitiation of vata.

Thus ends the description of the sour drugs. [140]

Drugs having saline taste:

सैन्धव सौवर्चल काल विड पाक्यानूपकूप्यवालुकैलमौलक सामुद्र रोमकौद्भिदौषरपाटेयकपांशुजान्येवम्प्रकाराणि चान्यानि लवणवर्ग परिसङ्ख्यातानि, एतान्यम्लोपहितान्युष्णोदकोपहितानि वा स्नेहवन्ति सुखोष्णं बस्तिं वातविकारिणे विधिज्ञो विधिवद्ददद्यात्‌|
इति लवणस्कन्धः||१४१||

The following belong to the group of saline drugs:

Saindhava (rock salt)

Sauvarcala (sonchal salt which is obtained by boiling alkalines like Soda with Emblic myrobatans)

Kala (a kind of black, factitious and purgative salt)

Vida (a kind of factitious salt, procured by boiling earth impregnated with saline particular, kind of fetid salt used medicinally as a tonic aperients)

Pakya (a type of salt prepared by evaporating earth and water from marshy land)

Anupa (a type of salt prepared by evaporating earth and water from marshy land)

Kupya (a type of salt prepared by evaporating well water)

Valukaila (a type of black salt prepared artificially)

Maulaka (a type of black salt prepared artificially)

Samudra (sea-salt)

Romaka (salt obtained from saline salt or from Sambar Lake)

Audbhida (salt obtained from saline soil)

Pateyaka (Poitu salt)

Pamsuja (salt prepared from saline clay)

The above-mentioned ones and such other substances are mixed with sour things or hot water and added with fat. What luke-warm this mixture is carefully administered as enema by an expert physician to a patient suffering from diseases due to the vitiation of Vata. Thus ends the description of the group saline drugs. [141]

Drugs having pungent taste:

पिप्पलीपिप्पलीमूलहस्तिपिप्पलीचव्यचित्रकशृङ्गवेरमरिचाजमोदार्द्रकविडङ्गकुस्तुम्बुरुपीलुतेजोवत्येलाकुष्ठ-
भल्लातकास्थिहिङ्गुनिर्यासकिलिममूलकसर्षपलशुनकरञ्जशिगुकमधुशिगुकखरपुष्पभूस्तृणसुमुखसुरसकुठेरकार्जक-
गण्डीरकालमालकपर्णासक्षवकफणिज्झकक्षारमूत्रपितानीति; एषामेवंविधानां चान्येषां कटुकवर्गपरिसङ्ख्यातानामौषधद्रव्याणां छेद्यानि
खण्डशश्छेदयित्वा भेद्यानि चाणुशो भेदयित्वा गोमूत्रेण सह साधयित्वोपसंस्कृत्य यथावन्मधुतैललवणोपहितं सुखोष्णं बस्तिं
श्लेष्मविकारिणे विधिज्ञो विधिवद्ददद्यात्|
इति कटुकस्कन्धः||१४२||

The following belong to the group of pungent drugs:

Pippali (Piper longum Linn)

Root of Pippali

Hasti pippali (Scindapsus officinalis Schott)

Chavya (Piper chaba Hunter)

Chitraka (Plumbago zeylanica Linn)

Srngavera (dried Rhizome of Zingiber officinale Rosc)

Maricha (Piper nigrum Linn)

Ajamoda (Trachyspermum roxburghianum Sprague)

Ardaka (Zingiber officinale Rosc)

Vidanga (Embelia ribes Burm f)

Kustumburu (Corriandrum sativum Linn)

Pilu (Salvadora persica Linn)

Tejovati (Zanthoxylum alatum Roxb)

Ela (Elettaria cardamomum Maton)

Kustha (Saussurea lappa C. B Clarke)

Nuts of Bhallataka (Semecarpus anacardium Linn f)

Resinous exudation of Hingu (Ferula narthex Boiss)

Kilima (Cedrus deodara Loud)

Mulaka (Raphanus sativus Linn)

Sarsapa (Brassica nigra Koch)

Lasuna (Allium sativum Linn)

Karanja (Pongamia pinnata Meer)

Sigruka (Moringa oleifera lam)

Madhusigruka (a variety of Moringa oleifera lam)

Kharapuspa (Achyranthes aspera Linn)

Bhustrna

Various types of Basisls, Viz. Sumukha, Surasa, Kutheraka, Arjaka, Gandiraka, Alamalaka, Parnasa, Ksavaka and

Phanijjhaka
Alkaline, urines and biles

The above-mentioned ones and such others belonging to the group of pungent drugs is cut and pierced into small pieces and boiled witj cow- urine. After they are filtered, they are added with honey, oil and salt as per requirements. An expert physician should properly administer this luke-warm mixture as enema to a patient suffering from diseases caused by the vitiation of Kapha.

Thus ends the description of the group of pungent drugs. [142]

Drugs having bitter taste:
चन्दन नलद कृतमाल नक्तमाल निम्ब तुम्बुरु कुटज हरिद्रा दारुहरिद्रा मुस्त मूर्वा किराततिक्तक कटुकरोहिणी त्रायमाणा- कारवेल्लिका करीर करवीर केबुक कठिल्लक वृष मण्डूकपर्णी कर्कोटक वार्ताकु कर्कश काकमाची काकोदुम्बरिकासुषव्यतिविषा- पटोल कुलक पाठा गुडूची वेत्राग्र वेतस विकङ्कत बकुल सोमवल्क सप्तपर्ण सुमनार्कावल्गुज वचा तगरागुरु वालकोशीराणीति, एषामेवंविधानां चान्येषां तिक्तवर्ग परिसङ्ख्याता नामौषध द्रव्याणां छेद्यानि खण्डशश्छेदयित्वा भेद्यानि चाणुशो भेदयित्वा प्रक्षाल्य पानीयेनाभ्यासिच्य साधयित्वोपसंस्कृत्य यथावन्मधुतैललवणोपहितं सुखोष्णं बस्तिं श्लेष्मविकारिणे विधिज्ञो विधिवद्ददद्यात्, शीतं तु मधुसर्पिभ्यामपसंसृज्य पित्तविकारिणे विधिज्ञो विधिवद्ददद्यात्| इति तिक्तस्कन्धः||१४३||

The following belong to the group of bitter drugs:
Chandana (Santalum album Linn)
Nalada (Nardostachys jatamansi DC)
Krtamala (Cassia fistula Linn)
Naktamala (Pongamia pinnata Meer)
Nimba (Azadirachta indica A. Juss)
Tumburu (Zanthoxylum alatum Roxb)
Kutaja (Holarrhena antidysenterica Wall)
Haridra (Curcuma longa linn)
Daruharidra (Berberis aristata DC)
Musta (Cyperus rotundus Linn)
Murva (Clematis triloba Heyne ex Roth)
Kiratatiktaka (Swertia chirata Buch-Ham)
Katukarohini (Picrorhiza kurroa Royle)
Trayamana (Gentiana kurroo Royle)
Karavellika (Momordica charantia Linn)
Karira
Karavira (Nerium indicum Mill)
Keduka
Kathillaka (Boerhavia diffusa Linn)
Vrsa (Adhathoda vasica Nees)
Mandukaparni (Centella asiatica Urban)
Karkotaka
Vartaku
Karkasa
Kakamaci (Solanum nigrum Linn)
Kakodumbarika
Susavi
Ativisa (Aconitum heterophyllum Wall)

Patola (Trichosanthes dioica Linn)
Kulaka
Patha (Cissampelos pareira Linn)
Guduchi (Tinospora cordifolia)
Tender shoots of vetra
Vetasa
Vikankata
Bakula (Mimusops elengi Linn)
Somavalka (Acacia catechu Willd)
Saptaparna (Alstonia scholaris R. Br)
Sumana
Arka (Calotropis gigantea R. Br ex Ait)
Avalguja (Psoralea corylifolia Linn)
Vaca (Acorus calamus Linn)
Tagara (Valeriana wallichii DC)
Aguru (Aquilaria agallocha Roxb)
Valaka (Pavonia odorata Wiltd)
Usira (Vetiveria zizanioides Nash)

The above-mentioned ones and such others belonging to the group of bitter drugs are cut or pierced into small pieces, washed, added with water and boiled. After it is filtered, this decoction is added with honey, oil and salt as per requirements. An expert physician should properly administer this luke- warm mixture as enema to a patient suffering from diseases caused by the vitiation of kapha. To a patient suffering from diseases due to the vitiation of Pitta, the expert physician should administer this mixture along with honey and ghee as enema after it is cooled down. [143]

Drugs having astringent taste:

प्रियङ्ग्वनन्तामास्थ्यम्बष्ठकीकट्वङ्गलोध्र मोचरस समङ्गा धातकीपुष्प पद्मा पद्मकेशर जम्ब्वाम्र प्लक्ष वट- कपीतनोदुम्बराश्वत्थ भल्लातकास्थ्यश्मन्तक शिरीष शिंशपा सोमवल्क तिन्दुक प्रियाल बदर खदिर- सप्तपर्णाश्वकर्णस्यन्दनार्जुनारिमेदैलवालुक परिपेलव कदम्ब शल्लकी जिङ्गिनी काश कशेरुक राजकशेरुकट्फलवंश- पद्मकाशोकशालधवसर्ज भूर्ज शण खरपुष्पापुरशमी माचीकवरकतुङ्गाजकर्णस्फूर्जक बिभीतक कुम्भीपुष्करबीज- बिसमृणाल ताल खर्जूर तरुणानीति, एषामेवंविधानां चान्येषां कषाय वर्ग परिसङ्ख्यातानामौषधद्रव्याणां छेद्यानि खण्डशश्छेदयित्वा भेद्यानि चाणुशो भेदयित्वा प्रक्षाल्य पानीयेनाभ्यासिच्य साधयित्वोपसंस्कृत्य यथावन्मधुतैललवणोपहितं सुखोष्णं बस्तिं श्लेष्मविकारिणे विधिज्ञो विधिवद्दद्यात्, शीतं तु मधुसर्पिभ्र्यामुपसंसृज्य पित्तविकारिणे दद्यात्।

इति कषायस्कन्धः ॥१४४॥

The following belong to the group of astringent drugs:
Priyangu (Callicarpa macrophylla Vahl)
Ananta (Hemidesmus indicus RB)
Stones of Amra (Mangifera indica Linn)
Ambasthaki (Cissampelos pareira Linn)
Katvanga (Oroxylum indicum Vent)
Lodhra (Symplocos racemosa Roxb)
Mocarasa (Salmalia malabarica Schott and Endl)
Samanga (Mimosa pudica Linn)
Flowers of Dhataki (Woodfordia fruticosa Kurz)
Padma (Nelumbo nucifera Gaertn)

Stamens of Padma
Jambu (Syzygium cumini Skeels)
Amra (Mangifera indica Linn)
Plaksa (Ficus lacor Buch-Ham)
Vata (Ficus bengalensis Linn)
Kapitana
Udumbara (Ficus racemosa Linn)
Asvattha (Ficus religiosa Linn)
Nuts of Bhallataka (Semecarpus anacardium Linn f)
Asmantaka
Sirisa (Albizia lebbeck Benth)
Simsapa (Dalbergia sissoo Roxb)
Somavalka (a variety of Acacia catechu Willd)
Tinduka
Priyala
Badara (Zizyphus jujuba Lam)
Khadira (Acacia catechu Willd)
Saptaparna (Alstonia scholaris R. Br)
Asvakarna
Syandana
Arjuna (Terminalia arjuna W. and A)
Arimeda
Elavaluka
Paripwlava
Kadamba (Anthocephalus indicus A Rich)
Sallaki (Boswellia serrata Roxb)
Jingini
Kasa (Saccharum spontaneum Linn)
Kaseruka
Rajakaseru
Kathala
Vamsa (Bambusa arundinacea Retx)
Padmaka (Prunus cerasoides D. Don)
Asoka (Saraca asoka Linn)
Sala (Shorea robusta Gaertn f)
Dhava
Bhurja
Sana
Kharapuspa (Achyranthes aspera Linn)
Kharapuspa (Achyranthes aspera Linn)
Pura (Commiphora mukul Engl)
Sami
Macika (Cedrus deodara Loud)
Varaka
Tunga (Calophyllum inophyllum Linn)
Ajakarna
Sphurjaka
Bibhitaka (Terminalia belerica roxb)

Kumbhi
Seed of lotus rhizome of lotus stalk of lotus
Sprouts of Tala
Sprouts of Kharjura (Phoenix sylvestris Roxb)

The above-mentioned ones and such others belonging to the group of astringent drugs are cut or pierced into small pieces, washed, added with water and boiled. After it is filtered, this decoction is added with honey. Oil and salt as per the requirement

An expert physician should properly administer this luke- warm mixture as enema to a patient suffering from diseases due to the vitiation of Kapha. To a patient suffering from diseases due to the vitiation of Pitta, the expert physician should administer this mixture along with honey and ghee, as enema after it is cooled down. [114]

तत्र श्लोकाः:-
षड्वर्गाः परिसङ्ख्याता य एते रसभेदतः|
आस्थापनमभिप्रेत्य तान्विद्यात्सार्वयौगिकान्||१४५||
सर्वशो हि प्रणिहिताः सर्वरोगेषु जानता|
सर्वान्रोगान्नियच्छन्ति येभ्य आस्थापनं हितम्||१४६||
To sum up: -The six groups of drugs enumerated on the basis of their tastes can be used as corrective for patients suffering from diseases which are curable by such types of enema. An expert physician should cure all such diseases as are amenable to corrective enema therapy by administering enema composed of all some of the useful drugs enumerated under a group. [145- 146]

येषां येषां प्रशान्त्यर्थं ये ये न परिकीर्तिताः|
द्रव्यवर्गा विकाराणां तेषां ते परिकोपकाः||१४७||
इत्येते षडास्थापनस्कन्धा रसतोऽनुविभज्य व्याख्याताः||१४८||
Each group of drugs alleviates particular Doshas as mentioned above, other Doshas not mentioned against a given of drugs get aggravated by that group of drugs.

Thus, the six groups of drugs for corrective enema classified on the basis of their tastes are explained. [147-148]

Selection of drugs:
तेभ्यो भिषग्बुद्धिमान् परिसङ्ख्यातमपि यद्यद्द्रव्यमयौगिकं मन्येत, तत्तदपकर्षयेत्; यद्यच्चानुक्तमपि यौगिकं मन्येत, तत्तद्विदध्यात्; वर्गमपि वर्गेणोपसंसृजेदेकमेकेनानेकेन वा युक्तिं प्रमाणीकृत्य|
प्रचरणमिव भिक्षुकस्य बीजमिव कर्षकस्य सूत्रं बुद्धिमतामल्पमप्यनल्पज्ञानाय भवति; तस्माद्बुद्धिमतामूहापोहवितर्काः, मन्दबुद्धेस्तु यथोक्तानुगमनमेव श्रेयः| यथोक्तं हि मार्गमनुगच्छन् भिषक् संसाधयति कार्यमनतिमहत्त्वाद्वा विनिपातयत्यनतिहृस्वत्वादुदाहरणस्येति||१४९||

A wise physician should discard such trom groups as are not found in the treatment of a particular disease. At the same time, even if some other drugs which are not mentioned above, but are found useful in the treatment of a disease, he should add them to the group concerned. If the rationale of the therapy for the treatment of a disease so demands, the drugs of some other groups may also be added to those of another group.

Like the hand-ful of rice collected as alms by a mendicant or the seeds of grains to be used by a farmer, these terse aphorisms stand a Wiseman in good stead as a source of vast- amount of knowledge. An intelligent physician uses these aphorisms as a guide to understand many other things by reasoning and implications.

A physician possessing lesser intelligence would of course follow only what is described here. In view of the fact that things described here are not too brief to allow any ambiguity, a physician would not commit any serious mistakes, even if he follows only what is stated here by way of illustrations. [149]

Drugs for anuvasana type of enema:

अतः परमनुवासनद्रव्याण्यनुव्याख्यास्यामः|

अनुवासनं तु स्नेह एव|

स्नेहस्तु द्विविधः- स्थावरात्मकः, जङ्गमात्मकश्च|

तत्र स्थावरात्मकः स्नेहस्तैलमतैलं च|

तद्द्वयं तैलमेव कृत्वोपदेक्ष्यामः, सर्वतस्तैलप्राधान्यात्|

जङ्गमात्मकस्तु वसा, मज्जा, सर्पिरिति|

तेषां तैल वसा मज्ज सर्पिषां यथापूर्वं श्रेष्ठं वात श्लेष्म विकारेष्वनुवासनीयेषु,

यथोत्तरं तु पित्तविकारेषु, सर्व एव वा सर्वविकारेष्वपि योगमुपयान्ति संस्कार विधि विशेषादिति||१५०||

We shall now expound the drugs used in Anuvasana type of (unctuous) enema, Anuvasana type of enema is composed of fats. Fats are two types, depending upon their sources, viz. vegetables and animals. Vegetable oils may be obtained from Tila (Sesamum indicum Linn) or form other such oil-bearing plants.

Both these types of oil will be described by a single term 'Taila' (lit meaning the oil extracted from the seeds of 'Tila i.e Sesamum indicum Linn) because the oil extracted from Tila is the most important of all oils, muscle fat, marrow and ghee constitute the fats of animal origin. The preceding one's bear superiority over the succeeding ones as ingredients of unctuous enema for the treatment of diseases caused by Vata and Kapha. On the other hand, the treatment of diseases due to Pitta. When processed in a specific manner, all of them are, however, useful in all types of diseases. [150]

Drugs of errhines:

शिरोविरेचन द्रव्याणि पुनरपामार्ग पिप्पली मरिच विडङ्ग शिगु शिरीष तुम्बुरु पिल्वजाज्यमोदावार्ताकीपृथ्वीकैलाहरेणुकाफलानि च, सुमुख सुरस कुठेरक गण्डीरकालमालक पर्णास क्षवक फणिज्झक हरिद्रा शृङ्गवेर मूलक लशुन तर्कारी सर्षप पत्राणि च, अर्कालर्क कुष्ठ नागदन्ती वचापामार्ग श्वेता ज्योतिष्मती गवाक्षी गण्डीर पुष्प्य वाक्पुष्पी वृश्चिकाली वयस्थातिविषामूलानि च, हरिद्रा शृङ्गवेर मूलक लशुन कन्दाश्च, लोध्र मदन सप्तपर्ण निम्बार्क पुष्पाणि च, देवदार्वगुरु सरल शल्लकी जिङ्गिन्यसन हिङ्गुनिर्यासाश्च, तेजोवती वराङ्गेङ्गुदी शोभाञ्जनक बृहती कण्टकारिकात्वचश्चेति| शिरोविरेचनं सप्तविधं, फल-पत्र-मूल-कन्द-पुष्प-निर्यास-त्वगाश्रयभेदात्|

लवण कटु तिक्त कषायाणि चेन्द्रियोपशयानि तथाऽपराण्यनुक्तान्यपि द्रव्याणि यथायोगविहितानि शिरोविरेचनार्थमुपदिश्यन्त इति||१५१||

The following drugs help in the elimination of Doshas from the head (errhines):

Fruits of

Apamarga (Achyranthes aspera Linn)

Pippali

Marica (Piper nigum Linn)

Vidanga (Embelia ribes)

Sigru (Moringa oleifera Lam)

Sirisa

Tumburu

Pilu

Ajaji (Cuminum cyminum Linn)

Ajamoda (Trachyspermum roxburghianum sprague)

Vartaki

Prthvika (Nigella sativa Linn)

Ela (Elettaria cardamomum)
Harenuka

Leaves of
Various types of basils, viz, Sumukha, surasa, Kutheraka, Gandira, kalamalakam Parnasa, ksavaka and Phanijjhaka
Srngavera (Curcuma longa Linn)
Srngavera (Zingiber officinale Rose)
Mulaka (Raphanus sativus Linn)
Lasuna (Allium sativum Linn)
Tarkari
Sarsapa (Brassica nigra Koch)

Roots of
Arka (Calotropis gigantea R. Br. Ex Ait)
Alarka (A type of Arka)
Kustha (Saussurea lappa C.B Clarke)
Nagadanti, (a variety f Baliospermum montanum muell- Arg)
Vaca (Acorus calamus Linn)
Apamarga (Achyranthes aspera Linn)
Sveta (white variety of Clitoria ternatea Linn)
Jyotismati (Celastrus paniculatus Willd)
Gavaksi
Gandirapuspi
Avakpuspi
Vrcikali
Vayastha (Bacopa monnieri Pennell)
Ativisa (Aconitum heterophyllum Wall)

Rhizomes etc of
Haridra (Curcuma longa Linn)
Srngavera (Zingiber officinale Rose)
Mulaka (Raphanus sativus Linn)
Lasuna (Allium sativum Linn)

Flowers of
Lodhra (Symplocos racemosa Roxb)
Masana (Randia dumetorum Lam)
Saptaparna (Alstonia scholaris R. Br)
Nimbi (Azadirachta indica A. Juss)
Arka (Calotropis gigantea R. Br. Ex Ait)

Resinous exudations of
Devadaru (Cedrus deodara Loud)
Aguru (Aquilaria agallocha Roxb)
Sarala (Pinus roxburghii Sergent)
Sallaki (Boswellia serrata Roxb)
Jingini
Asana (Pterocarpus marsupium)

Hingu (Ferula narthex Boiss)

Barks of
Tejovati
Varanga
Ingudi
Sobhanjanaka
Brhati
Kantakarika

Thus, articles used as errhines are classified into seven types, depending upon their source, viz, Fruit, leaf, root, rhizome, flower, resinous exudation and bark. Such of the saline, pungent and bitter drugs as are soothing to the sense organs and other which are not enumerated here but have similar Properties may also be used (as errhines) for the elimination of Doshas from the head. [151]

तत्र श्लोकाः-
लक्षणाचार्यशिष्याणां परीक्षा कारणं च यत्|
अध्येयाध्यापनविधी सम्भाषा विधिरेव च||१५२||
षड्भिरूनानि पञ्चाशद्वादमार्गपदानि च|
पदानि दश चान्यानि कारणादीनि तत्त्वतः||१५३||
सम्प्रश्नश्च परीक्षादेर्नवको वमनादिषु|
भिषग्जितीये रोगाणां विमाने सम्प्रकाशितः||१५४||
To sum up: - examination of the text, the preceptor and the disciple, objects of such examination, procedure for study, teaching and deliberations in a seminar, forty – four terms concreting the arguments in seminar., ten other terms, viz, cause etc. Nine queries about examination etc. drugs used for emesis etc- all these topics are discussed in this chapter on the "Determination of the Specific Requirements for the treatment of Diseases". [152-154]

बहुविधमिदमुक्तमर्थजातं बहुविधवाक्यविचित्रमर्थकान्तम्|
बहुविधशुभशब्दसन्धियुक्तं बहुविधवादनिसूदनं परेषाम्||१५५||
इमां मतिं बहुविधहेतुसंश्रयां विजज्ञिवान् परमतवादसूदनीम्|
न सज्जते परवचनावमर्दनैर्न शक्यते परवचनैश्च मर्दितुम्||१५६||
दोषादीनां तु भावानां सर्वेषामेव हेतुमत्|
मानात् सम्यग्विमानानि निरुक्तानि विभागशः||१५७||
Thus, the various aspects of the specific Determination have been explained, decorated with a variety of sentences elegant with relevant meanings, endowed with the conjunction of the various auspicious terms and with powers to nullify the various arguments put-forth by opponents. One who is well acquainted with the contents of this chapter based on the various principles of causality and with powers to nullify the arguments put forth by opponents would not surrender to the views of opponents nor can he ever be defeated by the specific Determinations classified according to the measurement of the therapeutic aspects like the Doshas etc. are described here with apt arguments. [155-157]

इत्यग्निवेशकृते तन्त्रे चरक प्रतिसंस्कृते विमानस्थाने
रोगभिषग्जितीयविमानं नामाष्टमोऽध्यायः||८||
Thus, ends the eight chapter on "The Determination of the specific requirements for the Treatment of Diseases" of the Vimana Section of Agnivesha's work as redacted by Charaka. [8]

शारीरस्थानम् Shareera Sthanam

17

Shareerasthana Chapter 1 Katidha Purusheeyam

Empirical Soul

अथातः कतिधापुरुषीयं शारीरं व्याख्यास्यामः||१||

इति ह स्माह भगवानात्रेयः||२||

We shall now explore the chapter dealing with the several of the "Empirical Soul" etc, conducive to the understanding of the constitution of the body. Thus said Lord Atreya [1-2]

Queries of Agnivesha:

कतिधा पुरुषो धीमन्! धातुभेदेन भिद्यते|

पुरुषः कारणं कस्मात्, प्रभवः पुरुषस्य कः||३||

What are the divisions of the 'Empirical Soul' according to the division of Dhatus (elements)?

Why is the "Empirical Soul' considered to be the cause of the body?

What is the origin of "Empirical Soul"?

किमज्ञो ज्ञः, स नित्यः किं किमनित्यो निदर्शितः|

प्रकृतिः का, विकाराः के, किं लिङ्गं पुरुषस्य च||४||

Is he wise (perceivable) or ignorant (non-perceivable)? Is he eternal or ephemeral?

What is the constitution? What are deformities / derivatives? What are the symptoms (characteristics) of the soul?

निष्क्रियं च स्वतन्त्रं च वशिनं सर्वगं विभुम्|

वदन्त्यात्मानमात्मज्ञाः क्षेत्रज्ञं साक्षिणं तथा||५||

Those who have expertise in spiritual science describe the "Empirical Soul" as

- devoid of action
- independent
- having self control
- absolutely free
- all pervasive
- knower of the body and
- a witness / spectator

निष्क्रियस्य क्रिया तस्य भगवन्! विद्यते कथम्|

स्वतन्त्रश्चेदनिष्टासु कथं योनिषु जायते||६||

When is the "Empirical Soul" devoid of action; how does action emanate from him?

When he is independent why does he take origin from (among the) undesired wombs / undesirable species?

वशी यद्यसुखैः कस्मादभावैराक्रम्यते बलात्|

सर्वाः सर्वगतत्वाच्च वेदनाः किं न वेति सः||७||

If the soul is under self-control (has gained control over all his senses) why is he forcibly enveloped by (influenced by) the emotions? (It means to tell 'If he is absolutely free, how is He overpowered with miserable ideals?')

If he is everywhere, is He not aware of all miseries of everyone?

न पश्यति विभुः कस्माच्छैलकुड्यतिरस्कृतम्|

क्षेत्रज्ञः क्षेत्रमथवा किं पूर्वमिति संशयः||८||

If He is omnipresent, how does He not visualise things interrupted by (beyond) the hills and walls?

Which comes first- the body or the knower of the body (soul)? There is always confusion about this.

ज्ञेयं क्षेत्रं विना पूर्वं क्षेत्रज्ञो हि न युज्यते|

क्षेत्रं च यदि पूर्वं स्यात् क्षेत्रज्ञः स्यादशाश्वतः||९||

Kshetra (body) is the one which needs to be known. If there is no knower then it is no use telling 'kshetrajna (the one who resides in the kshetra i.e., soul)'. This is because if there is kshetra only then there will be a knower of kshetra. If we first accept the existence of kshetra, we might have to accept that kshetrajna (soul) is anitya (impermanent, transient).

साक्षिभूतश्च कस्यायं कर्ता ह्यन्यो न विद्यते|

स्यात् कथं चाविकारस्य विशेषो वेदनाकृतः||१०||

If there doesn't exist another doer to do the actions apart from atma (soul) then to what and who is the soul 'the witness / observer' of (then whom does the soul observe or form a witness to)? It means to say that when someone does the actions, the other person who observes these actions would be considered as witness or observer. But we call the soul as an observer / witness of the actions. If there is no other doer of action other than the soul, then whom does the soul observe?

The soul is regarded as 'devoid of deformities', then how does this soul experience 'happiness and grief'?

अथ चार्तस्य भगवंस्तिसृणां कां चिकित्सति|

अतीतां वेदनां वैद्यो वर्तमानां भविष्यतीम्||११||

भविष्यन्त्या असम्प्राप्तिरतीताया अनागमः|

साम्प्रतिक्या अपि स्थानं नास्त्यर्तेः संशयो ह्यतः||१२||

Out of the three types of pain / miseries of a patient, i.e., The last one, the present one and the future one, which one should the physician treat?

The future pains / miseries are not in existence (not yet been manifested) therefore there is no question of treating them.

The past pains / miseries do not exist and will not recur.

The pains / miseries of the present time (which exist right now) are momentary and don't behave in a fixed way and so in the absence of continuity, it is not amenable to any treatment.

So, the above-mentioned doubt always exists i.e., 'which pains / miseries should the physician treat?'

कारणं वेदनानां किं, किमधिष्ठानमुच्यते|

क्व चैता वेदनाः सर्वा निवृत्तिं यान्त्यशेषतः||१३||

सर्ववित् सर्वसन्न्यासी सर्वसंयोगनिःसृतः|

एकः प्रशान्तो भूतात्मा कैर्लिंगैरुपलभ्यते||१४||

What are the causative factors of miseries (diseases)?

What are the sites of their manifestation?

Where do all these miseries sub- merge after their cure

What are the signs which help in the recognition of the "Empirical Soul" which is omnipresent, all –renouncing, devoid of all contacts, only one and tranquil?

इत्यग्निवेशस्य वचः श्रुत्वा मतिमतां वरः|
सर्वं यथावत् प्रोवाच प्रशान्तात्मा पुनर्वसुः||१५||

Master Punarvasu, the most learned one and wise among the other lot after hearing patiently all the questions asked by Agnivesha gave suitable replies to all the queries.

Different concepts about Purusha:
खादयश्चेतनाषष्ठा धातवः पुरुषः स्मृतः|
चेतनाधातुरप्येकः स्मृतः पुरुषसञ्ज्ञकः||१६||

Purusha comprises six Dhatus (elements), i.e.
- five Maha bhutas (in their subtle form) i.e., ether, wind, fire, water and earth
- soul / consciousness
Even the element of consciousness alone constitutes Purusha. [16]

Another concept of Purusha comprising twenty-four factors:
पुनश्च धातुभेदेन चतुर्विंशतिकः स्मृतः|
मनो दशेन्द्रियाण्यर्थाः प्रकृतिश्चाष्टधातुकी||१७||

Purusha is again said to be made up of 24 dhatus / tattvas (entities). They are –
Manas – mind – 1
Indriyas – sense organs and organs of action (motor organs) together – 10 in number. They are –
a. 5 jnanendriyas i.e., sense organs – eyes, ears, nose, tongue and skin
b. 5 karmendriyas i.e., motor organs – i.e., organs of speech, hands, legs (feet), anus and penis
Indriyartha – objects of sense organs – 5 in number i.e., vision / sight, sound, smell, taste and touch
Prakriti – 8 in number –
- Avyakta – primordial element
- Mahat – intellect
- Ahamkara – ego
- Panchamahabhuta – 5 elements of nature – earth, wind, water, fire, ether [17]

Proof of Existence of Mind and its attributes:
लक्षणं मनसो ज्ञानस्याभातो भाव एव च|
सति ह्यात्मेन्द्रियार्थानां सन्निकर्षे न वर्तते||१८||
वैवृत्यान्मनसो ज्ञानं सान्निध्यात्तच्च वर्तते|
अणुत्वमथ चैकत्वं द्वौ गुणौ मनसः स्मृतौ||१९||

The two main characteristics of the mind are –
- Gaining the knowledge of something (understanding something)
- Not gaining the knowledge of something (not understanding something)
These two are opposite characteristics but both belong to the mind. This is the reason why one understands something at a given point of time and sometimes he doesn't understand something else. This proves the existence of the mind as a separate sense organ. One doesn't get the knowledge of anything when the soul, sense organs and sense objects are associated. This is because the mind is absent in the association. So, when there is no contact of the mind with the soul, sense organs and sense objects one does not understand things. On the other hand, one can understand anything when the mind gets associated with the soul, sense organs and sense objects.
Below mentioned are the qualities of the mind –
- Minuteness / Atomicity and
- Oneness [18-19]

Objects of Mind:

चिन्त्यं विचार्यमूह्यं च ध्येयं सङ्कल्प्यमेव च|
यत्किञ्चिन्मनसो ज्ञेयं तत् सर्वं ह्यर्थसञ्ज्ञकम्||२०||

इन्द्रियाभिग्रहः कर्म मनसः स्वस्य निग्रहः|
ऊहो विचारश्च, ततः परं बुद्धिः प्रवर्तते||२१||

Below mentioned are the subjects of the mind –

- To think – what to do and what not and focusing on those things which need thought process
- To analyse / consider– example, 'I would be benefited if I do this, I would be at loss if I do this.' etc
- To guess / imagination / hypothesis – example, to think 'this would be the end result of any action taking'
- To meditate – upon whatever needs to be meditated upon / giving attention or pondering upon
- Determination / willful decision – example, taking a decision after properly analyzing every fragment of the action in terms of qualities and faults and determining 'since this is beneficial it shall be considered'
- Anything which can be known or understood by the mind (without the help of the sense organs) are considered as subject matters of the mind.

Functions of the mind – Below mentioned are the functions of the mind –
- Controlling the sense organs
- Controlling self / self restraint
- Imagining / making hypothesis and
- Analysis / consideration

Beyond that flourishes the domain of intellect. [20-21]

Process of perception

इन्द्रियेणेन्द्रियार्थो हि समनस्केन गृह्यते|
कल्प्यते मनसा तूर्ध्वं गुणतो दोषतोऽथवा||२२||

जायते विषये तत्र या बुद्धिर्निश्चयात्मिका|
व्यवस्यति तया वक्तुं कर्तुं वा बुद्धिपूर्वकम्||२३||

When the mind gets associated with the sense organs, the sense organs would perceive their respective sense objects. The mind later would analyze the objects and decide and ascertain whether they are advantageous (should be accepted) or disadvantageous (should be rejected).

The intellect which determines (the specific properties of the object impels a (sane) individual to speak or act intelligently. [22-23]

Composition of sense-organs:

एकैकाधिकयुक्तानि खादीनामिन्द्रियाणि तु|
पञ्च कर्मानुमेयानि येभ्यो बुद्धिः प्रवर्तते||२४||

The five sense faculties are made up of all the five Mahabhutas but among the five elements of nature only one element will be predominant in each sense organ. Fire element is predominant in the eye, water element in the tongue, earth element in nose, ether in ears and wind element in the skin. They are inferred from their five respective actions which serve as agents for the manifestation of the intellect. [24]

Motor- organs and their functions:

हस्तौ पादौ गुदोपस्थं वागिन्द्रियमथापि च|
कर्मेन्द्रियाणि पञ्चैव पादौ गमनकर्मणि||२५||

पायूपस्थं विसर्गार्थं हस्तौ ग्रहणधारणे|
जिह्वा वागिन्द्रियं वाक् च सत्या ज्योतिस्तमोऽनृता||२६||

Motor organs are five in number i.e., hands, feet, anus, phallus and the organ of speech (tongue). Feet are useful in locomotion, anus and phallus for voiding and hands for collection and holding. The tongue represents the organ of speech. Speech is of two kinds, viz, true and false. The former (true speech) can be compared to light which illuminates the worldly life and the life after death and the latter (false speech) to darkness which creates confusion. [25-26]

Attributes of five Mahabhutas

महाभूतानि खं वायुरग्निरापः क्षितिस्तथा।

शब्दः स्पर्शश्च रूपं च रसो गन्धश्च तद्गुणाः ||२७||

The five Mahabhutas are Akasha (ether), vayu (wind), Agni (fire), Jala (water) and Prthvi (earth). Their attributes are sound, touch, vision, taste and smell respectively. [27]

Mahabhutas & their attributes:

तेषामेकगुणः पूर्वो गुणवृद्धिः परे परे।

पूर्वः पूर्वगुणश्चैव क्रमशो गुणिषु स्मृतः ||२८||

Of the five Mahabhutas mentioned above, the first one (i.e., Akasha) has only one attribute. The number of attributes in the succeeding Mahabhutas goes on increasing successively. The attributes of the preceding ones are added to the succeeding ones respectively. [28]

Characteristics of Mahabhutas:

खरद्रवचलोष्णत्वं भूजलानिलतेजसाम्।

आकाशस्याप्रतीघातो दृष्टं लिङ्गं यथाक्रमम् ||२९||

लक्षणं सर्वमेवैतत् स्पर्शनेन्द्रियगोचरम्।

स्पर्शनेन्द्रियविज्ञेयः स्पर्शो हि सविपर्ययः ||३०||

Below mentioned are the characteristics of the five elements of nature –

Sl No Mahabhuta (Name of the element of nature) Characteristic feature Meaning

1 Prithvi – Earth Kharatva Roughness

2 Jala - Water Dravatva Liquidity

3 Vayu – Wind / Air Chalatva Mobility

4 Tejas - Fire Ushnatva Heat

5 Akasha – Ether Apratighata Not being obstructed

All these characteristics are perceived by the tactile sense organ / sense organ of touch (skin). Just like the tactile sense organ i.e., skin perceives touch sensation, it also perceives 'absence of touch'. [29-30]

गुणाः शरीरे गुणिनां निर्दिष्टाश्चिह्नमेव च|३१|

The qualities of the subtle and minute bhutas (sound, touch, sight etc sensory objects / perceptions) residing in the body will also be identified and known as the qualities of the mahabhutas (gross elements). [31- 1]

अर्थाः शब्दादयो ज्ञेया गोचरा विषया गुणाः ||३१||

The sound etc qualities which are perceived by the sense organs and are also the subjects of the sense organs are called as 'arthas' i.e., sense objects / objects perceivable by the sense organs. [31?]

Perceptive Faculty:

या यदिन्द्रियमाश्रित्य जन्तोर्बुद्धिः प्रवर्तते।

याति सा तेन निर्देशं मनसा च मनोभवा ||३२||

भेदात् कार्येन्द्रियार्थानां बह्व्यो वै बुद्धयः स्मृताः।

आत्मेन्द्रियमनोर्थानामेकैका सन्निकर्षजा ||३३||

अङ्गुल्यङ्गुष्ठतलजस्तन्त्रीवीणानखोद्भवः।

दृष्टः शब्दो यथा बुद्धिर्दृष्टा संयोगजा तथा ||३४||

The wisdom or intellect is associated with the sense organs for perception of sensory objects and also to understand them. The intellect gets the name of the sense organ with which it is associated at the time of perception of that particular sense object.

Examples,

Chakshusha Buddhi – the intellect associated with the eye – helps in perception of visual objects

Shravana Buddhi – the intellect associated with the ear, - helps in perception of sound

Spaarshana Buddhi – the intellect associated with the skin – helps in perception of touch

Raasana Buddhi – the intellect associated with the tongue – helps in perception of taste

Ghrana Buddhi – the intellect associated with nose – helps in perception of smell

Manasa Buddhi – the intellect associated with mind – helps in perception of the knowledge coming through various senses touching with the mind – responsible for mental perceptions like anxiety, sorrow etc.

Why do different types of the above-mentioned intellects exist?

Perceptual faculties / intellects are of several types. This is because the actions are of different kinds and the objects of sense organs are also of many kinds. The intellects depend on these factors i.e. various kinds of actions and sense objects. All these types of intellect are manifested due to its association with soul, sense organs, and mind and sense objects. This means to say that any type of knowledge is obtained only when all these faculties are associated in a close knitted loop.

Examples for 'manifestation of intellect in different forms'

The sound of click is produced by the friction between finger and thumb, just like the clap is produced when the hands (palms) collide with each other, and just like the tunes are produced from the association of guitar, its string and the nails (of the fingers). All these sounds are totally different from each other. Just like this due to the different types of combinations of the soul, mind, sense organs and the objects of sense organs – different kinds of intellect are produced / manifested. Just like the sounds are formed due to the combinations of what gives origin to them, the intellect also forms due to the combination and association of soul, mind, sense organs and sense objects. If these are not associated the intellect is not manifested. [32-34]

Purusha as coordinator

बुद्धीन्द्रियमनोर्थानां विद्याद्योगधरं परम्‌।
चतुर्विंशतिको ह्येष राशिः पुरुषसञ्ज्ञकः॥३५॥

Rasi Purusha (Individual formed by collective amalgamation of 24 elements) – We should consider the soul to be the one who has adorned the combination of (associated with the combination of) intellect, senses (sense organs), mind and the objects of the sense organs. Therefore Avyakta (soul) is the co-ordinator par-excellence of perceptual faculty, sense organs, mind and the objects of sense. The combination of the above mentioned (Verses 17-35) twenty four elements is known as Purusha. Being associated with 24 elements, the soul is called as chaturvimshati purusha or rashi purusha. [35]

Contact of Purusha because of Gunas:

रजस्तमोभ्यां युक्तस्य संयोगोऽयमनन्तवान्‌।
ताभ्यां निराकृताभ्यां तु सत्त्ववृद्ध्या निवर्तते॥३६॥

The contact of Purusha with 24 elements continues as long as he is influenced by Rajas and Tamas. The moment he gets rid of Rajas and Tamas he is freed from contacts by virtue of the dominance of Sattva. [36]

Knowledge of Purusha:

अत्र कर्म फलं चात्र ज्ञानं चात्र प्रतिष्ठितम्‌।
अत्र मोहः सुखं दुःखं जीवितं मरणं स्वता॥३७॥
एवं यो वेद तत्त्वेन स वेद प्रलयोदयौ।
पारम्पर्यं चिकित्सां च ज्ञातव्यं यच्च किञ्चन॥३८॥

It is in this combination of 24 elements which is known as Purusha, action, fruit of action, knowledge, ignorance, happiness, misery, life, death and ownership are established. One, who dually knows this, knows the life, death, continuity of the body i.e. the sequence of the cycle of birth and death with rebirth followed by death, treatment (Physical and spiritual) of diseases manifested in the current life time and also the methods to attain freedom from the vicious cycle of life and death and attain salvation and all other knowable objects. [37-38]

Purusha as a causative factor:

भास्तमः सत्यमनृतं वेदाः कर्म शुभाशुभम्।

न स्युः कर्ता च बोद्धा च पुरुषो न भवेद्यदि॥३९॥

नाश्रयो न सुखं नार्तिर्न गतिर्नागतिर्न वाक्।

न विज्ञानं न शास्त्राणि न जन्म मरणं न च॥४०॥

न बन्धो न च मोक्षः स्यात् पुरुषो न भवेद्यदि।

कारणं पुरुषस्तस्मात् कारणज्ञैरुदाहृतः॥४१॥

न चेत् कारणमात्मा स्याद्भादयः स्युरहेतुकाः।

न चैषु सम्भवेज् ज्ञानं न च तैः स्यात् प्रयोजनम्॥४२॥

The arguments in support of existence of the soul - If the doer, the one who experiences and the one who knows everything i.e., Purusha were not there, talent / knowledge and ignorance or light and darkness, truth or falsehood, the Vedas, good or bad action, could not exist. If the existence of purusha is not believed then the abode of the soul i.e., this body too would not have existed. There would also be no happiness, misery, movement / the soul leaving the body (salvation), immobility / rebirth, speech, knowledge, scriptures, birth, death, bondage or salvation. So, Purusha is recognised as a cause (of creation) by those well versed in the theory of causality.

If Purusha is not recognised as a cause, the above would be left without a cause. There would be no consciousness, nor any utility of theirs. [39-42]

Baseless talks:

कृतं मृद्दण्डचक्रैश्च कुम्भकाराद्ऋते घटम्।

कृतं मृत्तृणकाष्ठैश्च गृहकारादिवना गृहम्॥४३॥

यो वदेत् स वदेद्देहं सम्भूय करणैः कृतम्।

विना कर्तारम ज्ञानाद्युक्त्यागमबहिष्कृतः॥४४॥

This pot has been made by the combination of mud, stick and wheel without the involvement of the potter.

This house has been constructed by the combination of mud, straw, beams, bamboo and sticks without the involvement of an engineer.

Only a person who can tell these things would tell that the body has been created by the combination of 23 elements without the involvement and association of the soul.

It is only an ignorant person devoid of rational outlook and scriptural knowledge who can make such statements. [43-44]

Causality of Purusha:

कारणं पुरुषः सर्वैः प्रमाणैरुपलभ्यते।

येभ्यः प्रमेयं सर्वेभ्य आगमेभ्यः प्रमीयते॥४५॥

Nastika- view – opinions contradicting the eternity of the Soul

न ते तत्सदृशास्त्वन्ये पारम्पर्यसमुत्थिताः।

सारूप्याद्ये त एवेति निर्दिश्यन्ते नवा नवाः॥४६॥

भावास्तेषां समुदयो निरीशः सत्त्वसञ्ज्ञकः।

कर्ता भोक्ता न स पुमानिति केचिद्व्यवस्थिताः॥४७॥

There are no permanent entities as such. No object which exists is permanent. They are formed new and afresh after the previously existing objects which appear similar to them have been destroyed. This means to tell that they are produced afresh each time. They appear to be the same objects because of similarity of type and form between them. It is the people and schools of thought who believe in these concepts who tell that the living beings are devoid of soul. It is the living beings and not the soul as such is doers and enjoyers of action. This view is held by some schools of thought (Buddhists etc). [46-47]

Defects in the above said theory

तेषामन्यैः कृतस्यान्ये भावा भावैर्नवाः फलम्‌|
भुञ्जते सदृशाः प्राप्तं यैरात्मा नोपदिश्यते||४८||

According to them (i.e the pronouncers of the above theory, viz. Buddhists who do not believe in the existence of a permanent entity as Soul) the results of action performed by one would be enjoyed by some other similar (momentary entities) [48]

Causality of Purusha emphasised:

करणान्यान्यता दृष्टा कर्तुः कर्ता स एव तु|
कर्ता हि करणैर्युक्तः कारणं सर्वकर्मणाम्||४९||

The doer of action, for example a sculptor / engineer might use different equipment to accomplish his action, but the doer is the same. He is an efficient cause of all actions by the virtue of his possession and command of the various instruments. Just like this, the soul is only one, he performs many actions through different instruments i.e., organs of the body. So, the doer is only one but he can accomplish various actions and become the cause of them when he is accomplished with many instruments of actions and has command over them. [49]

Additional Proofs for causality of Purusha:

निमेषकालाद्भावानां कालः शीघ्रतरोऽत्यये|
भग्नानां न पुनर्भावः कृतं नान्यमुपैति च||५०||
मतं तत्त्वविदामेतद्यस्मातस्मात्‌ स कारणम्‌|
क्रियोपभोगे भूतानां नित्यः पुरुषसञ्ज्ञकः||५१||

Physical elements get destroyed at a rate faster than the twinkling of an eye; those destroyed do not come back to their original form again and the results of the deeds (like Yajna) of one individual are not enjoyed by another individual. The learned ones are therefore of the view that there is a permanent entity known as Purusha who is a causative factor for the action entity known as enjoyment of its fruits. [50-51]

Proof of the existence of soul:

अहङ्कारः फलं कर्म देहान्तरगतिः स्मृतिः|
विद्यते सति भूतानां कारणे देहमन्तरा||५२||

In living beings, a factor other than the body (i.e the soul) is responsible for ego, the fruits of action in the form of pleasure or pain, engagement in action, transmigration i.e., the soul moving from one body to the other and memory of the individual. [52]

Paramatman and Rashi Purusha:

प्रभवो न ह्यनादित्वादिद्यते परमात्मनः|
पुरुषो राशिसञ्ज्ञस्तु मोहेच्छाद्वेषकर्मजः||५३||

As the supreme Soul doesn't have any beginning, so there is nothing which can give birth to the soul (no birth as such can be ascribed to him). Of course, the empirical Soul (Purusha) who represents the combination of 24 elements is born out of trance, desire, hatred / enviousness and action. [53]

Process of perception:

आत्मा ज्ञः करणैर्योगाज् ज्ञानं त्वस्य प्रवर्तते|
करणानामवैमल्यादयोगाद्वा न वर्तते||५४||
पश्यतोऽपि यथाऽऽदर्शे सङ्क्लिष्टे नास्ति दर्शनम्|
तत्त्वं जले वा कलुषे चेतस्युपहते तथा||५५||

The empirical Soul is endowed with the power of perception and has knowledge of everything. It perceives things when it gets associated with the sense organs (sense faculties, mind and intellect). If these instruments of perception are either absent (not in association with the Empirical Soul) or impeded, then there will be no perception. One cannot get the real reflected picture of an image from a mirror which is covered with dirt or from water which is muddy. Similar is the case when the mind etc. gets afflicted. [54-55]

Coordination of various factors for perception:

करणानि मनो बुद्धिर्बुद्धिकर्मेन्द्रियाणि च|
कर्तुः संयोगजं कर्म वेदना बुद्धिरेव च||५६||
नैकः प्रवर्तते कर्तुं भूतात्मा नाश्नुते फलम्|
संयोगाद्वर्तते सर्वं तमृते नास्ति किञ्चन||५७||

The instruments of knowledge are mind, intellect, sense organs and organs of action. Their association with the Doer (Empirical Soul) results in action, sensations like pleasure and pain and knowledge / understanding. The empirical Soul alone (in the absence of instruments of knowledge) does neither initiate action nor enjoy the fruit of action. Combination of all these factors is responsible for the manifestation of all actions. If the association between the soul and the other elements doesn't occur no actions take place. [56-57]

Empirical Soul and Manifestations:

न ह्येको वर्तते भावो वर्तते नाप्यहेतुकः|
शीघ्रगत्वात्स्वभावात्त्वभावो न व्यतिवर्तते||५८||

The empirical Soul not alone but accompanied with instruments of knowledge is responsible for the manifestation of things that exist. Things do not manifest without their causal factors. Then we get a question: do void / non-existence of things too have causes? The answer is no. The process of decay on the other hand being too quick in succession does not need any cause as such. [58]

Absolute Soul and Empirical Soul:

अनादिः पुरुषो नित्यो विपरीतस्तु हेतुजः|
सदकारणवन्नित्यं दृष्टं हेतुजमन्यथा||५९||

Absolute Soul doesn't have a beginning (origin) and therefore is eternal. The Empirical Soul (i.e the combination of 24 elements) being caused by something (i.e., causes like ignorance, desire, hatred, action, righteousness and unrighteousness etc) is not so i.e it has a beginning and is ephemeral.

All that exists without cause is eternal. This means to say that anything which can be known in all the time lines (past, present and future) and do not have any causes which produce them is eternal. Anything produced from a cause is ephemeral i.e., anything which exists and which is produced by other causes is ephemeral. [59]

तदेव भावादग्राह्यं नित्यत्व न कुतश्चन|
भावाज्ज्ञेयं तदव्यक्तमचिन्त्यं व्यक्तमन्यथा||६०||
अव्यक्तमात्मा क्षेत्रज्ञः शाश्वतो विभुरव्ययः|
तस्मादयदन्यतदव्यक्तं, वक्ष्यते चापरं द्वयम्||६१||
व्यक्तमैन्द्रियकं चैव गृह्यते तद्यदिन्द्रियैः|
अतोऽन्यत् पुनरव्यक्तं लिङ्गग्राह्यमतीन्द्रियम्||६२||

The absolute Soul cannot be perceived by anything, for eternity is not caused by anything. So, the absolute Soul is unmanifested and imperceptible. The manifested creation is of course otherwise i.e., those things which are known through their manifestation i.e., the purusha made up of 24 elements is emphereal, manifested and percieved.

The absolute Soul is unmanifested, knower of creation, eternal, universal and indestructible. The manifested creation (Empirical Soul) is of course otherwise. Another way of distinguishing manifested things from the unmanifested one is that the former can be perceived by sense faculties. The latter is transcendental in nature and is imperceptible; it can only be inferred (rather than received) i.e., is beyond the perception of senses. [60-62]

Twenty- four Elements:

खादीनि बुद्धिरव्यक्तमहङ्कारस्तथाऽष्टमः।
भूतप्रकृतिरुद्दिष्टा विकाराश्चैव षोडश॥६३॥
बुद्धीन्द्रियाणि पञ्चैव पञ्च कर्मेन्द्रियाणि च।
समनस्काश्च पञ्चार्था विकारा इति सञ्ज्ञिताः॥६४॥

Eight Prakritis - The five subtle elements (Sabdanmatra, Sparsatanmatra, Rupatanmatra, Rasatanmatra and Gandhatanmatra), Buddhi (intellect), Avyakta (Prakrti or nature) and Ahamkara (ego) are the eight sources of creation.

Sixteen Vikritis - Transformations (vikara) are sixteen in number. They are - five sense faculties, five motor faculties, mind and five mahabhutas i.e. elements of nature. [63-64]

Ksetra and Ksetrajna:

इति क्षेत्रं समुद्दिष्टं सर्वमव्यक्तवर्जितम्।
अव्यक्तमस्य क्षेत्रस्य क्षेत्रज्ञमृषयो विदुः॥६५॥

All these elements taken together, except the unmanifested one (avyakta) is known as Ksetra i.e corpus. The unmanifested one is known as Ksetrajna (knower of the corpus). [65]

Process of creation:

जायते बुद्धिरव्यक्तादबुद्ध्याऽहमिति मन्यते।
परं खादीन्यहङ्कारादुत्पद्यन्ते यथाक्रमम्॥६६॥
ततः सम्पूर्णसर्वाङ्गो जातोऽभ्युदित उच्यते।६७।

The intellect (buddhi) originates from Avyakta (unmanifested, soul). Ego (Ahamkara) manifests from intellect (buddhi). From Ego the subtle forms of five Mahabhutas i.e. tanmatras get manifested i.e. akasha etc. Later the vikaras i.e., 16 transformations are formed in order. The empirical Soul thus manifested in its entirety is regarded as born. [66-67]

Process of dissolution:

पुरुषः प्रलये चेष्टैः पुनर्भावैर्वियुज्यते॥६७॥
अव्यक्ताद्व्यक्ततां याति व्यक्ताद्व्यक्ततां पुनः।
रजस्तमोभ्यामाविष्टश्चक्रवत् परिवर्तते॥६८॥
येषां द्वन्द्वे परा सक्तिरहङ्कारपराश्च ये।
उदयप्रलयौ तेषां न तेषां ये त्वतोऽन्यथा॥६९॥

During the time of destruction of the age, the Purusha (soul) again dissociates himself from all the manifestations meant for his enjoyment, viz, Buddhi etc. The five elements get absorbed into their subtle forms i.e., tanmatras. The tanmatras and eleven senses (5 sense organs, 5 motor organs and mind) get absorbed into the ego. The ego gets dissolved into the intellect and the intellect gets absorbed into the avyakta (the unmanifested). The universe is created from the unmanifested stage to the manifested one during creation, and then absorbed back again from the manifested stage to the unmanifested one during total annihilation.

Those who are attached to rajas and Tamas and those who are egoistic repeatedly undergo the process and vicious cycle of birth and death; others do not. Those indulged in and attached to the dualties like desire, hatred, selfishness, intoxication, lust, anger etc and those who are enveloped by egoism will be born and will also die i.e., they are put into the cycle of life and death. Those who are free from raja and tama qualities and also from egoism and erroneous knowledge will not be afflicted by the vicious cycle of life and death (would attain salvation). [67-69]

Proofs for the existence of absolute soul:

प्राणापानौ निमेषाद्या जीवनं मनसो गतिः|

इन्द्रियान्तरसञ्चारः प्रेरणं धारणं च यत्||७०||

देशान्तरगतिः स्वप्ने पञ्चत्वग्रहणं तथा|

दृष्टस्य दक्षिणेनाक्ष्णा सव्येनावगमस्तथा||७१||

इच्छा द्वेषः सुखं दुःखं प्रयत्नश्चेतना धृतिः|

बुद्धिः स्मृतिरहङ्कारो लिङ्गानि परमात्मनः||७२||

यस्मात् समुपलभ्यन्ते लिङ्गान्येतानि जीवतः|

न मृतस्यात्मलिङ्गानि तस्मादाहुर्महर्षयः||७३||

शरीरं हि गते तस्मिन् शून्यागारमचेतनम्|

पञ्चभूतावशेषत्वात् पञ्चत्वं गतमुच्यते||७४||

The following is the proof of the existence of the absolute soul:

Inspiration and expiration

Twinkling / blinking of the eye

Life

Mental perception (e.g. arriving at a far distant place like Pataliputra in imagination)

Shift from one object of sense organ to another (e.g shift from visual perception to tactual perception)

Mobility and stability of mind

Journey to another country in dreams

Anticipation of death

Knowledge of something visualised in the right eye by the left eye

Desire, hatred, happiness, misery, effort, consciousness, stability, intellect, memory and ego

All these are signs of the living person. These signs are not available in a dead body. So they are considered to be the proof for the existence of the absolute Soul. When that soul departs, the body becomes vacant and is deprived of consciousness; only the five Mahabhutas remain. So, a dead person is said to have attained the state of five Mahabhutas (Panchatatva). [70-74]

Mind and Soul:

अचेतनं क्रियावच्च मनश्चेतयिता परः|

युक्तस्य मनसा तस्य निर्दिश्यन्ते विभोः क्रियाः||७५||

चेतनावान् यतश्चात्मा ततः कर्ता निरुच्यते|

अचेतनत्वाच्च मनः क्रियावदपि नोच्यते||७६||

The mind is devoid of consciousness but has action. It is the soul which lends consciousness to the mind. When the soul gets associated with the mind, the actions done by the mind residing in the soul (in association with the soul) will be considered as the actions done by the soul. The soul has consciousness. Therefore, it is said to be the agent of action (one who does / is responsible for all action). Even though it possesses action the mind is said to be devoid of action since it is devoid of consciousness. [75-76]

Responsibility for transmigration:

यथास्वेनात्मनाऽऽत्मानं सर्वः सर्वासु योनिषु|

प्राणैस्तन्त्रयते प्राणी नह्यन्योऽस्त्यस्य तन्त्रकः||७७||

The soul will take itself from itself into different species (as a life element in different species of life) in accordance with the results of the actions done by self (previously). None else is responsible for the transmigration of living being from one species to another [77]

Freedom of action of the soul:

वशी तत् कुरुते कर्म यत् कृत्वा फलमश्नुते।
वशी चेतः समाधत्ते वशी सर्वं निरस्यति॥७८॥

The soul is absolutely free to act as he pleases. He is however obliged to enjoy the fruits of his action. He is also free to control his mind and to get rid of the results of good or bad acts of his own. [78]

Limitation in the power of perception of soul:

देही सर्वगतोऽप्यात्मा स्वे स्वे संस्पर्शनेन्द्रिये।
सर्वाः सर्वाश्रयस्थास्तु नात्माऽतो वेत्ति वेदनाः॥७९॥

Even though, soul is all pervasive, his sensations are limited to the body in which he resides. He can only perceive the sensations of only that body adorned by its own sense organ of touch - skin (he perceives the sensations in the body in which he resides depending on the contact of the sense organs with their respective sense objects). His sense organs (sense organs of the body in which he resides) cannot reach the body of other living beings. This is the reason the soul cannot perceive all sensations experienced by the other bodies. [79]

Omnipresence of Soul:

विभुत्वमत एवास्य यस्मात् सर्वगतो महान्।
मनसश्च समाधानात् पश्यत्यात्मा तिरस्कृतम्॥८०॥
नित्यानुबन्धं मनसा देहकर्मानुपातिना।
सर्वयोनिगतं विद्यादेकयोनावपि स्थितम्॥८१॥

The soul is omnipresent because he pervades the entire universe and is great. Since he is bound inside a single body (in spite of being omnipresent) his sensory perceptions are limited (to only the body in which he resides). His field of action is limited to the body alone (though he is all pervasive and present in all bodies) because of his regular and contact with the mind which performs all the actions of that body. When the soul gradually gets the mind under its control, it can perceive things in spite of (spatial, temporal or material) those things being obstructed (beyond the wall, screen or mountain) or hidden by something else. Since the soul is constantly associated with the mind involved in all actions of the body and since he cannot see the things beyond obstructions (due to constant association with the mind) the soul should be considered to be present in only one body in spite of knowing that he is all pervasive (present in all bodies). [80-81]

Beginning lessness of Soul:

आदिर्नास्त्यात्मनः क्षेत्रपारम्पर्यमनादिकम्।
अतस्तयोरनादित्वात् किं पूर्वमिति नोच्यते॥८२॥

The soul is beginningless and so is the process of evolution of the various elements. Thus, it is not possible to determine as to which one precedes the other. [82]

Soul as witness:

ज्ञः साक्षीत्युच्यते नाज्ञः साक्षी त्वात्मा यतः स्मृतः।
सर्वे भावा हि सर्वेषां भूतानामात्मसाक्षिकाः॥८३॥

It is only he who knows things can stand as a witness. The one who doesn't know anything and the inert things like stone etc cannot become witness of anything (Things cannot be witnessed by unconscious objects like stone). So, all attributes, actions etc., of Bhutas are witnessed by the Soul (who alone is knower of things). [83]

Sensations and Soul:

नैकः कदाचिद्भूतात्मा लक्षणैरुपलभ्यते।
विशेषोऽनुपलभ्यस्य तस्य नैकस्य विद्यते॥८४॥
संयोगपुरुषस्येष्टो विशेषो वेदनाकृतः।
वेदना यत्र नियता विशेषस्तत्र तत्कृतः॥८५॥

The absolute Soul is one and only one. He is inaccessible by any signs or symptoms. Being inaccessible he has no sensation. It is only the contractual or the empirical soul who has sensations. For, these sensations do not constitute the attributes of the soul as such. They in fact arise out of the contacts (of the sense organs with their objects) [84-85]

Treatment of diseases of past, present and future:

चिकित्सति भिषक् सर्वास्त्रिकाला वेदना इति।
यया युक्त्या वदन्त्येके सा युक्तिरुपधार्यताम्॥८६॥
पुनस्तच्छिरसः शूलं ज्वरः स पुनरागतः।
पुनः स कासो बलवांश्छर्दिः सा पुनरागता॥८७॥
एभिः प्रसिद्धवचनैरतीतागमनं मतम्।
कालश्चायमतीतानामर्तीनां पुनरागतः॥८८॥
तमर्तिकालमुद्दिश्य भेषजं यत् प्रयुज्यते।
अतीतानां प्रशमनं वेदनानां तदुच्यते॥८९॥
आपस्ताः पुनरागुर्मा याभिः शस्यं पुरा हतम्।
यथा प्रक्रियते सेतुः प्रतिकर्म तथाऽऽश्रये॥९०॥
पूर्वरूपं विकाराणां दृष्ट्वा प्रादुर्भविष्यताम्।
या क्रिया क्रियते सा च वेदनां हन्त्यनागताम्॥९१॥
पारम्पर्यानबन्धस्तु दुःखानां विनिवर्तते।
सुखहेतूपचारेण सुखं चापि प्रवर्तते॥९२॥
न समा यान्ति वैषम्यं विषमाः समतां न च।
हेतुभिः सदृशा नित्यं जायन्ते देहधातवः॥९३॥
युक्तिमेतां पुरस्कृत्य त्रिकालां वेदनां भिषक्।
हन्तीत्युक्तं चिकित्सा तु नैष्ठिकी या विनोपधाम्॥९४॥

The principle, on which the treatment of diseases pertaining to the past, present and future is based, is as follows:

Diseases of the past

Recurrence of headache, fever, cough and vomiting establishes the fact that diseases of the past do relapse. Some evey say 'the time of occurrence of the various diseases of the past' has come once again. The therapeutic devices meant for alleviating such recurring diseases by considering the past history (of such diseases) and also the time period of their occurrence (recurrence) are considered as the 'treatment of the diseases of the past'.

Diseases of the future

In order to prevent the flood waters from damaging the crops as they did in the past, a dam was constructed as a preventive measure. Similarly, some therapeutic devices are designed and the medicines are prescribed to prevent certain diseases which are likely to attack living beings in future after having considered the premonitory symptoms of the diseases and inferring the time of occurrence of pain or disease. This treatment relates to prevention of future diseases.

Diseases of the present

The successive continuity of aliments is checked by treatment conducive to the continuity of happiness and health is established. When one takes the treatments which would establish happiness and health and also would avoid taking the causative factors which would cause diseases, the diseases are not formed. And the diseases would get destroyed by themselves. Since the person is also taking the treatments which would establish health and happiness, health and happiness too would be established. Since the etiological factors are kept away, the diseases which could occur in future too are aborted in their premature stages and hence the health will be established. Due to the constant practice of intake of the causes (things) which would establish happiness and health, the state of equilibrium of tissues and body components will be established. When this state is maintained, the person would enjoy comprehensive health.

The state of equilibrium of Dhatus is not disturbed nor is the imbalanced state of dhatus brought to normalcy without the involvement of some causative factors. It is the causative factors which determine the equilibrium or imbalance of the Dhatus.

So, a physician treats the diseases pertaining to the past, present and future. [86- 94]

Desires & miseries:

उपधा हि परो हेतुर्दुःखदुःखाश्रयप्रदः|
त्यागः सर्वोपधानां च सर्वदुःखव्यपोहकः||९५||
कोषकारो यथा ह्यंशूनुपादत्ते वधप्रदान् |
उपादत्ते तथाऽर्थेभ्यस्तृष्णामज्ञः सदाऽऽतुरः||९६||
यस्त्वग्निकल्पानर्थान् ज्ञो ज्ञात्वा तेभ्यो निवर्तते|
अनारम्भादसंयोगात् दुःखं नोपतिष्ठते||९७||

Naishtiki Chikitsa – Absolute eradication of miseries is called nishtha. The treatments done to achieve this are called naishtiki chikitsa. The secret of success of this treatment is 'elimination of upadha' i.e., an abnormal thirst called desire which keeps one attached to this materialistic world and is a cause of all miseries. Desire is the root cause of all miseries. Elimination of desire is the eradication of all miseries.

The agony of birth and death (cycle of birth and death) is the greatest misery and the body is the abode of miseries. Therefore rejection / elimination of all kinds of upadha – desires is the best method of keeping away all diseases.

A silk-worm produces and weaves around it the silk threads which would cause its death. Similarly, an ignorant person, bound with worldly miseries, provides for himself and weaves around him the 'threads of death' of desire arising out of the various objects. A wise person who abstains from the objects of senses, considering them as dangerous as burning fire, would keep himself detached from the rajas and tamas qualities. He will not indulge himself in any actions which will push him to adorn this physical body to experience the fruits of those actions i.e., he would keep himself out of desires and materialistic attachments. By not beginning the actions which would keep him attached to the desires and attachments to the materialistic world and consequently being not embedded in the physical body he will get freedom from the miseries. [94-97]

Cause of miseries:

धीधृतिस्मृतिविभ्रंशः सम्प्राप्तिः कालकर्मणाम्|
असात्म्यार्थागमश्चेति ज्ञातव्या दुःखहेतवः||९८||

Impairment of intellect, courage (patience) and memory, advent of the maturity (of the result) of time and action and unwholesome contact with the objects of senses is considered to be the causative factors for miseries. [98]

Impairment of intellect:

विषमाभिनिवेशो यो नित्यानित्ये हिताहिते|
ज्ञेयः स बुद्धिविभ्रंशः समं बुद्धिर्हि पश्यति||९९||

If something eternal is viewed as ephemeral and something harmful, and vice versa, this is indicative of the impairment of intellect, for the Intellect normally views things as they are. [99]

Impairment of Patience:

विषयप्रवणं सत्वं धृतिभ्रंशान्न शक्यते|
नियन्तुमहितादर्थाद्धृतिर्हि नियमात्मिका||१००||

A mind indulging in worldly enjoyments cannot be restrained from harmful objects due to the impairment of courage / patience. It is patience which can restrain the mind (from its harmful objects). [100]

Impairment of memory:

तत्त्वज्ञाने स्मृतिर्यस्य रजोमोहावृतात्मनः|
भ्रश्यते स स्मृतिभ्रंशः स्मर्तव्यं हि स्मृतौ स्थितम्||१०१||

If memory is impaired due to a person being overcome by Rajas and tamas, this is known as the impairment of memory. Normally memory contains everything memorable. [101]

Intellectual Blashphemy:

धीधृतिस्मृतिविभ्रष्टः कर्म यत् कुरुतेऽशुभम्|
प्रज्ञापराधं तं विद्यात् सर्वदोषप्रकोपणम्||१०२||
उदीरणं गतिमतामुदीर्णानां च निग्रहः|
सेवनं साहसानां च नारीणां चातिसेवनम्||१०३||
कर्मकालातिपातश्च मिथ्यारम्भश्च कर्मणाम्|
विनयाचारलोपश्च पूज्यानां चाभिधर्षणम्||१०४||
ज्ञातानां स्वयमर्थानामहितानां निषेवणम्|
परमौन्मादिकानां च प्रत्ययानां निषेवणम्||१०५||
अकालादेशसञ्चारौ मैत्री सङ्क्लिष्टकर्मभिः|
इन्द्रियोपक्रमोक्तस्य सद्वृत्तस्य च वर्जनम्||१०६||
ईर्ष्यामानभयक्रोधलोभमोहमदभ्रमाः|
तज्जं वा कर्म यत् क्लिष्टं क्लिष्टं यद्देहकर्म च||१०७||
यच्चान्यदीदृशं कर्म रजोमोहसमुत्थितम्|
प्रज्ञापराधं तं शिष्टा ब्रुवते व्याधिकारणम्||१०८||

A person whose intellect, courage / patience and memory are impaired; the actions he does will be untowards and bad. These inauspicious or bad actions done by the person are called prajnaparadha i.e., intellectual blasphemy. This intellectual blasphemy aggravates all the Doshas i.e., the physical doshas (vata, pitta and kapha) and the mental doshas (rajas and tamas).

Forcible stimulation of natural urges (when they are not manifested) and suppression of the manifested ones (which are about to get expelled), exhibition of undue strength – being over adventurous in comparison to one's capacity / strength, over indulgence in sexual act, negligence of the time of treatment, inadequate, excessive and abnormal use of cleansing therapies – emesis, purgation, decoction enemas, oil enemas and errhines, loss of modesty and good conduct, disrespect for respectable ones, enjoyment of harmful sense objects purposefully i.e. sound, touch, sight, taste and smell, resorting to the intense causative factors which are responsible for the causative of madness, untimely movements / roaming around in restricted / prohibited places, friendship with persons of bad actions, avoidance of the healthy activates described in Sutra 10: 19:28, malice, vanity, fear, anger, greed, ignorance, intoxication and bewilderment or bad actions arising out of any of them or other physical evil acts arising out of Rajas and Tamas constitute intellectual blasphemy leading to the causation of various ailments. [102-108]

Intellectual blasphemy& mind:

बुद्ध्या विषमविज्ञानं विषमं च प्रवर्तनम्|
प्रज्ञापराधं जानीयान्मनसो गोचरं हि तत्||१०९||

Intellectual pseudo-conception (perception of improper knowledge by the intellect or information which is not 'as its is') and improper conduct (intellect getting indulged in actions in an improper way) represent intellectual blasphemy. (This is known as intellectual blasphemy as) alt this falls under the purview of the mind. [109]

Temporal diseases:

निर्दिष्टा कालसम्प्राप्तिर्व्याधीनां व्याधिसङ्ग्रहे|

चयप्रकोपप्रशमाः पित्तादीनां यथा पुरा||११०||
मिथ्यातिहीनलिङ्गाश्च वर्षान्ता रोगहेतवः|
जीर्णभुक्तप्रजीर्णान्नकालाकालस्थितिश्च या||१११||
पूर्वमध्यापराह्णाश्च रात्र्या यामास्त्रयश्च ये|
एषु कालेषु नियता ये रोगास्ते च कालजाः||११२||

Ailments caused due to changes in time / seasons are already described in Sutra 17: 114. It has been explained there, how Pitta and other Doshas get accumulated, aggravated and alleviated (depending on seasonal variation).

Erroneous, excessive and inadequate use / manifestation of the seasons cause dosha imbalances and cause diseases pertaining to those seasons.

Pitta, kapha and vata get aggravated during digestion, immediately after consumption of food and after complete digestion of food respectively and cause diseases in accordance with the aggravation of doshas.

Pitta, kapha and vata get aggravated due to food getting processed in abnormal time, untimely consumption of food and untimely digestion of food respectively and cause related diseases.

Kapha, Pitta and Vata get aggravated in the early hours of the morning, afternoon and evening respectively.

Kapha, Pitta and Vata get aggravated in the first, second and third parts of the night and cause diseases accordingly.

The doshas naturally get aggravated during these time periods and the diseases which get manifested during these times are called Kalaja diseases i.e., diseases caused due to the impact of time (and related dosha imbalance corresponding to that time). [110-112]

Examples of Temporal diseases;
अन्येद्युष्को द्व्यहग्राही तृतीयकचतुर्थकौ|
स्वे स्वे काले प्रवर्तन्ते काले ह्येषां बलागमः||११३||

Diseases like Anyedyuska (quotidian fever which occurs at a fixed time every day), Dvyahagrahi (reverse quotidian fever), and Trtiya (tertian fever which which occurs at an interval of two days) manifest themselves at fixed hours as they get strength only at such hours. [113]

Time of treatment of temporal diseases:
एते चान्ये च ये केचित् कालजा विविधा गदाः|
अनागते चिकित्स्यास्ते बलकालौ विजानता||११४||

Physician acquainted with the strength of time of occurrence of diseases should treat this and other similar diseases prior to their actual manifestation. [114]

Natural diseases:
कालस्य परिणामेन जरामृत्युनिमित्तजाः|
रोगाः स्वाभाविका दृष्टाः स्वभावो निष्प्रतिक्रियः||११५||

The diseases arising out of temporal factors that bring about old age and death are to be considered as natural ones, and natural manifestations are irremediable. [115]

Actions of past life and diseases:
निर्दिष्टं दैवशब्देन कर्म यत् पौर्वदेहिकम्|
हेतुस्तदपि कालेन रोगाणामुपलभ्यते||११६||

The action performed in the previous life which is known as Daiva (fate) also constitutes causative factors for the manifestation of diseases in due course of time. [116]

Cure of karmaja Diseases:
न हि कर्म महत् किञ्चित् फलं यस्य न भुज्यते|
क्रियाघ्नाः कर्मजा रोगाः प्रशमं यान्ति तत्क्षयात्||११७||

There is no major action (performed in the previous life) which does not lead to the corresponding results. Diseases arising out of such actions are not amenable to any therapeutic measures. They are cured only after the results of past action are exhausted i.e fully enjoyed [117]

Unwholesome contacts with Senses:

अत्युग्रशब्दश्रवणाच्छ्रवणात् सर्वशो न च|
शब्दानां चातिहीनानां भवन्ति श्रवणाज्जडाः||११८||
परुषोद्भीषणाशस्ताप्रियव्यसनसूचकैः|
शब्दैः श्रवणसंयोगो मिथ्यासंयोग उच्यते||११९||
असंस्पर्शोऽतिसंस्पर्शो हीनसंस्पर्श एव च|
स्पृश्यानां सङ्ग्रहेणोक्तः स्पर्शनेन्द्रियबाधकः||१२०||
यो भूतविषवातानामकालेनागतश्च यः|
स्नेहशीतोष्णसंस्पर्शो मिथ्यायोग स उच्यते||१२१||
रूपाणां भास्वतां दृष्टिर्विनश्यत्यतिदर्शनात्|
दर्शनाच्चातिसूक्ष्माणां सर्वशश्चाप्यदर्शनात्||१२२||
द्विष्टभैरवबीभत्सदूरातिशिलष्टदर्शनात् [१] |
तामसानां च रूपाणां मिथ्यासंयोग उच्यते||१२३||
अत्यादानमनादानमोकसात्म्यादिभिश्च यत्|
रसानां विषमादानमल्पादानं च दूषणम्||१२४||
अतिमृद्वतितीक्ष्णानां गन्धानामुपसेवनम्|
असेवनं सर्वशश्च घ्राणेन्द्रियविनाशनम्||१२५||
पूतिभूतविषदिवष्टा गन्धा ये चाप्यनार्तवाः|
तैर्गन्धैर्घ्राणसंयोगो मिथ्यायोगः स उच्यते||१२६||
इत्यसात्म्यार्थसंयोगस्त्रिविधो दोषकोपनः|१२७|

1. Inadequate, excessive or erroneous contact of auditory sense
The auditory sense faculty is impaired by the hearing of excessively loud sounds or low sound or not hearing the sounds at all. Hearing in excess of rough, terrifying, inauspicious or disliked sounds or sounds which indicate misery, disaster or death constitute the wrong utilization of the auditory sense organ.

2. Inadequate, excessive or erroneous contact of tactile sense
Inadequate, excessive or erroneous utilization of the organ of touch i.e., skin can cause skin disorders of various kinds.
Touching the touchable things in an inadequate way (deficit exposure) or not touching them at all is considered as deficit contact of the organ of touch.
Touching the touchable things in an excessive way (excessive exposure) or touching too hot or too cold things in excess is considered as excessive contact of the organ of touch.
Both these decrease the strength of the sense organ of touch.
Untimely contact with poisonous germs (?), Poisonous wind, and unctuous, cold and hot substances constitute wrong –utilization of tactile sensation.

3. Inadequate, excessive or erroneous contact of visual sense
Inadequate, excessive or erroneous utilization of sense organ of visual perception i.e., eyes can cause different eye disorders.
Seeing dazzling objects in excess is considered as excessive contact of the sense organ of vision i.e., eyes.
Seeing extremely subtle and smaller things in excess or by absolute non-utilization of visual faculty is considered as deficit contact of the sense organ of vision.
Seeing undesirable, terrific, despicable, objects and objects placed at a distance or in close proximity excessively - constitutes the wrong- utilization of visual faculty. Vision is also impaired by the contact of the visual faculty with

faint objects.

All these three will either make the vision weak or destroy the vision permanently.

4. Inadequate, excessive or erroneous contact of gustatory (taste) sense

Inadequate, excessive or erroneous utilization of the sense organs of taste perception i.e., tongue can cause different taste related disorders.

Consuming any particular taste in excess is considered as excessive contact of the sense organ of taste - tongue.

Consuming any one, two or three tastes or not at all taking them or taking them in less quantity is considered as deficit contact of the sense organ of taste.

Taking the tastes against one's compatibility / suitability, or taking the tastes in an erratic way i.e., Sometimes consuming a taste and some other taste at some other time, or taking one taste in excess and other tastes in lesser proportions is considered as erroneous contact of sense organs of taste.

All these three are harmful for the body.

5. Inadequate, excessive or erroneous contact of olfactory (smell) sense

Inadequate, excessive or erroneous utilization of sense organs of smell perception i.e., nose can cause different smell related disorders.

Taking too mild a smell or not smelling anything at all is considered as deficit contact of organ of smell.

Taking too strong / sharp smell is considered as excessive contact of the organ of smell.

Inhalation of smell of putrefied objects, germs and poisonous as well as unseasonal smell constitutes wrong-utilization of olfactory faculty.

These are the three types of unwholesome contact of senses with their respective objects which aggravate the Doshas. [118-127]

Unwholesomeness:

असात्म्यमिति तद्विद्याद्यन्न याति सहात्मताम्||१२७||

A thing which is not conducive to the body is regarded as Asatmya or unwholesome. [127]

Aindriyaka diseases:

मिथ्यातिहीनयोगेभ्यो यो व्याधिरुपजायते|

शब्दादीनां स विज्ञेयो व्याधिरैन्द्रियको बुधैः||१२८||

When a disease is caused by wrong utilization, excessive utilization and inadequate utilization (non-utilization) of sense faculties it is known as "Aindriyaka" i.e a disease caused by the impairment of senses. [128]

वेदनानामशान्तानामित्येते हेतवः स्मृताः|

सुखहेतुः समस्त्वेकः समयोगः सुदुर्लभः||१२९||

These are the factors responsible for miseries. Equitable utilization (of time, intellect and objects of sense faculties) brings about happiness. This equitable utilization is difficult to attain. [129]

Four-fold combination:

नेन्द्रियाणि न चैवार्थाः सुखदुःखस्य हेतवः|

हेतुस्तु सुखदुःखस्य योगो दृष्टश्चतुर्विधः||१३०||

सन्तीन्द्रियाणि सन्त्यर्था योगो न च न चास्ति रुक्|

न सुखं, कारणं तस्माद्योग एव चतुर्वधः||१३१||

Neither the sense organs nor their objects alone can bring about happiness or miseries. Proper utilization of sense organs will lead to happiness and health. On the other hand, the other three forms of utilization of sense organs i.e., erroneous, excessive or deficit / non utilization are responsible for miseries / diseases. Even if there are sense organs and their objects present, there would be neither disease nor any happiness unless there is association between the sense organs and their objects. So, this combination itself constitutes a causative factor for happiness and miseries.

[130-131]

Factors responsible for happiness & miseries:

नात्मेन्द्रियं मनो बुद्धिं गोचरं कर्म वा विना|
सुखदुःखं, यथा यच्च बोद्धव्यं तत्तथोच्यते||१३२||

As a matter of fact no happiness or misery can be caused without the Soul, the sense organs, mind, intellect, and objects of sense. It is only the four-fold combination which is relevant as a causative factor of happiness and miseries (that is to say the wholesome combination is required to be adhered to and the unwholesome one to be given up for the maintenance of good health). [132]

Two types of contacts:

स्पर्शनेन्द्रियसंस्पर्शः स्पर्शो मानस एव च|
द्विविधः सुखदुःखानां वेदनानां प्रवर्तकः||१३३||

Tactile contact and mental contact are the two types of contacts which bring about happiness and miseries. [133]

Happiness & miseries caused by Lust:

इच्छाद्वेषात्मिका तृष्णा सुखदुःखात् प्रवर्तते|
तृष्णा च सुखदुःखानां कारणं पुनरुच्यते||१३४||
उपादत्ते हि सा भावान् वेदनाश्रयसञ्ज्ञकान्|
स्पृश्यते नानुपादाने नास्पृष्टो वेति वेदनाः||१३५||

Happiness and miseries bring about lust in the form of likes and dislikes respectively. Then again, this lust is responsible for happiness and miseries. It is lust which gathers factors, which serve as substrata for happiness and misery. Unless such factors are gathered, there will be no contact whatsoever and there can be no happiness or miseries without such contact. [134-135]

Sites of sensations:

वेदनानामधिष्ठानं मनो देहश्च सेन्द्रियः|
केशलोमनखाग्रान्नमलद्रवगुणैर्विना||१३६||

The mind and the body together with the sense organs exclusive of Kesha (hair), Loman (small hair), tip of the nail, ingested food, excreta, excretory fluids and objects of sense are the sites of manifestation of happiness and miseries. [136]

Yoga & Moksha:

योगे मोक्षे च सर्वासां वेदनानामवर्तनम्|
मोक्षे निवृत्तिर्निःशेषा योगो मोक्षप्रवर्तकः||१३७||

Recurrence of all sensation is checked through Yoga and Moksha. The absolute eradication of sensation is attained through Moksa. The Yoga is a means to attain Moksha. [137]

What is Yoga?

आत्मेन्द्रियमनोर्थानां सन्निकर्षात् प्रवर्तते|
सुखदुःखमनारम्भादात्मस्थे मनसि स्थिरे||१३८||
निवर्तते तदुभयं वशित्वं चोपजायते|
सशरीरस्य योगज्ञास्तं योगमृषयो विदुः||१३९||

Happiness and miseries are felt due the contact of the Soul, the sense organs, mind and the objects of senses. Both these types of sensations disappear when the mind is concentrated and contained in the Soul because no actions happen when this happens. The person would then gain control over his mind and senses. The body and mind attain supernatural powers. The sages well versed in this science call this state as Yoga. [138-139]

Eight super-natural powers of Yogin:

आवेशश्चेतसो ज्ञानमर्थानां छन्दतः क्रिया|
दृष्टिः श्रोत्रं स्मृतिः कान्तिरिष्टतश्चाप्यदर्शनम्||१४०||
इत्यष्टविधमाख्यातं योगिनां बलमैश्वरम्|
शुद्धसत्त्वसमाधानात्तत् सर्वमुपजायते||१४१||

Entering other's body

Thought reading

Doing things at will

Super-natural vision

Supernatural audition

Miraculous memory

Uncommon brilliance and

Invisibility when so desired - these are the eight supernatural powers attained by those practising Yoga. All this is achieved through the purity of the mind (free from Rajas and Tamas). [140-141]

Salvation:

मोक्षो रजस्तमोऽभावात् बलवत्कर्मसङ्क्षयात्|
वियोगः सर्वसंयोगैरपुनर्भव उच्यते||१४२||

Moksha or salvation is nothing but an absolute detachment of all contacts by virtue of the absence of Rajas and Tamas in the mind and annihilation of effects of potent past actions. This is a state after which there will be no more physical or mental contacts. [142]

Means for attainment of Moksha:

सतामुपासनं सम्यगसतां परिवर्जनम्|
व्रतचर्योपवासौ च नियमाश्च पृथग्विधाः||१४३||
धारणं धर्मशास्त्राणां विज्ञानं विजने रतिः|
विषयेष्वरतिर्मोक्षे व्यवसायः परा धृतिः||१४४||
कर्मणामसमारम्भः कृतानां च परिक्षयः|
नैष्क्रम्यमनहङ्कारः संयोगे भयदर्शनम्||१४५||
मनोबुद्धिसमाधानमर्थतत्त्वपरीक्षणम्|
तत्त्वस्मृतेरुपस्थानात् सर्वमेतत् प्रवर्तते||१४६||

The following serves as means to attainment of Moksha:

Due devotion to noble Souls

Keeping away / ending of the company of wicked / bad people

Observing sacred vows and rituals

Fasting

Pursuit of the rules of good conduct

Compliance with scriptural prescriptions

Scriptural knowledge

Liking for lonely living

Detachment from the objects of sense

Striving for moksha (Salvation)

Absolute mental control and holding on to courage

Abstinence from the performance of acts leading to good and sinful effects

Annihilation of the effects of past-actions

Desire to get away from the worldly trap
Absence of egoistic disposition
Being afraid of contacts of the Soul, with the mind, intellect, senses etc
Concentration of the mind and intellect in the Soul and
Review of spiritual facts
All this can be attained by virtue of the constant remembering of the fact that the Soul is different from the body and the latter has nothing to do with the former. [143-146]

Aid to Memory:

स्मृतिः सत्सेवनाद्यैश्च धृत्यन्तैरुपजायते|
स्मृत्वा स्वभावं भावानां स्मरन् दुःखात् प्रमुच्यते||१४७||

The regime prescribed in verses above, beginning with devotion to the noble persons and ending with absolute mental control (items 1-10) serve as an aid to good memory if one only remembers the real nature of things, he gets rid of miseries. [147]

Causative factors of memory:

वक्ष्यन्ते कारणान्यष्टौ स्मृतिर्यैरुपजायते|
निमित्तरूपग्रहणात् सादृश्यात् सविपर्ययात्||१४८||
सत्त्वानुबन्धादभ्यासाज्ज्ञानयोगात् पुनः श्रुतात्|
दृष्टश्रुतानुभूतानां स्मारणात् स्मृतिरुच्यते||१४९||

The following are the factors that bring about a good memory:
Knowledge of cause (of a thing and event etc)
Knowledge of form (e.g., after seeing Gavaya in the forest one remembers a cow having a similar form)
Knowledge of similarity (e.g., on seeing a son one remembers his father having similar form)
Knowledge of contrast (e.g having seen an ugly form one remembers a beautiful form)
Concentration of mind
Repletion
Attainment of metaphysical knowledge and
Subsequent partial communication of an event
A memory is nothing but the remembrance of things directly perceived, heard (from scriptures) or experienced earlier. [148-149]

Power of Memory for Salvation:

एतत्तदेकमयनं मुक्तैर्मोक्षस्य दर्शितम्|
तत्त्वस्मृतिबलं, येन गता न पुनरागताः||१५०||
अयनं पुनराख्यातमेतद्योगस्य योगिभिः|
सङ्ख्यातधर्मैः साङ्ख्यैश्च मुक्तैर्मोक्षस्य चायनम्||१५१||

The power of metaphysical memory constitutes the best way of liberation, as shown by the liberated ones. Persons following this way do not come back to worldly traps. This is again the best way to the attain Yoga (communion with God) as well as Moksha (salvation). This is what the Yogins, the virtuous ones, the followers of the Sankhya system, and the liberated ones say. [150-151]

Real knowledge:

सर्व कारणवद्दुःखमस्वं चानित्यमेव च|
न चात्मकृतकं तद्धि तत्र चोत्पद्यते स्वता||१५२||
यावन्नोत्पद्यते सत्या बुद्धिर्नैतदहं यया|
नैतन्ममेति विज्ञाय ज्ञः सर्वमतिवर्तते||१५३||

Anything that has a cause constitutes misery, it is alien and ephemeral. It is not produced by the soul (Atman); but one has got a feeling of its ownership until one has got a real knowledge to the effect that this is something different from him; and is not his own. As soon as one knows it, he gets rid of all (miseries). [152-153]

Attainment of final renunciation:

तस्मिंश्चरमसन्न्यासे समूलाः सर्ववेदनाः|
ससञ्ज्ञाज्ञानविज्ञाना निवृत्तिं यान्त्यशेषतः||१५४||

As soon as the final renunciation in respect of all subsequent actions is attained, the very consciousness together with its final causes in the form of indeterminate, determinate or scriptural knowledge is completely eradicated. [154]

The state thereafter:

अतः परं ब्रह्मभूतो भूतात्मा नोपलभ्यते|
निःसृतः सर्वभावेभ्यश्चिह्नं यस्य न विद्यते|
ज्ञानं ब्रह्मविदां चात्र नाज्ञस्तज्ज्ञातुमर्हति||१५५||

When all kinds of pains end, when all kinds of knowledge cease to exist, and when the individual soul merges with the greater soul, there will be no existence of emphereal / individual souls. Therefore, he will not be available in any form. He will be free from all the entities (8 prakriti and 16 vikriti) and he does not even leave any indication (inspiration, expiration etc) of his Existence. This is what that well versant in the knowledge of Brhman says. It is impossible for an ignorant person to know this. [155]

To sum up:

तत्र श्लोकः:-

प्रश्नाः पुरुषमाश्रित्य त्रयोविंशतिरुत्तमाः|
कतिधापुरुषीयेऽस्मिन्निर्णीतास्तत्त्वदर्शिना||१५६||

In this chapter on "the various division of the Empirical Soul etc., as conducive to the understanding of the body" 23 important questions regarding the Empirical Soul have been answered by the enlightened seer. [156]

इत्यग्निवेशकृते तन्त्रे चरकप्रतिसंस्कृते शारीरस्थाने कतिधापुरुषीयं शारीरं नाम प्रथमोऽध्यायः||१||

Thus ends the first chapter on "the Divisions of the Empirical Soul etc, as conducive to the understanding of the body" of the Sharira section of Agnivesha's work as redacted by Charaka. [1]

18

Shareerasthana Chapter 2 Atulya Gotreeya Shareeram

Embryological Development

अथातोऽतुल्यगोत्रीयं शारीरं व्याख्यास्यामः||१||

इति ह स्माह भगवानात्रेयः||२||

We shall now explore the chapter on the development of embryos caused by the union of males and females of mutually different clans. Thus said Lord Atreya. [1-2]

Query about semen:

अतुल्यगोत्रस्य रजःक्षयान्ते रहोविसृष्टं मिथुनीकृतस्य|

किं स्याच्चतुष्पात्प्रभवं च षड्भ्यो यत् स्त्रीषु गर्भत्वमुपैति पुंसः||३||

When a man belonging to a different clan cohabits in a lonely place with a woman after her menstruation, the man ejaculates something composed of four Mahabhutas (elements of nature), has six tastes, and which results in conception in a woman. What is it? [3]

Composition of semen:

शुक्रं तदस्य प्रवदन्ति धीरा यद्धीयते गर्भसमुद्भवाय|

वाय्वग्निभूम्यब्गुणपादवत्तत् षड्भ्यो रसेभ्यः प्रभवश्च तस्य||४||

This thing which is implanted for the formation of embryos is known as Sukra or semen / sperm. This is composed of wind, fire, water and earth elements in the state of their excellence. All these factors individually share one fourth of the attributes of each of the Mahabhutas. Semen is also formed from the food comprising all the 6 tastes in balanced proportions. [4]

Queries about embryo:

सम्पूर्णदेहः समये सुखं च गर्भः कथं केन च जायते स्त्री|

गर्भ चिरादिवन्दति सप्रजाऽपि भूत्वाऽथवा नश्यति केन गर्भः||५||

What are the factors responsible for the development of the body of the embryo in its entirety? How does the delivery of the child take place in the proper time? How does the delivery take place with ease? Why does conception delay even in a fertile woman? Why does the foetus get destroyed after its formation? [5]

Factors responsible for easy delivery of a healthy foetus etc:

शुक्रासृगात्माशयकालसम्पद् यस्योपचारश्च हितैस्तथाऽन्नैः |

गर्भश्च काले च सुखी सुखं च सञ्जायते सम्परिपूर्णदेहः||६||

योनिप्रदोषान्मनसोऽभितापाच्छुक्रासृगाहारविहारदोषात्|

अकालयोगाद्बलसङ्क्षयाच्च गर्भं चिरादिवन्दति सप्रजाऽपि||७||

असृङ्गिरुद्धं पवनेन नार्यां गर्भं व्यवस्यन्त्यबुधाः कदाचित्|
गर्भस्य रूपं हि करोति तस्यास्तदसृगस्रवि विवर्धमानम्||८||
तदग्निसूर्यश्रमशोकरोगैरूष्णान्नपानैरथवा प्रवृत्तम्|
दृष्ट्वाऽसृगेकं न च गर्भसञ्ज्ञं केचिन्नरा भूतहृतं वदन्ति||९||
ओजोशनानां रजनीचराणामाहारहेतोर्न शरीरमिष्टम्|
गर्भं हरेयुर्यदि ते न मातुर्लब्धावकाशा न हरेयुरोजः||१०||

The foetus gets delivered easily in time in its well developed form and without any pain, if

- the sperms are not contaminated and are enriched with good qualities,

- the ovum is healthy and of good quality,

- the soul adorned with the effects of good deeds done in the previous births rearing to get associated with the zygote

- the uterus is health and in excellent condition to accept conception of the child

- conception taking place in the fertile period and

- when the woman takes wholesome diet and lifestyle activities during the period of pregnancy which ensures proper nourishment of the fetus

Even in a fertile woman, there is delay in conception because of

- the defects in the uterus – diseases of vagina and uterus,

- mental afflictions, and

- defects in sperms or ovum,

- improper / inadequate diet and regimens,

- union / conception in inappropriate time (infertile period) and

- weakness of the body of the woman as caused by diseases, consumption of less / inadequate food or malnutrition

When the flow of menstrual blood in a woman gets obstructed by the vitiated vata, the blood gradually accumulates in the uterus and produces signs of pregnancy. The ignorant consider it as real pregnancy.

Due to exposure to fire and the sun, exhaustion, grief, affliction with disease and intake of hot diet and drinks, the blood which has accumulated in the uterus starts flowing again. Seeing this and since the foetal parts are not found some people declare that the foetus has been taken away by evil spirits who move at night time and feed on ojus i.e. essence of all the tissues of the body.

Because parts of the foetus are not found there, some people say that the foetus has been taken out by the evil spirits who move at night and live on ojas. Further, if the evil spirit can take away the foetus, having obtained entrance into the mother's body, it could have easily eaten Ojas in her body leading to her death also. Therefore it is illogical to tell that the fetus has been taken away by the evil spirits. [6-10]

Query about the sex and number of foetus:
कन्यां सुतं वा सहितौ पृथग्वा सुतौ सुते वा तनयान् बहून् वा|
कस्मात् प्रसूते सुचिरेण गर्भमेकोऽभिवृद्धिं च यमेऽभ्युपैति||११||

What is the reason for a woman to give birth to:

A female child

A male child

Twins of male and female children

Twins of female children

Twins of male children and

Many children at a time

Why is the delivery of a foetus delayed? Why does only one out of a twin grow well? [11]

Factors responsible for sex determination twins etc:
रक्तेन कन्यामधिकेन पुत्रं शुक्रेण तेन द्विविधीकृतेन|
बीजेन कन्यां च सुतं च सूते यथास्वबीजान्यतराधिकेन||१२||

शुक्राधिकं द्वैधमुपैति बीजं यस्याः सुतौ सा सहितौ प्रसूते|
रक्ताधिकं वा यदि भेदमेति द्विधा सुते सा सहिते प्रसूते||१३||
भिनति यावद्बहुधा प्रपन्नः शुक्रार्तवं वायुरतिप्रवृद्धः|
तावन्त्यपत्यानि यथाविभागं कर्मात्मकान्यस्ववशात् प्रसूते||१४||
आहारमाप्नोति यदा न गर्भः शोषं समाप्नोति परिस्रुतिं वा|
तं स्त्री प्रसूते सुचिरेण गर्भं पुष्टो यदा वर्षगणैरपि स्यात्||१५||
कर्मात्मकत्वादि्विषमांशभेदाच्छुक्रासृजोर्वृद्धिमुपैति कुक्षौ|
एकोऽधिको न्यूनतरो द्वितीय एवं यमेऽप्यभ्यधिको विशेषः||१६||

Dominance of ovum during the conception results in the procreation of a female child.

When there is predominance of sperm a male child is born.

During the process of union, when the vayu divides the zygote into 2 equal halves, the portion in which there is predominance of sperm will become male and the portion in which there is predominance of ovum will become female child. In this form of twins there is one male and one female child.

When both the divisions are predominant in sperm then twin male children are formed.

When both the divisions are predominant with ovum, then twin female children are formed.

When the excessively aggravated Vata brings about many divisions of the sperm and ovum i.e. zygote, many children are born; their number depends upon the number of divisions. This is not under the control of the individual himself; this happens due to one's action during previous life.

When the foetus does not get nutrition and when the foetus is emaciated or there is exudation (due to threatening abortion), then the woman delivers after a long time and it may even take several years for the proper development and delivery of the foetus.

Depending upon the action in the past life of an individual the sperm and ovum may undergo uneven division during conception leading to the formation of twins and this may result in the better growth of one foetus than the other in the uterus leading to their inequality. [12-16]

Query about sex abnormality:

कस्मादि्द्विरेताः पवनेन्द्रियो वा संस्कारवाही नरनारिषण्डौ|
वक्री तथेष्याभिरतिः कथं वा सञ्जायते वातिकषण्डको वा||१७||

What are the reasons for Dviretas (hermaphrodism), Pavanedriyatva (aspermia), samskaravahi (Anaphrodisa), male sterility, female sterility, Vakri (hypospadia), irsjabhirati (mixoscopia) and Vatikasandaka (eviration) of the procreation? [17]

Factors responsible for sex abnormality:

बीजात् समांशादुपतप्तबीजात् स्त्रीपुंसलिङ्गी भवति द्विरेताः|
शुक्राशयं गर्भगतस्य हत्वा करोति वायुः पवनेन्द्रियत्वम्||१८||
शुक्राशयद्वारविघट्टनेन संस्कारवाहं कुरुतेऽनिलश्च|
मन्दाल्पबीजावबलावहर्षौ क्लीबौ च हेतुर्विकृतिद्वयस्य||१९||
मातुर्व्यवायप्रतिघेन वक्री स्याद्बीजदौर्बल्यतया पितुश्च|
ईर्ष्याभिभूतावपि मन्दहर्षावीष्याँरतेरेव वदन्ति हेतुम्||२०||
वात्यग्निदोषाद्वृषणौ तु यस्य नाशं गतौ वातिकषण्डकः सः|
इत्येवमष्टौ विकृतिप्रकाराः कर्मात्मकानामुपलक्षणीयाः||२१||

When that portion of the sperm and ovum of parents which is responsible for the creation of the genitals of the foetus is vitiated and these sperm and ovum undergo equal division, then the offspring becomes a hermaphrodite. Such offspring will have the characteristic features of both the sexes.

If the testicles of the foetus are afflicted with Vata, then the offspring becomes aspermic.

When vitiated vata obstructs the seminal passages the offspring becomes samskaravaka i.e. anaphrodisiac.

When there is union of man and woman who are debilitated, having less arousal, low libido, and deficit sperms and ovum respectively will give rise to either male or female sterility respectively.

Weakness in sperms of the male partner and irregular posture or lack of interest in sex of the female partner during coitus makes the offspring hypospadiac.

Reduced passion (interest in sex) and increased jealousy amongst the partners (man and woman indulged in sex) produces mixoscopia in the offspring.

Being affected with Vayu and agni (pitta), if the testicles of the foetus get destroyed, then there is eviration in the offspring.

These are the eight types of sexual abnormalities. They are caused by the effects of the misdeeds in the previous life of the individual. [18-21]

Query about signs of conception etc:

गर्भस्य सद्योऽनुगतस्य कुक्षौ स्त्रीपुन्नपुंसामुदरस्थितानाम्|
किं लक्षणं? कारणमिष्यते किं सरूपतां येन च यात्यपत्यम्||२२||

What are the signs of conception which have just taken place? What are the signs to indicate if the foetus in the womb is a boy, girl or a eunuch? What are the reasons for a child to resemble some body? [22]

Signs of conception etc:

निष्ठीविका गौरवमङ्गसादस्तन्द्राप्रहर्षौ हृदये व्यथा च|
तृप्तिश्च बीजग्रहणं च योन्यां गर्भस्य सद्योऽनुगतस्य लिङ्गम्||२३||
सव्याङ्गचेष्टा पुरुषार्थिनी स्त्री स्त्रीस्वप्नपानाशनशीलचेष्टा|
सव्यात्गर्भा न च वृत्तगर्भा सव्यप्रदुग्धा स्त्रियमेव सूते||२४||
पुत्रं त्वतो लिङ्गविपर्ययेण व्यामिश्रलिङ्गा प्रकृतिं तृतीयाम्|
गर्भोपपत्तौ तु मनः स्त्रिया यं जन्तुं व्रजेत्तत्सदृशं प्रसूते||२५||
गर्भस्य चत्वारि चतुर्विधानि भूतानि मातापितृसम्भवानि|
आहारजान्यात्मकृतानि चैव सर्वस्य सर्वाणि भवन्ति देहे||२६||
तेषां विशेषाद्बलवन्ति यानि भवन्ति मातापितृकर्मजानि|
तानि व्यवस्येत् सदृशत्वहेतुं सत्त्वं यथानूकमपि व्यवस्येत्||२७||

Signs of conception which has just taken place are

- salivation / feel to spit often,
- heaviness in the body,
- prostration / tiredness in the body parts,
- drowsiness,
- horripilation / feeling goose-bumps,
- cardiac distress,
- satisfaction in sex / feeling as if the stomach is full in spite of not having taken the food
- non-elimination of the ejaculated semen from the uterus / conception (implantation of the zygote)

Signs of pregnancy indicating the presence of female child in the womb

It should be inferred that the child in the mother's womb is definitely a female if the pregnant woman –

- prefers to work using left part of her body i.e. left upper and lower limbs
- wants company of men with desire for sexual intimacy
- sees women / girls in her dreams
- wishes to have foods and liquids carrying feminine names
- has all her activities, attitude and speech resembling that of a woman
- whose left part of her abdomen looks raised because the conception has taken place in the left side of the womb
- whose shape of the uterus (foetus) is not round but is elongated
- in whom the breast milk first manifests in her left breast

The woman having these signs would definitely deliver a female child.

Signs of pregnancy indicating the presence of male child in the womb

It should be inferred that the child in the mother's womb is definitely a male if the pregnant woman has the signs opposite to those mentioned above (signs indicating the presence of female child in the womb). The woman having these signs would definitely deliver a male child.

Signs of pregnancy indicating the presence of eunuch child in the womb

It should be inferred that the child in the mother's womb is definitely a eunuch if the pregnant woman presents with combined signs of both the above said types (signs indicating the presence of female and male child in the womb). The woman having these signs would definitely deliver a eunuch child.

The child resembles those persons and things about which the mother thinks in her mind during conception.

There are also other reasons for this similarity –

The child resembles the parents because the foetus and all body parts of the foetus are formed by the four elements of nature i.e. air / wind, fire, water and earth elements. Each of these elements are of 4 types i.e. – those formed from the mother (ovum), those formed from the father (sperm), those formed from the diet of the mother i.e. pregnant woman and those formed or accompanying the soul (which enters the foetus). The shape of the foetus depends on which among these factors is predominant at the time of conception. The quality of mind of the foetus i.e. sattva, rajas and tamas are determined upon the characteristics which the mind has imbibed and carried from the memories of the previous birth and the species from which the mind carries these qualities. [23-27]

Query about abnormality on foetus etc:

कस्मात् प्रजां स्त्री विकृतां प्रसूते हीनाधिकाङ्गीं विकलेन्द्रियां वा|

देहात् कथं देहमुपैति चान्यमात्मा सदा कैरनुबध्यते च||२८||

Why does a woman give birth to an abnormal offspring with deficient or excess limbs or impaired sensory and motor organs? How does the soul transmigrate from one body to another? With whom is it always attached? [28]

Factors responsible for abnormality in foetus:

बीजात्मकर्माशयकालदोषैर्मातुस्तथाऽऽहारविहारदोषैः|

कुर्वन्ति दोषा विविधानि दुष्टाः संस्थानवर्णेन्द्रियवैकृतानि||२९||

वर्षासु काष्टाश्मघनाम्बुवेगास्तरोः सरित्स्रोतसि संस्थितस्य|

यथैव कुर्युर्विकृतिं तथैव गर्भस्य कुक्षौ नियतस्य दोषाः||३०||

Because of the defects in seeds (sperms, ovum), actions associated with the soul, uterus, time and food as well as regimen of the mother, Doshas get vitiated in different kinds and this results in the impairment of the shape, colour and sensory as well as motor organs of the offspring. As a tree standing in the current of a river gets afflicted by the forceful downward movement of wood, stone pieces and water during the rainy season, the foetus in the uterus of the mother also gets afflicted with the vitiated Doshas. [29-30]

Atman-its transmigration:

भूतैश्चतुर्भिः सहितः सुसूक्ष्मैर्मनोजवो देहमुपैति देहात्|

कर्मात्मकत्वान्न तु तस्य दृश्यं दिव्यं विना दर्शनमस्ति रूपम्||३१||

स सर्वगः सर्वशरीरभृच्च स विश्वकर्मा स च विश्वरूपः|

स चेतनाधातुरतीन्द्रियश्च स नित्ययुक् सानुशयः स एव ||३२||

रसात्ममातापितृसम्भवानि भूतानि विद्याद्दश षट् च देहे|

चत्वारि तत्रात्मनि संश्रितानि स्थितस्तथाऽऽत्मा च चतुर्षु तेषु||३३||

भूतानि मातापितृसम्भवानि रजश्च शुक्रं च वदन्ति गर्भे|

आप्याय्यते शुक्रमसृक् च भूतैर्यैस्तानि भूतानि रसोद्भवानि||३४||

भूतानि चत्वारि तु कर्मजानि यान्यात्मलीनानि विशन्ति गर्भम्|

स बीजधर्मा ह्यपरापराणि देहान्तराण्यात्मनि याति याति॥३५॥
रूपादिध रूपप्रभवः प्रसिद्धः कर्मात्मकानां मनसो मनस्तः।
भवन्ति ये त्वाकृतिबुद्धिभेदारजस्तमस्तत्र च कर्म हेतुः॥३६॥

Being guided by the associated past actions (of previous birth) the soul who travels with the help of the mind, transmigrates from one body to another along with the four subtle Bhutas – elements of nature.

This Soul cannot be perceived by any other sense except the divine vision. He is omnipresent; he can enter into any physique; he can perform any action and can take any shape; he is the conscious element; he is beyond any sensory perception; and it is due to his association with the intellect etc. that he gets involved in attachment etc.

In the body of living beings, there are sixteen types of Bhutas. They are derived from Rasa (digestive product of mother's food), Soul (those accompanying Him), mother and father. Four of these Bhutas accompany the Soul and the Soul himself depends upon four of them for his existence. Bhutas from the mother and father are derived through their ovum and sperm. It is the Rasa (digestive product of food) which provides nourishment in the form of Bhutas to the sperm and ovum.

The four Bhutas which get fused (constantly associated) with the Soul to enter into the foetus are the products of the past actions. Continuity of the migration of Bhutas is maintained as the Soul who is like a seed (and who is responsible for several incarnations) transmigrates from one body to another.

It is a fact that in individuals having the association of past action, the physique and the mind are respectively derived from the physique and mind of his past life. The dissimilarity in the shape and intellectual faculties is caused by the Rajas, Tamas and the nature of the past actions. [31-36]

Factors responsible for keeping the Soul attached:

अतीन्द्रियैस्तैरतिसूक्ष्मरूपैरात्मा कदाचिन्न वियुक्तरूपः।
न कर्मणा नैव मनोमतिभ्यां न चाप्यहङ्कारविकारदोषैः॥३७॥
रजस्तमोभ्यां हि मनोऽनुबद्धं ज्ञानं विना तत्र हि सर्वदोषाः।
गतिप्रवृत्त्योस्तु निमित्तमुक्तं मनः सदोषं बलवच्च कर्म॥३८॥

The Soul can never dissociate himself from the transitory and excessively subtle Bhutas or from the effects of the past actions or from the mind and the intellect or from ego and other morbid factors.

The mind is constantly associated with Rajas and Tamas. This will keep one associated with the actions. All the doshas and morbidity would envelope and influence the mind until one attains spiritual knowledge. The mind associated with rajas and tamas qualities (morbid mind) and strong action (with strongly determined results) are responsible for transmigration of the Soul from one body to another and for the individual's inclination to do virtuous or vicious work. [37-38]

Query about diseases:

रोगाः कुतः संशमनं किमेषां हर्षस्य शोकस्य च किं निमित्तम्।
शरीरसत्त्वप्रभवा विकाराः कथं न शान्ताः पुनरापतेयुः॥३९॥

What are the causative factors of diseases? What are their curatives? What is the cause of happiness? What is the cause of sorrow? How can the recurrence of psychosomatic diseases be prevented after their manifestation? [39]

Factors for causation and alleviation of diseases:

प्रज्ञापराधो विषमास्तथाऽर्था हेतुस्तृतीयः परिणामकालः।
सर्वामयानां त्रिविधा च शान्तिर्ज्ञानार्थकालाः समयोगयुक्ताः॥४०॥

Causative factors of diseases are:
- Intellectual blasphemy
- Unwholesome contact with senses and
- Seasonal variations
All diseases can be cured in three ways, viz,

- Proper usage of knowledge
- wholesome contact of sense organs with sense objects / proper usage of senses and
- seasonal normality / proper usage of seasons [40]

Causes of happiness and misery and their cessation:

धर्म्याः क्रिया हर्षनिमित्तमुक्तास्ततोऽन्यथा शोकवशं नयन्ति।

शरीरसत्त्वप्रभवास्तु रोगास्तयोरवृत्त्या न भवन्ति भूयः॥४१॥

Righteous acts are responsible for happiness and unrighteous acts for misery. The body and the mind are the seats of diseases. When the association of mind and body permanently gets dissociated with the soul, the diseases of the body and mind will get cured and also cease to recur. [41]

Cessation of continuity of body and mind:

रूपस्य सत्त्वस्य च सन्ततिर्या नोक्तस्तदादिर्नहि सोऽस्ति कश्चित्।

तयोरवृत्तिः क्रियते पराभ्यां धृतिस्मृतिभ्यां परया धिया च॥४२॥

According to scriptures, there is no beginning of the mind and the body. The continuity of the mind and the body is broken only when the individual is in possession of the excellent courage and spiritual knowledge of power of meditation, memory and sattvik intellect. [42]

Factors responsible for non-affliction by diseases:

सत्याश्रये वा द्विविधे यथोक्ते पूर्वं गदेभ्यः प्रतिकर्म नित्यम्।

जितेन्द्रियं नानुपतन्ति रोगास्तत्कालयुक्तं यदि नास्ति दैवम्॥४३॥

One does not get afflicted with diseases even during the existence of the body and the mind which are the seats of diseases, if before the manifestation of diseases, he takes recourse to preventive therapeutic measures and abstains from intellectual blasphemy and unwholesome contact with senses, provided the manifestation of the diseases at that time is not predetermined by the fruits of his previously done actions i.e., karma / daivam. [43]

Daiva and Purusakara:

दैवं पुरा यत् कृतमुच्यते तत् तत् पौरुषं यत्त्विह कर्म दृष्टम्।

प्रवृत्तिहेतुर्विषमः स दृष्टो निवृत्तिहेतुर्हि समः स एव॥४४॥

The effect of what is done during the previous life is known as Daiva. The effect of what is done during the present life is known as Purushakara. The non-righteous deeds of the previous life expose one to diseases; if however, they are righteous, then the individual remains free from diseases. [44]

Methods for prevention of seasonal diseases:

हैमन्तिकं दोषचयं वसन्ते प्रवाहयन् ग्रैष्मिकमभ्रकाले।

घनात्यये वार्षिकमाशु सम्यक् प्राप्नोति रोगानृतुजान्न जातु ॥४५॥

Doshas accumulated during Hemanta (December- February) should be eliminated in the month of Chaitra (March- April). Those accumulated during summer (April- June) should be eliminated in the month of Shravana (July- August) and those accumulated during the rainy season (August- October) are eliminated in the month of Margashira (November- December). [45]

Factors responsible for keeping a person free from diseases:

नरो हिताहारविहारसेवी समीक्ष्यकारी विषयेष्वसक्तः।

दाता समः सत्यपरः क्षमावानाप्तोपसेवी च भवत्यरोगः॥४६॥

मतिर्वचः कर्म सुखानुबन्धं सत्त्वं विधेयं विशदा च बुद्धिः।

ज्ञानं तपस्तत्परता च योगे यस्यास्ति तं नानुपतन्ति रोगाः॥४७॥

One who resorts to wholesome diet and regimens, who enters into action after proper observation, who is unattached to the pleasure drawn from the satisfaction of sensory objects, who is given to charity, impartiality, truthfulness and forgiveness and who is at service of learned people, seldom gets afflicted with diseases.

Diseases do not afflict an individual who is endowed with excellence of thoughts, speech and acts which are ultimately blissful, independent thinking, clear understanding, knowledge, observance of spiritual prescriptions and love for meditation. [46-47]

तत्र श्लोकः|
इहाग्निवेशस्य महार्थयुक्तं षट्त्रिंशकं प्रश्नगणं महर्षिः|
अतुल्यगोत्रे भगवान् यथावन्निर्णीतवान् ज्ञानविवर्धनार्थम्||४८||

To sum up: -

With regard to enlightenment Lord Atreya has properly replied to thirty six important queries of Agnivesha in this chapter on "the development of embryo caused by the union of males and females of mutually different clans. " [48]

इत्यग्निवेशकृते तन्त्रे चरकप्रतिसंस्कृते शारीरस्थानेऽतुल्यगोत्रीयं शारीरं नाम द्विवतीयोऽध्यायः||२||

Thus ends the second chapter on the development of embryo caused by the union of males and females and females of mutually different clan, of the Sharira section of Agnivesha's work as redacted by Charaka. [2]

19

Shareerasthana Chapter 3
Khuddika Garbhavakranti Shareeram

Formation of embryo

अथातः खुड्डिकां गर्भावक्रान्तिं शारीरं व्याख्यास्यामः||१||

इति ह स्माह भगवानात्रेयः||२||

Now we shall explore the minor chapter on "the formation of embryos as conducive to the understanding of the body". Thus said Lord Atreya [1-2]

Factors responsible for procreation:

पुरुषस्यानुपहतरेतसः स्त्रियाश्चाप्रदुष्टयोनिशोणितगर्भाशयाया यदा भवति संसर्गः ऋतुकाले, यदा चानयोस्तथायुक्ते संसर्गे शुक्रशोणितसंसर्गमन्तर्गर्भाशयगतं जीवोऽवक्रामति सत्त्वसम्प्रयोगात्तदा गर्भोऽभिनिर्वर्तते, स सात्म्यरसोपयोगादरोगोऽभिवर्धते सम्यगुपचारैश्चोपचर्यमाणः, ततः प्राप्तकालः सर्वेन्द्रियोपपन्नः परिपूर्णशरीरो बलवर्णसत्त्वसंहननसम्पदुपेतः सुखेन जायते समुदयादेषां भावानां- मातृजश्चायं गर्भः पितृजश्चात्मजश्च सात्म्यजश्च रसजश्च, अस्ति च खलु सत्त्वमौपपादुकमिति होवाच भगवानात्रेयः||३||

When a man with unimpaired sperm and a woman with unaffiliated genital tract, ovum and uterine bed cohabit during the period of fertilization, the Jiva (Soul) along with the mind descends into the zygote (combined form of the sperm and ovum) lodged inside the uterus. This results in the formation of the embryo.

Following this, the embryo grows without hindrance and in a healthy way, being nourished by the wholesome Rasa i.e. the nutrition coming from the mother and as a result of the pregnant woman following all the prescribed regimens during pregnancy.

Thereafter the foetus formed with all the sensory and motor organs, and properly developed body with all limbs and body parts intact and fully formed, and endowed with the excellence of strength, complexion, mental faculties and compactness gets delivered in proper time i.e. 9th or 10th month of gestation. This occurs due to the combination of the factors derived from the following sources –

- Mother
- Father
- Soul
- Wholesomeness
- Rasa (digestive product of the mother's food)
- Mind

The embryo also associates the mind and soul with a new body (transmigration of soul). Thus said Lord Atreya [3]

Bharadvaja's objection:

नेति भरद्वाजः, किं कारणं- न हि माता न पिता नात्मा न सात्म्यं न पानाशनभक्ष्यलेह्योपयोगा गर्भं जनयन्ति, न च परलोकादेत्य गर्भे
सत्त्वमवक्रामति (१)|४|

'No', said Bharadvaja, because neither mother nor father, nor wholesomeness, nor the utilization of drinkables, eatables, chewables or lickables can produce a foetus. It is also not correct to say that the mind transmigrates from another world to take part in the formation of the foetus. [4-I]

यदि हि मातापितरौ गर्भं जनयेतां, भूयस्यः स्त्रियः पुमांसश्च भूयांसः पुत्रकामाः, ते सर्वे पुत्रजन्माभिसन्धाय मैथुनधर्ममापद्यमानाः पुत्रानेव
जनयेयुर्दुहितृर्वा दुहितृकामाः, न तु काश्चित् स्त्रियः केचिद्वा पुरुषा निरपत्याः स्युरपत्यकामा [१] वा परिदेवेरन् (२)|४|

If parents are responsible for the formation of the foetus many men and women who are keenly desirous of sons can produce them by resorting to cohabitation. Similarly those who desire daughters can get them. None of the men or women would be devoid of children and none would grieve for not having a child. [4-II]

न चात्माऽऽत्मानं जनयति|

यदि ह्यात्माऽऽत्मानं जनयेज्जातो वा जनयेदात्मानमजातो वा, तच्चोभयथाऽप्ययुक्तम्|

न हि जातो जनयति सत्त्वात्, न चाजातो जनयत्यसत्त्वात्, तस्मादुभयथाऽप्यनुपपत्तिः|

तिष्ठतु तावदेतत्|

यद्ययमात्माऽऽत्मानं शक्तो जनयितुं स्यात्, न त्वेनमिष्टास्वेव कथं योनिषु जनयेद्वशिनमप्रतिहतगतिं कामरूपिणं
तेजोबलवर्णसत्त्वसंहननसमुदितमजरमरुजममरम्; एवंविधं ह्यात्माऽऽत्मानमिच्छत्यतो वा भूयः (३)|४|

Atman (soul) is not produced by another Atman. If this is to be accepted, we would get a doubt 'does the soul manifest by itself and then produce itself or does it produce itself without getting manifested?' Both these propositions are untenable.

The soul which is born already exists. Therefore he cannot create himself.

The soul which is unborn also cannot create another soul. This is because an unborn soul is non-existent and in such condition cannot create another soul.

Therefore the proposition that the soul creates an embryo is untenable both ways. Let us consider the problem from another angle.

If the Soul is capable of reproducing Himself, then how is it that He does not choose a desirable womb endowed with lordship, unrestrained movement, capacity to have forms as he pleases, wherein he would be endowed with strength, speed, beautiful colour and complexion, mental faculties, compactness and having freedom from aging, disease and death? The Soul wants Himself to be like this or even better. [4-III]

असात्म्यजश्चायं गर्भः|

यदि हि सात्म्यजःस्यात्, तर्हि सात्म्यसेविनामेवैकान्तेन प्रजा स्यात्, असात्म्यसेविनश्च निखिलेनानपत्याः स्युः, तच्चोभयमुभयत्रैव दृश्यते
(४)|४|

Wholesomeness is not responsible for the formation of the foetus. Had it been so, only those who resort to wholesomeness should get children and the remaining ones who resort to unwholesomeness should never get a child but both the types of people are found to be equally successful or unsuccessful in getting children. [4-IV]

अरसजश्चायं गर्भः|

यदि हि रसजः स्यात्, न केचित् स्त्रीपुरुषेष्वनपत्याः स्युः, न हि कश्चिदस्त्येषां यो रसान्नोपयुङ्क्ते; श्रेष्ठरसोपयोगिनां चेद्गर्भा जायन्त
इत्यभिप्रेतमिति, एवं सत्याजौरभ्रमार्गमायूरगोक्षीरदधिघृतमधुतैलसैन्धवेक्षुरसमुद्गशालिभृतानामेवैकान्तेन प्रजा स्यात्,
श्यामाकवरकोद्दालककोरदूषककन्दमूलभक्षाश्च निखिलेनानपत्याः स्युः, तच्चोभयमुभयत्र दृश्यते (५)|४|

The foetus is not formed of Rasa (digestive product of food). If it is true then no man or woman would remain childless. None of them live without Rasa (digestive product of food). If the intention here is that individuals having the excellence of Rasa should have children, then only those who take meat soup of goat, sheep, deer, and peacock, milk, curd and ghee of the cow, honey, oil, rock salt, sugarcane juice, Mudga (Phaseolus Mungo Linn) and Sali rice for nourishment should get children and the others who take Syamaka, Varaka, Uddaklaka, Korasusa (type of corn, rhizomes and roots) should always be deprived of a progeny. But both the types of people are equally successful or unsuccessful in getting children [4-V]

न खल्वपि परलोकादेत्य सत्त्वं गर्भमवक्रामति; यदि ह्येनमवक्रामेत्, नास्य किञ्चित् पौर्वदेहिकं स्यादविदितमश्रुतमदृष्टं वा, स च तच्च न किञ्चिदपि स्मरति (६)||४||

तस्मादेतद्ब्रूमहे- अमातृजश्चायं गर्भोऽपितृजश्चानात्मजश्चासात्म्यजश्चारसजश्च, न चास्ति सत्त्वमौपपादुकमिति (होवाच भरद्वाजः)||४||

The mind does not come from the world (from the previous birth) beyond to enter into the foetus. If it does so, nothing of its past life should remain unknown, unheard and unseen by him. But actually it does not remember any such things. The mind actually on getting associated with the sense organs would reflect the knowledge of various objects. The mind if coming from the other world / previous birth should remember and have known the memories of things and subjects from the past and that is not the truth.

Therefore, I say, the foetus is not formed out of the mother, father, Soul, wholesomeness or Rasa (digestive product of food). It is also not correct to say that the mind transmigrates from another world to take birth in the formation of the foetus. Thus said Bharadvaja [4]

Atreya's decision:

नेति भगवानात्रेयः, सर्वेभ्य एभ्यो भावेभ्यः समुदितेभ्यो गर्भोऽभिनिर्वर्तते||५||

Lord Atreya said, "no the foetus is formed out of the combination of all these factors". [5]

Factors derived from mother:

मातृजश्चायं गर्भः|

न हि मातुर्विना गर्भोत्पत्तिः स्यात्, न च जन्म जरायुजानाम्|

यानि खल्वस्य गर्भस्य मातृजानि, यानि चास्य मातृतः सम्भवतः सम्भवन्ति, तान्यनुव्याख्यास्यामः; तद्यथा- त्वक्च लोहितं च मांसं च मेदश्च नाभिश्च हृदयं च क्लोम च यकृच्च प्लीहा च वृक्कौ च बस्तिश्च पुरीषाधानं चामाशयश्च पक्वाशयश्चोतरगुदं चाधरगुदं च क्षुद्रान्त्रं च स्थूलान्त्रं च वापा च वपावहनं चेति (मातृजानि)||६||

The foetus is produced out of the mother. Without, mother there is no possibility of conception and birth of viviparous creatures. We shall hereafter describe those organs which are derived from the maternal source (from ovum) and which are found because of the existence of the mother.

They are skin, blood, flesh, fat, umbilicus, heart, Kloman (right lung), liver, spleen, kidneys, bladder, rectum, stomach, Pakvashaya (colon), upper and lower parts of the anus, small intestine, large intestine, mesentery and omentum, (these are the organs derived from maternal source). [6]

Factors derived from father:

पितृजश्चायं गर्भः|

नहि पितुरृते गर्भोत्पत्तिः स्यात्, न च जन्म जरायुजानाम्|

यानि खल्वस्य गर्भस्य पितृजानि, यानि चास्य पितृतः सम्भवतः सम्भवन्ति, तान्यनुव्याख्यास्यामः; तद्यथा- केशश्मश्रुनखलोमदन्तास्थिसिरास्नायुधमन्यः शुक्रं चेति (पितृजानि)||७||

The foetus is produced from the father (from sperm). Without father there is no possibility of conception and birth of viviparous creatures. We shall hereafter describe those organs which are derived from paternal source, (from sperm) and which are formed because of the existence of the father.

They are hair of the head, hair of the face, nail, and small hairs of the body, teeth, bones, veins, ligaments, arteries and semen. (These are the organs derived from paternal source) [7]

Atman as a Source:

आत्मजश्चायं गर्भः|

गर्भात्मा ह्यन्तरात्मा यः, तं 'जीव' इत्याचक्षते शाश्वतमरुजमजरममरमक्षयमभेद्यमच्छेद्यमलोऽयं विश्वरूपं विश्वकर्माणमव्यक्तमनादिमनिधनमक्षरमपि|

स गर्भाशयमनुप्रविश्य शुक्रशोणिताभ्यां संयोगमेत्य गर्भत्वेन जनयत्यात्मनाऽऽत्मानम्, आत्मसञ्ज्ञा हि गर्भे|

तस्य पुनरात्मनो जन्मानादित्वान्नोपपद्यते, तस्मान्न जात एवायमजातं गर्भं जनयति, अजातो ह्ययमजातं गर्भं जनयति; स चैव गर्भः कालान्तरेण बालयुवस्थविरभावान् प्राप्नोति, स यस्यां यस्यामवस्थायां वर्तते तस्यां तस्यां जातो भवति, या त्वस्य पुरस्कृतातस्यां जनिष्यमाणश्च, तस्मात् स एव जातश्चाजातश्च युगपद्भवति; यस्मिंश्चैतदुभयं सम्भवति जातत्वं जनिष्यमाणत्वं च स जातो जन्यते, स चैवानागतेष्ववस्थान्तरेष्वजातो जन्ययत्यात्मनाऽऽत्मानम्|

सतो ह्यवस्थान्तरगमनमात्रमेव हि जन्म चोच्यते तत्र तत्र वयसि तस्यां तस्यामवस्थायां; यथा- सतामेव शुक्रशोणितजीवानां प्राक् संयोगाद्गर्भत्वं न भवति, तच्च संयोगाद्भवति; यथा- सतस्तस्यैव पुरुषस्य प्रागपत्यात् पितृत्वं न भवति, तच्चापत्याद्भवति; तथा सतस्तस्यैव गर्भस्य तस्यां तस्यामवस्थायां जातत्वमजातत्वं चोच्यते||८||

The foetus is produced out of the Soul. The Antaratman (Soul inside the animal body) is the same as garbhatman (Soul in the foetus). This is known as Jiva or animated Soul.

According to religious scriptures,

- This Soul is eternal.
- He does not get afflicted by diseases.
- He does not undergo the process of aging.
- He does not succumb to death.

He does not undergo diminution.

- He cannot be penetrated.
- He cannot be cut. He cannot get irrupted.
- He is omnipresent and omnipotent.
- He is invisible.
- He is without the beginning and end, and
- He is unchangeable.

On entering the uterus and getting associated with the sperm and ovum (zygote) the life element will take the form of 'foetus made up of six elements'. In the foetus the life element will take the designation and name of 'atma' – the soul. Since the soul doesn't have a beginning (origin) the soul doesn't take its birth. In spite of the soul not being manifested (not having taken birth) it will create (pour life into) the foetus composed of six elements. The same foetus during the course of time attains the state of childhood, youth and old age. According to the stage in which he is, he will be considered to have taken origin (birth) at that particular stage and coming to the stage which has not been manifested it will be said that he will be manifested in the upcoming stage in future. This means to tell that he is considered to be unborn or in the process of taking birth. Therefore, he is both born and unborn simultaneously.

In such situations where the Soul is considered to be both born or being born he produces that state of life after having taken birth himself. In other situations, where that state of the body (Soul), is yet to come, the soul is considered to produce him without being born.

In those particular ages (stages of growth) i.e. types of growth as well as in these particular states (situations) of growth as well as in these particular states (situations) of living beings, the change of the state of the associated body, is considered to be the birth of Atman. The sperm, ovum and life element (atma) are available but until they get associated with each other in the uterus they will not get the name 'garbha – i.e., foetus'. When these three components get associated, they will get the name as 'foetus'. Similarly the state of 'mere existence from the beginning' doesn't qualify a person to be called as a father unless he has a child. It is only after the birth of his child that a man will be called as 'father' of that child. Similarly, the existent foetus (Soul) can be considered to be born or unborn depending upon the state attained or 'yet to be attained' by him. [8]

Guiding factors:

न खलु गर्भस्य न च मातुर्न पितुर्न चात्मनः सर्वभावेषु यथेष्टकारित्वमस्ति; ते किञ्चित् स्ववशात् कुर्वन्ति, किञ्चित् कर्मवशात्, क्वचिच्चैषां करणशक्तिर्भवति, क्वचिन्न भवति।

यत्र सत्त्वादिकरणसम्पत्तत्र यथाबलमेव यथेष्टकारित्वम्, अतोऽन्यथा विपर्ययः।

न च करणदोषादकरणमात्मासम्भवति गर्भजनने, दृष्टं चेष्टा योनिरैश्वर्य मोक्षश्चात्मविद्भिरात्मायत्तम्।

नह्यन्यः सुखदुःखयोः कर्ता।

न चान्यतो गर्भो जायते जायमानः, नाङ्कुरोत्पत्तिरबीजात्।।९।।

Mother, father and Soul independently cannot satisfy the entire requirement for the formation of a foetus. They themselves do certain things independently and some other things they do because of the force of the actions of the previous life.

They possess the ability to do certain things themselves. For some other things, they do not have that ability. They would do some actions with the help of the essential tools in the form of mind, senses and intellect. When these tools do not possess excellent qualities and are weak they will not be capable of doing the actions as per their choice and liberty.

It is only when these factors (mother, father, soul) are added with the excellence of other factors like mind, sense organs, sperm, ovum etc., depending upon the actions in the previous life, they will be able to render the actions as per their strength and as they want them to be done and also have the capacity to manifest things by themselves.

On the contrary if the mind etc entities are not adorned by good qualities i.e. if they are defective the person becomes enveloped and influenced by rajas and tamas qualities. He will start doing undesired and abnormal (nonerighteous) actions. Because of defects in these factors, the soul (devoid of such instruments in their normal state) cannot help in the formation of a foetus. He will also not be capable of taking birth in desired species.

It is not wise to think that the soul which fails to create a foetus when mind, intellect etc are defective is not the creator of the foetus. It is well known that spiritual individuals, who have realized a Soul of their own, can enter into the desired womb, attain great things and attain salvation. These people have also considered that atma or soul himself is responsible for salvation i.e. freedom from the vicious cycle of life and death.

There is none else who is responsible for the happiness and sorrow of the individual other than the soul (only the soul is responsible for one's happiness and sorrow). The foetus is not formed by anything else being born. Germination is not possible from anything else other than the seeds. Therefore the life element in the foetus will not come from any inert things; the life process is imparted by the life element atma i.e. soul itself. [9]

Factors derived from Atman:

यानि तु खल्वस्य गर्भस्यात्मजानि, यानि चास्यात्मतः सम्भवतः सम्भवन्ति, तान्यनुव्याख्यास्यामः तद्यथा- तासु तासु योनिष्तूत्पत्तिरायुरात्मज्ञानं मन इन्द्रियाणि प्राणापानौ प्रेरणं धारणमाकृतिस्वरवर्णविशेषाः सुखदुःखे इच्छाद्वेषौ चेतना धृतिर्बुद्धिः स्मृतिरहङ्कारः प्रयत्नश्चेति (आत्मजानि)।।१०।।

We shall hereafter describe those aspects of the individual which are derived from the Soul and which are formed because of the existence of Soul. They are – taking birth in such and such wombs (human, animal, bird etc), life span (having less, moderate or more lifespan), self-realisation, mind, senses, to take things into and to excrete things out of the body (breathe in and breathe out), stimulation / motivation (to the senses), to behold (the information), characteristic shape, voice and colour / complexion of the individual, desire for happiness and sorrow, liking and disliking, consciousness, courage, intellect, memory, egoism and efforts. All these aspects of the individual are derived from the Soul. [10]

Factors derived from Satmya:

सात्म्यजश्चायं गर्भः।

नह्यसात्म्यसेवित्वमन्तरेण स्त्रीपुरुषयोर्वन्ध्यत्वमस्ति, गर्भेषु वाऽप्यनिष्टो भावः।

यावत् खल्वसात्म्यसेविनां स्त्रीपुरुषाणां त्रयो दोषाः प्रकुपिताः शरीरमुपसर्पन्तो न शुक्रशोणितगर्भाशयोपघातायोपपद्यन्ते, तावत् समर्था

गर्भजननाय भवन्ति।

सात्म्यसेविनां पुनः स्त्रीपुरुषाणामनुपहतशुक्रशोणितगर्भाशयानामृतकाले सन्निपतितानां जीवस्यानवक्रमणाद्गर्भा न प्रादुर्भवन्ति।

नहि केवलं सात्म्यज एवायं गर्भः, समुदयोऽत्र कारणमुच्यते।

यानि खल्वस्य गर्भस्य सात्म्यजानि, यानि चास्य सात्म्यतः सम्भवतः सम्भवन्ति, तान्यनुव्याख्यास्यामः; तद्यथा-आरोग्यमनालस्यमलोलुपत्वमिन्द्रियप्रसादः स्वरवर्णबीजसम्पत् प्रहर्षभूयस्त्वं चेति (सात्म्यजानि)।।११।।

The foetus is produced from out of the wholesomeness. Without consumption of unwholesome foods and things man or woman would not become sterile / impotent. There would also not occur deformities or morbidity / defects in the foetus. When the men and women would consume unwholesome foods and things they would vitiate the doshas. If these vitiated doshas put into circulation reach the sperms, ovum and uterus and contaminate them they would not be capable of procreating offspring. Men and women would be capable of procreating offspring as long as the sperms, ovum and uterus are not afflicted by the vitiated circulating doshas (vitiated by the consumption of unwholesome things). This is because in people who consume wholesome foods sperms, ovum and uterus would be healthy.

Even during the fertile period, during the union (sexual) of the men and women who are given with wholesome things and whose sperms, ovum and uterus are unimpaired, do not produce the offspring if the soul responsible for the formation of the foetus doesn't enter into the uterus. This is because the foetus is not formed just by consumption of wholesome foods but by the combination of factors.

Here we explain the aspects of the individual are derived from wholesomeness and are manifested because of the existence of such wholesomeness. They are the state of freedom from diseases, laziness and greed, clarity of senses, excellence of voice, colour and semen and calmness of mind. These aspects of the individual are derived from wholesomeness. [11]

Factors derived from Satmya:

रसजश्चायं गर्भः।

न हि रसादृते मातुः प्राणयात्राऽपि स्यात्, किं पुनर्गर्भजन्म।

न चैवासम्यगुपयुज्यमाना रसा गर्भमभिनिर्वर्तयन्ति, न च केवलं सम्यगुपयोगादेव रसानां गर्भाभिनिर्वृत्तिर्भवति, समुदायोऽप्यत्र कारणमुच्यते।

यानि तु खल्वस्य गर्भस्य रसजानि, यानि चास्य रसतः सम्भवतः सम्भवन्ति, तान्यनुव्याख्यास्यामः; तद्यथा-शरीरस्याभिनिर्वृत्तिरभिवृद्धिः प्राणानुबन्धस्तृप्तिः पुष्टिरुत्साहश्चेति (रसजानि)।।१२।।

The foetus is produced from Rasa (digestive product of the mother's food). Without Rasa even the mother will not live, what to speak of the formation of the foetus in her womb (the foetus also will not live). When the nutrition / nourishment are not proper it doesn't help in the formation / development of the foetus.

Conversely, a foetus is not formed simply by the employment of proper nourishment. Here also the combination of the factors is responsible for the production of the foetus.

We shall hereafter describe those aspects of the individual which are produced due to proper nutrition. They are - manifestation and growth (in height of the body), continuity of the strength, satisfaction, plumpness and enthusiasm. These aspects of the individual are derived from Rasa [12]

Factors derived from Sattva:

अस्ति खलु सत्त्वमौपपादुकं; यज्जीवं स्पृक्शरीरेणाभिसम्बध्नाति, यस्मिन्नपगमनपुरस्कृते शीलमस्य व्यावर्तते, भक्तिर्विपर्यस्यते, सर्वेन्द्रियाण्युपतप्यन्ते, बलं हीयते, व्याधय आप्याय्यन्ते, यस्माद्धीनः प्राणाञ्जहाति, यदिन्द्रियाणामभिग्राहकं च 'मन' इत्यभिधीयते; तत्त्रिविधमाख्यायते- शुद्धं, राजसं, तामसमिति।

येनास्य खलु मनो भूयिष्ठं, तेन द्विवतीयायामाजातौ सम्प्रयोगो भवति; यदा तु तेनैव शुद्धेन संयुज्यते, तदा जातेरतिक्रान्ताया अपि स्मरति।

स्मार्तं हि ज्ञानमात्मनस्तस्यैव मनसोऽनुबन्धादनुवर्तते, यस्यानुवृत्तिं पुरस्कृत्य पुरुषो 'जातिस्मर' इत्युच्यते।

यानि खल्वस्य गर्भस्य सत्त्वजानि, यान्यस्य सत्त्वतः सम्भवतः सम्भवन्ति, तान्यनुव्याख्यास्यामः; तद्यथा- भक्तिः शीलं शौचं द्वेषः स्मृतिर्मोहस्त्यागो मात्सर्यं शौर्यं भयं क्रोधस्तन्द्रोत्साहस्तैक्ष्ण्यं मार्दवं गाम्भीर्यमनवस्थितत्वमित्येवमादयश्चान्ये, ते सत्त्वविकारा यानुत्तरकालं सत्त्वभेदमधिकृत्योपदेक्ष्यामः।

नानाविधानि खलु सत्वानि, तानि सर्वाण्येकपुरुषे भवन्ति, न च भवन्त्येककालम्, एकं तु प्रायोवृत्त्याऽऽह ||१३||

Mind is also the connecting link which connects the Soul with the physical body. The mind would enter another (new) body along with the soul and establishes a relationship with that body. This means to tell that the mind establishes its relationship with the gross body with the help of the subtle body of the soul. So, on the eve of death when the mind starts leaving the body, there occurs a change in the normal behaviour and inclinations, the sense organs are disturbed, strength diminishes and living beings are attacked with diseases.

Living beings devoid of mind breathe their last because the sense organs derive their inspiration from nothing but mind.

The mind which indulges the sense organs in their respective sense objects and also controls them is of three kinds. They are Sattvika, Rajasa and Tamasa. The mind dominated by any of the above mentioned attributes in one life follows in the subsequent life as well. When the individual is endowed with the Sattvika type of mind from previous life he can remember things of the past incarnation. Because of this power to recall things of the past, incantation, the individual is called "Jatismara".

We shall hereafter describe those aspects of individuals which are derived from mind and which are manifested because of the existence of mind. They are liking, conduct, purity, enmity, memory, attachment, detachment, jealousy, valour, fear, anger, drowsiness, enthusiasm, sharpness, softness, seriousness, instability and such other manifestations of the mind which will be described later while discussing the various types of mind. All of them occur in the man but all of them are not manifested at the same time. An individual is said to belong to that particular type of mind by which he is dominated. [13]

Embryo- conglomeration of several factors:

एवमयं नानाविधानामेषां गर्भकराणां भावानां समुदायादभिनिर्वर्तते गर्भः; यथा- कूटागारं नानाद्रव्यसमुदायात्, यथा वा- रथो नानारथाङ्गसमुदायात्; तस्मादेतदवोचाम- मातृजश्चायं गर्भः, पितृजश्च, आत्मजश्च, सात्म्यजश्च, रसजश्च, अस्ति च सत्वमौपपादुकमिति (होवाच भगवानात्रेयः)||१४||

As a Kutagara (round shaped cottage used for administering hot fomentation therapy) is constructed from out of various types of construction materials and just like a chariot is constructed from out of various parts, similarly the embryo is formed from out of various types of procreative factors.

Therefore we assert that the foetus is formed from various factors, i.e. mother (ovum), father (sperm), soul, wholesomeness and rasa (digestive product of mother's food). The mind serves as the connecting link. Thus said Lord Atreya. [14]

Observations of Bharadvaja:

भरद्वाज उवाच- यद्ययमेषां नानाविधानां गर्भकराणां भावानां समुदायादभिनिर्वर्तते गर्भः कथमयं सन्धीयते, यदि चापि सन्धीयते कस्मात् समुदायप्रभवः सन् गर्भो मनुष्यविग्रहेण जायते, मनुष्यश्च मनुष्यप्रभव उच्यते; तत्र चेदिष्टमेतद्यस्मान्मनुष्यो मनुष्यप्रभवस्तस्मादेव मनुष्यविग्रहेण जायते, यथा- गौर्गोप्रभवः, यथा- चाश्वोऽश्वप्रभव इति; एवं सति यदुक्तमग्रे समुदायात्मक इति तदयुक्तम्|

यदि च मनुष्यो मनुष्यप्रभवः, कस्माज्जडान्धकुब्जमूकवामनमिम्मिनव्यङ्गोन्मत्तकुष्ठिकिलासिभ्यो जाताः पितृसदृशरूपा न भवन्ति|

अथात्रापि बुद्धिरेव स्यात्- स्वेनैवायमात्मा चक्षुषा रूपाणि वेति, श्रोत्रेण शब्दान्, घ्राणेन गन्धान्, रसनेन रसान्, स्पर्शनेन स्पर्शान्, बुद्ध्या बोद्धव्यमित्यनेन हेतुना न जडादिभ्यो जाताः पितृसदृशा भवन्ति|

अत्रापि प्रतिज्ञाहानिदोषः स्यात्, एवमुक्ते ह्यात्मा सतिस्विन्द्रियेषु ज्ञः स्यादसत्स्वज्ञः; यत्र चैतदुभयं सम्भवति ज्ञत्वमज्ञत्वं च, सविकारश्चात्मा |

यदि च दर्शनादिभिरात्मा विषयान् वेति, निरिन्द्रियो दर्शनादिविरहादज्ञः स्यात्, अज्ञत्वादकारणम्, अकारणत्वाच्च नात्मेति वागवस्तुमात्रमेतद्वचनमनर्थं स्यादिति (होवाच भरद्वाजः)||१५||

Bharadvaja said: "if the foetus is formed out of the conglomeration of these various procreative factors, then how do they get united? Their conglomeration apart, how is that the union of these factors results in the production of a creature in the form of a human being? If you opine and argue that since man is born from another man, just like the cow is born from another cow and the horse is born from another horse and hence takes the shape and form of human being, then the statement made earlier that the man is formed by the combination of six factors shall not be accepted / relevant.

If it is to be believed that man is created by another man, then why the child born to parents who are dull, blind, hunch-backed, mute, dwarf, lisping suffering from freckles, insanity, Kustha (obstinate skin diseases including leprosy) and Kilasa (leucoderma) does not carry the defects of his parents?

If it is argued that the Soul sees things by His own eyes, hears by His own ears, smells by His own nose, tastes by His Own tongue, touches by His own skin, understands by His own Intellect and because of this individuals born of dumb etc; do not carry the defects of their parents (because it is not the sense organs of parents but those of the Soul which takes part in procreation)? This is because the soul is independent, he will perceive things through his sense organs and independently form these sense organs, therefore the progeny of blind will not be blind, and the progeny of deaf will not be deaf.

If we accept that the Soul understands things with the help of sense organs i.e. by vision etc. that will also mean to say that in the absence of these sense organs, He won't be able to know and understand things. This also means that the soul is both a knower and non-knower. Does that mean that the soul is faulty?

If we say that the soul gains knowledge through the sense organs, does that mean that in the absence of sense organs the soul would become non-knower? Does that mean that because of the absence of the power to know things, he cannot serve as a causative factor and if He is not a causative factor, will be ridiculed as a story. (Thus said Bharadvaj). [15]

Atreya's observations:

आत्रेय उवाच- पुरस्तादेतत् प्रतिज्ञातं- सत्त्वं जीवं स्पृक्शरीरेणाभिसम्बध्नातीति|

यस्मात्तु समुदायप्रभवः सन् स गर्भो मनुष्यविग्रहेण जायते, मनुष्यो मनुष्यप्रभव इत्युच्यते, तद्वक्ष्यामः- भूतानां चतुर्विधा योनिर्भवति-जराय्वण्डस्वेदोद्भिदः|

तासां खलु चतसृणामपि योनीनामेकैका योनिरपरिसङ्ख्येयभेदा भवति, भूतानामाकृतिविशेषापरिसङ्ख्येयत्वात्|

तत्र जरायुजानामण्डजानां च प्राणिनामेते गर्भकरा भावा यां यां योनिमापद्यन्ते, तस्यां तस्यां योनौ तथातथारूपा भवन्ति; यथा-कनकरजततताम्रत्रपुसीसकान्यासिच्यमानानि तेषु तेषु मधूच्छिष्टविग्रहेषु, तानि यदा मनुष्यबिम्बमापद्यन्ते तदा मनुष्यविग्रहेण जायन्ते, तस्मात् समुदायप्रभावः सन् गर्भो मनुष्यविग्रहेण जायते; मनुष्यश्च मनुष्यप्रभव उच्यते, तद्योनित्वात्||१६||

Lord Atreya said, "It has already been concluded that the mind is responsible for the union of the Soul with the physical body. A human being is considered to be a Soul with the physical body. A human being is considered to be a causative factor for the production of another human being simply because the foetus is composed of the conglomeration of various factors which produce a human form.

Thus, there are four species of living beings, viz, viviparous, oviparous, Svedaja (living- beings born of hot moisture) and Udbhija (living- beings born piercing earth). Each of these four species is of innumerable types. This is because of the innumerable of distinctive features they possess.

The species of the first two categories take their specific forms depending on the contact of the causative factors of the foetus with the wombs of the specific species just like the gold, silver, copper, tin and lead melted and poured into various designs of bee-works take respective forms.

Similarly, when the foetus formed due to the conglomeration of various factors occupying the womb of human beings, they would take the human form and shape because of the effect of human species. A human being is considered to be a product of a human being because he belongs to the same species. [16]

Factors for hereditary defects:

यच्चोक्तं- यदि च मनुष्यो मनुष्यप्रभवः, कस्मान्न जडादिभ्यो जाताः पितृसदृशरूपा भवन्तीति; तत्रोच्यते- यस्य यस्य ह्यङ्गावयवस्य बीजे बीज भाग उपतप्तो भवति, तस्य तस्याङ्गावयवस्य विकृतिरुपजायते, नोपजायते चानुपतापात्; तस्मादुभयोपपत्तिरप्यत्र|

सर्वस्य चात्मजानीन्द्रियाणि, तेषां भावाभावहेतुर्दैवं; तस्मान्नैकान्ततो जडादिभ्यो जाताः पितृसदृशरूपा भवन्ति||१७||

A question was also raised that if the human being is a product of another human being, why is the progeny of a dull human being not always dull? The reply is that if the part of the seed (sperm or ovum) which is responsible for the formation of a particular organ is vitiated, this will result in the vitiation of that respective organ. If it is not vitiated, there would be no vitiation of the respective organs either.

So both the possibilities are there (i.e. the respective organs of the progeny may or may not be vitiated depending upon the vitiation or otherwise of the part of the seed responsible for the formation of such organs). As a matter of fact, the sense organs of all living beings are born out of the Soul and their existence or otherwise are determined by fate i.e. the result of the past action. So, the offspring of the dull parents do not invariably resemble their parents. [17]

Knowledge of Soul though sense organs:

न चात्मा सत्स्विन्द्रियेषु ज्ञः, असत्सु वा भवत्यज्ञः; न ह्यसत्त्वः कदाचिदात्मा, सत्त्वविशेषाच्चोपलभ्यते ज्ञानविशेष इति||१८||

It is not that the Soul is endowed with consciousness only when he is possessed of sense organs and is devoid of consciousness otherwise. The soul can never be separated from the mind, and so, He is always endowed with consciousness. [18]

Thus it is said:

भवन्ति चात्र-

न कर्तुरिन्द्रियाभावात् कार्यज्ञानं प्रवर्तते|

या क्रिया वर्तते भावैः सा विना तैर्न वर्तते||१९||

जानन्नपि मृदोऽभावात् कुम्भकृन्न प्रवर्तते|२०|

The soul is never devoid of consciousness of course, he cannot respond to the various actions in the absence of the sense organs. So it is not possible to perform any act without the presence of sense organs as it is not possible for a potter to work if he does not have the required quantity of mud irrespective of his knowledge regarding the production of a pitcher. [19-20]

Concentration of mind for proper examination:

श्रूयतां चेदमध्यात्ममात्मज्ञानबलं महत्||२०||

इन्द्रियाणि च सङ्क्षिप्य मनः सङ्क्षिप्य चञ्चलम्|

प्रविश्याध्यात्ममात्मज्ञः स्वे ज्ञाने पर्यवस्थितः||२१||

सर्वत्रावहितज्ञानः सर्वभावान् परीक्षते|२२|

Listen to this spiritual wisdom which is of immense help for the attainment of the knowledge of Soul.

One should control his sense organs as well as fickle mind and keep himself established in his own self after knowing the real nature of the Soul and attaining the height of spiritual wisdom.

Thus, with this knowledge undisturbed in all situations, he will be able to examine all aspects (of the science of medicine) [20-21]

गृह्णीष्व चे(वे)दमपरं भरद्वाज विनिर्णयम्||२२||

निवृत्तेन्द्रियवाक्चेष्टः सुप्तः स्वप्नगतो यदा|

विषयान् सुखदुःखे च वेति नाज्ञोऽप्यतः स्मृतः||२३||

नात्मज्ञानादृते चैकं ज्ञानं किञ्चित् प्रवर्तते|

न ह्येको वर्तते भावो वर्तते नाप्यहेतुकः||२४||

Try to understand this point also, O! Bharadvaja, Even if somebody has lost some of his sense organs_ vocal and motor faculties, in a dream he does experience the various objects of sense happiness, miseries etc., he cannot, therefore, be treated as a creature devoid of consciousness. There cannot be any knowledge without knowledge of the Soul.

Nothing can move alone unless prompted by an efficient cause to do so. [22-24]

तस्माज्ज्ञः प्रकृतिश्चात्मा द्रष्टा कारणमेव च|

सर्वमेतद्भरद्वाज निर्णीतं जहि संशयम्||२५||

So, get rid of all doubts.

O! Bharadvaja, I have explained to you everything about the Soul. The Soul is omniscient, primary cause, seer and efficient cause. [25]

तत्र श्लोकौ-
हेतुर्गर्भस्य निर्वृत्तौ वृद्धौ जन्मनि चैव यः|
पुनर्वसुमतिर्या च भरद्वाजमतिश्च या||२६||
प्रतिज्ञाप्रतिषेधश्च विशदश्चात्मनिर्णयः|
गर्भावक्रान्तिमुद्दिश्य खुड्डीकां तत्प्रकाशितम्||२७||

To sum up: -

In the minor chapter on the formation of embryo as conducive to the understanding of the body, the following topics are discussed:

Factors responsible for the formation, growth and delivery of the embryo;

The views of Punarvasu and Bharadvaja on this topic

The attack on the conclusions (by Bharadvaja) and

A detailed exposition of the nature of the Soul [26-27]

इत्यग्निवेशकृते तन्त्रे चरकप्रतिसंस्कृते शारीरस्थाने खुड्डीकागर्भावक्रान्तिशारीरं नाम तृतीयोऽध्यायः||३||

Thus ends the third minor chapter of Sharira Section the "Formation of Embryo as conductive to Understanding of the Body" of Agnivesha's work as redacted by Charaka. [3]

20

Shareerasthana Chapter 4 Mahatim Garbhavakranti Shareeram

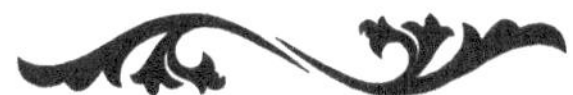

Formation of Embryo

अथातो महतीं गर्भावक्रान्तिं शारीरं व्याख्यास्यामः||१||

इति ह स्माह भगवानात्रेयः||२||

We shall now explore the major chapter on the formation of the Embryo as conducive to the understanding of the body. Thus said Lord Atreya [1-2]

Important Topics discussed in this chapter:

यतश्च गर्भः सम्भवति, यस्मिंश्च गर्भसञ्ज्ञा, यदि्वकारश्च गर्भः, यया चानुपूर्व्याऽभिनिर्वर्तते कुक्षौ, यश्चास्य वृद्धिहेतुः, यतश्चास्याजन्म भवति, यतश्च जायमानः कुक्षौ विनाशं प्राप्नोति, यतश्च कात्स्न्र्येनाविनश्यन् विकृतिमापद्यते, तदनुव्याख्यास्यामः||३||

We shall now discuss the origin of the embryo, its definition, its composition, and its successive development in the womb, the cause of its growth, the cause of the non-manifestation of the embryo, the cause of destruction of the embryo in the womb and the cause of its morbidity without complete destruction. [3]

Factors composing the foetus:

मातृतः पितृत आत्मतः सात्म्यतो रसतः सत्त्वत इत्येतेभ्यो भावेभ्यः समुदितेभ्यो गर्भः सम्भवति|

तस्य ये येऽवयवा यतो यतः सम्भवतः सम्भवन्ति तान् विभज्य मातृजादीनवयवान् पृथक् पृथगुक्तमग्रे||४||

The embryo is formed out of the combination of parents, the Soul, wholesomeness, Rasa (digestive product of mother's food) and mind. The sources of the respective organs / phenomena like ovum etc. have already been described in greater detail. [4]

Definition of term "Garbha":

शुक्रशोणितजीवसंयोगे तु खलु कुक्षिगते गर्भसञ्ज्ञा भवति||५||

The union of sperm, ovum and the Soul in the wombs is designed as an embryo. [5]

Six elements composing the foetus:

गर्भस्तु खल्वन्तरिक्षवाय्वग्नितोयभूमिविकारश्चेतनाधिष्ठानभूतः|

एवमनया युक्त्या पञ्चमहाभूतविकारसमुदायात्मको गर्भश्चेतनाधिष्ठानभूतः; स ह्यस्य षष्ठो धातुरुक्तः||६||

The embryo is formed by the five Mahabhutas. Viz, Akasha - ether, Vayu – air / wind, Agni - fire, Jala – water and Prthvi – earth and it serves as the receptacle of consciousness. Applying this principle, the foetus represents the combination of five Mahabhutas i.e., five elements of nature and a receptacle of consciousness. The consciousness or soul represents the sixth element of the embryo. [6]

Process of conception:

यया चानुपूर्व्याऽभिनिर्वर्तते कुक्षौ तां व्याख्यास्यामः- गते पुराणे रजसि नवे चावस्थिते शुद्धस्नातां स्त्रियमव्यापन्नयोनिशोणितगर्भाशयामृतुमतीमाचक्ष्महे|

तया सह तथाभूतया यदा पुमानव्यापन्नबीजो मिश्रीभावं गच्छति, तदा तस्य हर्षोदीरितः परः शरीरधात्वात्मा शुक्रभूतोऽङ्गादङ्गात् सम्भवति|

स तथा हर्षभूतेनात्मनोदीरितश्चाधिष्ठितश्च बीजरूपो धातुः पुरुषशरीरादभिनिष्पत्त्योचितेन पथा गर्भाशयमनुप्रविश्यार्तवेनाभिसंसर्गमेति||७||

Now we shall explain the order in which the embryo develops in the womb. A woman not suffering from sterility attains the state of fertility after the period of menstruation is over and the formation of fresh blood (inside the uterus) begins, provided she has had a purificatory bath and her genital tract, ovum and the uterus are in excellent condition.

If a man with his sperm unimpaired, cohabits with such a woman, his semen which constitutes the essence of the tissue elements of his body, comes out from each and every organ. The semen consisting of sperms impelled by the organs is ejaculated from the body of the man and enters the uterus through the woman's genital tract and finally unites with the ovum. [7]

Union of Atman:

तत्र पूर्वं चेतनाधातुः सत्त्वकरणो गुणग्रहणाय प्रवर्तते; स हि हेतुः कारणं निमित्तमक्षरं कर्ता मन्ता वेदिता बोद्धा द्रष्टा धाता ब्रह्मा विश्वकर्मा विश्वरूपः पुरुषः प्रभवोऽव्ययो नित्यो गुणी ग्रहणं प्रधानमव्यक्तं जीवो ज्ञः पुद्गलश्चेतनावान् विभुर्भूतात्मा चेन्द्रियात्मा चान्तरात्मा चेति|

स गुणोपादानकालेऽन्तरिक्षं पूर्वतरमन्येभ्यो गुणेभ्य उपादत्ते, यथा- प्रलयात्यये सिसृक्षुर्भूतान्यक्षरभूत आत्मा सत्त्वोपादानः पूर्वतरमाकाशं सृजति, ततः क्रमेण व्यक्ततरगुणान् धातून् वाय्वादिकांश्चतुरः; तथा देहग्रहणेऽपि प्रवर्तमानः पूर्वतरमाकाशमेवोपादत्ते, ततः क्रमेण व्यक्ततरगुणान् धातून् वाय्वादिकांश्चतुरः|

सर्वमपि तु खल्वेतद्गुणोपादानमणुना कालेन भवति||८||

First of all, the conscious element i.e., the Soul endowed with mental equipment i.e., the mind unites with the Mahabhutas i.e., elements of nature. He is known by various names as mentioned below –

- hetu (concomitant cause)
- karana (non-constituent cause)
- nimita (Effective cause)
- akshara (the indestructible one)
- karta (the Agent / the doer)
- manta (the Thinker)
- vedita (the knower)
- boddha (the intelligent one)
- drasta (one who sees, the visionary)
- dhata (the Supporter)
- brahma (the creator)
- vishvakarman (the Builder of the universe)
- visvarupa (the prototype of the universe)
- purusa (the supreme person)
- prabhava (the source of origin)
- avyaya (the indestructible)
- nitya (the eternal)
- guni (the receptacle of mahabhutas)
- grahana (one having capacity to collect / unite the mahabhutas so as to form the body)
- pradhana (the main or predominant one)

- avyakta (the non-manifested one)
- jiva (the one who keeps the living beings in a living condition)
- jna (the conscious one)
- pudgala (the one who goes / jumps from one body to the other)
- cetanavan (one having the consciousness / power to sense)
- vibhu (omnipresent)
- bhutatma (empirical soul)
- indriyatman (organic soul) and
- antraratman (inner soul)

The soul, first of all, unites with Akasha before uniting with the other Bhutas. This is like the creation of Akasha by God / greater soul after the period of deluge. A God, the indestructible one, equipped with the mind creates Akasha first, and then the other Bhutas whose attributes are more and more manifested successively i.e., vayu, agni etc. Similarly, the Soul, desirous of creating another body, first of all, unites with the Akasha, and then with other four Bhutas whose attributes are more and more manifested successively i.e., vayu, agni etc. All this action (association of the Soul with the five mahabhutas) takes place in a very short time. [8]

Manifestations during first month:

स सर्वगुणवान् गर्भत्वमापन्नः प्रथमे मासि सम्मूर्च्छितः सर्वधातुकलुषीकृतः खेटभूतो भवत्यव्यक्तविग्रहः सदसद्भूताङ्गावयवः||९||

When accompanied with all the attributes, the Soul takes the form of an embryo. During the first month of gestation, it takes the form of jelly because of the intimate mixture of the five Mahabhutas (which get develop in the subsequent months as the tissue elements, i.e., Rasa etc, of the body). During this month, the embryo bears no particular form and the organs of the embryo are both manifest and latent. [9]

Characteristics during second month:

द्विवतीये मासि घनः सम्पद्यते पिण्डः पेश्यर्बुदं वा|

तत्र घनः पुरुषः, पेशी स्त्री, अर्बुदं नपुंसकम्||१०||

During the second month of generation, the embryo takes a compact form in the shape of a knot, elongated muscle or tumour (round and elevated).
- The knot shaped embryo leads to the production of male foetus.
- The muscle shaped embryo leads to the formation of a female foetus.
- The tumour shaped embryo leads to the formation of a eunuch. [10]

Manifestations during third month

तृतीये मासि सर्वेन्द्रियाणि सर्वाङ्गावयवाश्च यौगपद्येनाभिनिर्वर्तन्ते||११||

During the third month, all the senses and limbs along with their organs manifest themselves simultaneously. [11]

Factors derived from various sources:

तत्रास्य केचिदङ्गावयवा मातृजादीनवयवान् विभज्य पूर्वमुक्ता यथावत्|

महाभूतविकारप्रविभागेन त्विदानीमस्य तांश्चैवाङ्गावयवान् कांश्चित् पर्यायान्तरेणापरांश्चानुव्याख्यास्यामः|

मातृजादयोऽप्यस्य महाभूतविकारा एव|

तत्रास्याकाशात्मकं शब्दः श्रोत्रं लाघवं सौक्ष्म्यं विवेकश्च, वाय्वात्मकं स्पर्शः स्पर्शनं रौक्ष्यं प्रेरणं धातुव्यूहनं चेष्टाश्च शारीर्यः, अग्न्यात्मकं रूपं दर्शनं प्रकाशः पक्तिरौष्ण्यं च, अबात्मकं रसो रसनं शैत्यं मार्दवं स्नेहः क्लेदश्च, पृथिव्यात्मकं गन्धो घ्राणं गौरवं स्थैर्य मूर्तिश्चेति||१२||

The description of some of the limbs and organs of the foetus have already been described under various headings such as those derived from mother, those derived from father etc (vide Sharira 3: 6- 18). Different aspects of some of these limbs and organs, and some more will now be described here in a different way of classification, in accordance to their manifestation based on the modifications of various mahabhutas (which form those limbs and organs). In fact, organs derived from mother etc, are nothing but the modifications of the Mahabhutas.

- Sound, the sense organ of sound, lightness, minuteness / subtleness and distinction are derived from Akasha.
- Touch, the sense of touch, roughness, impulsion, formation of different tissues and actions of the body are derived from Vayu.
- Sight, the sense of vision, brightness, digestion and production of heat in the body are derived from Agni.
- Taste, the sense of taste, coldness, softness, unctuousness and dampness (wetness) are derived from Jala.
- Smell, the sense of smell, heaviness, steadiness, and form are derived from Prthvi. [12]

Individual and Universe:

एवमयं लोकसम्मितः पुरुषः|

यावन्तो हि लोके मूर्तिमन्तो भावविशेषास्तावन्तः पुरुषे, यावन्तः पुरुषे तावन्तो लोके इति; बुधास्त्वेवं द्रष्टुमिच्छन्ति||१३||

Thus, the individual is an epitome of the universe. All the material and spiritual phenomena of the universe are present in the individual. Similarly, all those present in the individual are also contained in the universe. This is how the wise desire to perceive [13]

एवमस्येन्द्रियाण्यङ्गावयवाश्च यौगपद्येनाभिनिर्वर्तन्तेऽन्यत्र तेभ्यो भावेभ्यो येऽस्य जातस्योत्तरकालं जायन्ते; तद्यथा- दन्ता व्यञ्जनानि व्यक्तीभावस्तथायुक्तानि चापराणि|

एषा प्रकृतिः, विकृतिः पुनरतोऽन्यथा|

सन्ति खल्वस्मिन् गर्भे केचिन्नित्या भावाः, सन्ति चानित्याः केचित्|

तस्य य एवाङ्गावयवाः सन्तिष्ठन्ते, त एव स्त्रीलिङ्गं पुरुषलिङ्गं नपुंसकलिङ्गं वा बिभ्रति|

तत्र स्त्रीपुरुषयोर्ये वैशेषिका भावाः प्रधानसंश्रया गुणसंश्रयाश्च, तेषां यतो भूयस्त्वं ततोऽन्यतरभावः|

तद्यथा- क्लैब्यं भीरुत्वमवैशारद्यं मोहोऽनवस्थानमधोगुरुत्वमसहनं शैथिल्यं मार्दवं गर्भाशयबीजभागस्तथायुक्तानि चापराणि स्त्रीकराणि, अतो विपरीतानि पुरुषकराणि, उभयभागावयवा नपुंसककराणि भवन्ति||१४||

Thus, the senses and organs of the foetus are simultaneously manifested except those that are manifested only after birth. For example, teeth, secondary sexual characteristics like bread and breasts, signs of puberty like the production of semen and ovum and such other traits are developed later. This is normal and anything other than this is abnormal. In this foetus, there are some characteristics which are permanent and some others are temporary. These permanent characteristics determine the masculine, feminine or neutral character of the foetus. The characteristics features which determine its male or female sex are either of spiritual or material (Bhautika derived from sperm and ovum) nature. Sex deference is caused by the dominance of one or the other of these factors. For example:
- Weakness
- Timidity
- Lack of wisdom
- Ignorance
- Unsteadiness
- Heaviness of lower limbs
- Intolerance
- Slackness
- Softness

Presence of the uterus and ovary and other characteristic features determine the female sex; opposite traits determine the male sex and in a female sex; opposite traits determine the male sex and, in a eunuch, both these traits are equally present. [14]

Bi cardiac state:

तस्य यत्कालमेवेन्द्रियाणि सन्तिष्ठन्ते, तत्कालमेव चेतसि वेदना निर्बन्धं प्राप्नोति; तस्मातदा प्रभृति गर्भः स्पन्दते, प्रार्थयते च जन्मान्तरानुभूतं यत् किञ्चित्, तद्द्वैहृदय्यमाचक्षते वृद्धाः|

मातृजं चास्य हृदयं मातृहृदयेनाभिसम्बद्धं भवति रसवाहिनीभिः संवाहिनीभिः; तस्मात्तयोस्ताभिर्भक्तितः संस्पन्दते |

तच्चैव कारणमवेक्षमाणा न द्वैहृदय्यस्य विमानितं गर्भमिच्छन्ति कर्तुम्|

विमानने ह्यस्य दृश्यते विनाशो विकृतिर्वा|
समानयोगक्षेमा हि तदा भवति गर्भेण केषुचिदर्थेषु माता|
तस्मात् प्रियहिताभ्यां गर्भिणीं विशेषणोपचरन्ति कुशलाः||१५||

As soon as senses are manifested in the embryo, its mind starts experiencing feelings like pleasure and grief. This is the reason why the foetus starts responding to and getting adjusted to being comfortable with pleasure and also to keep away from grief and pains. It will also start desiring comfortable feelings that it has experienced since many previous births. The desires of the foetus are exhibited in the form of desires of the mother.

This condition wherein the child's heart is associated with that of the mother according to the wise is known as Dauharda or bi-cardiac state.

The heart of the foetus which is derived from the maternal source is connected with the mother's heart through the channels carrying nutrient material.

These channels connecting the foetus and the mother carry the desires of the child to the mother and those of the mother to the child. It is with this perspective that the wise and experienced people advise not to ignore or reject the desires of the mother. This is because if these wishes are ignored or rejected, they may cause destruction or deformity in the foetus.

So, the wise people insist that the pregnant woman shall be attended with special care so as to fulfil her favourite desires and useful needs.[15]

Signs of bi cardiac slate:

तस्या गर्भोपपत्तेर्वैहृदय्यस्य च विज्ञानार्थं लिङ्गानि समासेनोपदेक्ष्यामः|

उपचारसाधनं ह्यस्य ज्ञाने, ज्ञानं च लिङ्गतः, तस्मादिष्टो लिङ्गोपदेशः|

तद्यथा- आर्तवादर्शनमास्यसंस्रवणमन्ननाभिलाषश्छर्दिररोचकोऽम्लकामता च विशेषेण श्रद्धाप्रणयनमुच्चावचेषु भावेषु गुरुगात्रत्वं चक्षुषोर्ग्लानिः स्तनयोः स्तन्यमोष्ठयोः स्तनमण्डलयोश्च काष्ण्यर्मत्यर्थं श्वयथुः पादयोरीषल्लोमराज्युद्गमो योन्याश्चाटालत्वमिति गर्भे पर्यागते रूपाणि भवन्ति||१६||

Now we shall explain in brief the signs and symptoms that are indicative of pregnancy as well the bi-cardiac condition. The knowledge of signs and symptoms facilitate the management of these conditions. Therefore, it is necessary to explain their signs and symptoms. They are as follows:

- Stoppage of menstruation
- Excessive salivation
- Loss of appetite
- Vomiting
- Anorexia
- Liking for sour foods
- Liking for all types of foods - both wholesome and unwholesome
- Heaviness of the body
- Feeling of heaviness in the eyes
- Appearance of milk in breasts
- Appearance of excessive darkness in the lips and the areola of breasts
- Slight oedema of feet
- Appearance of small hairs and
- Dilation of vagina [16]

Satisfaction of her desires:

सा यद्यदिच्छेत्तत्तदस्यै दद्यादन्यत्र गर्भोपघातकरेभ्यो भावेभ्यः||१७||

The mother should be given whatever she wants during this period except perhaps those that are harmful for the foetus [17]

Factors injurious to foetus:

गर्भोपघातकरास्त्विमे भावा भवन्तिः; तद्यथा- सर्वमतिगुरूष्णतीक्ष्णं दारुणाश्च चेष्टाः; इमांश्चान्यानुपदिशन्ति वृद्धाः-देवतारक्षोऽनुचरपरिरक्षणार्थं न रक्तानि वासांसि बिभृयान्न मदकराणि मद्यान्यभ्यवहरेन्न यानमधिरोहेन्न मांसमश्नीयात् सर्वेन्द्रियप्रतिकूलांश्च भावान् दूरतः परिवर्जयेत्, यच्चान्यदपि किञ्चित् स्त्रियो विद्युः॥१८॥

The following are the factors inflicting injury to the foetus:

All things that are very heavy, hot and sharp and

Violent actions like sexual intercourse

Wise men also prescribe the following precautionary measures with a view to avoid any injury to the foetus:

- With a view to be saved of the Gods, Rakshasas (devils) and their followers, she should not use red apparel
- She should not take intoxicant wines
- She should not take meat
- She should not be far away from things as are unwholesome to the senses and
- She should avoid all such things as advised by (experienced) ladies. [18]

Embryonic defects by ignoring her desires:

तीव्रायां तु खलु प्रार्थनायां काममहितमप्यस्यै हितेनोपहितं दद्यात् प्रार्थनाविनयनार्थम्|

प्रार्थनासन्धारणादि्ध वायुः प्रकुपितोऽन्तःशरीरमनुचरन् गर्भस्यापद्यमानस्य विनाशं वैरूप्यं वा कुर्यात्॥१९॥

If the longing is very strong, then even things which are harmful can be given by neutralizing their injurious effects through processing or adding wholesome things. This is necessary with a view to satisfying the desires. By the suppression of the longings, the vata gets vitiated, moves inside the body, and destroys or deforms the foetus in the formative stage. [19]

Developments during fourth month:

चतुर्थे मासि स्थिरत्वमापद्यते गर्भः, तस्मात्तदा गर्भिणी गुरुगात्रत्वमधिकमापद्यते विशेषेण॥२०॥

During the fourth month of gestation, the foetus stabilised. Therefore, at that time, pregnant women specifically experience excessive heaviness in her body. [20]

Manifestations during fifth month:

पञ्चमे मासि गर्भस्य मांसशोणितोपचयो भवत्यधिकमन्येभ्यो मासेभ्यः, तस्मात्तदा गर्भिणी कार्श्यमापद्यते विशेषेण॥२१॥

There is an excessive increase of flesh and blood of the foetus during the fifth month of gestation in comparison to other months. Therefore, at that time the pregnant woman grows excessively thinner. [21]

Developments during sixth month:

षष्ठे मासि गर्भस्य बलवर्णोपचयो भवत्यधिकमन्येभ्यो मासेभ्यः, तस्मात्तदा गर्भिणी बलवर्णहानिमापद्यते विशेषेण॥२२॥

There is an excessive increase in the strength and complexion of the foetus during the sixth month of generation in comparison to the other months of gestation. Therefore, at that time the pregnant woman loses her strength and complexion considerably. [22]

Developments during seventh month:

सप्तमे मासि गर्भः सर्वैर्भावैराप्याय्यते, तस्मात्तदा गर्भिणी सर्वाकारैः क्लान्ततमा भवति॥२३॥

There is an all-round development of the foetus during the seventh month of gestation. Therefore, a pregnant woman becomes exceedingly deficient in all aspects of her health in the 7th gestational month. [23]

Manifestations during eight months:

अष्टमे मासि गर्भश्च मातृतो गर्भतश्च माता रसहारिणीभिः संवाहिनीभिर्मुहुर्मुहुरोजः परस्परत आददाते गर्भस्यासम्पूर्णत्वात् |

तस्मात्तदा गर्भिणीमुहुर्मुहुर्मुदा युक्ता भवति मुहुर्मुहुश्च म्लाना, तथा गर्भः; तस्मात्तदा गर्भस्य जन्म व्यापत्तिमद्भवत्योजसोऽनवस्थितत्वात् |

तं चैवार्थमभिसमीक्ष्याष्टमं मासमगण्यमित्याचक्षते कुशलाः||२४||

During the eight months of gestation, the Ojas formed in the body of the foetus moves to the body of the mother and vice versa through the channels carrying nourishment from the mother to the foetus because of the immaturity of the foetus.

Therefore, at that time the pregnant woman often has a wavering feeling of joy and sorrow. Similar is the condition of the foetus. It is because of this unsteadiness of the Ojas that the delivery of the foetus during this month is considered to be dangerous and risky. In view of this, experts advise that even the reckoning of the eight months of pregnancy should be avoided. This is because if the pregnant woman is constantly aware that she is running through the eighth month of pregnancy she will always be in fear, the fear may also lead to abnormal increase of vata which might consequently cause damage to the foetus. This may further lead to foetal anomalies. [24]

Time of delivery:

तस्मिन्नेकदिवसातिक्रान्तेऽपि नवमं मासमुपादाय प्रसवकालमित्याहुरादशमान्मासात्|
एतावान् प्रसवकालः, वैकारिकमतः परं कुक्षाववस्थानं गर्भस्य||२५||

Even the first day after this eight month i.e., from the first day of the ninth month till the end of the tenth month is known as the period of parturition. Normally delivery takes place during this period. Retention of the foetus in the pelvis thereafter is abnormal. [25]

एवमनयाऽऽनुपूर्व्याऽभिनिर्वर्तते कुक्षौ||२६||

The following factors help in the growth of the foetus in the pelvis of the mother:

Factors for growth of foetus:

मात्रादीनां खलु गर्भकराणां भावानां सम्पदस्तथा वृत्तस्य सौष्ठवान्मातृतश्चैवोपस्नेहोपस्वेदाभ्यां कालपरिणामात् स्वभावसंसिद्धेश्च कुक्षौ वृद्धिं प्राप्नोति||२७||

The below mentioned factors are responsible for the growth of the foetus –

Excellence of the factors responsible for the production of the foetus which include –

- Maternal factor (ovum
- Paternal factor (sperm)
- Soul
- Wholesomeness
  Digestive product of the mother's food and
- Mind
     Other factors –
- Proper regimen by the mother during pregnancy
- Availability of nourishment and heat through Upasneha (transudation) and (conduction) respectively
- Proper time and
- Instinctive or natural tendencies [27]

Factors responsible for absence of birth:

मात्रादीनामेव तु खलु गर्भकराणां भावानां व्यापत्तिनिमित्तमस्याजन्म भवति||२८||

Because of the defects in the factors responsible for the production of the foetus i.e., mother (ovum), father (sperm) etc., there is no birth of the child. [28]

Death or delay in delivery of the foetus:

ये ह्यस्य कुक्षौ वृद्धिहेतुसमाख्याता भावास्तेषां विपर्ययादुदरे विनाशमापद्यते, अथवाऽप्यचिरजातः स्यात्||२९||

The foetus gets destroyed in the pelvis (of the mother) or there is delay in delivery if factors contrary to the ones described for its growth are present. [29]

Causes of deformity in a female child:

यतस्तु कात्स्न्र्येनाविनश्यन् विकृतिमापद्यते, तदनुव्याख्यास्यामः- यदा स्त्रिया दोषप्रकोपणोक्तान्यासेवमानाया दोषाः प्रकुपिताः शरीरमुपसर्पन्तः शोणितगर्भाशयावुपपद्यन्ते , न च कात्स्न्र्येन शोणितगर्भाशयौ दूषयन्ति, तदेयं गर्भं लभते स्त्री; तदा तस्य गर्भस्य मातृजानामवयवानामन्यतमोऽवयवो विकृतिमापद्यत एकोऽथवाऽनेके, यस्य यस्य ह्यवयवस्य बीजे बीजभागे वा दोषाः प्रकोपमापद्यन्ते, तं तमवयवं विकृतिराविशति।

यदा ह्यस्याः शोणिते गर्भाशयबीजभागः प्रदोषमापद्यते, तदा वन्ध्यां जनयति; यदा पुनरस्याः शोणिते गर्भाशयबीजभागावयवः प्रदोषमापद्यते, तदा पूतिप्रजां जनयति; यदा त्वस्याः शोणिते गर्भाशयबीजभागावयवः स्त्रीकराणां च शरीरबीजभागानामेकदेशः प्रदोषमापद्यते, तदा स्त्र्याकृतिभूयिष्ठामस्त्रियं वार्तां नाम जनयति, तां स्त्रीव्यापदमाचक्षते||३०||

Factors which lead to deformity and not complete destruction are now being described.

If the woman conceives when her ovum and uterus were not completely vitiated but simply afflicted by the circulating Doshas aggravated because of her indulgence in Dosha aggravating regimens, one or many of the organs of the foetus derived from the maternal source (ovum) i.e., skin, blood etc., get deformed. In the ovum (bija) or whichever part of the ovum (bija bhaga / bijamsha) responsible for the formation of a particular organ the doshas get vitiated, deformity would occur in those ovum / parts of the ovum. Consequently, the corresponding organs derived from these Bijas and Bijabhagas get deformed.

When the Bija bhaga (part of the bija) in the ovum of the mother which is responsible for the production of the uterus is excessively vitiated, then she gives birth to a sterile child. When the Bijabhagavayava (a fraction of the part of the Bija) in the ovum of the mother which is responsible for the production of the uterus is excessively vitiated, then she gives birth to a foul / fetid smelling child i.e., Puti praja (who delivers dead foetus- c.f commentary).

When the Bijabhagavayava which is responsible for the production of the uterus and also the portions of the Bijabhagas which are responsible for the production of organs that characterize a female, i.e., breasts, genital organ, hair etc. in the ovum of the mother gets excessively vitiated then she gives birth to a child who is not a complete female but only having the feminine characteristics in abundance - such a type of child is known as Varta. These deformities are caused by the vitiation of the ovum and are called as female deformities. [30]

Causes of deformity in a male child:

एवमेव पुरुषस्य यदा बीजे बीजभागः प्रदोषमापद्यते, तदा वन्ध्यं जनयति; यदा पुनरस्य बीजे बीजभागावयवः प्रदोषमापद्यते, तदा पूतिप्रजं जनयति; यदा त्वस्य बीजे बीजभागावयवः पुरुषकराणां च शरीरबीजभागानामेकदेशः प्रदोषमापद्यते, तदा पुरुषाकृतिभूयिष्ठमपुरुषं तृणपुत्रिकं नाम जनयति; तां पुरुषव्यापदमाचक्षते||३१||

Similarly, when the big / major part of the Bija which is responsible for the production of the sperm in the foetus is excessively vitiated, the child born would be sterile.

When the Bijabhagavayava (only a fraction of the part of the Bija) which is responsible for the production of the sperm is excessively vitiated, then this gives birth to a Putipraja (whose child dies before delivery).

When the Bijabhagavayava which is responsible for the production of sperm and also portions of the Bijabhagas which are responsible for the production of organs that characterise a male, are excessively vitiated, then this gives birth to a child who is not a complete male but only having masculine characteristics in abundance. Such a type of child is known as Trnaputrika.

These deformities are caused by the vitiation of the sperm and are called as male deformities. [31]

एतेन मातृजानां पितृजानां चावयवानां विकृतिव्याख्यानेन सात्म्यजानां रसजानां सत्त्वजानां चावयवानां विकृतिर्व्याख्याता भवति||३२||

Thus, the deformities of organs derived from the mother (ovum) and father (sperm) are explained. On the same line the deformities of the organs derived from Stamya (wholesomeness), Rasa (digestive product of the mother's food) and Sattva (mind) can be explained. [32]

Absolute soul:

निर्विकारः परस्त्वात्मा सर्वभूतानां निर्विशेषः; सत्त्वशरीरयोस्तु विशेषाद्विशेषोपलब्धिः||३३||

The absolute soul does not undergo any modification. Its presence in different types of creatures does not bear any distinction. It appears to have distinctions only on account of the specific features of the body and mind of different types of creatures. [33]

Doshas of the body & Mind:

तत्र त्रयः शरीरदोषा वातपित्तश्लेष्माणः, ते शरीरं दूषयन्ति; द्वौ पुनः सत्त्वदोषौ रजस्तमश्च, तौ सत्त्वं दूषयतः।

ताभ्यां च सत्त्वशरीराभ्यां दुष्टाभ्यां विकृतिरुपजायते, नोपजायते चाप्रदुष्टाभ्याम्॥३४॥

Now, there are three physical Doshas (vitiating elements), i.e., Vata, Pitta and Kapha - they vitiate the body. Again, there are two mental Doshas i.e., Rajas and Tamas - they vitiate the mind. Vitiation of the body and the mind result in the manifestation of diseases. No diseases are manifested without the vitiation of these doshas. [34]

Types of body:

तत्र शरीरं योनिविशेषाच्चतुर्विधमुक्तमग्रे॥३५॥

Depending upon the Yoni (mode of propagation) the body of animals is already described to be four types - c. F Sharira 3: 16 [35]

Types of minds:

त्रिविधं खलु सत्त्वं- शुद्धं, राजसं, तामसमिति।

तत्र शुद्धमदोषमाख्यातं कल्याणांशत्वात्, राजसं सदोषमाख्यातं रोषांशत्वात्, तामसमपि सदोषमाख्यातं मोहांशत्वात्।

तेषां तु त्रयाणामपि सत्त्वानामेकैकस्य भेदाग्रमपरिसङ्ख्येयं तरतमयोगाच्छरीरयोनिविशेषेभ्यश्चान्योन्यानुविधानत्वाच्च।

शरीरं ह्यपि सत्त्वमनुविधीयते, सत्त्वं च शरीरम्।

तस्मात् कतिचित्सत्त्वभेदाननूकाभिनिर्देशेन निदर्शनार्थमनुव्याख्यास्यामः॥३६॥

Mental faculty is of three types - Satvika, rajasa and Tamasa.

- The Sattvika one is free from defects as it is endowed with auspiciousness.

- The Rajasika type is defective because it promotes wrathful disposition.

- The Tamasika one is similarly defective because it suffers from ignorance.

Each of the three types of mental faculty is in fact of innumerable variety by permutations and combinations of the various factors relating to the body, species and mutual interactions.

Sometimes even the body follows the mind and vice versa. So, we shall now explain some of the varieties of mental faculties briefly by way of illustration. [36]

Different types of Sattvika individuals:

तद्यथा- शुचिं सत्याभिसन्धं जितात्मानं संविभागिनं ज्ञानविज्ञानवचनप्रतिवचनसम्पन्नं स्मृतिमन्तं कामक्रोधलोभमानमोहेष्र्याहर्षामर्षापेतं समं सर्वभूतेषु ब्राह्मं विद्यात् (१)।

इज्याध्ययनव्रतहोमब्रह्मचर्यपरमतिथिव्रतमुपशान्तमदमानरागद्वेषमोहलोभरोष प्रतिभावचनविज्ञानोपधारणशक्तिसम्पन्नमार्षं विद्यात् (२)।

ऐश्वर्यवन्तमादेयवाक्यं यज्वानं शूरमोजस्विनं तेजसोपेतमक्लिष्टकर्माणं दीर्घदर्शिनं धर्मार्थकामाभिरतमैन्द्रं विद्यात् (३)।

लेखास्थवृत्तं प्राप्तकारिणमसम्प्रहार्यमुत्थानवन्तं स्मृतिमन्तमैश्वर्यलम्भिनं व्यपगतरागेष्र्याद्वेषमोहं याम्यं विद्यात् (४)।

शूरं धीरं शुचिमशुचिद्वेषिणं यज्वानमम्भोविहाररतिमक्लिष्टकर्माणं स्थानकोपप्रसादं वारुणं विद्यात् (५)।

स्थानमानोपभोगपरिवारसम्पन्नं धर्मार्थकामनित्यं शुचिं सुखविहारं व्यक्तकोपप्रसादं कौबेरं विद्यात् (६)।

प्रियनृत्यगीतवादित्रोल्लापकश्लोकाख्यायिकेतिहासपुराणेषु कुशलं गन्धमाल्यानुलेपनवसनस्त्रीविहारकामनित्यमनसूयकं गान्धर्वं विद्यात् (७)।

इत्येवं शुद्धस्य सत्त्वस्य सप्तविधं भेदांश्च विद्यात् कल्याणांशत्वात्; तत्संयोगातु ब्राह्ममत्यन्तशुद्धं व्यवस्येत्॥३७॥

The Sattvika type of mental faculty is auspicious and is of seven categories. Their characteristic features are furnished in the statement given below:

1 Brahma (sharing the traits of Brahma) 1 Purity, love for truth, self-controlled

2 Power of discrimination, material and spiritual knowledge

3 Power of exposition, reply and memory

4 Freedom from passion, anger, greed, ego, ignorance, jealousy, dejection and intolerance and

5 Favourable disposition equally for all creatures.

2 Arsa (sharing the traits of Rshis) 1. Devotion to sacred rituals, study, sacred vows, oblations and celibacy

2 Hospitable disposition

3 Freedom from proved, ego, attachment, hatred, ignorance, greed and anger

4 Intellectual excellence and eloquence and

5 Power of understanding and retention

3 Anidra (sharing the traits of Lord Indra) 1 Lord-ship and authoritative speech

2 Performance of scared rituals

3 Bravery, strength and splendour

4 Freedom from mean acts

5 Farsightedness and

6 Devotion to virtuous acts, earning of wealth and proper satisfaction of desires

4 Yamya (sharing the traits of Yama) 1 Observance of the property of actions

2 Initiation of actions in time

3 Non- violability

4 Readiness for initiating action

5 Memory and lordship

6 Freedom from attachment, envy, hatred and ignorance

5 Varuna (sharing the traits of Varuna) 1 Bravery, patience, purity and dislike for impurity.

2 Observance of religious rites

3 Fondness for mean- acts and

4 Aversion for mean-acts and

5 Exhibition of anger and pleasure in proper place

6 Kauvera (sharing the traits of Kuvera) 1 Possession of station, honour, luxuries and attendance

2 Constant liking for virtuous acts wealth and satisfaction of desires

3 Purity and

4 Liking for pleasures of recreation

7 Gandharva (sharing the traits of Gandharva) 1 Fondness for dancing, singing, music and praise

2 Expertness in poetry, stories, historical narrations and epics

3 Constant fondness for scents, garlands, unguents apparel, association of woman and passion.

Of the seven types of Sattvika mental faculties described above, the one linked to Brahma is the purest. [37]

Different types of Rajasa individuals:

शूरं चण्डमसूयकमैश्वर्यवन्तमौपधिकं रौद्रमननुक्रोशमात्मपूजकमासुरं विद्यात् (१)।

अमर्षिणमनुबन्धकोपं छिद्रप्रहारिणं क्रूरमाहारातिमात्ररुचिमामिषप्रियतमं स्वप्नायासबहुलमीर्ष्युं राक्षसं विद्यात् (२)।

महाशनं स्त्रैणं स्त्रीरहस्काममशुचिं शुचिद्वेषिणं भीरुं भीषयितारं विकृतविहाराहारशीलं पैशाचं विद्यात् (३)।

क्रुद्धशूरमक्रुद्धभीरुं तीक्ष्णमायासबहुलं सन्त्रस्तगोचरमाहारविहारपरं सार्पं विद्यात् (४)।

आहारकाममतिदुःखशीलाचारोपचारमसूयकमसंविभागिनमतिलोलुपमकर्मशीलं प्रैतं विद्यात् (५)।

अनुषक्तकाममजस्रमाहारविहारपरमनवस्थितममर्षणमसञ्चयं शाकुनं विद्यात् (६)।

इत्येवं खलु राजसस्य सत्त्वस्य षड्विधं भेदांशं विद्यात्, रोषांशत्वात्॥३८॥

The Rajasika type of mental faculty represents wrathful disposition and is of six types. Their characteristic features are furnished in the statement given below:

Types of mental faculty Characteristic features of the individual

1 Asura 1 Bravery, cruelty, envy, lordship movement in disguise, terrifying appearance and ruthlessness and

2 Indulgence in self praise

2 Raksasa (sharing the traits of Raksasa) 1 Intolerance, consent anger, violence at weak points, cruelty gluttonous habits and fondness for non-vegetarian food

2 Excessive sleep and indolence and

3 Envious sleep and indolence

3 Paisaca (sharing the traits of Pisaca) 1 Gluttonous habit

2 Fondness for women

3 Liking for staying with women in lonely place

4 Unclean habits, disliking for cleanliness

5 Cowardice and terrifying disposition and

6 Resorting to abnormal diet and regimens

4 Sarpa (sharing the traits of Sarpa or Snake) 1 Bravery when in wrathful disposition and cowardice when not in wrathful disposition

2 Sharp reaction

3 Excessive indolence and

4 Walking, talking food and resorting to other regimens with a fearful disposition

5 Praita (sharing the traits of a Preta) 1 Excessive desire for food

2 Excessively painful disposition in character and past times

3 Enviousness and

4 Actions without discrimination excessive greediness and inaction

6 Sakuna (sharing the traits of a Sakuni or Bird) 1 Attachment with passion, excessive food and regimen, unsteadiness, ruthlessness and acquistiveness. [38]

Different types of Tamasa Individuals:

निराकरिष्णुममेधसं जुगुप्सिताचाराहरं मैथुनपरं स्वप्नशीलं पाशवं विद्यात् (१)।

भीरुमबुधमाहारलुब्धमनवस्थितमनुषक्तकामक्रोधं सरणशीलं तोयकामं मात्स्यं विद्यात् (२)।

अलसं केवलमभिनिविष्टमाहारे सर्वबुद्ध्यङ्गहीनं वानस्पत्यं विद्यात् (३)।

इत्येवं तामसस्य सत्त्वस्य त्रिविधं भेदांशं विद्यान्मोहांशत्त्वात्।।३९।।

The Tamasika type of mental faculty represents ignorant disposition and is of three types. Their characteristic features are furnished in the statement given below:

Type of mental faculty Characteristic features of the individual

1 Pasava (sharing the traits of animal) 1 Forbidding disposition

2 Lack of intelligence

3 Excessive sexual indulgence and sleep

2 Matsya (sharing the traits of fish) 1 Cowardice, lack of intelligence greediness for food, unsteadiness, constant passionate and wrathful disposition and

2 Fondness for constant movement and desire for water

3 Vanaspatya (sharing the traits of vegetable life) Indolence, indulgence in food, and defines of all the intellectual faculties. [39]

Innumerability of the types of mental faculties:

इत्यपरिसङ्ख्येयभेदानां त्रयाणामपि सत्त्वानां भेदैकदेशो व्याख्यातः; शुद्धस्य सत्त्वस्य सप्तविधो ब्रह्मर्षिशक्रयमवरुणकुबेरगन्धर्वसत्त्वानुकारेण, राजसस्य षड्विधो दैत्यपिशाचराक्षससर्पप्रेतशकुनिसत्त्वानुकारेण, तामसस्य त्रिविधः पशुमत्स्यवनस्पतिसत्त्वानुकारेण, कथं च यथासत्त्वमुपचारः स्यादिति।।४०।।

The three types of mental faculties have innumerable varieties.

- The sattvika type of mental faculty is of seven types depending upon the dispositions of Brahmi, Rsi, Indra, Yama, Varuna, Kubera and Gandharva.

- The Rajasa type of mental faculty is of six types upon the dispositions of Asura, Raksasa, Pisaca, Sarpa, Preta and

Sakuni.

- The Tamasa type of mental faculty is of three types depending upon the dispositions of Pashu (animal), Matsya (fish) and Vanaspati (vegetable life).

All these descriptions are made with a view to indicate the general mode of treatments that should be provided for these types of persons. [40]

केवलश्चायमुद्देशो यथोद्देशमभिनिर्दिष्टो भवति गर्भावक्रान्तिसम्प्रयुक्तः ; तस्य चार्थस्य विज्ञाने सामर्थ्य गर्भकराणां च भावानामनुसमाधिः, विधातश्च विघातकराणां भावानामिति||४१||

The description above is fully in keeping with the purpose with which the chapter was initiated i.e., to provide knowledge one can help resort to the factors which are responsible for the proper growth of the foetus and avoid such factors which come in the way of its proper development. [41]

To sum up:

तत्र श्लोकाः-

निमित्तमात्मा प्रकृतिर्वृद्धिः कुक्षौ क्रमेण च|
वृद्धिहेतुश्च गर्भस्य पञ्चार्थाः शुभसञ्ज्ञिताः||४२||
अजन्मनि च यो हेतुर्विनाशे विकृतावपि|
इमांस्त्रीनशुभान् भावानाहुर्गर्भविघातकान्||४३||
शुभाशुभसमाख्यातानष्टौ भावानिमान् भिषक्|
सर्वथा वेद यः सर्वान् स राज्ञः कर्तुमर्हति||४४||
अवाप्त्युपायान् गर्भस्य स एवं ज्ञातुमर्हति|
ये च गर्भविघातोक्ता भावास्तांश्चाप्युदारधीः||४५||

The following topics are discussed in this chapter:

The five auspicious factors, Viz., (a) instrumental cause, (b) Soul, (c) material cause, (d) gradual development of the foetus in the womb and, (e) factors responsible for the growth of the foetus in the womb.

The five inauspicious factors which are injurious to the foetus, viz (a) factors which are responsible for the prevention of conception and (b) destruction of or, (c) deformity in the foetus.

He who knows all aspects of all these eight factors which are auspicious for the foetus is fit to be a royal physician.

An intelligent physician should know those factors which help in the formation and growth of the foetus and also those which are responsible for the destruction of the foetus. [42-45]

इत्यग्निवेशकृते तन्त्रे चरकप्रतिसंस्कृते शारीरस्थाने महतीगर्भावक्रान्तिशारीरं नाम चतुर्थोऽध्यायः||४||

Thus ends the fourth major chapter of the Sharira section of "Formation of the Embryo" as conducive to the understanding of the body of Agnivesha's work as redacted by Charaka. [4]

21

Shareerasthana Chapter 5 Purusha Vichayam Shareeram

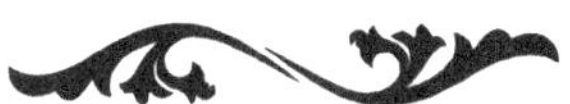

Individual and Universe

अथातः पुरुषविचयं शारीरं व्याख्यास्यामः||१||

इति ह स्माह भगवानात्रेयः||२||

Now we shall explore the chapter dealing with "the individual as an Epitome of the Universe" as conducive to the understanding of the body. Thus said Lord Atreya [1-2]

Individual – an epitome of universe:

पुरुषोऽयं लोकसम्मितः' इत्युवाच भगवान् पुनर्वसुरात्रेयः|

यावन्तो हि लोके (मूर्तिमन्तो) भावविशेषास्तावन्तः पुरुषे, यावन्तः पुरुषे तावन्तो लोके; इत्येवंवादिनं भगवन्तमात्रेयमग्निवेश उवाच- नैतावता वाक्येनोक्तं वाक्यार्थमवगाहामहे, भगवता बुद्ध्या भूयस्तरमतोऽनुव्याख्यायमानं शुश्रूषामह इति||३||

तमुवाच भगवानात्रेयः- अपरिसङ्ख्येया लोकावयविशेषाः, पुरुषावयविशेषा अप्यपरिसङ्ख्येयाः; तेषां यथास्थूलं कतिचिद्भावान् सामान्यमभिप्रेत्योदाहरिष्यामः, तानेकमना निबोध सम्यगुपवर्ण्यमानानग्निवेश!|

षड्धातवः समुदिताः 'पुरुष' इति शब्दं लभन्ते; तद्यथा- पृथिव्यापस्तेजो वायुराकाशं ब्रह्म चाव्यक्तमिति, एत एव च षड्धातवः समुदिताः 'पुरुष' इति शब्दं लभन्ते||४||

An individual is an epitome of the universe as all material and spiritual phenomena of the universe are present in the individual and all those present in the individual are also contained in the universe.

"Thus said Punarvasu Atreya. Then Agnivesha enquired, "We cannot grasp the idea contained in this aphoristic statement from your enlightened self. "Lord Atreya replied, "Innumerable are the specific parts of the universe and so are innumerable the specific parts of an individual. I will explain to you some of the gross phenomena common to the universe as well as the individual, listen to me attentively Agnivesha. Purusha is nothing but the combination of the six Dhatus, i.e. Prthvi - earth, Jala - water, Teja / Agni – fire, Vayu – air / wind, Akasha – ether and Brahman – the soul. [3-4]

Identity of factors in individual with those of universe:

तस्य पुरुषस्य पृथिवी मूर्तिः, आपः क्लेदः, तेजोऽभिसन्तापः, वायुः प्राणः, वियत् सुषिराणि, ब्रह्म अन्तरात्मा|

यथा खलु ब्राह्मी विभूतिर्लोके तथा पुरुषेऽप्यान्तरात्मिकी विभूतिः, ब्रह्मणो विभूतिर्लोके प्रजापतिरन्तरात्मनो विभूतिः पुरुषे सत्वं, यस्त्विन्द्रो लोके स पुरुषेऽहङ्कारः, आदित्यस्त्वादानं, रुद्रो रोषः, सोमः प्रसादः, वसवः सुखम्, अश्विनौ कान्तिः, मरुदुत्साहः, विश्वेदेवाः सर्वेन्द्रियाणि सर्वेन्द्रियार्थाश्च, तमो मोहः, ज्योतिर्ज्ञानं, यथा लोकस्य सर्गादिस्तथा पुरुषस्य गर्भाधानं, यथा कृतयुगमेवं बाल्यं, यथा त्रेता तथा यौवनं, यथा द्वापरस्तथा स्थाविर्य, यथा कलिरेवमातुर्य, यथा युगान्तस्तथा मरणमिति|

एवमेतेनानुमानेनानुक्तानामपि लोकपुरुषयोरवयवविशेषाणामग्निवेश! सामान्यं विद्यादिति||५||

Prthvi constitutes the form of man,

Jala – constitutes the moisture,

Tejas – constitutes the heat,

Vayu – constitutes the life element / élan Vitae,

Akasha – constitutes all the porous parts and

Brahman – constitutes the internal Soul.

Identity of the various universal phenomena as present in the individual is given below:

Universal Phenomena Corresponding phenomena in man

1,2 Potentially of the Brahman symbolised by Daksha Prajapati 1,2 Potentially of the internal Soul symbolised by the mind

3 Indra 3 Ahamkara (ego)

4 Aditya 4 Accumulation

5 Rudra 5 Anger

6 Soma (Moon) 6 Pleasure

7 Vasus 7 Happiness

8 The Asvins 8 complexion

9 Marut 9 enthusiasm

10 Visvedeva 10 All the senses and objects of senses.

11 Tamas (darkness) 11 Ignorance

12 Jyothi (light) 12 Knowledge

13 Beginning of creation 13 Impregnation

14 Krta age 14 Childhood

15 Treta age 15 Youth

16 Dvapara age 16 Middle age

17 Kali age 17 Old age

18 Deluge 18 Death

The above description is given only by way of illustration. There are many other phenomena common to the universe and man which can be understood by inference, O! Agnivesha. [5]

Utility of the knowledge of the Individual as an epitome of Universe:

एवंवादिनं भगवन्तमात्रेयमग्निवेश उवाच- एवमेतत् सर्वमनपवादं यथोक्तं भगवता लोकपुरुषयोः सामान्यम्|

किन्न्वस्य सामान्योपदेशस्य प्रयोजनमिति||६||

भगवानुवाच- शृण्वग्निवेश! सर्वलोकमात्मन्यात्मानं च सर्वलोके सममनुपश्यतः सत्या बुद्धिः समुत्पद्यते|

सर्वलोकं ह्यात्मनि पश्यतो भवत्यात्मैव सुखदुःखयोः कर्ता नान्य इति|

कर्मात्मकत्वाच्च हेत्वादिभिर्युक्तः सर्वलोकोऽहमिति विदित्वा ज्ञानं पूर्वमुत्थाप्यतेऽपवर्गायेति|

तत्र संयोगापेक्षीलोकशब्दः|

षड्धातुसमुदायो हि सामान्यतः सर्वलोकः||७||

Agnivesha again asked Lord Atreya, "All that you have said about the identity of phenomena present in the universe and man is true without any exception. But then how is this statement relevant in the context of medicine?".

Lord Atreya replied, "Listen to me O! Agnivesha. One who sees equality in the entire universe in his own self, and his own self in the entire universe is in possession of true knowledge. Such a person experiencing the entire universe in his own self believes that none but his own self is responsible for happiness and miseries. The individual self being subordinate to his own action indulges in various activities only when impelled by hetu (cause) etc. As soon as he realises his identity with the entire universe, he is in possession of true knowledge which stands him in good stead in getting salvation.

The term "Loka" implies here a combination of several factors. A congregation of six Dhatus constitutes the entire universe consisting of all creatures. [6-7]

Miseries and happiness of the Individual:

तस्य हेतुः, उत्पत्तिः, वृद्धिः, उपप्लवः, वियोगश्च।

तत्र हेतुरुत्पत्तिकारणं, उत्पत्तिर्जन्म, वृद्धिराप्यायनम्, उपप्लवो दुःखागमः, षड्धातुविभागो वियोगः सजीवापगमः स प्राणनिरोधः स भङ्गः स लोकस्वभावः।

तस्य मूलं सर्वोपप्लवानां च प्रवृत्तिः, निवृत्तिरुपरमः।

प्रवृत्तिर्दुःखं, निवृत्तिः सुखमिति यज्ज्ञानमुत्पद्यते तत् सत्यम्।

तस्य हेतुः सर्वलोकसामान्यज्ञानम्।

एतत्प्रयोजनं सामान्योपदेशस्येति॥८॥

An individual has a Hetu (cause), Utpatti (birth), Vrddhi (growth), Upaplava (Decay) and Viyoga (dissolution). Hetu is the cause of manifestation, Utpatti is birth, Vrddhi is growth, Upaplava is insulation or attainment of the natural state.

His attachment to the various actions constitutes a causative factor of all his miseries and detachment a causative factor of cessation of all miseries. Realisation of the fact that 'attachment leads to miseries' and 'detachment leads to happiness' is considered as the real knowledge.

This knowledge can be achieved only by virtue of the realisation of the identity of the universe and man. This is the object of instruction relating to the identity of the universe and man. [8]

Cause of attachment and method of detachment:

अथाग्निवेश उवाच- किम्मूला भगवन्! प्रवृत्तिः, निवृत्तौ च क उपाय इति॥९॥

भगवानुवाच- मोहेच्छाद्वेषकर्ममूला प्रवृत्तिः।

तज्जा ह्यहङ्कारसङ्गसंशयाभिसम्प्लवाभ्यवपातविप्रत्ययाविशेषानुपायास्तरुणमिव द्रुममतिविपुलशाखास्तरवोऽभिभूय पुरुषमवतत्यैवोतिष्ठन्ते; यैरभिभूतो न सतामतिवर्तते।

तत्रैवञ्जातिरूपवित्तवृत्तबुद्धिशीलविद्याभिजनवयोवीर्यप्रभावसम्पन्नोऽहमित्यहङ्कारः, यन्मनोवाक्कायकर्म नापवर्गाय स सङ्गः, कर्मफलमोक्षपुरुषप्रेत्यभावादयः सन्ति वा नेति संशयः, सर्वावस्थास्वनन्योऽहमहं स्रष्टा स्वभावसंसिद्धोऽहमहं शरीरेन्द्रियबुद्धिस्मृतिविशेषराशिरिति ग्रहणमभिसम्प्लवः, मम मातृपितृभ्रातृदारापत्यबन्धुमित्रभृत्यगणो गणस्य चाहमित्यभ्यवपातः, कार्याकार्यहिताहितशुभाशुभेषु विपरीताभिनिवेशो विप्रत्ययः, ज्ञाज्ञयोः प्रकृतिविकारयोः प्रवृत्तिनिवृत्योश्च सामान्यदर्शनमविशेषः, प्रोक्षणानशनाग्निहोत्रत्रिषवणाभ्युक्षणावाहनयाजनयजनयाचनसलिलहुताशनप्रवेशादयः समारम्भाः प्रोच्यन्ते ह्यनुपायाः।

एवमयमधीधृतिस्मृतिरहङ्काराभिनिविष्टः सक्तः ससंशयोऽभिसम्प्लुतबुद्धिररभ्यवपतितोऽन्यथादृष्टिरविशेषग्राही विमार्गगतिर्निवासवृक्षः सत्त्वशरीरदोषमूलानां सर्वदुःखानां भवति।

एवमहङ्कारादिभिर्दोषैर्भ्राम्यमाणो नातिवर्तते प्रवृत्तिं, सा च मूलमघस्य॥१०॥

Thereafter Agnivesha asked, "What is the cause of attachment and what are the factors responsible for detachment?" Lord Atreya said, "Attachment is caused by ignorance, desire, hatred and purposeful action. Ahamkara, Sanga, Samshaya, abhisamplava, abhyavapata, Vipratyaya, avisesa and Anupaya also arise out of attachment.

These factors arising out of attachment would encroach and envelope an individual, overcome (dominate) him and become all powerful just like a big tree with many long branches dominate (overcome) and overgrow a small tree and become all powerful and encroaching. These factors engulf an individual to such an extent that he would find it impossible to free himself from the clutches of ignorance etc worldly habits.

Ahamkara represents an egoistic feeling. It is to tell 'I belong to the best clan, I am endowed with the best of appearance, wealth, goodness, character, great intelligence, great conduct, good family / lineage, youth, valour / potency and influence.

Sanga represents that mental, vocal or bodily action which is not conducive to the attainment of salvation.

Samsaya stands for doubt regarding the existence of the result of the past action, salvation, soul, life after death, reincarnation / rebirth etc.

Abhisamplava – includes imbibing or establishing the other's quality. It can be considered as the mistaken perception of identifying one's soul with one's body. Example – making statements like 'in any given situation, I am second to none (I am the ultimate)', or 'I am the creator of everything' or 'I am a self established and accomplished person by nature' or 'I am a combination of body, sense organs, intelligence and memory'.

Abhyavapata – It includes showing possessiveness towards the things indifferent to self and which doesn't belong to self. It is a sense of ownership. Example – 'telling I have father, mother, wife, progeny, relatives, friends and servants and I belong to them'.

Vipratyaya – includes 'contrasting belief' like considering a desirable act as undesirable, something beneficial as non-beneficial or harmful and the acts and things which are auspicious as inauspicious and vice versa.

Avishesha – is the lack of distinction when a person becomes incapable of making distinction between consciousness and unconsciousness, nature and its modifications, attachment and non-attachment (detachment).

Anupaya – includes religious rituals which are inefficient. These rituals include –

- Proksana – consecration
- Anashana – fasting / starvation
- Agnihotra – oblation to the fire
- Trishavana – performing sacrifice thrice a day while worshipping soma
- Abhyukshana – wetting
- Aavahana – invocation
- Yajana – leading or guiding sacrificial rituals
- Yajna – fire sacrifice
- Yachana – begging
- Salila hutashana praveshah – entering into water and fire

The person becomes an abode of all miseries and is also trapped in the vicious cycle of life and death and will not attain salvation if –

- he is devoid of intellect, restraint and memory
- is egoistic and self centred
- is attached to objects, persons and actions
- is incapable of distinguishing between what is good and what is bad
- is unable to distinguish between self (soul) and the physical body

The well-being of the purusha – individually and also socially - is the source of salvation from all kinds of miseries which eventually is also the ultimate goal of Ayurveda.

Salvation and ways and means of attaining it:

निवृत्तिरपवर्गः; तत् परं प्रशान्तं तत्तदक्षरं तद्ब्रह्म स मोक्षः॥११॥

तत्र मुमुक्षूणामुदयनानि व्याख्यास्यामः।

तत्र लोकदोषदर्शिनो मुमुक्षोरादित एवाचार्याभिगमनं, तस्योपदेशानुष्ठानम्, अग्नेरेवोपचर्या, धर्मशास्त्रानुगमनं, तदर्थावबोधः, तेनावष्टम्भः, तत्र यथोक्ताः क्रियाः, सतामुपासनम्, असतां परिवर्जनम्, असङ्गतिर्दुर्जनेन, सत्यं सर्वभूतहितमपरुषमनतिकाले परीक्ष्य वचनं, सर्वप्राणिषु चात्मनीवावेक्षा, सर्वासामस्मरणमसङ्कल्पनमप्रार्थनमनभिभाषणं च स्त्रीणां, सर्वपरिग्रहत्यागः, कौपीनं प्रच्छादनार्थं, धातुरागनिवसनं, कन्थासीवनहेतोः सूचीपिप्पलकं, शौचाधानतोर्जलकुण्डिका, दण्डधारणं, भैक्षचर्यार्थं पात्रं, प्राणधारणार्थमेककालमग्राम्यो यथोपपन्नोऽभ्यवहारः, श्रमापनयनार्थं शीर्णशुष्कपर्णतृणास्तरणोपधानं, ध्यानहेतोः कायनिबन्धनं, वनेष्वनिकेतवासः, तन्द्रानिन्द्रालस्यादिकर्मवर्जनं, इन्द्रियार्थेष्वनुरागोपतापनिग्रहः, सुप्तस्थितगतप्रेक्षिता हारविहारप्रत्यङ्गचेष्टादिकेष्वारम्भेषु स्मृतिपूर्विका प्रवृत्तिः, सत्कारस्तुतिगर्हावमानक्षमत्वं, क्षुत्पिपासायासश्रमशीतोष्णवातवर्षासुखदुःखसंस्पर्शसहत्वं, शोकदैन्यमानोद्वेगमदलोभरागेष्याभयक्रोधादिभिरसञ्चलनम्, अहङ्कारादिष्वपसर्गसञ्ज्ञा, लोकपुरुषयोः सर्गादिसामान्यावेक्षणं, कार्यकालात्ययभयं, योगारम्भे सततमनिर्वेदः, सत्त्वोत्साहः, अपवर्गाय धीधृतिस्मृतिबलाधानं; नियमनमिन्द्रियाणां चेतसि, चेतस आत्मनि, आत्मनश्च; धातुभेदेन शरीरावयवसङ्ख्यानमभीक्ष्णं, सर्वं कारणवद्दुःखमस्वमनित्यमित्यभ्युपगमः, सर्वप्रवृत्तिष्वघसञ्ज्ञा, सर्वसन्न्यासे सुखमित्यभिनिवेशः; एष मार्गोऽपवर्गाय, अतोऽन्यथा बध्यते; इत्युदयनानि व्याख्यातानि॥१२॥

Detachment is salvation.

It is Para (absolute).

It is Prasanta (Serene).

It is Akshara (immutable).

It is Brahman.

It is Moksha (Emancipation),

We shall now explain the ways and means of getting salvation. From the very beginning the following constitute the conduct and behaviour of a man who has realised the defects of the world and who is desirous of getting salvation:

Visit to the preceptor i.e. the one imparting instructions on salvation

To carry out his instructions

Exclusive service to the fire

To follow the prescriptions of religious scriptures

To understand the meaning of such scriptures

To have patience as prescribed in scriptures

To perform acts as prescribed in scriptures

Devotion to the noble

To keep away from the company of the wicked

Dissociation with the wicked

To make statement which are true, useful for all creatures and not harsh; such statements should be made after proper examination at appropriate time

To look at all creatures as if they represent himself

Avoidance of all contacts including remembering, thinking, requesting and talking with woman

Avoidance of all acquisitions

Wearing of Kaupina (loin- cloth)

Wearing of saffron coloured dress

Having a needle case for the sewing of robe

Having a water pot for maintaining cleanliness

Having sacred Danda (stick)

Having sacred begging bowel

Taking prescribed food only once a day just to preserve his life

Having a bed consisting of dry leaves, grass etc, just for rest

Use of Yogapatta (a wooden resting plank) for meditation

Living in the woods without having any home

Avoidance of drowsiness, sleep, laziness etc

Avoidance of attachment and hatred towards the objects of sense organs

Initiating actions like sleeping, staying, going, seeing, eating, enjoying, movement of all various limbs (with a sense of recollection of the nature of his own soul etc)

Maintenance of serenity in the face of honour, praise, criticism and insult

To stand the onslaught of hunger, thirst, efforts, labour, cold, heat, wind, rains, happiness, miseries and sensory contacts non-disturbance by sorrow, miseries, respect, perturbation, vanity, greed, attachment, envy, fear, anger etc

To view pride etc, as disturbing factors

To remember the identical nature of creation etc, of the self and the universe

To be afraid of postponing actions conducive to salvation

To have confidence in yogic practices

To be optimistic about spiritual attainments

To direct intelligence, patience, memory and strength for salvation

Restraint of sense organs in the mind (so as not to allow them to move towards external objects) restraint of the mind in the self and finally of the self in himself

Realisation of different organs of the body as composed of Dhatus (tissue elements)

To realise that belonging to self

To view all attached actions as sinful and

To consider renunciation as a potent factor for happiness

This is the gateway to salvation. One finds himself in bondage otherwise. Thus the ways and means to salvation are explained. [11-12]

Thus it is said:-

भवन्ति चात्र-

एतैरविमलं सत्त्वं शुद्ध्युपायैर्विशुध्यति।
मृज्यमान इवादर्शस्तैलचेलकचादिभिः||१३||
ग्रहाम्बुदरजोधूमनीहारैरसमावृतम्।
यथार्कमण्डलं भाति भाति सत्त्वं तथाऽमलम्||१४||
ज्वलत्यात्मनि संरुद्धं तत् सत्त्वं संवृतायने।
शुद्धः स्थिरः प्रसन्नार्चिर्दीपो दीपाशये यथा||१५||

The vitiated mind gets purified by these purifying factors as a mirror is cleaned with the help of oil-cloth, hair etc. Just like the Sun dazzles when it is not covered by Rahu, cold, dust, smoke and fog, the mind too shines when it is in a state of purity.

While restrained in the soul with his movement obscured, the mind, pure and stable, shines just like the lamp shines with bright flame in the lamp case. [13-15]

शुद्धसत्त्वस्य या शुद्धा सत्या बुद्धिः प्रवर्तते।
यया भिनत्यतिबलं महामोहमयं तमः||१६||
सर्वभावस्वभावज्ञो यया भवति निःस्पृहः।
योगं यया साधयते साङ्ख्यः सम्पद्यते यया||१७||
यया नोपैत्यहङ्कारं नोपास्ते कारणं यया।
यया नालम्बते किञ्चित् सर्वं सन्न्यस्यते यया||१८||
याति ब्रह्म यया नित्यमजरं शान्तमव्ययम् [१] ।
विद्या सिद्धिर्मतिर्मेधा प्रज्ञा ज्ञानं च सा मता||१९||

A person with his mind pure, is in possession of true wisdom

- which dispels the excessively thick darkness caused by ignorance,
- which brings about detachment and knowledge about the nature of all things,
- which is conducive to the attainment of yogic power,
- which renders an individual wise,
- which brings about freedom from vanity and detachment from the causative factors of miseries,
- which renders an individual free from hopes,
- which brings about renunciation and
- which serves as a means to attainment of Brahman, the Eternal, Immutable, Tranquil and Indestructible

It is this wisdom which is known as Vidya (learning), Siddhi (accomplishment), Mati (Jnana (knowledge). [16-19]

Effect of identification of the individual with the Universe

लोके विततमात्मानं लोकं चात्मनि पश्यतः।
परावरदृशः शान्तिर्ज्ञानमूला न नश्यति||२०||

If one realises himself as spread in the entire universe and the entire universe spreads in him, he is indeed in possession of transcendental and worldly vision. His serenity of mind based on wisdom does never feed away. [20]

Cessation of contacts:

पश्यतः सर्वभावान् हि सर्वावस्थासु सर्वदा।
ब्रह्मभूतस्य संयोगो न शुद्धस्योपपद्यते||२१||

When a person visualises the presence of everything in all situations, he is one with Brahma, the absolute. He no longer has any contacts with the various and sinful acts. [21]

Liberation from bondage:

नात्मनः करणाभावाल्लिङ्गमप्युपलभ्यते।

स सर्वकरणायोगान्मुक्त इत्यभिधीयते।।२२।।

It is not possible even to characterize the liberated Soul because he has no contact whatsoever with mental or other sense faculties. So, being detached of all sensory contacts, he is considered to be a liberated Soul. [22]

Synonyms of "Santi (Liberation)"

विपापं विरजः शान्तं परमक्षरमव्ययम्।

अमृतं ब्रह्म निर्वाणं पर्यायैः शान्तिरुच्यते।।२३।।

एतत्तत् सौम्य! विज्ञानं यज्ज्ञात्वा मुक्तसंशयाः।

मुनयः प्रशमं जग्मुर्वीतमोहरजःस्पृहाः।।२४।।

Shanti (Liberation) is synonymous with Vipapa (free from sinful acts), Viraja (free from attachments), Santa (serene), Para (absolute), Aksara (indestructible), Avyaya (immutable), and Amrita (extinction of all miseries). This is spiritual knowledge after knowing which, the sages get freedom from all doubts, ignorance, attachment and desires attain the state of Prasama (absolute tranquillity) i.e. salvation. [23-24]

तत्र श्लोकौ-

सप्रयोजनमुद्दिष्टं लोकस्य पुरुषस्य च।

सामान्यं मूलमुत्पत्तौ निवृत्तौ मार्ग एव च।।२५।।

शुद्धसत्त्वसमाधानं सत्या बुद्धिश्च नैष्ठिकी।

विचये पुरुषस्योक्ता निष्ठा च परमर्षिणा।।२६।।

To sum up: -

In this chapter with 'the individual as an epitome of the universe', the sage has described the following topics:

The common origin of the universe and the individual together with purpose behind the knowledge of such a common knowledge.

Attainment of the pure state of the mind

Virtuous intellect conducive to the attainment of salvation and

Salvation [25-26]

इत्यग्निवेशकृते तन्त्रे चरकप्रतिसंस्कृते शारीरस्थाने पुरुषविचयशारीरं नाम पञ्चमोऽध्यायः।।५।।

Thus ends the fifth chapter dealing with "the Individual as an Epitome of the universe as conducive to the understanding of the body" of the Sharira section of Agnivesha's work as redacted by Charaka. [5]

22

Shareerasthana Chapter 6
Shareera Vichayam Shareeram

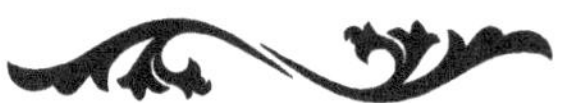

Constitution of Physique

अथातः शरीरविचयं शारीरं व्याख्यास्यामः॥१॥

इति ह स्माह भगवानात्रेयः॥२॥

We shall now expound the chapter on 'knowledge of the details of the Body" as conducive to its understanding. Thus said Lord Atreya [1-2]

Utility of the detailed knowledge of body:

शरीरविचयः शरीरोपकारार्थमिष्यते।

ज्ञात्वा हि शरीरतत्त्वं शरीरोपकारकरेषु भावेषु ज्ञानमुत्पद्यते।

तस्माच्छरीरविचयं प्रशंसन्ति कुशलाः॥३॥

Detailed knowledge of body:

Detailed knowledge of the human body is conducive to the wellbeing of the individual. Understanding of the factors that constitute the body provides knowledge regarding the factors which are responsible for its well being. It is because of this that experts praise the knowledge of the details of the body (and insist that one has a thorough knowledge of the same). [3]

Composition of body - results of their concordance & discordance:

तत्र शरीरं नाम चेतनाधिष्ठानभूतं पञ्चमहाभूतविकारसमुदायात्मकं समयोगवाहि ।

यदा ह्यस्मिन् शरीरे धातवो वैषम्यमापद्यन्ते तदा क्लेशं विनाशं वा प्राप्नोति।

वैषम्यगमनं हि पुनर्धातूनां वृद्धिह्रासगमनमकात्स्न्येर्न प्रकृत्या च॥४॥

The body which is maintained in a state of equilibrium represents the conglomeration of factors derived from five Mahabhutas and this is the site of manifestation of consciousness. When Dhatus in this body becomes conflicting then there is disease or destruction (of the body). Aggravation or diminution of dhatus either partially or in their entirety constitutes this discordance. [4]

यौगपद्येन तु विरोधिनां धातूनां वृद्धिह्रासौ भवतः।

यद्धि यस्य धातोर्वृद्धिकरं तत्ततो विपरीतगुणस्य धातोः प्रत्यवायकरं सम्पद्यते॥५॥

Dhatus having mutually opposite qualities undergo increase and decrease simultaneously. A thing which increases a particular Dhatu is also responsible for the decrease of the Dhatu having opposite qualities. [5]

Maintaining equilibrium of Dhatus is the object of treatment:

तदेव तस्माद्भेषजं सम्यगवचार्यमाणं युगपन्न्यूनातिरिक्तानां धातूनां साम्यकरं भवति, अधिकमपकर्षति न्यूनमाप्याययति॥६॥

Therefore, medical therapies when properly administered simultaneously bring both the reduced and increased

Dhatus to their normal state by reducing the increased ones and increasing the reduced ones. [6]

Maintenance of equilibrium of Dhatus:

एतावदेव हि भैषज्यप्रयोगे फलमिष्टं स्वस्थवृत्तानुष्ठाने च यावद्धातूनां साम्यं स्यात्|

स्वस्था ह्यपि धातूनां साम्यानुग्रहार्थमेव कुशला रसगुणानाहारविकारांश्च पर्यायेणेच्छन्त्युपयोक्तुं सात्म्यसमाज्ञातान्; एकप्रकारभूयिष्ठांश्चोपयुञ्जानास्तद्विपरीतकरसमाज्ञातया चेष्टया सममिच्छन्ति कर्तुम्||७||

While administering therapies and also while resorting to regimens for the maintenance of positive health, equilibrium of Dhatus is sought for as the 'end result'.

Even healthy persons should properly use wholesome food with appropriate taste and attributes and also foods processed properly with an intention to maintain the equilibrium of Dhatus.

After taking the food dominated by particular attributes, it is desirable to neutralize their effects by resorting to the regimens which are contradictory to them. [7]

Instructions for maintaining equilibrium:

देशकालात्मगुणविपरीतानां हि कर्मणामाहारविकाराणां च क्रियोपयोगः सम्यक्, सर्वातियोगसन्धारणम्, असन्धारणमुदीर्णानां च गतिमतां, साहसानां च वर्जनं, स्वस्थवृत्तमेतावद्धातूनां साम्यानुग्रहार्थमुपदिश्यते||८||

Equilibrium of dhatus provides positive health. To maintain this equilibrium one should follow the below mentioned advices –

- One should properly resort to such actions and take such foods which are contrary to the locality, season and physical constitution of the individual. For example, one should indulge in sleep while living in a desert; one should resort to exercise during the spring season; an individual with a fatty body should resort to exercise and vigil in excess.
- One should refrain from excessive utilization, wrong utilization and non-utilization of the time, intellect and objects of senses.
- One should not suppress manifested urges and
- One should refrain from exhibiting strength beyond one's real capacity. [8]

Food and Dhatus:

धातवः पुनः शारीराः समानगुणैः समानगुणभूयिष्ठैर्वाऽप्याहारविकारैरभ्यस्यमानैर्वृद्धिं प्राप्नुवन्ति, ह्रासं तु विपरीतगुणैर्विपरीतगुणभूयिष्ठैर्वाऽप्याहारैरभ्यस्यमानैः||९||

Dhatus (tissue elements) inside the body of the individual get increased by the habitual use of food preparations which are either of similar attributes or are dominated by such attributes. Habitual use of foods having opposite qualities or having the dominance of such opposite qualities reduces the Dhatus. [9]

Attributes of Dhatus in the Body:

तत्रेमे शरीरधातुगुणाः सङ्ख्यासामर्थ्यकराः; तद्यथा-

गुरुलघुशीतोष्णस्निग्धरूक्षमन्दतीक्ष्णस्थिरसरमृदुकठिनविशदपिच्छिलश्लक्ष्णखरसूक्ष्मस्थूलसान्द्रद्रवाः|

तेषु ये गुरवस्ते गुरुभिराहारविकारगुणैरभ्यस्यमानैराप्याय्यन्ते, लघवश्च ह्रसन्ति; लघवस्तु लघुभिराप्याय्यन्ते, गुरवश्च ह्रसन्ति|

एवमेव सर्वधातुगुणानां सामान्ययोगाद्वृद्धिः, विपर्ययाद्ध्रासः|

तस्मान्मांसमाप्याय्यते मांसेन भूयस्तरमन्येभ्यः शरीरधातुभ्यः, तथा लोहितं लोहितेन, मेदो मेदसा, वसा वसया, अस्थि तरुणास्थ्ना, मज्जा मज्ज्ञा, शुक्रं शुक्रेण, गर्भस्त्वामगर्भेण||१०||

Guru (heaviness)

Laghu (lightness)

Shita (coldness)

Usna (heat)

Snigdha (unctuousness)

Ruksa (roughness)

Manda (dullness)

Tiksna (sharpness)

Sthira (immobility)

Sara (mobility / flow)

Mrdu (softness)

Kathina (hardness)

Visassa (non sliminess)

Picchila (sliminess)

Suksma (minuteness)

Sthula (bulkiness, stoutness)

Sandra (density) and

Drava (liquidity)

These are the twenty attributes of body tissues which account for their increase or decrease. By the habitual use of heavy food preparations the Dhatus which are heavy (having heaviness attribute / quality) get increased, and those which are light (having lightness attribute / quality) get reduced. Similarly by the continued use of lighter foods the tissues which are light get increased and the tissues which are heavy get decreased.

Similarly, all Dhatus get increased by the use of substances having similar properties and get reduced by the use of those having opposite properties. Following the same principle - by consumption of meat the muscle tissues in the body would increase in comparison to the other tissues. Similarly blood tissue increases by blood, adipose tissue would increase by fat, consumption of muscle fat increases the same tissue i.e. muscle fat, consumption of cartilage increases bone tissue, the bone marrow tissue would increase on consumption of bone marrow, semen would increase on consumption of semen and the foetus would increase by consumption of amagarbha i.e. immature foetus such as an egg. [10]

Administration of ingredients having predominance of attributes:

यत्र त्वेवंलक्षणेन सामान्येन सामान्यवतामाहारविकाराणामसान्निध्यं स्यात्, सन्निहितानां वाऽप्ययुक्तत्वान्नोपयोगो घृणित्वादन्यस्माद्वा कारणात्, स च धातुरभिवर्धयितव्यः स्यात्, तस्य ये समानगुणाः स्युराहारविकारा असेव्याश्च, तत्र समानगुणभूयिष्ठानामन्यप्रकृतीनामप्याहारविकाराणामुपयोगः स्यात्।

तद्यथा- शुक्रक्षये क्षीरसर्पिषोरुपयोगो मधुरस्निग्धशीतसमाख्यातानां चापरेषां द्रव्याणां, मूत्रक्षये पुनरिक्षुरसवारुणीमण्डद्रवमधुराम्ललवणोपक्लेदिनां, पुरीषक्षये कुल्माषमाषकृष्कुण्डाजमध्ययवशाकधान्याम्लानां, वातक्षये कटुकतिक्तकषायरूक्षलघुशीतानां, पित्तक्षयेऽम्ललवणकटुक्षारोष्णतीक्ष्णानां, श्लेष्मक्षये स्निग्धगुरुमधुरसान्द्रपिच्छिलानां द्रव्याणाम्। कर्मापि यद्यस्य धातोर्वृद्धिकरं तत्तदासेव्यम्।

एवमन्येषामपि शरीरधातूनां सामान्यविपर्ययाभ्यां वृद्धिह्रासौ यथाकालं कार्यौ।

इति सर्वधातूनामेकैकशोऽतिदेशतश्च वृद्धिह्रासकराणि व्याख्यातानि भवन्ति॥११॥

If a particular tissue element is to be increased and the homologous dietary articles cannot be taken because of their non-availability, hateful disposition or any other cause, then food preparations of different nature but having the predominance of the attributes of the Dhatu to be promoted should be used. (Certain examples in this connection are given below)

When there is a deficiency of semen, milk, ghee and such other substances known to be sweet, unctuous and cold should be administered with a view to promote it.

For treating a patient suffering from the diminution of urine, sugarcane juice, Varuni type of wine, Manda (thin gruel) liquid things and substances having sweet, saline and sour tastes and of sticky nature are to be administered.

For treating a patient suffering from the diminution of faeces, Kulmasha (paste of barley mixed up with hot water and slightly boiled so as from a cake), Masha (Vigna mungo), Kuskunda (Mushroom), Ajamadhya (middle portion of the goat consisting of intestines and other abdominal viscera), yava (barley), leafy vegetables and Dhanyamla (sour fermented liquor from rice gruel) should give.

For the treatment of patients suffering from the diminution of Vata, substances having pungent, bitter and astringent tastes and dry, light and cooling properties should be administered.

For the treatment of patient suffering from the diminution of Pitta, substances having sour, saline and pungent tastes and alkaline, hot and sharp properties should be administered and

For the treatment of patients suffering from the diminution of Kapha, substances having sweet taste, unctuous, heavy, dense and slimy properties should be administered.

Even all those activities which would increase these dhatus should be resorted to. Similarly other Dhatus should also be either increased or decreased by the administration of homologous and non- homologous substances in appropriate time. Thus the factors which increase or decrease all the Dhatus are described – some Dhatus are individually described and for remaining Dhatus, the principle laid down here should be applied. [11]

Factors responsible for growth of body:

कात्स्न्र्येन शरीरवृद्धिधकरास्त्विमे भावा भवन्ति; तद्यथा- कालयोगः, स्वभावसंसिद्धिः, आहारसौष्ठवम्, अविघातश्चेति॥१२॥

The following factors are responsible for the growth of the body in its entirety.

1. Opportunity; for example, youth is the proper time for the growth of the individual. During young age, it is the specificity of the time which is responsible for the growth of the individual.

2. Favourable disposition of the nature; for example, results of the unseen (past) actions are also responsible for the growth of individual's body

3. Excellence of the properties of food and

4. Absence of inhibiting factors; for example, excessive indulgence in sex and mental affliction inhibits the growth of the individual's body [12]

Factors responsible for promotion of strength:

बलवृद्धिधकरास्त्विमे भावा भवन्ति।

तद्यथा- बलवत्पुरुषे देशे जन्म बलवत्पुरुषे काले च, सुखश्च कालयोगः, बीजक्षेत्रगुणसम्पच्च, आहारसम्पच्च, शरीरसम्पच्च, सात्म्यसम्पच्च, सत्त्वसम्पच्च, स्वभावसंसिद्धिश्च, यौवनं च, कर्म च, संहर्षश्चेति॥१३॥

The following factors are responsible for the promotion of strength:

- Birth in a country where people are naturally strong;
- Birth at a time when people naturally gain strength
- Favourable disposition of time (pleasant and moderate climate)
- Excellence of the qualities of the seed (sperm) and Ashaya (ovum and uterus) of the parents;
- Excellence of the ingested food
- Excellence of the physique
- Excellence of the Satmya (wholesomeness of various factors responsible for the maintenance of the body)
- Excellence of the mind
- Favourable disposition of the nature
- Exercise and
- Cheerful disposition [13]

Factors responsible for transformation of food:

आहारपरिणामकरास्त्विमे भावा भवन्ति।

तद्यथा- ऊष्मा, वायुः, क्लेदः, स्नेहः, कालः, समयोगश्चेति ॥१४॥

Heat (Pitta), Vata (air, wind), moisture, unctuousness, time of digestion and appropriate administration - these factors are responsible for the transformation (digestion, assimilation and metabolism) of food. [14]

Specific actions of transforming factors:

तत्र तु खल्वेषामूष्मादीनामाहारपरिणामकराणां भावानामिमे कर्मविशेषा भवन्ति।

तद्यथा- ऊष्मा पचति, वायुरुपकर्षति, क्लेदः शैथिल्यमापादयति, स्नेहो मार्दवं जनयति, कालः पर्याप्तिमभिनिर्वर्तयति, समयोगस्त्वेषां

परिणामधातुसाम्यकरः सम्पद्यते||१५||

Factors described in the above verse which are said to be responsible for transformation (digestion, assimilation and metabolism) perform the following specific action:
- Pitta (heat) digests
- Vata transports food nearer to Pitta for digestion
- Moisture loosens the food particles
- Unctuousness softness the ingredients
- Time bring about the maturity of the process of digestion and
- Appropriate administration of food brings about equilibrium of Dhatus [15]

Transformation of attributes:

परिणमतस्त्वाहारस्य गुणाः शरीरगुणभावमापद्यन्ते यथास्वमविरुद्धाः; विरुद्धाश्च विहन्युर्विहताश्च विरोधिभिः शरीरम्||१६|

During the process of transformation, the attributes of food ingredients assume the attributes of (or become homologous with) such of the tissue elements of the body as are not contradictory to nature. When they are contradictory, properties of one act against the other during the process of interaction resulting in the decay of the body [16]

Two categories of physical attributes:

शरीरगुणाः पुनर्द्विविधाः सङ्ग्रहेण- मलभूताः, प्रसादभूताश्च|

तत्र मलभूतास्ते ये शरीरस्याबाधकराः स्युः|

तद्यथा- शरीरच्छिद्रेषूपदेहाः पृथग्जन्मानो बहिर्मुखाः, परिपक्वाश्च धातवः, प्रकुपिताश्च वातपित्तश्लेष्माणः, ये चान्येऽपि केचिच्छरीरे तिष्ठन्तो भावाः शरीरस्योपघातायोपपद्यन्ते, सर्वास्तान्मले सञ्चक्ष्महे; इतरांस्तु प्रसादे , गुर्वादींश्च द्रवान्तान् गुणभेदेन, रसादींश्च शुक्रान्तान् द्रव्यभेदेन||१७||

Attributes of the body are again of two categories, viz. Prasada (pure substance) and Mala (impurities). Of them, those which cause obstruction or troubles in the body are called mala. Substances which are produced in various orifices and channels of the body, which are divergent forms and are in the process of being removed out of the body, the wastes / putrefied materials of the eyes, ears and nose, the blood and other tissues which have got suppurated and have acquired the form of pus, vitiated Vata, Pitta and Kapha and such other substances which while existing in the body causes its destruction belong to this category.

All of them come under the category of Mala (impurities) and the remaining is Prasada (Pure substance). The latter (prasada) are classified into seven categories i.e. the tissues beginning with Rasa (plasma) and ending with Shukra (semen). They can be classified into twenty categories on the basis of their attributes beginning with Gurutva (heaviness) and ending with Dravatva (fluidity). Therefore the seven tissues and twenty attributes (qualities) when are in a state of balance and not producing the diseases are considered as prasada bhaga i.e. pure substances of the body. [17]

Vitiation by Doshas:

तेषां सर्वेषामेव वातपित्तश्लेष्माणो दुष्टा दूषयितारो भवन्ति, दोषस्वभावात्|

वातादीनां पुनर्धार्त्वन्तरे कालान्तरे प्रदुष्टानां विविधाशितपीतीयेऽध्याये विज्ञानान्युक्तानि|

एतावत्येव दुष्टदोषगतिर्यावत् संस्पर्शनाच्छरीरधातूनाम्|

प्रकृतिभूतानां तु खलु वातादीनां फलमारोग्यम्|

तस्मादेषां प्रकृतिभावे प्रयतितव्यं बुद्धिमद्भिरिति||१८||

Of all these, Vata, Pitta and Kapha naturally have the capacity to vitiate things (tissues of the body). When these doshas get vitiated by exogenous factors they would vitiate the other elements of the body (including the tissues).

Signs and symptoms of the vitiation of various Dhatus in different times have already been described in the 28th chapter of Sutra section. Such are the manifestations of the vitiated Doshas when they come in contact with the tissue elements of the body.

When in normal state, Vata etc; are responsible for the maintenance of the health of the individual. So a wise man should try to keep the doshas in their normal state. [18]

भवति चात्र-
शरीरं सर्वथा सर्वं सर्वदा वेद यो भिषक्|
आयुर्वेदं स कात्स्र्न्येन वेद लोकसुखप्रदम्||१९||

The physician, who is always conversant with the various aspects of the entire body, is also very proficient in Ayurveda - which could bestow happiness and health to the entire universe. [19]

Query about foetus:
एवंवादिनं भगवन्तमात्रेयमग्निवेश उवाच श्रृतमेतद्यदुक्तं भगवता शरीराधिकारे वचः|
किन्नु खलु गर्भस्याङ्गं पूर्वमभिनिर्वर्तते कुक्षौ, कुतो मुखः कथं चान्तर्गतस्तिष्ठति, किमाहारश्च वर्तयति, कथम्भूतश्च निष्क्रामति, कैश्चायमाहारोपचारैर्जातः सद्यो हन्यते, कैर्व्याधिरभिवर्धते, किञ्चास्य देवादिप्रकोपनिमित्ता विकाराः सम्भवन्ति आहोस्विन्न, किञ्चास्य कालाकालमृत्व्योर्भावाभावयोर्भगवानध्यवस्यति, किञ्चास्य परमायुः, कानि चास्य परमायुषो निमित्तानीति||२०||

While Lord Atreya was imparting the above instructions, Agnivesha asked, "We have heard your expositions on the body. Now we would like to hear the following:

Which of the organs of the foetus is manifested first in the pelvis of the mother?

Where does the face of the foetus lie in the uterus and what posture does it maintain inside?

By which food is it nourished and how does it come out?

What are the foods and regimens which are responsible for its immediate death after birth?

What are the factors that help in the growth of the foetus without any disease?

Whether the diseases afflicting the foetus are caused by Gods etc or not?

What is your opinion regarding the timely or untimely death of the foetus?

What is the span of its life? and

What factors are responsible for the maintenance of the lifespan? "[20]

Views of Sages about 'organs to be formed first' in a foetus
तमेवमुक्तवन्तमग्निवेशं भगवान् पुनर्वसुरात्रेय उवाच- पूर्वमुक्तमेतद्गर्भावक्रान्तौ यथाऽयमभिनिर्वर्तते कुक्षौ, यच्चास्य यदा सन्तिष्ठतेऽङ्गजातम्|
विप्रतिवादास्तन्त्र बहुविधाः सूत्रकृतामृषीणां सन्ति सर्वेषां; तानपि निबोधोच्यमानान्- शिरः पूर्वमभिनिर्वर्तते कुक्षाविति कुमारशिरा भरद्वाजः पश्यति, सर्वेन्द्रियाणां तदधिष्ठानमिति कृत्वा; हृदयमिति काङ्कायनो बाह्लीकभिषक्, चेतनाधिष्ठानत्वात्; नाभिरिति भद्रकाप्यः, आहारागम इति कृत्वा; पक्वाशयगुदमिति भद्रशौनकः, गारुताधिष्ठानत्वात्; हस्तपादमिति बडिशः, तत्करणत्वात् पुरुषस्य; इन्द्रियाणीति जनको वैदेहः, तान्यस्य बुद्ध्यधिष्ठानानीति कृत्वा; परोक्षत्वादचिन्त्यमिति मारीचिः कश्यपः; सर्वाङ्गाभिनिर्वृत्तिर्युगपदिति धन्वन्तरिः; तदुपपन्नं, सर्वाङ्गानां तुल्यकालाभिनिर्वृत्तत्वाद्धृदयप्रभृतीनाम्|
सर्वाङ्गानां ह्यस्य हृदयं मूलमधिष्ठानं च केषाञ्चिद्भावानाम्, नच तस्मात् पूर्वाभिनिर्वृत्तिरेषां; तस्माद्धृदयप्रभृतीनां सर्वाङ्गानां तुल्यकालाभिनिर्वृत्तिः, सर्वे भावा ह्यन्योन्यप्रतिबद्धाः; तस्माद्यथाभूतदर्शनं साधु||२१||

Lord Punarvasu Atreya replied to Agnivesha, "In the fourth chapter of this section dealing with the formation of embryos, the manner in which the foetus is formed in the uterus of the mother and the mode of manifestation of its various organs are already described. But there are various types of controversies on such problems among all the sages who are authors in the subject. They are enumerated below:

Sl No Name of the sage Opinion regarding the first organ of the foetus formed / manifested

1 Kumarashira Bharadvaja observed that the head of the foetus is first manifested in the uterus because it is the receptacle of all sense organs

2 Kankayana, the physician from Bahlika, heart being the receptacle of consciousness is first formed

3 Bhadrakapya Nabhi (umbilicus) is first formed as it serves the means to provide nourishment to the foetus

4 Bhadrashaunaka rectum located near the colon is first formed since this is the site for Vata

5 Badisa hands and feet are first formed being the instruments of the individual for his activities

6 Janaka of Videha sense organs being the receptacles of senses are first formed

7 Marici Kasyapa it is not possible to make any statement about first formation of any organs as they cannot be observed directly

8 Dhanvantari all the organs are formed simultaneously

The view of Dhanvantari is correct as all the organs like heart etc. are (actually) formed simultaneously.

According to Atreya, it is true that the heart is the origin of all organs and the receptacle of certain phenomena. So the formation of all other organs does not take place before the formation of the heart. So, all these organs like heart etc are formed simultaneously. All phenomena are in fact inter-dependent. So the view of Dhanvantari is quite correct and should be acceptable by all. [21]

Posture of the foetus:

गर्भस्तु खलु मातुः पृष्ठाभिमुख ऊर्ध्वशिराः सङ्कुच्याङ्गान्यास्तेऽन्तःकुक्षौ ||२२||

The foetus lies in the uterus with its face towards the back of the mother, head upwards and limbs folded and wrapped up by the placenta. [22]

Thirst and hunger of foetus:

व्यपगतपिपासाबुभुक्षस्तु खलु गर्भः परतन्त्रवृत्तिर्मातरमाश्रित्य वर्तयत्युपस्नेहोपस्वेदाभ्यां गर्भाशये सदसद्भूताङ्गावयवः, तदनन्तरं ह्यस्य कश्चिल्लोमकूपायनैरुपस्नेहः कश्चिन्नाभिनाड्ययनैः|

नाभ्यां ह्यस्य नाडी प्रसक्ता, नाड्यां चापरा, अपरा चास्य मातुः प्रसक्ता हृदये, मातृहृदयं ह्यस्य तामपराभिसम्प्लवते सिराभिः स्यन्दमानाभिः ; स तस्य रसो बलवर्णकरः सम्पद्यते, स च सर्वरसवानाहारः|

स्त्रिया ह्यापन्नगर्भायास्त्रिधा रसः प्रतिपद्यते- स्वशरीरपुष्टये, स्तन्याय, गर्भवृद्धये च|

स तेनाहारेणोपष्टब्धः (परतन्त्रवृत्तिर्मातरमाश्रित्य) वर्तयत्यन्तर्गतः||२३||

The foetus is free from thirst and hunger. It is dependent upon the mother for all its activities. It lives upon the nourishment by the process of Upasneha (exudation) and Upasveda (conduction of heat). Some of its organs are well manifested and some others are not so. It draws nourishment by the process of exudation sometimes through the holes in the hair follicles and sometimes through the channels of umbilical cord.

The umbilical cord of the foetus is attached to the umbilicus and the placenta to the umbilical cord. The placenta is in turn connected with the heart of the mother. The heart of the mother floods the placenta (with nourishment) by the pulsating vessels. This rasa (nutritive fluid) promotes strength and complexion of the foetus because it is composed of all the tastes.

Rasa (digestive product of food) of the pregnant woman serves three purposes i.e.

1. Nourishment of her own body

2. Lactation and

3. Growth and development of the foetus being supported by that food

The foetus that is dependent upon the mother keeps living inside (the uterus). [23]

Process of delivery:

स चोपस्थितकाले जन्मनि प्रसूतिमारुतयोगात् परिवृत्यावाक्शिरा निष्क्रामत्यपत्यपथेन, एषा प्रकृतिः, विकृतिः पुनरतोऽन्यथा|

परं त्वतः स्वतन्त्रवृत्तिर्भवति||२४||

During the time of delivery, the foetus turns its head downloads by virtue of the Prasuti Maruta (Vayu which regulates the process of delivery) and gets delivered through the vaginal path. This is the normal situation. Situations other than this constitute abnormality. After delivery the child is free in its movement. [24]

Factors responsible for proper growth of foetus:

तस्याहारोपचारौ जातिसूत्रीयोपदिष्टावविकारकरौ चाभिवृद्धिकरौ भवतः||२५||

ताभ्यामेव च विषमसेविताभ्यां जातः सद्य उपहन्यते तरुरिवाचिरव्यपरोपितो वातातपाभ्यामप्रतिष्ठितमूलः||२६||

The diet and regimen described in the 8th chapter of this section, if adopted, promotes the growth of foetus without causing any morbidity.

The same diet and regimens inappropriately administered might destroy the foetus immediately after birth as the wind and sun destroy a planted tree whose roots are not yet firmly established. [25-26]

Justifications for the existence of diseases caused by divine displeasure:

आप्तोपदेशादद्भुतरूपदर्शनात् समुत्थानलिङ्गचिकित्सितविशेषाच्चादोषप्रकोपानुरूपा देवादिप्रकोपनिमित्ता विकाराः समुपलभ्यन्ते||२७||

Can diseases in the foetus be caused due to the displeasure of Gods and other divine entities?

It might be possible. The reasons / proofs are as mentioned below –

- The description of the same has been given by the wise persons and authors in various treatises

- Sight of unexpected events like super- natural strength, knowledge, charm etc

- Specific nature of the etiologic, signs, symptoms and treatment and

- There are certain diseases which do not correspond to the aggravation of any of these Doshas [27]

Timely and Untimely death:

कालाकालमृत्य्वोस्तु खलु भावाभावयोरिदमध्यवसितं नः- "यः कश्चिन् म्रियते स काल एव म्रियते, न हि कालच्छिद्रमस्ति" इत्येके भाषन्ते|

तच्चासम्यक्|

न ह्यच्छिद्रता सच्छिद्रता वा कालस्योपपद्यते, कालस्वलक्षणस्वभावात्|

तत्राहुरपरे- यो यदा म्रियते स तस्य नियतो मृत्युकालः; स सर्वभूतानां सत्यः, समक्रियत्वादिति|

एतदपि चान्यथाऽर्थग्रहणम्|

न हि कश्चिन्न म्रियत इति समक्रियः|

कालो ह्यायुषः प्रमाणमधिकृत्योच्यते|

यस्य चेष्टं यो यदा म्रियते स तस्य मृत्युकाल इति, तस्य सर्वे भावा यथास्वं नियतकाला भविष्यन्ति; तच्च नोपपद्यते, प्रत्यक्षं ह्यकालाहारवचनकर्मणां फलमनिष्टं, विपर्यये चेष्टं; प्रत्यक्षतश्चोपलभ्यते खलु कालाकालव्यक्तिस्तासु तास्ववस्थासु तं तमर्थमभिसमीक्ष्य, तद्यथा- कालोऽयमस्य व्याधेराहारस्यौषधस्य प्रतिकर्मणो विसर्गस्य, अकालो वेति|

लोकेऽप्येतद्भवति- काले देवो वर्षत्यकाले देवो वर्षति, काले शीतमकाले शीतं, काले तपत्यकाले तपति, काले पुष्पफलमकाले च पुष्पफलमिति|

तस्मादुभयमस्ति- काले मृत्युरकाले च; नैकान्तिकमत्र|

यदि ह्यकाले मृत्युर्न स्यान्नियतकालप्रमाणमायुः सर्वं स्यात्; एवं गते हिताहितज्ञानमकारणं स्यात्, प्रत्यक्षानुमानोपदेशाश्चाप्रमाणानि स्युर्ये प्रमाणभूताः सर्वतन्त्रेषु, यैरायुष्याण्यनायुष्याणि चोपलभ्यन्ते|

वाग्वस्तुमात्रमेतद्वादमृषयो मन्यन्ते- नाकाले मृत्युरस्तीति||२८||

Our views on the existence and non-existence of timely and untimely death are as follows:

"Whosoever dies would die on time because time has no void whatsoever (time is moving constantly without interruption)". This is what some scholars say. But this is not correct. Time having or not having void, both are incorrect. Time has a distinct feature of its own which does not admit any void or absence thereof in its definition.

Some others say "Whenever one dies, he dies at the appointed hour of death. Being free from hatred or attachment, time deals equally with all creatures (so death always occurs at the predestined moment)," this also is simply distortion of facts.

The fact that everybody dies does not prove the equality in temporal actions.

If it is said that the time when one dies is the time predetermined for this death, then every movement of life as and when it occurs can be taken as pre-determined in respect of time. But this also is not true. According to this theory all actions should happen at a fixed and predetermined time. But this will not happen as a rule. Even practically we can see that untimely food; speech and action will yield worse outcomes and when the same are done timely the effects will be good and desirable.

One can also observe by means of direct perception manifestation of various factors depending upon their timely or untimely action. For example, such and such is the opportune or inopportune time for such and such diseases, food, medicine, therapy and remission.

Even a layman talks in these terms, such as, it rains on time or otherwise; it is cold or hot on time or otherwise; flowers and fruits of the tree have occurred in time of otherwise. So both the things equally hold good. Therefore, death occurs in time. If there was no untimely death, then the span of every one would have been fixed and therefore the knowledge of wholesome and unwholesome objects would be of no use at all. The source of knowledge like perception, inference and verbal testimony accepted in all scriptures would cease to be sources of knowledge because all these sources of knowledge clearly prove that there are factors which are conducive to longevity and otherwise so the statement of some Rshis to the effect that untimely death cannot occur is confined to words only (and not to facts). [28]

Factors responsible for maintenance of normal span of life:

वर्षशतं खल्वायुषः प्रमाणमस्मिन् काले||२९||

तस्य निमित्तं प्रकृतिगुणात्मसम्पत् सात्म्योपसेवनं चेति||३०||

In the Kali age the normal span of life (of human beings) is one hundred years.

The factors responsible for the maintenance (of the normal span) of life are:

- Prakrti Sampat i.e. state of balance and excellence of Doshas in the constitution of the individual
- Guna Sampat i.e. excellence of the compactness of the body and excellence of hereditary qualities; and
- Atmasampt i.e. virtuous acts conducive to longevity. [29-30]

तत्र श्लोकाः:-

शरीरं यद्यथा तच्च वर्तते क्लिष्टमामयैः|

यथा क्लेशं विनाशं च याति ये चास्य धातवः||३१||

वृद्धिह्रासौ यथा तेषां क्षीणानामौषधं च यत्|

देहवृद्धिकरा भावा बलवृद्धिकराश्च ये||३२||

परिणामकरा भावा या च तेषां पृथक् क्रिया|

मलाख्याः सम्प्रसादाख्या धातवः प्रश्न एव च||३३||

नवको निर्णयश्चास्य विधिवत् सम्प्रकाशितः|

तथ्यः शरीरविचये शारीरे परमर्षिणा||३४||

To sum up:

The following nine topics are duly discussed by the great sage in this chapter on the "Knowledge of the Details of the Body" is conducive to its understanding:

Definition of Sharira (body) the way how it is afflicted leading to disease and destruction:

Increase or decrease of Dhatus

Treatment of deficient Dhatus

Factors responsible for the growth of body

Factors responsible for the digestion and metabolism of food

Factors which help in the digestion and metabolism of food

The mode of action of each of the above mentioned factors

Mala (impurities) and Prasada (Pure) type of Dhatus and

various queries [31-34]

इत्यग्निवेशकृते तन्त्रे चरकप्रतिसंस्कृते शारीरस्थाने शरीरविचयशारीरं नाम षष्ठोऽध्यायः||६||

Thus ends the sixth chapter of Sharira section on "the knowledge of the Details of the Body as conducive to its understanding "of Agnivesha's work as redacted by Charaka. [6]

23

Shareerasthana Chapter 7
Shareera Samkhya Shareeram

Enumeration of organs

अथातः शरीरसङ्ख्याशारीरं व्याख्यास्यामः||१||

इति ह स्माह भगवानात्रेयः||२||

We shall now explore the chapter on "the enumeration of the organs as conducive to the understanding of the human body". Thus said Lord Atreya [1-2]

Query about organs of body:

शरीरसङ्ख्यामवयवशः कृत्स्नं शरीरं प्रविभज्य सर्वशरीरसङ्ख्यानप्रमाण ज्ञानहेतोर्भगवन्तमात्रेयमग्निवेशः पप्रच्छ||३||

With a view to ascertain the number and measurement of the entire body by classifying the body according to its component organs, Agnivesha asked Lord Atreya to enumerate the organs of the body. [3]

Six layers of skin:

तमुवाच भगवानात्रेयः- शृणु मत्तोऽग्निवेश! सर्वशरीरमाचक्षाणस्य यथा प्रश्नमेकमना यथावत्|

शरीरे षट् त्वचः; तद्यथा- उदकधरा त्वग्बाह्या, दिवतीया त्वसृग्धरा, तृतीया सिध्मकिलाससम्भवाधिष्ठाना, चतुर्थी दद्रुकुष्ठसम्भवाधिष्ठाना, पञ्चमी त्वलजीविद्रधिसम्भवाधिष्ठाना, षष्ठी तु यस्यां छिन्नायां ताम्यत्यन्ध इव च तमः प्रविशति यां चाप्यधिष्ठायारूंषि जायन्ते पर्वसु कृष्णरक्तानि स्थूलमूलानि दुश्चिकित्स्यतमानि च; इति षट् त्वचः|

एताः षडङ्गं शरीरमवतत्य तिष्ठन्ति||४||

Lord Atreya replied, "Listen to me attentively O! Agnivesha! I shall describe the entire body in appropriate manner as per your questions"

There are six layers of skin as follows:

First one is the external layer which is known as Udaka-Dhara (containing / made up of a watery substance of Lymph).

The second layer is Asrgdara (containing blood, capillaries)

The third layer is the site for the manifestation of Sidhma (a type of dermatosis) and Kilasa (Leucoderma)

The fourth layer is the site for the manifestation of Dadru (ring-worm) and Kustha (obstinate skin diseases including leprosy)

The fifth Layer is the site for the manifestation of Alaji (boil) and Vidradhi (abscess).

The sixth layer is that by the excision of which the individual gets trembling and enters into darkness (gets fainting) like a blind man. In this layer the boils manifest in the joints which are blackish red in colour and are deep rooted. Such boils are extremely difficult to treat. These are the six layers of the skin by which the entire body along with its six organs (parts) remain covered. [4]

Parts of the body:

तत्रायं शरीरस्याङ्गविभागः; तद्यथा- द्वौ बाहू, द्वे सक्थिनी, शिरोग्रीवम्, अन्तराधिः, इति षडङ्गमङ्गम्||५||

The body is divided into six parts, viz. Two upper limbs, head including neck and the trunk. (These are the six parts of the body). [5]

Number of bones:

त्रीणि षष्टीनि शतान्यस्थ्नां सह दन्तोलूखलनखेन |

तद्यथा- द्वात्रिंशद्दन्ताः, द्वात्रिंशद्दन्तोलूखलानि, विंशतिर्नखाः, षष्टिः पाणिपादाङ्गुल्यस्थीनि, विंशतिः पाणिपादशलाकाः, चत्वारि पाणिपादशलाकाधिष्ठानानि, द्वे पार्ष्ण्योरस्थिनी, चत्वारः पादयोर्गुल्फाः, द्वौ मणिकौ हस्तयोः, चत्वार्यरत्न्योरस्थीनि, चत्वारि जङ्घयोः, द्वे जानुनी, द्वे जानुकपालिके, द्वावूरुनलकौ, द्वौ बाहुनलकौ, द्वावंसौ, द्वे अंसफलके, द्वावक्षकौ, एकं जत्रु, द्वे तालुके, द्वे श्रोणिफलके, एकं भगास्थि, पञ्चचत्वारिंशत् पृष्ठगतान्यस्थीनि, पञ्चदश ग्रीवायां, चतुर्दशोरसि, द्वयोः पार्श्वयोश्चतुर्विंशतिः पर्शुकाः, तावन्ति स्थालकानि, तावन्ति चैव स्थालकार्बुदानि, एकं हन्वस्थि, द्वे हनुमूलबन्धने, एकास्थि नासिकागण्डकूटललाटं, द्वौ शङ्खौ, चत्वारि शिरःकपालानीति; एवं त्रीणि षष्टीनि शतान्यस्थ्नां सह दन्तोलूखलनखेनेति||६||

Along with teeth, sockets of teeth and nails, bones in the body are 360 in number. They are as follows:

Teeth- 32

Sockets of teeth- 32

Nails – 20

Phalangeal bones of hands and feet- 60

Meta phalangeal bones of hands and feet- 20

Six bones which from the base to support the meta phalangeal bones of hands & feet- 4

Parshni (bones of heels or calcaneus)-2

Gulpha (ankle bones) - 4

Mani (wrist bones) - 2

Aratni (bones of forearms) - 4

Jangha (bones of legs) - 4

Janu (bones of knees) - 2

Janu Kapala (knee caps) -2

Hollow bones of thighs (femurs)-2

Hollow bones of arms (humerus) - 2

Amsa (bones of the Shoulder)-2

Amsaphalaka (shoulder blades) - 2

Aksaka (clavicles) - 2

Jatru (windpipe) - 2

Talu (palate bones) - 2

Bhagasthi (public bone) - 2

Bhagasthi (public bone) - 1

Bones of the back - 45

Bone of the neck - 15

Bone of chest - 14

Bones of the sides (ribs) - 24

Sockets (for ribs) - 24

Tubercles in the sockets (for ribs) - 24

Hanvasthi or Jawbone (lower) - 1

Hanumula Bandhana (bones which keep the lower jaw locked up) -2

Bone constituting of cheeks and forehead - 1

Sankha (temporal bones) -2

Sirah kapala (pan shaped bones of the head) - 4

Thus the 360 bones including teeth, sockets of bones and nails are accounted for. [6]

Sensory and motor organs:

पञ्चेन्द्रियाधिष्ठानानि; तद्यथा- त्वग्, जिह्वा, नासिका, अक्षिणी, कर्णौ च|

पञ्च बुद्धीन्द्रियाणि; तद्यथा- स्पर्शनं, रसनं, घ्राणं, दर्शनं, श्रोत्रमिति|

पञ्च कर्मेन्द्रियाणि; तद्यथा- हस्तौ, पादौ, पायुः, उपस्थः, जिह्वा चेति||७||

हृदयं चेतनाधिष्ठानमेकम||८||

There are five organs of senses i.e.

- Skin

- Tongue

- Nose

- Two eyes and

- Two ears

These are five sense faculties i.e.

- Tactile

- Gustatory

- Olfactory

- Visual and

- Auditory

There are five motor organs i.e.

- Two hands

- Two feet

- Anus

- Sex organs and

- Tongue

The site of consciousness is only one, i.e. the heart. [7-8]

Resorts of life:

दश प्राणायतनानि; तद्यथा- मूर्धा, कण्ठः, हृदयं, नाभिः, गुदं, बस्तिः, ओजः, शुक्रं, शोणितं, मांसमिति|

तेषु षट् पूर्वाणि मर्मसङ्ख्यातानि||९||

There are ten resorts of life, viz,

- Head

- Throat

- Heart

- Umbilicus

- Anus

- Bladder

- Ojas

- Semen

- Blood and

- Flesh

Of them the first six organs are known as Marma (vital organs) [9]

Visceras:

पञ्चदश कोष्ठाङ्गानि; तद्यथा- नाभिश्च, हृदयं च, क्लोम च, यकृच्च, प्लीहा च, वृक्कौ च, बस्तिश्च, पुरीषाधारश्च, आमाशयश्च, पक्वाशयश्च, उत्तरगुदं च, अधरगुदं च, क्षुद्रान्त्रं च, स्थूलान्त्रं च, वपावहनं चेति||१०||

Kosthangas (viscera in the thorax and abdomen) are fifteen in number. They are

- Nabhi (umbilicus)

- Hrdaya (heart)
- Kloman (lungs)
- Yakrt (liver)
- Pliha (spleen)
- Vrkkau (two kidneys)
- Basti (urinary bladder)
- Purisadhara (pelvic colon)
- Amashaya (stomach)
- Pakvashaya (colon)
- Uttaraguda (rectum)
- Adharaguda (anus)
- Ksudrantra (small intestine)
- Sthulantra (large intestine) and
- Vapavahana (omentum). [10]

Pratyangas or sub-parts of body:

षट्पञ्चाशत् प्रत्यङ्गानि षट्स्वङ्गेषूपनिबद्धानि, यान्यपरिसङ्ख्यातानि पूर्वमङ्गेषु परिसङ्ख्यायमानेषु, तान्यन्यैः पर्यायैरिह प्रकाश्यानि भवन्ति|

तद्यथा- द्वे जङ्घापिण्डिके, द्वे ऊरुपिण्डिके, द्वौ स्फिचौ, द्वौ वृषणौ, एकं शेफः, द्वे उखे, द्वौ वङ्क्षणौ, द्वौ कुकुन्दरौ, एकं बस्तिशीर्षम्, एकमुदरं, द्वौ स्तनौ, द्वौ श्लेष्मभुवौ , द्वे बाहुपिण्डिके, चिबुकमेकं, द्वावोष्ठौ, द्वे सृक्कण्यौ, द्वौ दन्तवेष्टकौ, एकं तालु, एका गलशुण्डिका, द्वे उपजिह्विके, एका गोजिह्विका, द्वौ गण्डौ, द्वे कर्णशष्कुलिके, द्वौ कर्णपुत्रकौ, द्वे अक्षिकूटे, चत्वार्यक्षिवर्त्मानि, द्वे अक्षिकनीनिके, द्वे भ्रुवौ, एकाऽवटुः, चत्वारि पाणिपादहृदयानि||११||

In the six Angas (parts of the body) there are about 56 Pratyngas (sub-parts). They were not described before while enumerating the six parts of the body. They are enumerated below following a different mode of classification:
- Janghapindika (calves) - 2
- Urupindika (muscular portion of the thigh) - 2
- Sphik (buttocks) - 2
- Vrsana (testicles) - 2
- Sepha (phallus) - 1
- Ukha (Elevations bordering axillae) - 2
- Vanksana (groins) - 2
- Kukundara (hips) - 2
- Vastisirsa (pelvis) - 1
- Udara- (abdomen) - 1
- Stana (breasts) - 2
- Slesmabhu (tonsils) - 2
- Bahupidika (muscular portion of arms – 2)
- Cibuka (chin) - 1
- Ostha(lips) - 2
- Srkkani (angles of the mouth - 2)
- Dantavestaka (gums) - 2
- Talu (Palate) - 1
- Galasundika (uvula) - 1
- Upajihvika (ear holes) - 2
- Gojhva (tongue or the organs of the ear) - 2
- Ganda (cheeks) - 2
- Karnasaskulika (ear holes) - 2

- Karnaputraka (external portion of the ear) - 2
- Aksikuta (orbit of eye) - 2
- Aksivartma (eye bids) - 4
- Aksikaninuka (medial angles of the eyes near the nose) - 2
- Bhru (eye brows) - 2
- Avatu (thyroid) - 1
- Panipadahrdaya (soles of hands and feet) - 4 [11]

Major orifices:

नव महन्ति छिद्राणि- सप्त शिरसि, द्वे चाधः||१२||
एतावद्दृश्यं शक्यमपि निर्देष्टुम्||१३||

There are nine major orifices - seven in the head and two below:
The above are the visible factors and are capable of description. [12-13]

Enumeration of other organs:

अनिर्देश्यमतः परं तर्क्यमेव|
तद्यथा- नव स्नायुशतानि, सप्त सिराशतानि, द्वे धमनीशते, चत्वारि पेशीशतानि, सप्तोत्तरं मर्मशतं, द्वे सन्धिशते, एकोनत्रिंशत्सहस्राणि नव च शतानि षट्पञ्चाशत्कानि सिराधमनीनामणुशः प्रविभज्यमानानां मुखाग्रपरिमाणं, तावन्ति चैव केशश्मश्रुलोमानीति|
एतद्यथावत्सङ्ख्यातं त्वक्प्रभृति दृश्यं, तर्क्यमतः परम्|
एतदुभयमपि न विकल्पते, प्रकृतिभावाच्छरीरस्य||१४||

Beyond what is described above can be ascertained from inference only. They are enumerated below:
- Snayu (sinew / ligaments) – 900
- Sira (veins) – 700
- Dhamani (arteries) - 200Muscles – 400
- Marma (vital parts in the body) – 107
- Joints – 200
- Terminals of the fine ramifications of the veins and arteries- 29956
- Kesha(hair), Smashru (beard and moustaches) and loma (small hair) – 2994

Tvak (skin) etc., enumerated above are properly visible and the number of the remaining can be ascertained by inference only. Both these categories do not undergo any variation during the normal state of the individual's body. [14]

Measurement of liquid constituents of body:

यत्त्वञ्जलिसङ्ख्येयं तदुपदेक्ष्यामः; तत् परं प्रमाणमभिज्ञेयं, तच्च वृद्धिह्रासयोगि, तर्क्यमेव|
तद्यथा- दशोदकस्याञ्जलयः शरीरे स्वेनाञ्जलिप्रमाणेन, यत् प्रच्यवमानं पुरीषमनुबध्नात्यतियोगेन तथा मूत्रं रुधिरमन्यांश्च शरीरधातून्, यत् सर्वशरीरचरं बाह्या त्वग्बिभर्ति, यत् त्वगन्तरे व्रणगतं लसीकाशब्दं लभते, यच्चोष्मणाऽनुबद्धं लोमकूपेभ्यो निष्पतत् स्वेदशब्दमवाप्नोति, तदुदकं दशाञ्जलिप्रमाणं; नवाञ्जलयः पूर्वस्याहारपरिणामधातोः, यं 'रस' इत्याचक्षते; अष्टौ शोणितस्य, सप्त पुरीषस्य, षट् श्लेष्मणः, पञ्च पित्तस्य, चत्वारो मूत्रस्य, त्रयो वसायाः, द्वौ मेदसः, एको मज्जायाः, मस्तिष्कस्यार्धाञ्जलिः, शुक्रस्य तावदेव प्रमाणं, तावदेव श्लैष्मिकस्यौजस इति|
एतच्छरीरतत्त्वमुक्तम्||१५||

Substance of the body which can be measured by volume taking Anjali (space created by joining both the hands in the form of a cup) as a unit are now being described. The measurement described here pertains to the ideal standard. These substances can undergo variation in the form of increase or decrease in a normal individual and this can be ascertained by inference.

Measurement of these substances are given below:

Substances and Measurement in terms of Anjali of the individual whose substances are being measured

Udaka (watery portion / aqueous element) a substance which is seen mixed with faeces during the occurrence of diarrhoea; it is also found in association with urine, blood, and other tissue elements of the body. It is spread all over the body with its site in the external skin. Inside the skin, it is known as Lasika (lymph) which exudes through ulcers. When the body becomes hot, it comes out from hair follicles in the form of sweat - 10

Rasa which is the first product of the ingested food after it is metabolised - 9

Blood - 8

Faeces - 7

Kapha - 6

Pitta - 5

Urine - 4

Vasa (muscle fat) - 3

Medas (fat) - 2

Majja (bone-marrow) - 1

Mastiska (the fat) like substance inside the skull) - 1/2

Shukra (semen) - ½

Shlaismika type of Ojas - 1/2

Thus the various factors in the body are described. [15]

Mahabhautic predominance in various constituents:

तत्र यदि्वशेषतः स्थूलं स्थिरं मूर्तिमद्गुरुखरकठिनमङ्गं नखास्थिदन्तमांसचर्मवर्चःकेशश्मश्रुलोमकण्डरादि तत् पार्थिवं गन्धो घ्राणं च; यद्द्रवसरमन्दस्निग्धमृदुपिच्छिलं रसरुधिरवसाकफपित्तमूत्रस्वेदादि तदाप्यं रसो रसनं च; यत् पित्तमूष्मा च यो या च भाः शरीरे तत् सर्वमाग्नेयं रूपं दर्शनं च; यदुच्छ्वासप्रश्वासोन्मेषनिमेषाकुञ्चनप्रसारणगमनप्रेरणधारणादि तद्वायवीयं स्पर्शः स्पर्शनं च; यदि्विक्तं यदुच्यते महान्ति चाणूनि स्रोतांसि तदान्तरीक्षं शब्दः श्रोत्रं च; यत् प्रयोक्तृ तत् प्रधानं बुदि्धर्मनश्च|

इति शरीरावयवसङ्ख्या यथास्थूलभेदेनावयवानां निर्दिष्टा||१६||

These organs are dominated by one or other of the Mahabhutas. Their specific characteristics are given below:

Mahabhautika predominance and Respective organs with their specific characteristics

Parthiva (dominated by Prithvi Mahabhuta – earth element) - 1 - Organs which are gross, stable, having forms, heavy, rough and hard like nail, bone, teeth, flesh, skin, faeces, hair, smasru (moustache)

Smell (of the body) and

Olfactory faculty

Apya (dominated by Jala Mahabhuta – water element) - 1 - Factors in the body which are liquid, mobile, slow, unctuous, soft and slimy like Rasa (Plasma), Rudira (blood), Vasa (muscle fat), Kapha, pitta, urine and sweat

Gustatory faculty

Agneya (dominated by Agnimahabhuta – fire element) - 1 - All factors like pitta, temperature and lustre of the body

Colours (of different factors in the body) and

Visual faculty

Vayaviya (dominated by Vayu mahabhuta – air / wind element) - 1 - Bodily phenomena like inhalation, exhalation, opening and closing of eyes, contraction, impelling and retention

Factors of the body which are known by touch and

Tactile faculty

Antariksha (dominated by Akasha mahabhuta – ether element) - 1 - Factors of the nature of void, speaking (voice), gross and subtle channels

Sounds (excluding speech) emanating from different organs of the body and

Auditory faculty

The soul, the intellect & the mind while stimulating the various sense organs towards their objects are dominated by the qualities of the respective sense organs.

Thus the body divided into various gross organs is merited. [16]

Innumerability of organs of body:

शरीरावयवास्तु परमाणुभेदेनापरिसङ्ख्येया भवन्ति, अतिबहुत्वादतिसौक्ष्म्यादतीन्द्रियत्वाच्च|

तेषां संयोगविभागे परमाणूनां कारणं वायुः कर्मस्वभावश्च||१७||

Paramanus are the minute cells / units of the body and they cannot be counted because (1) they are beyond sensory perception. These Paramanus make up the organs of the body. Based on the innumerability of the paramanus, the number of organs of the body is also considered as innumerable. Vayu, the specific nature of the results of the past action and the basic nature associated with these Paramanus are responsible for their union and disjunction. [17]

Knowledge of organs of the body- salvation:

तदेतच्छरीरं सङ्ख्यातमनेकावयवं दृष्टमेकत्वेन सङ्गः, पृथक्त्वेनापवर्गः|

तत्र प्रधानमसक्तं सर्वसत्तानिवृत्तौ निवर्तते इति||१८||

When this body composed of various parts is perceived as one unit, this leads to attachment; when the various composing factors are viewed as separate from each other, this leads to salvation. Of the various parts, the Soul is unattached. When He dissociates Himself from all (favourable and unfavourable) manifestations, there is salvation (from the worldly affairs). [18]

तत्र श्लोकौ-

शरीरसङ्ख्यां यो वेद सर्वावयवशो भिषक्|

तद्ज्ञाननिमितेन स मोहेन न युज्यते||१९||

अमूढो मोहमूलैश्च न दोषैरभिभूयते|

निर्दोषो निःस्पृहः शान्तः प्रशाम्यत्यपुनर्भवः||२०||

The physician, who knows the number of various components of the body in their entirety, does not associate himself with illusion which is caused by ignorance. Because of the absence of illusion he does not get afflicted with the faults (of such illusion) and being free from faults, he becomes unattached and peaceful which leads to the prevention of his rebirth. [19-20]

इत्यग्निवेशकृते तन्त्रे चरकप्रतिसंस्कृते शारीरस्थाने शरीरसङ्ख्याशारीरं नाम सप्तमोऽध्यायः||७||

Thus ends the seventh chapter of Sharira Section on "The Enumeration of Organs as conducive to the understanding of the human body" of Agnivesha's work as redacted by Charaka [7]

24

Shareerasthana Chapter 8
Jatisutreeyam Shareeram

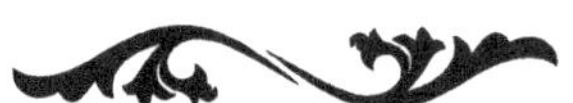

Method of Procreation

अथातो जातिसूत्रीयं शारीरं व्याख्यास्यामः||१||

इति ह स्माह भगवानात्रेयः||२||

We shall now explore the chapter on "The method of Procreation "as conducive to the understanding of the human body. Thus said Lord Atreya [1-2]

Method of procreating excellent progeny:

स्त्रीपुंसयोर्व्यापन्नशुक्रशोणितगर्भाशययोः श्रेयसीं प्रजामिच्छतोस्तदर्थाभिनिर्वृत्तिकरं कर्मोपदेक्ष्यामः||३||

Now we shall explain the method by which the man with unimpaired semen and, the woman with unimpaired ovum and uterus desirous of an excellent progeny can achieve their objective [3]

Preparatory measures:

अथाप्येतौ स्त्रीपुंसौ स्नेहस्वेदाभ्यामुपपाद्य, वमनविरेचनाभ्यां संशोध्य, क्रमेण प्रकृतिमापादयेत्|

संशुद्धौ चास्थापनानुवासनाभ्यामुपाचरेत्; उपाचरेच्च मधुरौषधसंस्कृताभ्यां घृतक्षीराभ्यां पुरुषं, स्त्रियं तु तैलमाषाभ्याम्||४||

The couple is treated with oleation and sudation therapies and thereafter the Doshas from their body is eliminated by the administration of Vamana (emesis) and Virechana (Purgation) therapies. Then the patient is brought to normalcy stage (by administering a prescribed diet).

After the elimination of Doshas, the couple is administered with Asthapana (corrective / decoction / cleansing) and anuvasana (unctuous) types of enemas. Man should also be administered ghee and milk boiled with Drugs having sweet taste. The woman is given til oil and Masha (Black gram / Phaseolus Radiatus Linn) to eat. [4]

Cohabitation:

ततः पुष्पात् प्रभृति त्रिरात्रमासीत ब्रह्मचारिण्यधःशायिनी, पाणिभ्यामन्नमजर्जरपात्रादभुञ्जाना, न च काञ्चिन्मृजामापद्येत|

ततश्चतुर्थेऽहन्येनामुत्साद्य सशिरस्कं स्नापयित्वा शुक्लानि वासांस्याच्छादयेत् पुरुषं च|

ततः शुक्लवाससौ स्रग्विणौ सुमनसावन्योन्यमभिकामौ संवसेयातां स्नानात् प्रभृति युग्मेष्वह:सु पुत्रकामौ, अयुग्मेषु दुहितृकामौ||५||

न च न्युब्जां पार्श्वगतां वा संसेवेत|

न्युब्जाया वातो बलवान् स योनिं पीडयति, पार्श्वगताया दक्षिणे पार्श्वे श्लेष्मा स च्युतः पिदधाति गर्भाशयं, वामे पार्श्वे पित्तं तदस्याः पीडितं विदहति रक्तं शुक्रं च, तस्मादुत्ताना बीजं गृह्णीयात्; तथाहि यथास्थानमवतिष्ठन्ते दोषाः|

पर्याप्ते चैनां शीतोदकेन परिषिञ्चेत्|

तत्रात्यशिता क्षुधिता पिपासिता भीता विमनाः शोकार्ता क्रुद्धाऽन्यं च पुमांसमिच्छन्ती मैथुने चातिकामा वा न गर्भं धत्ते, विगुणां वा प्रजां जनयति|

अतिबालामतिवृद्धां दीर्घरोगिणीमन्येन वा विकारेणोपसृष्टां वर्जयेत्|

• 262 •

पुरुषेऽप्येत एव दोषाः|

अतः सर्वदोषवर्जितौ स्त्रीपुरुषौ संसृज्येयाताम्||६||

सञ्जातहर्षौ मैथुने चानुकूलाविष्टगन्धं स्वास्तीर्णं सुखं शयनमुपकल्प्य मनोज्ञं हितमशनमशित्वा नात्यशितौ दक्षिणपादेन पुमानारोहेत् वामपादेन स्त्री||७||

तत्र मन्त्रं प्रयुञ्जीत- "अहिरसि आयुरसि सर्वतः प्रतिष्ठाऽसि धाता त्वा ददतु विधाता त्वा दधातु ब्रह्मवर्चसा भव" इति|

"ब्रह्मा बृहस्पतिर्विष्णुःसोमःसूर्यस्तथाऽश्विनौ|

भगोऽथ मित्रावरुणौ वीरं ददतु मे सुतम्"

इत्युक्त्वा संवसेयाताम्||८||

For three days, right from the day of onset of menstruation, the woman should -

- observe celibacy

- sleep on the ground

- take food from an unbroken vessel kept in her hands and

- should never clean her body

On the fourth day

- she should use unction

- take head-bath and wear white apparel

- her husband should also adopt the same regimen

- both of them wearing white apparel for each other should enter into cohabitation

- if a male child is desired, they should meet on the odd days

During intercourse, the woman should not assume a prone posture (face downwards). She should also not be prone over the man who is supine nor should she be on her side. If she maintains a prone posture during cohabitation then Vata gets aggravated and afflicts her uterus. This might cause disorders of vagina and uterus.

If she remains in her right-side during intercourse then Kapha which remains in that side gets displaced and blocks the uterus. Left side is the abode of Pitta. If pressure is put on that side during intercourse, then the ovum and the sperm get burnt up. Therefore, the woman should receive seed while lying on her back. In this posture Doshas remain in their respective sites and will also not produce any complication.

After the completion of intercourse, she is sprinkled / given a bath with cold water. The below mentioned factors prevents conception or produces a deformed child in a woman during intercourse –

- intake of food in excess

- fasting

- thirst

- fear

- dejection

- grief

- anger

- desire for another man

- excessive desire for intercourse

One should not indulge in intercourse with a woman who is too young or old, who is suffering from a chronic disease or afflicted with any other disease. Similarly, a woman should not indulge in intercourse with a man having the same defects. Therefore, the couple desirous of having healthy progeny should ensure that they are free from all such defects before entering into the sexual act.

The couple having excitement for intercourse should take relishing and wholesome food (not in excess), and arrange for a bed which is pleasant, scented, well spread and comfortable, The man should ascend this bed with his right leg first and the woman with her left leg first.

Then this Mantra (incantation) is recited. "Oh foetus, you are the serpent God (vibrant like Sun God), you are my life, you are my reputation, and you constitute the support of everything. May the God, the saviour of the world, protects you, May the creator protect and maintain you. Be equipped with Brahmavarcas. May Brahma, Brhaspati,

Vishnu, Soma, Surya, the Asvins, Bhaga, Mitra and Varuna provide me with a brave male child in this foetus. Having recited this Mantra, they should enter into intercourse. [5-8]

Regimens for a son of excellent qualities:

चेदेवमाशासीत- बृहन्तमवदातं हर्यक्षमोजस्विनं शुचिं सत्त्वसम्पन्नं पुत्रमिच्छेयमिति, शुद्धस्नानात् प्रभृत्यस्यै मन्थमवदातयवानां मधुसर्पिर्भ्यां संसृज्य श्वेताया गोः सरूपवत्सायाः पयसाऽऽलोड्य राजते कांस्ये वा पात्रे काले काले सप्ताहं सततं प्रयच्छेत् पानाय।

प्रातश्च शालियवान्नविकारान् दधिमधुसर्पिर्भिः पयोभिर्वा संसृज्य भुञ्जीत, तथा सायमवदातशरणशयनासनपानवसनभूषणा च स्यात्।

सायं प्रातश्च शश्वच्छ्वेतं महान्तं वृषभमाजानेयं वा हरिचन्दनाङ्गदं पश्येत्।

सौम्याभिश्चैनां कथाभिर्मनोनुकूलाभिरुपासीत।

सौम्याकृतिवचनोपचारचेष्टांश्च स्त्रीपुरुषानितरानपि चेन्द्रियार्थानवदातान् पश्येत्।

सहचर्यश्चैनां प्रियहिताभ्यां सततमुपचरेयुस्तथा भर्ता।

न च मिश्रीभावमापद्येयातामिति।

अनेन विधिना सप्तरात्रं स्थित्वाऽष्टमेऽहन्याप्लुत्यादिभिः सशिरस्कं सह भर्त्रा अहतानि वस्त्राण्याच्छादयेदवदातानि, अवदाताश्च स्रजो भूषणानि च बिभृयात्।।९।।

If she desires to have a son with a massive body, white complexioned with the strength like that of a lion, with vigour, purity and strong mind, then from the first day of her purificatory bath (after the menstruation) she is given Mantha (thin gruel) prepared with white barley by boiling it with the milk of a white cow having a white calf and mixing it with ghee and honey in a silver or bronze vessel to drink every morning and evening continuously for one week.

In the morning and also in the evening one should consume rice or food preparations prepared with barley flour mixed with curds, honey, ghee or milk. In the evening, sleep on white mattress / bed sheets (bed covered with white cloth) placed in a white coloured house / apartment, and use white coloured drinks (milk, juice, buttermilk etc) and wear white coloured apparel and ornaments. In the morning and evening, she should continuously look at a white and corpulent bull, a white horse belonging to an appreciable clan or white sandalwood or she is entertained with pleasing and favourite stories.

The woman should see and be in the company of men and women with good personalities, pleasing words and refined behaviour and actions, and pleasant objects of senses i.e., sounds, touch, objects of vision, tastes and smell. Her friends too should behave in a good and pleasant way with her. The husband of the woman too should conduct himself with decent behaviour with her. They should also not get intimate physically for seven days. After having adopted the above regimens for seven nights, she along with her husband should take a complete bath including the head and should wear white and unturned apparel as well as white garlands and ornaments. [9]

Vedic rites for procreating a child of desire qualities:

तत ऋत्विक् प्रागुत्तरस्यां दिश्यगारस्य प्राग्प्रवणमुदक्प्रवणं वा प्रदेशमभिसमीक्ष्य, गोमयोदकाभ्यां स्थण्डिलमुपलिप्य, प्रोक्ष्य चोदकेन, वेदीमस्मिन् स्थापयेत्।

तां पश्चिमेनाहतवस्त्रसञ्चये श्वेतार्षभे वाऽप्यजिन उपविशेद् ब्राह्मणप्रयुक्तः, राजन्यप्रयुक्तस्तु वैयाघ्रे चर्मण्यानडुहे वा, वैश्यप्रयुक्तस्तु रौरवे बास्ते वा।

तत्रोपविष्टः पालाशीभिरैङ्गुदीभिरौदुम्बरीभिर्माधूकीभिर्वा समिद्भिरग्निमुपसमाधाय, कुशैः परिस्तीर्य, परिधिभिश्च परिधाय, लाजैः शुक्लाभिश्च गन्धवतीभिः सुमनोभिरुपकिरेत्।

तत्र प्रणीयोदपात्रं पवित्रपूतमुपसंस्कृत्य सर्पिराज्यार्थं यथोक्तवर्णानाजानेयादीन् समन्ततः स्थापयेत्।।१०।।

ततः पुत्रकामा पश्चिमतोऽग्निं दक्षिणतो ब्राह्मणमुपविश्यान्वालभेत सह भर्त्रा यथेष्टं पुत्रमाशासाना।

ततस्तस्या आशासानाया ऋत्विक् प्रजापतिमभिनिर्दिश्य योनौ तस्याः कामपरिपूरणार्थं काम्यामिष्टिं निर्वर्तयेद् 'विष्णुर्योनिं कल्पयतु' इत्यनयर्चा।

ततश्चैवाज्येन स्थालीपाकमभिघार्य त्रिर्जुहुयाद्यथाम्नायम्।

मन्त्रोपमन्त्रितमुदपात्रं तस्यै दद्यात् सर्वोदकार्थान् कुरुष्वेति।

ततः समाप्ते कर्मणि पूर्वं दक्षिणपादमभिहरन्ती प्रदक्षिणमग्निमनुपरिक्रामेत् सह भर्त्रा।

ततो ब्राह्मणान् स्वस्ति वाचयित्वाऽऽज्यशेषं प्राश्नीयात् पूर्वं पुमान्, पश्चात् स्त्री; न चोच्छिष्टमवशेषयेत्।

ततस्तौ सह संवसेयातामष्टरात्रं, तथाविधपरिच्छदावेव च स्यातां, तथेष्टपुत्रं जनयेताम्||११||

या तु स्त्री श्यामं लोहिताक्षं व्यूढोरस्कं महाबाहुं च पुत्रमाशासीत, या वा कृष्णं कृष्णमृदुदीर्घकेशं शुक्लाक्षं शुक्लदन्तं तेजस्विनमात्मवन्तम्; एष एवानयोरपि होमविधिः|

किन्तु परिबर्हो वर्णवर्जं स्यात्|

पुत्रवर्णानुरूपस्तु यथाशीरेव तयोः परिबर्होऽन्यः कार्यः स्यात्||१२||

शूद्रा तु नमस्कारमेव कुर्यात् (देवाग्निद्विजगुरुतपस्विसिद्धेभ्यः)||१३||

या या च यथाविधं पुत्रमाशासीत तस्यास्तस्यास्तां तां पुत्राशिषमनुनिशम्य तांस्ताञ्जनपदान्मनसाऽनुपरिक्रामयेत्|

ततो या या येषां येषां जनपदानां मनुष्याणामनुरूपं पुत्रमाशासीत सा सा तेषां तेषां जनपदानां मनुष्याणामाहारविहारोपचारपरिच्छदाननुविधत्स्वेति वाच्या स्यात्|

इत्येतत् सर्वं पुत्राशिषां समृद्धिकरं कर्म व्याख्यातं भवति||१४||

Then the priest should select a suitable place. The place should have sloping towards the east or the north. This place is smeared with cow dung mixed with water.

There, an altar is erected after sprinkling the water. He (the priest) should thereafter be seated towards the west of the altar.

- If he is invited by a Brahmana, he should sit on a cushion prepared of untorn (fresh) clothes or the hide of a white bull.

- If he is invited by a Ksatriya he should sit on the hide of a tiger or a bullock.

- If invited by a Vaishya he should sit on the hide of an antelope or a he-goat.

The priest should then offer the wood of one of the below mentioned to the fire in the form of oblation –

- Palasha (Butea monosperma Kuntze)

- Ingudi (Balanites aegyptiaca Delile)

- Udumbara (Ficus racemosa Linn), or

- Madhuka (Madhuca indica J.F Gmel)

Then the altar is covered with Kusha (Desmostachya bipinnata Stapf), and it is bound by the four big sticks of Palasha (Butea monosperma Kuntze). Between the altar and the boundary created around it, parched / puffed rice and white fragrant flowers should be spread out. The priest should take the sacred water pot, purified with sacred Mantras and get the ghee purified for the sake of oblation and then bring the steed etc. The shelter constructed around the altar should be decorated with garlands of white flowers.

As described above all the things should be placed all around the altar.

The woman along with her husband desirous of having a son (child) should sit towards the west of the sacred fire and towards the south of the priest, should perform the sacred rites and should express her desire to have the progeny of excellent quality.

After she has expressed her desire, the priest should respectfully remember Prajapati and with a view to fulfilling the desired progeny in her womb, should offer Kamya type of oblation (to the fire), reciting the Mantra (may Lord Vishnu fulfil her desire in the womb)- Rigveda – 10: 148:8.

[May lord Vishnu prepare the womb; May Lord Tvastr make the respective forms; may Lord Prajapati spray the sperm: May Lord Dhatr protects your (wife's) womb]. Immediately thereafter the priest should prepare the Sthali Paka (caru i.e., rice cooked with ghee) and offer it three times as oblation to the fire as prescribed in the Vedas.

He should then hand over the water vessel impregnated with Mantras to her and say "You should use this for all purposes for which water is required". On completion of these sacred rites, she should take a round of the sacred fire along with her husband with her right step preceding the other one. Then other Brahmanas assembled there should recite auspicious hymns. Thereafter the husband should consume the remaining portion of ghee used for sacrifice (fire sacrifice ritual) enchanted by auspicious hymns by the Brahmanas. Later the wife should consume the same ghee (another portion). The entire ghee should be consumed by the couple without leaving out even a small quantity (should not be wasted). Thereafter they should have intercourse for eight nights. They should continue to use the same type of apparel in order to procreate a son of desired qualities.

A woman who desires to have a son of bluish complexion, red eyes, elevated chest and long arms or who desires to have a son of black complexion having black, soft and long hair, white eyes, white teeth, brilliance and self-control should perform the same sacred rite as mentioned above.

But the variation will be only with regard to the colour of the apparel used. The woman desirous of having a child bearing particular body color should also wear apparel of the same colour.

A woman of shudra caste should live in a house, wear clothes, ornaments and garlands, use seating, bedding, foods and drinks having forms and colors which she would desire to have it in her child. She should offer only obeisance to the Gods, fire, Brahmanas, preceptors, ascetics and Siddhas (those who have attained perfection).

The woman is asked to visit a country or region of her choice in her mind depending on which 'country-man' would she wishes her son to resemble. She should also be asked to adopt the food, regimen, manners and apparel of the people of those countries whom she wishes her son to resemble.

Thus, the regimens to be followed by a woman desirous of having a son of her choice have been explained. [10-14]

Other factors responsible for the complexion of progeny:

न खलु केवलमेतदेव कर्म वर्णवैशेष्यकरं भवति|

अपि तु तेजोधातुरप्युदकान्तरिक्षधातुप्रायोऽवदातवर्णकरो भवति, पृथिवीवायुधातुप्रायः कृष्णवर्णकरः, समसर्वधातुप्रायः श्यामवर्णकरः||१५||

It is not that only the above-mentioned factors are responsible for begetting a child of a specific colour. Even the Agni mahabhuta when associated with Jala and Akasha Mahabhutas also produce white complexion.

Agni associated with Prthvi and Vayu produces black complexion and with all the Mahabhutas in equal proportion, it produces blue complexion. [15]

Mental faculty of the progeny:

सत्त्ववैशेष्यकराणि पुनस्तेषां तेषां प्राणिनां मातापितृसत्त्वान्यन्तर्वत्न्याः श्रुतयश्चाभीक्ष्णं स्वोचितं च कर्म सत्त्वविशेषाभ्यासश्चेति||१६||

The following factors determine the state of the mental faculty of the child:

- The mental faculty of parents
- The sounds, words and conversations (music etc) heard repeatedly by the pregnant woman;
- Actions performed by the embryo in his previous life and
- Frequent practice and indulgence in a particular type of mental faculty by the progeny in his previous life (being used to the qualities of sattva, raja or tama mind faculties in the previous birth will be carried by the mind into its consecutive births) [16]

Importance of purification of body of the couple:

यथोक्तेन विधिनोपसंस्कृतशरीरयोः स्त्रीपुरुषयोर्मिश्रीभावमापन्नयोः शुक्रं शोणितेन सह संयोगं समेत्याव्यापन्नमव्यापन्नेन योनावनुपहतायामप्रदुष्टे गर्भाशये गर्भमभिनिर्वर्तयत्येकान्तेन|

यथा- निर्मले वाससि सुपरिकल्पिते रञ्जनं समुदितगुणमुपनिपातादेव रागमभिनिर्वर्तयति, तद्वत्; यथा वा क्षीरं दध्नाऽभिषुतमभिषवणादिवहाय स्वभावमापद्यते दधिभावं, शुक्रं तद्वत्||१७||

When a man and woman copulate after purifying their bodies according to the methods prescribed above, the unimpaired sperm unites with the unimpaired ovum in the unimpaired womb lying within an unimpaired genital tract. Then this definitely results in the formation of an embryo.

Just like a spotless clean cloth becomes colored on coming in contact with coloring substance, just like the milk abandons its original form and gets converted into curds when it comes in contact with few drops of curd, the sperm on coming in contact with ovum (and getting associated with it) forms the embryo. [17]

Sexual characteristics of Progeny:

एवमभिनिर्वर्तमानस्य गर्भस्य स्त्रीपुरुषत्वे हेतुः पूर्वमुक्तः|

यथा हि बीजमनुपतप्तमुप्तं स्वां स्वां प्रकृतिमनुविधीयते व्रीहिर्वा व्रीहित्वं यवो वा यवत्वं तथा स्त्रीपुरुषावपि यथोक्तं हेतुविभागमनुविधीयेते||१८||

Factors responsible for bringing about masculine or feminine characteristics in the embryo have already been described. An unimpaired seed sown (in a fertile land) germinates bearing its own characteristic features, e.g paddy from paddy seed and barley from barley seed. So, the male and female characteristics of the embryo are determined by those of the parents. (c f Sarira , 2:12). [18]

Pumsavana:

तयोः कर्मणा वेदोक्तेन विवर्तनमुपदिश्यते प्राग्व्यक्तीभावात् प्रयुक्तेन सम्यक्|

कर्मणां हि देशकालसम्पदुपेतानां नियतमिष्टफलत्वं, तथैतरेषामितरत्वम्|

तस्मादापन्नगर्भां स्त्रियमभिसमीक्ष्य प्राग्व्यक्तीभावाद्गर्भस्य पुंसवनमस्यै दद्यात्|

गोष्ठे जातस्य न्यग्रोधस्य प्रागुत्तराभ्यां शाखाभ्यां शुङ्गे अनुपहते आदाय द्वाभ्यां धान्यमाषाभ्यां सम्पदुपेताभ्यां गौरसर्षपाभ्यां वा सह दधिन प्रक्षिप्य पुष्येण पिबेत्, तथैवापराञ्जीवकर्षभकापामार्गसहचरकल्कांश्च युगपदेकैकशो यथेष्टं वाऽप्युपसंस्कृत्य पयसा, कुड्यकीटकं मत्स्यकं वोदकाञ्जलौ प्रक्षिप्य पुष्येण पिबेत्, तथा कनकमयान् राजतानायसांश्च पुरुषकानग्निवर्णानणुप्रमाणान् दधिन पयस्युदकाञ्जलौ वा प्रक्षिप्य पिबेदनवशेषतः पुष्येण, पुष्येणैव च शालिपिष्टस्य पच्यमानस्योष्माणमुपाघ्राय तस्यैव च पिष्टस्योदकसंसृष्टस्य रसं देहल्यामुपनिधाय दक्षिणे नासापुटे स्वयमासिञ्चेत् पिचुना|

यच्चान्यदपि ब्राह्मणा ब्रूयुराप्ता वा स्त्रियः पुंसवनमिष्टं तच्चानुष्ठेयम्|

इति पुंसवनानि||१९||

The procedure prescribed in the Vedas (Ayurveda) to be properly adopted to change the sex of the foetus before its manifestation is now being described.

These methods, if adopted, in association with the excellence of locality and time produce the desired effects invariably. If there is any variation in these, the results would become otherwise. Therefore, the pregnant woman is administered Pumsavana therapy (to beget a male child) before the manifestation of the sex of the foetus.

These recipes are given below:

During the conjunction of Pusya star (with moon), two fresh and intact buds from the branches of a Banyan tree grown in eastern or northern side, in a cow-shed, along with 2 grains of Masha i.e., black gram or white variety of mustard seeds should be ground in curds. This should be given for drinking to the pregnant woman.

Similarly, milk boiled with the paste of Jivaka (?), Rsabhaka (?), Apamarga (Achyranthes aspera Linn) and Sahacara (Barleria cristata Linn)) - all of them together or any one, two or three of them together as per requirement is given to the pregnant woman for the desired effect.

During Pusya conjunction, she should drink an Anjali (a handful of) of water added with Kudyakitaka (a type of small insect) or Matsyaka (a type of small fish).

During Pusya conjunction, she is made to drink without any remnant, an Anjali (a handful of) of curd, milk or water in which a small and dazzling (fire coloured) statue of a man prepared of gold, silver or iron made red hot on fire is dipped in.

During Pusya conjunction, she should inhale the steam coming out of the water boiled by adding flour of Shali rice. To this processed flour (shali rice paste formed after its cooking), water is added again. A cotton swab is dipped in this fluid. Later she should sleep resting her head on the threshold with head low. She should take the cotton swab dipped in rice flour water and squeeze it into her right nostril such that the drops enter the right part of the nose.

In addition to the above, other therapies as prescribed by Brahmanas and saintly ladies for Pumsavana (to beget a male child) are adopted.

Thus ends the Pumsavana rites. [9]

Measures for maintenance of pregnancy:

अत ऊर्ध्वं गर्भस्थापनानि व्याख्यास्यामः- ऐन्द्री ब्राह्मी शतवीर्या सहस्रवीर्याऽमोघाऽव्यथा शिवाऽरिष्टा वाट्यपुष्पी विष्वक्सेनकान्ता चेत्यासामोषधीनां शिरसा दक्षिणेन वा पाणिना धारणं, एताभिश्चैव सिद्धस्य पयसः सर्पिषो वा पानम्, एताभिश्चैव पुष्ये पुष्ये स्नानं, सदा च ताः समालभेत|

तथा सर्वासां जीवनीयोक्तानामोषधीनां सदोपयोगस्तैस्तैरुपयोगविधिभिः|

इति गर्भस्थापनानि व्याख्यातानि भवन्ति||२०||

Hereafter we shall describe the measures which help in the measure which help in the maintenance of pregnancy.

- Aindri (Citrullus colocynthis Schrad)
- Brahmi (Bacopa monnieri Pennel)
- Satavirya (Cynodon dactylon Pers)
- Sahasravirya (a variety of Durva)
- Amongha or patala (Stereospermum suaveolens DC)
- Avyatha or Guduci (Tinospora cordifolia Miers)
- Siva (Terminalia chebula Linn)
- Arista (Picrorhiza kurroa Royle ex Linn)
- Vatyapuspi or yellow variety of Bala (Sida cordifolia Linn)
- Visvaksenakanta or Priyangu (Callicarpa macrophylla Vahl)

All these medicines are worn (tied to) in the head or right hand (of the pregnant woman) and milk or ghee boiled with these drugs is taken (oral consumption) by her. She should take a bath in water boiled with these drugs during Pusya conjunction. She should also touch these drugs.

In the above manner all drugs included under Jivaniya group- vide Sutra, 4:8 should always be used by her. Thus, measures which help in the maintenance of pregnancy are described. [20]

Factors injurious to pregnancy:

गर्भोपघातकरास्त्विमे भावा भवन्ति; तद्यथा- उत्कटविषमकठिनासनसेविन्या वातमूत्रपुरीषवेगानुपरुन्धत्या दारुणानुचितव्यायामसेविन्यास्तीक्ष्णोष्णातिमात्रसेविन्याः प्रमिताशनसेविन्या गर्भो म्रियतेऽन्तः कुक्षेः, अकाले वा संसते, शोषी वा भवति; तथाऽभिघातप्रपीडनैः शवभ्रूकूपप्रपातदेशावलोकनैर्वाऽभीक्ष्णं मातुः प्रपतत्यकालेगर्भः, तथाऽतिमात्रसङ्क्षोभिभिर्यानैर्यानेन, अप्रियातिमात्रश्रवणैर्वा|

प्रततोतानशायिन्याः पुनर्गर्भस्य नाभ्याश्रया नाडी कण्ठमनुवेष्टयति, विवृतशायिनी नक्तञ्चारिणी चोन्मत्तं जनयति, अपस्मारिणं पुनः कलिकलहशीला, व्यवायशीला दुर्वपुष्पमहीकं स्त्रैणं वा, शोकनित्या भीतमपचितमल्पायुषं वा, अभिध्यात्री परोपतापिनिमीर्ष्युं स्त्रैणं वा, स्तेना त्वायासबहुलमतिद्रोहिणमकर्मशीलं वा, अमर्षिणी चण्डमौपधिकमसूयकं वा स्वप्ननित्या तन्द्रालुमबुधमल्पाग्निं वा, मद्यनित्या पिपासालुमल्पस्मृतिमनवस्थितचित्तं वा, गोधामांसप्राया शार्करिणमश्मरिणं शनैर्मेहिणं वा, वराहमांसप्राया रक्ताक्षं क्रथनमतिपरुषरोमाणं वा, मत्स्यमांसनित्या चिरनिमेषं स्तब्धाक्षं वा, मधुरनित्या प्रमेहिणं मूकमतिस्थूलं वा, अम्लनित्या रक्तपित्तिनं त्वगक्षिरोगिणं वा, लवणनित्या शीघ्रवलीपलितं खालित्यरोगिणं वा, कटुकनित्या दुर्बलमल्पशुक्रमनपत्यं वा, तिक्तनित्या शोषिणमबलमनुपचितं वा, कषायनित्या श्यावमानाहिनमुदावर्तिनं वा, यद्यच्च यस्य यस्य व्याधेर्निदानमुक्तं तत्तदासेवमानाऽन्तर्वत्नी तन्निमित्तविकारबहुलमपत्यं जनयति|

पितृजास्तु शुक्रदोषा मातृजैरपचारैर्व्याख्याताः|

इति गर्भोपघातकरा भावा भवन्त्युक्ताः |

तस्मादहितानाहारविहारान् प्रजासम्पदमिच्छन्ती स्त्री विशेषेण वर्जयेत्|

साध्वाचारा चात्मानमुपचरेदिध्दताभ्यामाहारविहाराभ्यामिति||२१||

The following factors cause impairment on pregnancy:
- seating which are uncomfortable, irregular and high
- forcibly withholding the urges of flatus, urination and defecation
- getting indulged in difficult exercises which doesn't suit one's capacity
- consumption of foods hot and sharp in nature
- consumption of foods in excessive or less quantity
- taking foods rich only in one or two tastes

The above-mentioned factors lead either to the death of the foetus inside the uterus, premature birth, abortion or cachexia of the foetus.

Other factors which lead to miscarriage or abortion –
- injury
- frequent pressure
- frequently looking inside abysses, deep wells and place of water fall
- travelling in the vehicles which are excessively uncomfortable (jerky)

- hearing of unbearable sounds in excess

Other harmful factors and their effects

1. constantly sleeping in supine position - by this the cord attached to the umbilicus of the foetus gets twisted around the neck

2. sleeping in open air and moving at night alone - this results in the production of an insane progeny (insanity is caused by the attack of evil spirits which get an access to the mother's body conveniently in such situations)

3. resorting to vocal abuses and physical assaults - they make the progeny epileptic

4. habitually resorting to sexual intercourse - it makes the progeny physically ill-formed, shameless and subjugated to women

5. constantly given to grief - this makes the progeny timid, thin / emaciated and short lived (less life span)

6. thinking ill of others - this makes the offspring anti-social, envious and subjugated to women

7. stealing other's property - makes the offspring exceedingly lazy, malicious and inactive

8. resorting to anger - this makes the offspring forceful, deceitful and jealous

9. constantly given to sleep - this makes the offspring drowsy, dull and deficient in digestive power

10. addiction to wine - The offspring suffers from thirst disorder, deficit memory and imbalance of mind

11. addiction to the intake of inguna flesh - the offspring suffers from diabetes, stones in the urinary bladder and dribbling of urine

12. addiction to the intake of pork - produces redness in eyes, sudden obstruction of breathing and excessive roughness of the hair in the offspring

13. addiction to fish - causes delayed closure of eyes or eyes which do not blink

14. addiction to intake of sweet things - makes the offspring suffer from prameha (obstinate urinary disorder including diabetes), muka (dumbness) and atisthaulya (excessive corpulence)

15. addiction to the intake of sour things - makes the offspring suffer from Raktapitta (a disease characterized by bleeding from different parts of the body)) and diseases of the skin and eyes

16. addition to the intake of salt - makes the offspring suffer from early skin wrinkles, graying of hairs and baldness

17. addiction to the intake of pungent things - this makes the offspring weak, deficient in semen or impotent / sterile

18. addiction to the intake of bitter things - makes the offspring cachectic, weak and emaciated

19. addiction to the intake of astringent things - makes the offspring gray in complexion, causes constipation and udavarta (typanitic)

20. regimens described as the causative factors for the various diseases - offspring also predominantly suffers from the diseases caused by such etiological factors.

Defects in the offspring caused by the vitiation of the sperm of the father are to be described on the same line as those of the mother. Thus, the factors responsible for the impairment of the pregnancy are described.

Thus, the parents, especially the mother, desirous of an offspring endowed with excellent quantities should refrain from unwholesome diet and regimens. They should perform virtuous acts and resort to diets and regimens which are beneficial. [21]

Line of treatment of a pregnant woman:

व्याधींश्चास्या मृदुमधुरशिशिरसुखसुकुमारप्रायैरौषधाहारोपचारैरुपचरेत्, न चास्या वमनविरेचनशिरोविरेचनानि प्रयोजयेत्, न रक्तमवसेचयेत्, सर्वकालं च नास्थापनमनुवासनं वा कुर्यादन्यत्रात्ययिकाद्व्याधेः|
अष्टमं मासमुपादाय वमनादिसाध्येषु पुनर्विकारेष्वात्ययिकेषु मृदुभिर्वमनादिभिस्तदर्थकारिभिर्वोपचारः स्यात्|
पूर्णमिव तैलपात्रमसङ्क्षोभयताऽन्तर्वत्नी भवत्युपचर्या||२२||

A physician should treat her ailments by means of drugs, diet and other regimens which are mostly soft, sweet, cold, pleasant and tender. She should not be administered emesis; purgation, head-purging errhines (nasal medication) and bloodletting therapies. Unless the disease is exceedingly serious, she should never be administered asthapana (corrective type of enema) and anuvasana (oleating type of enema). Emesis etc. may however, be given to the pregnant woman after the eight months of pregnancy, if there is any serious emergency. But these therapies or any such other therapies having similar action should be of very mild nature. Any such therapies here mean gargle, mouthwash or expectorant therapies should be done instead of emesis, suppositories should be administered instead of purgation therapy, oil pulling therapy over the head should be done instead of errhines. A pregnant woman is to be treated very cautiously as if one is walking with a pot full of oil in hand without letting a drop to fall. [22]

Abortion:

सा चेदपचाराद् द्वयोस्त्रिषु वा मासेषु पुष्पं पश्येन्नास्या गर्भः स्थास्यतीति विद्यात्; अजातसारो हि तस्मिन् काले भवति गर्भः||२३||

Miscarriage & its management:

सा चेच्चतुष्प्रभृतिषु मासेषु क्रोधशोकासूयेर्ष्याभयत्रासव्यवायव्यायामसङ्क्षोभसन्धारणविषमाशनशयनस्थानक्षुत्पिपासातियोगात् कदाहाराद्वा पुष्पं पश्येत्, तस्या गर्भस्थापनविधिमुपदेक्ष्यामः|

पुष्पदर्शनादेवैनां ब्रूयात्- शयनं तावन्मृदुसुखशिशिरास्तरणसंस्तीर्णमीषदवनतशिरस्कं प्रतिपद्यस्वेति|

ततो यष्टीमधुकसर्पिर्भ्या परमशिशिरवारिणी संस्थिताभ्यां पिचुमाप्लाव्योपस्थसमीपे स्थापयेतस्याः, तथा शतधौतसहस्रधौताभ्यां सर्पिर्भ्यामधोनाभेः सर्वतः प्रदिह्यात्, सर्वतश्च गव्येन चैनां पयसा सुशीतेन मधुकाम्बुना वा न्यग्रोधादिकषायेण वा परिषेचयेदधो नाभेः, उदकं वा सुशीतमवगाहयेत्, क्षीरिणां कषायद्रुमाणां च स्वरसपरिपीतानि चेलानि ग्राहयेत्, न्यग्रोधादिशुङ्गासिद्धयोर्वाक्षीरसर्पिषोः पिचुं ग्राहयेत्, अतश्चैवाक्षमात्रं प्राशयेत्, प्राशयेद्वा केवलं क्षीरसर्पिः, पद्मोत्पलकुमुदकिञ्जल्कांश्चास्यै समधुशर्करान् लेहार्थं दद्यात्, शृङ्गाटकपुष्करबीजकशेरुकान् भक्षणार्थं, गन्धप्रियङ्गुसितोत्पलशालूकोदुम्बरशलाटुन्यग्रोधशुङ्गानि वा पाययेदेनामाजेन पयसा, पयसा चैनां बलातिबलाशालिष्टिकेक्षुमूलकाकोलीशृतेन समधुशर्करं रक्तशालीनामोदनं मृदुसुरभिशीतलं भोजयेत्, लावकपिञ्जलकुरङ्गशम्बरशशहरिणैणकालपुच्छकरसेन वा घृतसुसंस्कृतेन सुखशिशिरोपवातदेशस्थां भोजयेत्, क्रोधशोकायासव्यवायव्यायामेभ्यश्चाभिरक्षेत्, सौम्याभिश्चैनां कथाभिर्मनोनुकूलाभिरुपासीत; तथाऽस्या गर्भस्तिष्ठति||२४||

If there is bleeding from the genital tract during the fourth month of pregnancy or thereafter due to excess of anger, grief, envy, jealousy, fear, terror, cohabitation, exercise, jerk, suppression of the manifested urges, improper food, wrong posture, hunger, thirst and intake of unwholesome food then following procedure is adopted for the maintenance of pregnancy:

Immediately after the manifestation of bleeding she is advised to lie down in head-low and elevated leg position on the bed covered with a soft, soothing, comfortable and cooling bed–sheet.

Thereafter, a cotton swab dipped in ghee mixed with the powder of Yastimadhu (Glycyrrhiza glabra Linn) which are kept inside excessively cold water is placed over the vagina.

Her entire body below the navel is smeared with Satadhauta-Ghrta (ghee washed for one hundred times) and Sahasradhauta Grtha (ghee washed for one thousand times).

Her entire body below the navel is sprinkled with excessively cold cow- milk, decoction of Yasthi madhu (licorice) and the decoction prepared of Nyagrodha (Ficus benghalensis Linn) etc.

She is bathed with cold water.

Cotton swabs dipped in the juice of Ksiri vrkshas (trees bearing milk / latex yielding trees) and trees having astringent taste are kept inside her vagina.

Cotton swabs dipped in the milk or ghee boiled with the sunga (bud) of Nyarodha (Ficus benghalensis) etc. may also be kept inside the vagina.

She may be given the milk or ghee boiled with the bud or Nyagrodha to be taken in the dose of an Aksa (12ml)

She may be given milk or ghee alone.

Pollens of Padma (Nelumbo nucifera Gaertn), Utpala (Nymphea alba Linn) and Kumuda (a variety of Utpala) along with honey and sugar may be given to her as linctus.

She should eat Srngataka (Trapa bispinosa Roxb), seeds of Puskara (Nelumbo nucifera Gaertn) and Kaseruka (Scripus grossus Linn f)

She may be given milk boiled with Priyangu (Callicarpa macrophylla Vahl), blue variety of Utpala (Nymphaea alba Linn) and buds of Nyagrodha (Ficus benghalensis Linn) to drink.

She is given to eat soft, fragrant and cold rice of red variety of Shali (Oryza sativa Linn) along with honey and sugar mixed with the milk boiled with Bala (Sida cordifolia Linn), Atibala (a variety of Bala), roots of Shali, swastika (a variety of Shali) and iksu (Saccharum officinarum Linn) and Kakoli.

She should reside in a comfortable place having cold breeze and take the rice prepared of red variety of Shali (Oryza sativa Linn) along with the meat soup of animals, viz Lava (common quail), Kapinjala (Gray bar), Sasa (Rabbit), Harina (black buck), ena (Antelope) and Kalapucchaka (Black tailed deer) well-seasoned with ghee.

She should refrain from anger, sorrow, exertion, sexual intercourse and exercise.

She is entertained with talks which are gentle and give pleasure to her mind. The above measures help in maintaining pregnancy. [24]

Miscarriage caused by Sama:

यस्याः पुनरामान्वयात् पुष्पदर्शनं स्यात्, प्रायस्तस्यास्तद्गर्भोपघातकरं भवति,
विरुद्धोपक्रमत्वात्तयोः||२५||

If bleeding appears because of the factors which are simultaneously responsible for the formation of Ama, this mostly leads to abortion because both of them (correction of bleeding and Ama formation) require mutually contradictory treatment. [25]

Upavistaka and Nagodara:

यस्याः पुनरुष्णतीक्ष्णोपयोगाद्गर्भिण्या महति सञ्जातसारे गर्भे पुष्पदर्शनं स्यादन्यो वा योनिस्रावस्तस्या गर्भो वृद्धिं न प्राप्नोति निःसुतत्वात्; स कालमवतिष्ठतेऽतिमात्रं, तमुपविष्टकमित्याचक्षते केचित्।

उपवासव्रतकर्मपरायाः पुनः कदाहारायाः स्नेहद्वेषिण्या वातप्रकोपणोक्तान्यासेवमानाया गर्भो वृद्धिं न प्राप्नोति परिशुष्कत्वात्; स चापि कालमवतिष्ठतेऽतिमात्रम्, अस्पन्दनश्च भवति, तं तु नागोदरमित्याचक्षते||२६||

Upavishtaka - Bleeding or any other form of uterine secretion may occur because of the intake of hot and sharp things by a pregnant woman in whom the vital elements of the foetus have been formed and the shape and form of the foetus too are in matured state.

Evidently this amounts to the loss of vital elements from its body through exudation, resulting in inhibition to the growth of foetus. Such a foetus remains inside the womb for a very long time. This condition is known by some experts as Upavistaka (prolonged gestation).

If the pregnant women resort to fasting and observance of religious rites, if there is malnutrition, if she has aversion to the intake of fats and if she resorts to such factors which might cause aggravation of vata, the foetus dries up and does not grow. Such a foetus remains in the womb of the mother for a very long period and there is no quacking of the foetus. This condition is known as Nagodara (Elephantine Gestation). [26]

Management of Upavistaka etc:

नार्योस्तयोरुभयोरपि चिकित्सितविशेषमुपदेक्ष्यामः:- भौतिकजीवनीयबृंहणीयमधुरवातहरसिद्धानां सर्पिषां पयसामागगर्भाणां चोपयोगो गर्भवृद्धिकरः; तथा सम्भोजनमेतैरेव सिद्धैश्च घृतादिभिः सुभिक्षायाः, अभीक्ष्णं यानवाहनापमार्जनावजृम्भणैरुपपादनमिति||२७||

We shall now explain the specific treatment for both the above-mentioned conditions of the pregnant woman.

She should use eggs, and ghee or milk boiled with Bhautika (drugs which are antagonistic to evil spirits and germs like Vaca) Guggulu, Mahapaisacika Ghrta- Vide Cikitsa, 9:45- 48), Jivaniya (vitalizing drugs), Brmhaniya (drugs promoting the corpulence of the body), madhura (drugs having sweet taste) and Vatahara (drugs which alleviate Vata) drugs for the growth of the foetus.

She should take ghee etc. boiled with the above-mentioned drugs when there is a good appetite.

This is supplemented by the frequent use of a (proper) conveyance for travelling, bath and geniculation. [27]

Treatment of Nagodara:

यस्याः पुनर्गर्भः प्रसुप्तो न स्पन्दते तां श्येनमत्स्यगवयशिखितामचूडतितित्तिरीणामन्यतमस्य सर्पिष्मता रसेन माषयूषेण वा प्रभूतसर्पिषा मूलकयूषेण वा रक्तशालीनामोदनं मृदुमधुरशीतलं भोजयेत्।

तैलाभ्यङ्गेन चास्या अभीक्ष्णमुदरबस्तिवङ्क्षणोरुकटीपार्श्वपृष्ठप्रदेशानीषदुष्णेनोपचरेत्||२८||

The patient whose foetus being inactive does not quicken, is given soft, sweet and cooling juice of red variety of Shali

(Oryza sativa Linn) along with the
meat soup of either of the animals and birds like falcon, fish, gayal cow, peacock, cock, and partridge mixed with ghee or with soup prepared of masha (Phaseolus mungo) or radish mixed with ghee in large quantities. Her abdomen, lower abdomen, groin, thighs, waist, sides of chest and back is frequently massaged with luke-warm oil. [28]

Treatment of ailments in eighth month:

यस्याः पुनरुदावर्तविबन्धः स्यादष्टमे मासे न चानुवासनसाध्यं मन्येत ततस्तस्यास्तद्विकारप्रशमनमुपकल्पयेन्निरूहम्|

उदावर्तो ह्युपेक्षितः सहसा सगर्भां गर्भिणीं गर्भमथवाऽतिपातयेत्|

तत्र वीरणशालिषष्टिककुशकाशेक्षुवालिकावेतसपरिव्याधमूलानां भूतीकानन्ताकाश्मर्यपरूषकमधुकमृद्वीकानां च पयसाऽर्धोदकेनोद्गमय्य रसं प्रियालबिभीतकमज्जतिलकल्कसम्प्रयुक्तमीषल्लवणमनत्युष्णं च निरूहं दद्यात्|

व्यपगतविबन्धां चैनां सुखसलिलपरिषिक्ताङ्गीं स्थैर्यकरमविदाहिनमाहारं भुक्तवतीं सायं मधुरकसिद्धेन तैलेनानुवासयेत्|

न्युब्जां त्वेनामास्थापनानुवासनाभ्यामुपचरेत्||२९||

If she suffers from Udavarta (an acute condition in the abdomen characterized by the retention of feces) along with constipation during the eight months of pregnancy, administration of anuvasana basti (unctuous enema) is considered to be unsuitable because of the association of ama in this condition. In this condition she is given with Niruha Basti (corrective enema). If neglected, Udavarta causes the death of the pregnant woman along with the foetus or of foetus alone.

A decoction is prepared by boiling the roots of Virana (Vetiveria zizanioides Nash), Shali (Oryza sativa Linn), Sastika (a type of Shali), Kusha (Desmostachya bipinnata Staff), Kasha (Saccharum spontaneum Linn), Iksuvalika (Asteracantha longifolia Nees), Vetasa (Salix caprea Linn), Parivyadha (a type of Vetasa), and Bhutika (Trachyspermum ammi Sprague), Ananta (Hemidesmus indicus R.B), Kashmarya (Gmelina glabra Linn), Parushaka (Grewia asiatica Linn), Madhuka (Glycyrrhiza glabra Linn) and Mrdvika. (Vitis vinifera Linn), in milk added with water half in quantity. To this decoction, the paste of Priyala (Buchanania lanzan Spreng), pulp inside the seed of Bibhitaka (Terminalia bellerica Roxb) and Tila (Sesamum indicum Linn) and a small quantity of salt is added. This mixture, when slightly warm, is administered as Niruha (corrective enema.).

After the constipation is relieved, her body is washed with water of pleasant temperature and she is given food which promotes stability and does not cause burning sensation. Thereafter, in the evening she is administered anuvasana basti (unctuons) type of enema prepared by boiling oil with the group of sweet drugs. Anuvasana and Niruha types of enemas are administered to her while she is in a prone posture. [29]

Signs and foetal death:

यस्याः पुनरुदावर्तविबन्धः स्यादष्टमे मासे न चानुवासनसाध्यं मन्येत ततस्तस्यास्तद्विकारप्रशमनमुपकल्पयेन्निरूहम्|

उदावर्तो ह्युपेक्षितः सहसा सगर्भां गर्भिणीं गर्भमथवाऽतिपातयेत्|

तत्र वीरणशालिषष्टिककुशकाशेक्षुवालिकावेतसपरिव्याधमूलानां भूतीकानन्ताकाश्मर्यपरूषकमधुकमृद्वीकानां च पयसाऽर्धोदकेनोद्गमय्य रसं प्रियालबिभीतकमज्जतिलकल्कसम्प्रयुक्तमीषल्लवणमनत्युष्णं च निरूहं दद्यात्|

व्यपगतविबन्धां चैनां सुखसलिलपरिषिक्ताङ्गीं स्थैर्यकरमविदाहिनमाहारं भुक्तवतीं सायं मधुरकसिद्धेन तैलेनानुवासयेत्|

न्युब्जां त्वेनामास्थापनानुवासनाभ्यामुपचरेत्||२९||

The foetus may die inside the womb of the woman due to

- Excessive accumulation of Doshas
- Excessive intake of sharp and hot things
- Suppression of the manifested urges of flatus, urine and stool,
- Maintenance of irregular posture in sitting, sleeping, standing, compression and injury
- Anger, grief, envy, fear, terror etc. And other activities which are beyond her strength and capacity

Symptoms death of foetus inside the womb –

- The woman's abdomen becomes still, rigid, extended, cold and hard as if a there is a stone inside
- Absence of quickening of the foetus
- Manifestation of excessive pain

- No manifestation of labour pain
- Absence of any secretion from the genital tract
- Sunken eyes
- Fainting
- Agonizing pain
- Giddiness
- Severe breathlessness
- Restlessness / excessive disliking for everything and
- Improper manifestation of natural urges
With these symptoms, the woman is diagnosed as carrying a dead foetus in her womb. [30]

Management of a woman with dead foetus:

तस्य गर्भशल्यस्य जरायुप्रपातनं कर्म संशमनमित्याहुरेके, मन्त्रादिकमथर्ववेदविहितमित्येके, परिदृष्टकर्मणा शल्यहर्त्रा हरणमित्येके|
व्यपगतगर्भशल्यां तु स्त्रियमामगर्भां सुरासीध्वरिष्टमधुमदिरासवानामन्यतममग्रे सामर्थ्यतः पाययेद्गर्भकोष्ठशुद्ध्यर्थमर्तिविस्मरणार्थं
प्रहर्षणार्थं च, अतः परं सम्प्रीणनैर्बलानुरक्षिभिरस्नेहसम्प्रयुक्तैर्यवाग्वादिभिर्वा तत्कालयोगिभिराहारैरुपचरेद्दोषधातुक्लेदविशोषणमात्रं
कालम्|
अतः परं स्नेहपानैर्बस्तिभिराहारविधिभिश्च दीपनीयजीवनीयबृंहणीयमधुरवातहरसमाख्यातैरुपचरेत्|
परिपक्वगर्भशल्यायाः पुनर्विमुक्तगर्भशल्यायास्तदहरेव स्नेहोपचारः स्यात्||३१||
To give relief to such a patient having a dead foetus in her womb, the following three methods are prescribed:
- Expulsion of the placenta
- Recitation of Mantras etc., as prescribed in the Atharva Veda and
- Removal of the dead foetus by surgical measure by an experienced surgeon
(The dead foetus inside the womb may either be a mature or an immature one).
If it is immature, after the removal of the dead foetus, she is given in the beginning to drink either of the Sura, Sidhu, Arista, Madhu, and Madira and Asava types of wine, in accordance with her capacity, for the purification of the sense of exhilaration. Thereafter, till the excessive moisture in Doshas and Dhatus are dried up, she is immediately given Yavagu (gruel) etc; which is palatable and strength promoting, without adding any fat into it. Thereafter she is treated with the administration of fats, enema and different types of diet which are Dipaniya (promoters of digestive power), Jivaniya (promoters of Vitality), Brmhaniya (promoters of corpulence), Madhura (sweet in taste in taste), and Vatahara (alleviators of Vata).
For a patient whose foetus has attained maturity before death fatty things are given immediately after the dead foetus is removed. [31]

Regimens for a pregnant woman:

परमतो निर्विकारमाप्याय्यमानस्य गर्भस्य मासे मासे कर्मोपदेक्ष्यामः|
प्रथमे मासे शङ्किता चेद्गर्भमापन्ना क्षीरमनुपस्कृतं मात्रावच्छीतं काले काले पिबेत्, सात्म्यमेव च भोजनं सायं प्रातश्च भुञ्जीत; दिवतीये मासे क्षीरमेव च मधुरौषधसिद्धं; तृतीये मासे क्षीरं मधुसर्पिभ्यर्मुपसंसृज्य; चतुर्थे मासे क्षीरनवनीतमक्षमात्रमश्नीयात्; पञ्चमे मासे क्षीरसर्पिः; षष्ठे मासे क्षीरसर्पिर्मधुरौषधसिद्धं; तदेव सप्तमे मासे|
तत्र गर्भस्य केशा जायमाना मातुर्विदाहं जनयन्तीति स्त्रियो भाषन्ते; तन्नेति भगवानात्रेयः, किन्तु गर्भोत्पीडनाद्वातपित्तश्लेष्माण उरः प्राप्य विदाहं जनयन्ति, ततः कण्डूरुपजायते, कण्डूमूला च किक्किसावाप्तिर्भवति|
तत्र कोलोदकेन नवनीतस्य मधुरौषधसिद्धस्य पाणितलमात्रं काले कालेऽस्यै पानार्थं दद्यात्, चन्दनमृणालकल्कैश्चास्याः स्तनोदरं विमृद्गीयात्, शिरीषधातकीसर्षपमधुकचूर्णैर्वा, कुटजार्जकबीजमुस्तहरिद्राकल्कैर्वा, निम्बकोलसुरसमञ्जिष्ठाकल्कैर्वा, पृष्टहरिणशशरुधिरयुतया त्रिफलया वा; करवीरपत्रसिद्धेन तैलेनाभ्यङ्गः; परिषेकः पुनर्मालतीमधुकसिद्धेनाम्भसा; जातकण्डूश्च कण्डूयनं वर्जयेत्त्वग्भेदवैरूप्यपरिहारार्थम्, असह्यायां तु कण्डवामुन्मर्दनोद्धर्षणाभ्यां परिहारः स्यात्; मधुरमाहारजातं वातहरमल्पमस्नेहलवणमल्पोदकानुपानं च भुञ्जीत|
अष्टमे तु मासे क्षीरयवागूं सर्पिष्मतीं काले काले पिबेत्; तन्नेति भद्रकाप्यः, पैङ्गल्याबाधो ह्यस्या गर्भमागच्छेदिति; अस्त्वत्र पैङ्गल्याबाध

इत्याह भगवान् पुनर्वसुरात्रेयः, न त्वेवैतन्न कार्यम्; एवं कुर्वती ह्यरोगाऽऽरोग्यबलवर्णस्वरसंहननसम्पदुपेतं ज्ञातीनामपि श्रेष्ठमपत्यं जनयति।

नवमे तु खल्वेनां मासे मधुरौषधसिद्धेन तैलेनानुवासयेत्।

अतश्चैवास्यास्तैलात् पिचुं योनौ प्रणयेद्गर्भस्थानमार्गस्नेहनार्थम्।

यदिदं कर्म प्रथमं मासं समुपादायोपदिष्टमानवमान्मासातेन गर्भिण्या गर्भसमये गर्भधारिणीकुक्षिकटीपार्श्वपृष्ठं मृदूभवति, वातश्चानुलोमः सम्पद्यते, मूत्रपुरीषे च प्रकृतिभूते सुखेन मार्गमनुपद्यते, चर्मनखानि च मार्दवमुपयान्ति, बलवर्णौ चोपचीयेते; पुत्रं चेष्टं सम्पदुपेतं सुखिनं सुखेनैषा काले प्रजायत इति||३२||

Now we shall describe the measures to be adopted month by month for the foetus which grows without any morbidity

First month:

If pregnancy is suspected she should take milk in adequate quantity regularly. This milk need not be boiled with anything and is taken when it is cold. She should take eat wholesome food in the morning and evening.

Second month

Milk is boiled with drugs having a sweet taste.

Third month:

Milk mixed with honey and ghee should be given.

Fourth month

Milk is given along with butter in one Karsa (12g) dose.

Fifth Month:

Ghee extracted directly from milk (without subjecting it to fermentation leading to the formation of curd) is given to her.

Sixth month:

Ghee taken out directly from milk and boiled with Madhurausadhis (drugs which are sweet in taste) is given.

Seventh month:

She is given the same medication prescribed for the sixth month.

According to the notion commonly prevalent among women, the mother during this month gets a burning sensation (in the chest) because of the growth of hair in the foetus but this is not correct according to Lord Atreya. According to him, three Doshas viz, Vata, Pitta and Kapha get into the chest because of the pressure of the foetus and this causes burning sensation there which leads to itching resulting in the formation of Kikkisa (Linea albicantes or white abdominal lines seen after pregnancy).

For the management of such a condition the following therapies are prescribed.

She is made to drink regularly one Tola (12g) of butter boiled with Madhurausadhi (certain selected drugs having sweet taste) along with decoction of Kola (Ziziphus jujuba LaM)

Her breasts and abdomen are anointed with

(i) the paste of Chandana (Santalum album Linn) and Mrnala (lotus stalk)

(ii) Powder of Sirisa (Albizia lebbeck Benth), Dhataki (Woodfordia fruticosa Kurz), Sarsapa (Brassica nigra Koch) and Madhuka (Glycyrrhiza glabra Linn) or

(iii) Paste of Kutaja (Holarrhena antidysenterica), Musta (Cyperus rotundus Linn), Haridra (Curcuma longa Linn), or

(iv) Paste of Nimba (Azadirachta indica A. Juss), Kola (Ziziphus jujuba Lam), surasa (Ocimum sanctum Linn) and Manjistha (Rubia cordifolia Linn) or

(v) Triphala (Terminalia chebula Linn, Terminalia belerica Roxb, and Emblica officinalis Gaertn) mixed with the blood of Prsata (spotted deer) and rabbit

Gentle massage is given with oil boiled with the leaves of Karavira (Nerium indicum Mill).

Water boiled with Malati (Aganosma dichotoma K.Schum) and Madhuka (Glycyrrhiza glabra Linn) is used for affusion.

When she feels the itching sensation, she should not scartch the part because it may injure the skin and disfigure it.

When the itching is intolerable, it is corrected by kneading and friction massage.

The ingredients of her food are sweet in taste and they alleviate Vata. The food is taken in small quantity without adding fat and salt. Water, in small quantity is used as Anupana (post- prandial drink).

Eight months:

During this month, she should regularly take milk and gruel added with ghee. This was not acceptable to Bhadrakapya. According to him this will cause Pingala (tawny) colouration of the eyes of the foetus. Lord Punarvasu Atreya replied, "Even if there is (twenty) coloration of the eyes of the foetus, it is not that this therapy should not be given. By doing this, the mother herself will keep good health and give birth to a child endowed with the excellence of health, strength, complexion, voice and compactness which will make him the best even among the children of the entire clan.

Ninth Month:

She is given Anuvasana Basti (unctuous enema) with the oil boiled with Madhurausasadhi (certain selected drugs having sweet taste).

Cotton swabs soaked in this oil are kept in the vagina for the oleation of the uterus and genital tract.

Benefits of monthly management

Adoption of the above-mentioned procedure for the management of the pregnant woman right from the first month up to the ninth month of pregnancy help in the following:

- Softening of placenta, pelvis, waist, sides of the chest and back

- Downward movement of Vata (flatus)

- Normalization of the urine and stool and their elimination with ease;

- Softening of her skin and nails

- Promotion of strength and complexion and

- Delivery with ease of desirable and healthy son (child) endowed with excellent qualities in proper time. [32]

Construction of maternity home:

प्राक् चैवास्या नवमान्मासात् सूतिकागारं कारयेदपहृतास्थिशर्कराकपाले देशे प्रशस्तरूपरसगन्धायां भूमौ प्राग्द्वारमुदग्द्वारं वा बैल्वानां काष्ठानां तैन्दुकैङ्गुदकानां भाल्लातकानां वार(रु)णानां खादिराणां वा; यानि चान्यान्यपि ब्राह्मणाः शंसेयुरथर्ववेदविदस्तेषां; वसनालेपनाच्छादनापिधानसम्पदुपेतं वास्तुविद्याहृदययोगाग्निसलिलोदूखलवर्चःस्थानस्नानभूमिमहानसमृतुसुखं च॥३३॥

Before the ninth month of her pregnancy, the maternity home is constructed in a place free from bones, gravels and pieces of earthen vessels. The soil of the locality should have excellent colour, taste and smell. Its doors should face towards the east or the north and the wood of Bilva (Aegle marmelos corr), Tinduka (Diospyros peregrina Gurke), Ingudi (Balanites aegyptiaca Delile), Bhallataka (Semecarpus anacardium Linn), Varana and Khadira (Acacia catechu Wild) are used for the construction of this maternity home.

Such other measures prescribed by the Brahmanas well versed with the Athrava Veda should also be adopted. This house is equipped with cloth, sheet and bed covers, fire place, water storage, place for pounding, lavatory, bath-room and kitchen is provided here as per the instructions laid down in Vastuvidya (Science of House building). It is air-conditioned to make it comfortable for the particular season. [33]

Drugs to be stored in Maternity home:

तत्र सर्पिस्तैलमधुसैन्धवसौवर्चलकालविड्लवणविड्ङ्गकुष्ठकिलिमनागर-पिप्पलीपिप्पलीमूलहस्तिपिप्पलीमण्डूकपर्ण्येलालाङ्गलीवचाचव्यचित्रकचिरबिल्व-हिङ्गुसर्षपलशुनकतककणकणिकानीपातसीबल्वजभूर्जकुलत्थमैरेयसुरासवाः सन्निहिताः स्युः; तथाऽश्मानौ द्वौ, द्वे कु(च)ण्डमुसले, द्वे उदूखले, खरवृषभश्च, द्वौ च तीक्ष्णौ सूचीपिप्पलकौ सौवर्णराजतौ, शस्त्राणि च तीक्ष्णायसानि, द्वौ च बिल्वमयौ पर्यङ्कौ, तैन्दुकैङ्गुदानि च काष्ठान्यग्निसन्धुक्षणानि, स्त्रियश्च बह्व्यो बहुशः प्रजाताः सौहार्दयुक्ताः सततमनुरक्ताः प्रदक्षिणाचाराः प्रतिपत्तिकुशलाः प्रकृतिवत्सलास्त्यक्तविषादाः क्लेशसहिन्योऽभिमताः, ब्राह्मणाश्चाथर्ववेदविदः; यच्चान्यदपि तत्र समर्थं मन्येत, यच्चान्यच्च ब्राह्मणा ब्रूयुः स्त्रियश्च वृद्धास्तत् कार्यम्॥३४॥

The following drugs are stored in the maternity home:

- Ghee
- Oil
- Honey
- Rock-salt
- Sonchal salt
- Black salt
- Vida salt
- Vidanga(Embelia ribes Burm.f)
- Kustha (Saussurea lappa C.B Clarke)
- Killima (Cedrus deodara Loud)
- Nagara (Zingiber officinale Rose)
- Pippali (Piper longum Linn)
- Root of Pippali (Piper longum)
- Hastipippali (Scindapsus officinalis Schott)
- Mandukaparni (Centella asiatica urban)
- Ela (Elettaria cardamomum Maton)
- Langali (Gloriosa superba Linn)
- Vaca (Acorus calamus Linn)
- Cavya (Piper chaba Hunter)
- Chitraka (Plumbago zeylanica Linn)
- Cirabilva (Pongamia pinnata Merr)
- Hingu (Ferula narthex Boiss)
- Sarsapa (Brassica nigra Koch)
- Lasuna (Alium sativum Linn)
- Kataka (Strychnos potatorum Linn F)
- Kana (also known as Kundaka)
- Kanika (having grains thicker than those of Kana)
- Nipa (Anthocephalus indicus A. Rich)
- Atasi (Linum usitatissimum Linn)
- Balvaja
- Bhurja (Betula utilis D. Don)
- Kulattha (Dolichos biflorus Linn)
- Maireya, Sura and Asava types of wine

In addition to the above, the following substances are kept there.

- Two grinding stones
- Two small pestles
- Two mortars
- One untamed Bull
- Two gold and silver cases for keeping needless
- Various surgical instruments which is sharp and prepared of metal
- Two bed-steeds made of Bilva (Aegle marmelos Corr)
- Wood of Tinduka (Diospyros peregrina Gurke) and Ingudi (Balanites aeyptica Delile) for fuel
- Number of female attendants who are multiparas, affectionate, constantly attached to love, free, from grief, tolerant of hardship and agreeable,
- Brahmins are well versed in the Atharva Veda.

Besides the above, whatever is found necessary and advised by the Brahmins and told ladies should also be kept there. [34]

Admission into maternity home:

ततः प्रवृत्ते नवमे मासे पुण्येऽहनि प्रशस्तनक्षत्रयोगमुपगते प्रशस्ते भगवति शशिनि कल्याणे कल्याणे च करणे मैत्रे मुहूर्ते शान्तिं हुत्वा गोब्राह्मणमग्निमुदकं चादौ प्रवेश्य गोभ्यस्तृणोदकं मधुलाजांश्च प्रदाय ब्राह्मणेभ्योऽक्षतान् सुमनसो नान्दीमुखानि च फलानीष्टानि दत्त्वोदकपूर्वमासनस्थेभ्योऽभिवाद्य पुनराचम्य स्वस्ति वाचयेत्|

ततः पुण्याहशब्देन गोब्राह्मणं समनुवर्तमाना प्रदक्षिणं प्रविशेत् सूतिकागारम्|

तत्रस्था च प्रसवकालं प्रतीक्षेत||३५||

At the onset of ninth month of pregnancy, on an auspicious day having the propitious moon in conjunction with a favourable constellation and during a propitious Karana (an astrological term indicating a division of the day) and Muhurta (an approximate time) oblation should be offered to the sacred fire for peace. Cows, Brahmanas, fire and water are brought to the maternity home in the first instance. Cows are given grass, water and fried paddy added with honey and the Brahmanas are given Aksata (unbroken grains of rice), flowers, and fruits like Kharjura (Dates / Phoenix sylvestris Roxb) which are indicative of good fortune.

The woman should take water and then, after prayers to the respected ones, sit properly. Thereafter she should perform Acamana (taking water in a manner prescribed for auspicious occasions) again and therefore others should recite auspicious Mantras. Then Punyaha (Lit auspicious day) Mantra is recited. Keeping the cow and the Brahmanas on right side, she should enter into the maternity home. There, she should wait for the delivery. [35]

Signs of impending delivery:

तस्यास्तु खल्विमानि लिङ्गानि प्रजननकालमभितो भवन्ति; तद्यथा- क्लमो गात्राणां, ग्लानिराननस्य, अक्ष्णोः शैथिल्यं, विमुक्तबन्धनत्वमिव वक्षसः, कुक्षेरवस्रंसनम्, अधोगुरुत्वं, वङ्क्षणबस्तिकटीकुक्षिपार्श्वपृष्ठनिस्तोदः, योनेः प्रसवणम्, अनन्नाभिलाषश्चेति; ततोऽनन्तरमावीनां प्रादुर्भावः, प्रसेकश्च गर्भोदकस्य||३६||

The following signs indicate the approach of the time of delivery.

- Exhaustion of the limbs
- Feeling of depression in the face
- Looseness in eyes
- Feeling in the chest as if a knot is being untied
- Feeling as if something is coming down from the pelvis
- Heaviness in the lower part of the body
- Pain in groin, region of baldder, pelvis, sides of the chest and back
- Onset of show from the gential tract and
- Loss of appetite

Thereafter true labour pain associated with the excretion of amniotic fluid starts. [36]

Management after onset of labour pain:

आवीप्रादुर्भावे तु भूमौ शयनं विदध्यान्मृद्वास्तरणोपपन्नम्|

तदध्यासीत सा|

तां ततः समन्ततः परिवार्य यथोक्तगुणाः स्त्रियः पर्युपासीरन्नाश्वासयन्त्यो वाग्भिर्ग्राहिणीयाभिः सान्त्वनीयाभिश्च||३७||

When the labour pain starts, a bed is prepared on the ground with soft material used as bed spread and she should be asked to sit over it. Female attendants having the above-mentioned qualities should thereafter remain all around her and console her with talks which are comforting and consoling to her. [37]

Management in case of delay in delivery:

सा चेदावीभिः सङ्क्लिश्यमाना न प्रजायेताथैनां ब्रूयात्- उत्तिष्ठ, मुसलमन्यतरं गृहीष्व, अनेनैतदुलूखलं धान्यपूर्णं मुहुर्मुहुरभिजहि मुहुर्मुहुरवजृम्भस्व चङ्क्रमस्व चान्तराऽन्तरेति; एवमुपदिशन्त्येके|

तन्नेत्याह भगवानात्रेयः|

दारुणव्यायामवर्जनं हि गर्भिण्याः सततमुपदिश्यते, विशेषतश्च प्रजननकाले प्रचलितसर्वधातुदोषायाः सुकुमार्या नार्या

मुसलव्यायामसमीरितो वायुरन्तरं लब्ध्वा प्राणान् हिंस्यात्, दुष्प्रतीकारतमा हि तस्मिन् काले विशेषेण भवति गर्भिणी; तस्मान्मुसलग्रहणं परिहार्यमृषयो मन्यन्ते, जृम्भणं चङ्क्रमणं च पुनरनुष्ठेयमिति|

अथास्यै दद्यात् कुष्ठैलालाङ्गलिकीवचाचित्रकचिरबिल्वचव्यचूर्णमुपघ्रातुं, सा तन्मुहुर्मुहुरुपजिघ्रेत्, तथा भूर्जपत्रधूमं शिंशपासारधूमं वा|

तस्याश्चान्तराऽन्तरा कटीपार्श्वपृष्ठसक्थिदेशानीषदुष्णेन तैलेनाभ्यज्यानुसुखमवमृद्नीयात् |

अनेन कर्मणा गर्भोऽवाक् प्रतिपद्यते||३८||

Some are of the view that if the delivery does not take place in spite of severe labour pain, the pregnant woman is instructed to get up and take up one of thepounding clubs (Pestles). With the help of this club, she should frequently strike the container / mortar filled up with corn. Simultaneously she should frequently resort to pendicilation and while doing so, according to them, she is asked to resort to circumambulation at intervals.

This proposition is not acceptable to Lord Atreya because pregnant women are invariably advised to avoid violent exercises, specially during the time of delivery, in the delicate body of the woman, all the Doshas and Dhatus are in a state of instability and if she resorts to exercise with the help of a club, Vayu gets aggravated, and finding an opportunity, it may destroy the life. Such a condition of a pregnant woman is too difficult to cure. Therefore, Rshis (sages) are of the view that pregnant woman should not resort to exercise with a club. Pendiculation and circumambulation can however be resorted to.

For inhalation she is given the powder of Kustha (Saussurea lappa C.B Clarke), ela (Elettaria cardamomum Maton), Langalika (Gloriosa superba Linn), Vacha (Acorus calamus Linn), chitraka (Plumbago zeylanica Linn), Cirabilva (Pongamia pinnata Merr) and Chavya (Piper chaba Hunter). She should inhale this powder frequently. Back of Bhuraj (Betula utilis D. Don) and the pith of Simshapa (Dalbergia sissoo Roxb) may be used for fumigation.

At intervals she is anointed with warm oil on her waist, sides of the chest, back and thighs and they are gently massaged. By doing this the foetus is brought downwards. [38]

Recitation of mantra:

स यदा जानीयादिवमुच्य हृदयमुदरमस्यास्त्वाविशति, बस्तिशिरोऽवगृह्णाति, त्वरयन्त्येनामाव्यः, परिवर्ततेऽधो [६] गर्भ इति; अस्यामवस्थायां पर्यङ्कमेनामारोप्य प्रवाहयितुमुपक्रमेत|

कर्णे चास्या मन्त्रमिममनुकूला स्त्री जपेत्-

'क्षितिर्जलं वियत्तेजो वायुर्विष्णुः प्रजापतिः|

सगर्भां त्वां सदा पान्तु वैशल्यं च दिशन्तु ते|

प्रसूष्व त्वमविक्लिष्टमविक्लिष्टा शुभानने!|

कार्तिकेयद्युतिं पुत्रं कार्तिकेयाभिरक्षितम्' इति||३९||

When a pregnant woman feels as if the foetus got separated from her heart and entered into the lower abdomen and had approached the area of Basti sira (brim of the pelvis), when the frequency of labour pain has increased and the foetus has turned and is coming downwards, the physician should at this stage, make her lie down over a bed-stead (specially prepared for the purpose). She should then be asked to strain so as to facilitate delivery. A woman favourably disposed to her should recite the following Mantra near her ears:

"(May the Prthvi, Akasha,Agni, Vayu, Vishnu and Prajapati protect the pregnant one at all the times and facilitate the delivery of the child. O! Auspicious one, may the delivery take place without any distresses either to you or to your son, who be endowed with brilliance of Lord Kartikeya and also be protected by him)". [39]

Duties of attendants:

ताश्चैनां यथोक्तगुणाः स्त्रियोऽनुशिष्युः- अनागतावीर्मा प्रवाहिष्ठाः; या ह्यनागतावीः प्रवाहते व्यर्थमेवास्यास्तत् कर्म भवति, प्रजा चास्या विकृता विकृतिमापन्ना च, श्वासकासशोषप्लीहप्रसक्ता वा भवति|

यथा हि क्षवथूद्गारवातमूत्रपुरीषवेगान् प्रयतमानोऽप्यप्राप्तकालान्न लभते कृच्छ्रेण वाऽप्यवाप्नोति, तथाऽनागतकालं गर्भमपि प्रवाहमाणा; यथा चैषामेव क्षवथ्वादीनां सन्धारणमुपघातायोपपद्यते, तथा प्राप्तकालस्य गर्भस्याप्रवाहणमिति|

सा यथानिर्देशं कुरुष्वेति वक्तव्या स्यात्|

तथा च कुर्वती शनैः पूर्व प्रवाहेत, ततोऽनन्तरं बलवत्तरम्|

तस्यां च प्रवाहमाणायां स्त्रियः शब्दं कुर्युः- 'प्रजाता प्रजाता धन्यं धन्यं पुत्रम्' इति|
तथाऽस्या हर्षणाप्याय्यन्ते प्राणाः||४०||

Ladies having the above mentioned (vide para-34) qualities should instruct her as follows:
"Do not strain in the absence of labour pain." Straining in the absence of labour pain does not serve any useful purpose. It causes morbidity and deformity in the foetus and produces diseases like Svasa (breathlessness), Kasa (cough), Sosa (consumption) and Pliha (enlargement of Spleen). As in the absence of natural urges, sneezing, eructation, passage of flatus, urination and defecation do not occur, if at all they occur, they do so with considerable difficulty and artificial efforts. Similarly, premature straining in the absence of natural (normal) labour pain does not produce the desired result. As the suppression of manifested urges of sneezing etc. leads to disastrous effects, so does the absence of straining while there is labour pain. She is asked to obey the instructions. While doing so, she should put strain slowly in the beginning and gradually increase the pressure, while she puts strain, female attendants should say aloud, "thanks, you have delivered a son". This gives her relief and joy, and adds to her regaining the vitality. {40}

Removal of Placenta:

यदा च प्रजाता स्यात्तदैवैनामवेक्षेत- काचिदस्या अपरा प्रपन्ना न वेति|
तस्याश्चेदपरा न प्रपन्ना स्यादथैनामन्यतमा स्त्री दक्षिणेन पाणिना नाभेरुपरिष्टाद्बलवन्निपीड्य सव्येन पाणिना पृष्ठत उपसङ्गृह्य तां सुनिर्धूतं निर्धुनुयात्|
अथास्याः पार्ष्ण्या श्रोणीमाकोटयेत्|
अस्याः स्फिचावुपसङ्गृह्य सुपीडितं पीडयेत्|
अथास्या बालवेण्या कण्ठतालु परिमृशेत्|
भूर्जपत्रकाचमणिसर्पनिर्मोकैश्चास्या योनिं धूपयेत्|
कुष्ठतालीसकल्कं बल्वजयूषे मैरेयसुरामण्डे तीक्ष्णे कौलत्थे व यूषे मण्डूकपर्णीपिप्पलीसम्पाके वा सम्प्लाव्य पाययेदेनाम्|
तथा सूक्ष्मैलाकिलिमकुष्ठनागर विडङ्गपिप्पलीकालागुरुचव्यचित्रकोपकुञ्चिकाकल्कं खरवृषभस्य वा जीवतो दक्षिणं कर्णमुत्कृत्य दृषदि जर्जरीकृत्य बल्वजक्वाथादीनामाप्लावनानामन्यतमे प्रक्षिप्याप्लाव्य मुहूर्तस्थितमुद्धृत्य तदाप्लावनं पाययेदेनाम्|
शतपुष्पाकुष्ठमदनहिङ्गुसिद्धस्य चैनां तैलस्य पिचुं ग्राहयेत्|
अतश्चैवानुवासयेत्|
एतैरेव चाप्लावनैः फलजीमूतेक्ष्वाकुधामार्गवकुटजकृतवेधनहस्तिपिप्पल्युपहितैरास्थापयेत्|
तदास्थापनमस्याः सह वातमूत्रपुरीषैर्निहरत्यपरामासक्तां वायोरेवाप्रतिलोमगत्वात् |
अपरां हि वातमूत्रपुरीषाण्यन्यानि चान्तर्बहिर्मार्गाणि सज्जन्ति||४१||

Immediately after delivery, she is examined for the placenta and it is confirmed if the placenta has come out or not. If the placenta does not come out, the following measures are adopted:
One of the female attendants should forcefully press her (patient's) abdomen (downwards) with her right hand from above the umbilical region while holding her (patient's) back by her left hand and then shake the body of the patient well.
The attendant with her heels should press the hip region of the patient.
The attendant should strongly press her butts with her hands.
Her throat is rubbed with the help of the braid of her hair.
Her vagina is fumigated by burning the bark of Bhurja (Betula utilis D. Don), Kacamani (Quartz) and slough of snake.
She is made to drink the paste of Kustha (Saussurea lappa C.B Clarke) and Talisa (Abies webbiana Lindl) mixed with either of the following:
- Decoction of Balvaja the scum of maireya or sura types of wine having an acute effect
- The decoction of Kulattha (Dolichos biflorus Liinn)
- Decoction of Mandukaparni (Centella asiatica Urban) and Pippali (Piper longum Linn)
A portion of the right ear of the untamed and alive bull is cut and smashed in a stone mortar, and this is added with

the paste of Suksmaila (Elettaria cardamomum Maton), Kilima (Cedrus deodara Loud), Kustha (Saussurea lappa C. B Clarke), Nagara (Zingiber officinale Rosc), and Vidanga (Embelia ribes burm f.), Pippali (Piper longum Linn), Kalaguru (black variety of Aquilaria agallocha Roxb), Chavya (Piper chaba Hunter), Chitraka (Plumbago zeylanica Linn) and Upakunchika (Nigella sativa Linn). The paste should then be soaked in the decoction of Balvaja (?) etc, described above and kept for some time. Then the paste is taken out and the liquid which has thus remained is given to her to drink.

The cotton swab soaked in oil boiled with Satapuspa (Foeniculum vulgare Mill), Kustha (Saussurea lappa. C.B Clarke), Madana (Randia dumetorum Lam) and Hingu (Ferula narthex Boiss) are kept in her genital tract. With this oil she is given Anuvasana Basti (unctuous enema).

The decoction of Balvaja (?) is mixed with the paste of Phala (Randia dumetorum Lam), Jimuta (Luffa echinata Roxb), Iksvaku (Lagenaria siceraria Standl), Dhamargava (Luffa cylindrica M. Roem), Kutaja (Holarrhena antidysenterica wall), Krtavedhana (Luffa acutangula Roxb), and Hastipippali (Scindapsus officinalis Schott) and used for Asthapana (corrective) type of enema. By this Asthapana, there will be downward movement of Vayu (in the abdomen) as a result of which along with flatus, urine and stool, the placenta also comes out. Flatus, urine and stool, and such other excreta as having a tendency to come out of the body during the normal course of events may get obstructed inside the abdomen resulting in the obstruction of the placenta from coming out. [41]

Management of new- born baby:

तस्यास्तु खल्वपरायाः प्रपतनार्थे कर्मणि क्रियमाणे जातमात्रस्यैव कुमारस्य कार्याण्येतानि कर्माणि भवन्ति; तद्यथा- अश्मनोः सङ्घट्टनं कर्णयोर्मूले, शीतोदकेनोष्णोदकेन वा मुखपरिषेकः, तथा स क्लेशविहतान् प्राणान् पुनर्लभेत|

कृष्णकपालिकाशूर्पेण चैनमभिनिष्पुणीयुर्यद्यचेष्टः स्याद् यावत् प्राणानां प्रत्यागमनम् (ततत् सर्वमेव कार्यम्)|

ततः प्रत्यागतप्राणं प्रकृतिभूतमभिसमीक्ष्य स्नानोदकग्रहणाभ्यामुपपादयेत्||४२||

अथास्य ताल्वोष्ठकण्ठजिह्वाप्रमार्जनमारभेताङ्गुल्या सुपरिलिखितनखया सुप्रक्षालितोपधानकार्पाससपिचुमत्या|

प्रथमं प्रमार्जितास्यस्य चास्य शिरस्तालु कार्पासपिचुना स्नेहगर्भेण प्रतिसञ्छादयेत्|

ततोऽस्यानन्तरं सैन्धवोपहितेन सर्पिषा कार्यं प्रच्छर्दनम्||४३||

While taking steps to bring out the placenta, the following measures are taken for the resuscitation of the foetus immediately after birth:

- Stinking of stones near the ears of the child

- Sprinkling with cold water (during summer) and warm water (during winter) on the face

By the above-mentioned measures, the child will gain vitality. The child had lost this vitality as a result of the strain caused by the pressure of the genital tract during the process of its delivery. If after this, there is no movement, then the child should be fanned with the help of black earthen plates until the child starts breathing. For this to happen, all the above-mentioned measures are required to be taken. When the respiration is established and the child attains normally, his excretory passages are cleaned with water and he is given a bath.

Thereafter his palate, lips, throat and tongue are wiped with attendant's fingers from which the nails are properly clipped off and which are well-cleansed and covered with cotton swabs. After cleaning his mouth, the Sirastalu (Anterior fontanelle in the head) of the child is covered with cotton swabs soaked with unctuous substances. Thereafter, the child is given to eat ghee mixed rock-salt for emesis. [42-23]

Separation of Umblical cord:

ततः कल्पनं नाड्याः|

अतस्तस्याः कल्पनविधिमुपदेक्ष्यामः- नाभिबन्धनात् प्रभृत्यष्टाङ्गुलमभिज्ञानं कृत्वा छेदनावकाशस्य द्वयोरन्तरयोः शनैर्गृहीत्वा तीक्ष्णेन रौक्मराजतायसानां छेदनानामन्यतमेनार्धधारेण छेदयेत्|

तामग्रे सूत्रेणोपनिबध्य कण्ठेऽस्य शिथिलमवसृजेत्|

तस्य चेन्नाभिः पच्येत, तां लोध्रमधुकप्रियङ्गुसुरदारुहरिद्राकल्कसिद्धेन तैलेनाभ्यज्यात्, एषामेव तैलौषधानां चूर्णेनावचूर्णयेत्|

इति नाडीकल्पनविधिरुक्तः सम्यक्||४४||

Thereafter the cord is separated (by cutting and ligature). Now the method of separating the cord is being described. The cord is marked at a Distance of eight Angulas (approximately 25.5 cm) from its root where it is attached with the navel. Both the sides of the help of an ardhadhara type of instrument (having very sharp edge), made of gold, silver or steel, the cord is carefully tied with the help of a thread and the ends of the thread is loosely tied to the neck of the foetus.

If there is suppuration of the umbilical cord, the oil boiled with the paste of Lodhra (Symplocos racemosa Roxb), Madhuka, Suradaru (Cedrus deodara Loud) and Haridra (Curcuma longa Linn) is applied. These very medicines which are prescribed to be used for the preparation of oil are made into powder and sprinkled over the suppurated umbilicus.

Thus, the proper method of the separation of umbilical cord is discussed. [44]

Defective separation of the cord:

असम्यक्कल्पने हि नाड्या आयामव्यायामोत्तुण्डिता-पिण्डलिका-विनामिका-विजृम्भिकाबाधेभ्यो भयम्|
तत्राविदाहिभिर्वातपित्तप्रशमनैरभ्यङ्गोत्सादनपरिषेकैः सर्पिर्भिश्चोपक्रमेत गुरुलाघवमभिसमीक्ष्य||४५||

Improper separation of the cord may cause the following morbidity due to the increase in length and breadth of the cord:
- Ayamottundiata (elevation of the umbilicus length wise)
- Vyayamottundiata (elevation of a circular ring around the breadth)
- Pindalika (formation of a circular ring around the umbilicus)
- Vinamika (elevation of the umbilicus in the periphery and depression in the centre) and
- Vijrmbhika (constant increase in the size of the umbilicus)
Carefully observing the seriousness or mildness of the afflicted Doshas, these conditions are treated by massage, unction and sprinkling of ghee prepared of drugs which are not irritative but alleviators of Vata and Pitta. [45]

Birth- rites:

अतोऽनन्तरं जातकर्म कुमारस्य कार्यम्|
तद्यथा- मधुसर्पिषी मन्त्रोपमन्त्रिते यथाम्नायं प्रथमं प्राशितुं दद्यात्|
स्तनमत ऊर्ध्वमेतेनैव विधिना दक्षिणं पातुं पुरस्तात् प्रयच्छेत्|
अथातः शीर्षतः स्थापयेदुदकुम्भं मन्त्रोपमन्त्रितम्||४६||

Thereafter the birth rites of the foetus as prescribed in the Vedas are performed, which are as follows:
- First of all, the child is given honey and ghee impregnated with Mantra prescribed for this purpose in the Vedas
- Thereafter, following the same procedure, milk from the right breast is given to the child first.
- An earthen jar filled with water is impregnated with Mantras and kept near the head of the child. [46]

Protection of new-born:

अथास्य रक्षां विदध्यात्- आदानीखदिरकर्कन्धुपीलुपरूषकशाखाभिरस्या गृहं समन्ततः परिवारयेत्|
सर्वतश्च सूतिकागारस्य सर्षपातसीतण्डुलकणकणिकाः प्रकिरेयुः|
तथा तण्डुलबलिहोमः सततमुभयकालं क्रियेतानामकर्मणः |
द्वारे च मुसलं देहलीमनु तिरश्चीनं न्यसेत्|
वचाकुष्ठक्षौमकहिङ्गुसर्षपातसीलशुनकणकणिकानां रक्षोघ्नसमाख्यातानां चौषधीनां पोट्टलिकां बद्ध्वा सूतिकागारस्योतरदेहल्यामवसृजेत्, तथा सूतिकायाः कण्ठे सप्त्रायाः, स्थाल्युदककुम्भपर्यङ्केष्वपि, तथैव च द्वयोर्द्वारपक्षयोः|
कणककण्टकेन्धनवानग्निस्तिन्दुककाष्ठेन्धनश्चाग्निः सूतिकागारस्याभ्यन्तरतो नित्यं स्यात्|
स्त्रियश्चैनां यथोक्तगुणाः सुहृदश्चानुश्चानुजागृर्युर्दशाहं द्वादशाहं वा|
अनुपरतप्रदानमङ्गलाशीःस्तुतिगीतवादित्रमन्नपानविशदमनुरक्तप्रहृष्टजनसम्पूर्णं च तद्वेश्म कार्यम्|
ब्राह्मणश्चाथर्ववेदवित् सततमुभयकालं शान्तिं जुहुयात् स्वस्त्ययनार्थं कुमारस्य तथा सूतिकायाः|

इत्येतद्रक्षाविधानमुक्तम्॥४७॥

Thereafter measures are taken for the protection of the child.

Branches of Adani, khadira (Acacia catechu Willd), Karkandhu (Ziziphus nummularia W.A), Pilu (Salvadora persica Linn) and Parusaka (Grewia asiatica Linn) are placed all around the maternity home. Grains of mustard, Atasi (Linum usitatissimum Linn), and broken rice is strewn in all places of the maternity home.

Till the name giving ceremony (which occurs on the 10th day after birth), Tandulabali homa (a type of Yajna in which rice is offered to the sacred fire) should be constantly performed both the times during the day. At the gate, a pestle is placed parallel to the threshold. Broken pieces of Vaca (Acorus calamus Linn), Kustha (Saussurea lappa C. B. Clarke), and Ksaumaka Hingu (Ferula narthex Boiss), Sarsapa (Brassica nigra Koch) Atasi (Linum usitatissimum Linn) and Lasuna (Allium sativum Linn) and such other drugs which are known to provide protection from the attacks of evil spirits (like Guggulu or Commiphora mukul Engl) is tied in a packet and hanged to the upper beam of the threshold of the maternity home.

Similar packets are made to hang in the neck of the mother and the child. They are kept in cooking vessels, water jars, cot and doors of on both the sides. Inside the maternity home, fire from the fuel of the thorn of Kanaka and wood of Tinduka (Diospyros peregrina Gurke) are constantly kept burning.

Female attendants having the attributes described in para 34 and friends of the lady should keep constant vigil by remaining awake for 10 or 12 days. The whole house is kept crowded with people who are pious, affectionate and happy, and engaged constantly in gifts, propitious blessings, praise, song, music, food and drinks. To bestow auspiciousness upon the mother and the child, Brahmans well versed with the Atharvaveda should constantly offer sacrifices in the sacred fire during both the times of the day.

Thus measures to be adopted for the protection of the mother and the child are described. [47]

Management of mother after delivery:

सूतिकां तु खलु बुभुक्षितां विदित्वा स्नेहं पाययेत् परमया शक्त्या सर्पिस्तैलं वसां मज्जानं वा सात्म्यीभावमभिसमीक्ष्य पिप्पलीपिप्पलीमूलचव्यचित्रकशृङ्गवेरचूर्णसहितम्।

स्नेहं पीतवत्याश्च सर्पिस्तैलाभ्यामभ्यज्य वेष्टयेदुदरं महताऽच्छेन वाससा; तथा तस्या न वायुरुदरे विकृतिमुत्पादयत्यनवकाशत्वात्।

जीर्णे तु स्नेहे पिप्पल्यादिभिरेव सिद्धां यवागूं सुस्निग्धां द्रवां मात्रशः पाययेत्।

उभयतःकालं चोष्णोदकेन च परिषेचयेत् प्राक् स्नेहयवागूपानाभ्याम्।

एवं पञ्चरात्रं सप्तरात्रं वाऽनुपाल्य क्रमेणाप्याययेत्।

स्वस्थवृत्तमेतावत् सूतिकायाः॥४८॥

Ghee, oil, Vasa (muscle fat) and Majja (bone-marrow), whichever is found suitable, is given along with the powder of Pippali (Piper longum Linn), root of Pippali, Chavya (Piper chaba Hunter), Chitraka (Plumbago zeylanica Linn) and Srngavera (Zingiber officinale Rose) to the mother after she feels hungry.

The quantity of it is in conformity with the strength of the mother. After the intake of fat, her abdomen is anointed with ghee and oil, and wrapped round tightly with a long and clean cloth. By doing so, Vayu does not cause any morbidity in her abdomen because of the absence of any empty space therein.

After the unctuous potion is digested, gruel prepared by boiling with Pippali etc. is given in proper quantity. This gruel is in liquid form and added with unctuous substances. Before the administration of unctuous substances and gruel, she is maintained like this for five to seven nights and then gradually nourished.

These are the measures for the maintenance of positive health of the mother who has recently delivered [48]

Line of treatment of her ailments:

तस्यास्तु खलु यो व्याधिरुत्पद्यते स कृच्छ्रसाध्यो भवत्यसाध्यो वा, गर्भवृद्धिक्षयितशिथिलसर्वधातुत्वात्, प्रवाहणवेदनाक्लेदनरक्तनिःसृतिविशेषशून्यशरीरत्वाच्च; तस्मातां यथोक्तेन विधिनोपचरेत्; भौतिकजीवनीयबृंहणीयमधुरवातहरसिद्धैरभ्यङ्गोत्सादनपरिषेकावगाहनान्नपानविधिभिर्विशेषतश्चोपचरेत्; विशेषतो हि शून्यशरीराः स्त्रियः प्रजाता भवन्ति॥४९॥

If she is afflicted with any disease in these situations, the condition becomes either difficult to cure or incurable because all the tissue elements of her body are diminished in quantity.

This is because the nutrition of the mother is utilized mostly for the growth of the foetus. Further her body is afflicted with emptiness because of the strain involved in labour pain and the loss of blood. This is treated according to the procedure already laid down. She is specifically treated by massage, sprinkling, bath, food, drink prepared with drugs which are Bhautika (alleviators of the effects of evil spirits and germs), Jivaniya (promoter of Vitality), Brimhaniya (promoter of corpulence), sweet in taste and Vatahara (alleviators of Vata) because the body of the woman specifically becomes empty after delivery. [49]

Rites for naming the child:

दशमे त्वहनि सपुत्रा स्त्री सर्वगन्धौषधैर्गौरसर्षपलोधैश्च स्नाता लघ्वहतशुचिवस्त्रं परिधाय पवित्रेष्टलघुविचित्रभूषणवती च संस्पृश्य मङ्गलान्युचितामर्चयित्वा च देवतां शिखिनः शुक्लवाससोऽव्यङ्गांश्च ब्राह्मणान् स्वस्ति वाचयित्वा कुमारमहतानां च वाससां सञ्चये प्राक्शिरसमुदक्शिरसं वा संवेश्य देवतापूर्व द्विजातिभ्यः प्रणमतीत्युक्त्वा कुमारस्य पिता द्वे नामनी कारयेन्नाक्षत्रिकं नामाभिप्रायिकं च|

तत्राभिप्रायिकं घोषवदाद्यन्तस्थान्तमूष्मान्तं वाऽवृद्धं त्रिपुरुषानुक्रमनवप्रतिष्ठितं, नाक्षत्रिकं तु नक्षत्रदेवतासमानाख्यं द्व्यक्षरं चतुरक्षरं वा||५०||

On the tenth day, the mother along with her son is bathed in water boiled with all fragrant drugs, white mustard seeds and Lodhra (Symplocos racemosa). Then she should wear light, untorn, and clean apparel and ornaments which are clean, describle, light and variegated. Thereafter, she should touch auspicious things and offer prayer to appropriate deities and fire, and take blessings from Brahmanas who are dressed with white apparel and who have no deformity of organs.

The child is kept over a bed of untorn new clothes with his head towards the east or the north. Then the father should say that the child is offering prayer to the deity and Brahmanas, and then give two names - one Naksatrika (based upon the constellation in which the child was born) and the other Abhiprayika (the name by which he would be called or known in the family or society). The second category of name should begin with a letter of Ghosa character (e.g G , Gh, J, Jh, D, dh, d, dh and b, bh- according to Cakrapani only voiced aspirated stops) and end with letters of Antyastha character (viz, ya, ra, la, and va) or Usma character (viz, sa, sa, sa and Ha). There should not be letters of vrddhi category (diphthongs) in this type of name and it is in conformity with the pattern of naming a child representaing three generations (father, grandfather and great grandfather). The name should also be a famous one.

The Naksatrika type of name should have similarity with that of the God who is ascribed to the constellation in which the child is born. It is composed of either two or four letters. [50]

Examination of the child to ascertain his span of life:

वृत्ते च नामकर्मणि कुमारं परीक्षितुमुपक्रमेतायुषः प्रमाणज्ञानहेतोः|

तत्रेमान्यायुष्मतां कुमाराणां लक्षणानि भवन्ति|

तद्यथा- एकैकजा मृद्वोऽल्पाः स्निग्धाः सुबद्धमूलाः कृष्णाः केशाः प्रशस्यन्ते, स्थिरा बहला त्वक्, प्रकृत्याऽतिसम्पन्नमीषत्प्रमाणातिवृत्तमनुरूपमातपत्रोपमं शिरः, व्यूढं दृढं समं सुश्लिष्टशङ्खसन्ध्यूर्ध्वव्यञ्जनसम्पन्नमुपचितं वलिभिरर्धचन्द्राकृति ललाटं, बहलौ विपुलसमपीठौ समौ नीचैर्वृद्धौ पृष्ठतोऽवनतौ सुश्लिष्टकर्णपुत्रकौ महाच्छिद्रौ कर्णौ, ईषत्प्रलम्बिन्यावसङ्गते समे संहते महत्यौ भ्रुवौ, समे समाहितदर्शने व्यक्तभागविभागे बलवती तेजसोपपन्ने स्वङ्गापाङ्गे चक्षुषी, ऋज्वी महोच्छ्वासा वंशसम्पन्नेषदवनताग्रा नासिका, महद्ऋजुसुनिविष्टदन्तमास्यम्, आयामविस्तारोपपन्ना श्लक्ष्णा तन्वी प्रकृतिवर्णयुक्ता जिह्वा, श्लक्ष्णं युक्तोपचयमूष्मोपपन्नं रक्तं तालु, महानदीनः स्निग्धोऽनादी गम्भीरसमुत्थो धीरः स्वरः, नातिस्थूलौ नातिकृशौ विस्तारोपपन्नावास्यप्रच्छादनौ रक्तावोष्ठौ, महत्यौ हनू, वृत्ता नातिमहती ग्रीवा, व्यूढमुपचितमुरः, गूढं जत्र पृष्ठवंशश्च, विप्रकृष्टान्तरौ स्तनौ, असम्पातिनी स्थिरे पार्श्वे, वृत्तपरिपूर्णायतौ बाहू सक्थिनी अङ्गुलयश्च, महदुपचितं पाणिपादं, स्थिरा वृत्ताः स्निग्धास्तामास्तुङ्गाः कूर्माकाराः करजाः, प्रदक्षिणावर्ता सोत्सङ्गा च नाभिः, उरस्त्रिभागहीना समा समुपचितमांसा कटी, वृत्तौ स्थिरोपचितमांसौ नात्युन्नतौ नात्यवनतौ स्फिचौ, अनुपूर्व वृत्तावुपचययुक्तावूरू, नात्युपचिते नात्यपचिते एणीपदे प्रगूढसिरास्थिसन्धी जङ्घे, नात्युपचितौ नात्यपचितौ गुल्फौ, पूर्वोपदिष्टगुणौ पादौ कूर्माकारौ, प्रकृतियुक्तानि वातमूत्रपुरीषगुह्यानि तथा स्वप्रजागरणायाससस्मितरुदितस्तनग्रहणानि, यच्च

किञ्चिदन्यदप्यनुक्तमस्ति तदपि सर्व प्रकृतिसम्पन्नमिष्टं, विपरीतं पुनरनिष्टम्‌|

इति दीर्घायुर्लक्षणानि||५१||

After performing the rites for giving a name to the child, he is examined with a view to ascertaining the span of his life. The following signs and symptoms are those of children having a long span of life:

Organs of the child and Characteristic features indicative of long span of life

Hair - Distant, soft, sparse, unctuous, firmly rooted and black

Skin - Thick and not loose

Head - Constitutionally of excellent type, slightly bigger in size (than the measurement furnished in Vimana 8: 117), proportionate with other parts of the body and resembling an umbrella in shape.

Forehead - Broad, strong, even, compact, having firm union with temporal bones, having three transverse lines, plump, having wrinkles and having the shape of a half moon.

Ears - Thick, large in size, having even lobes, equal in size, having elongations downwards, bent towards the back side, having compact tragus and having a big earhole.

Eye brows - Slightly hanging downwards, separated from each other, equal in size, compact and large in size.

Eyes - Equal in size , having fixed look, having equal in size, having fixed look, having clear cut divisions (of pupil, iris or black portion of the eye), strong, lustrous, beautiful and having beautiful Apanga (cornes of eyes)

Nose - Straight, capable of taking deep breath, well ridged, and slightly curved at the tip

Mouth - Big in size, straight and having (two rows of) compact teeth

Tongue

Having proper length and breadth, smooth, thin and endowed with natural colour

Palate - Smooth, plump, hot in touch and red in colour

Voice - Profound,not sluggish, sweet, having echo, deep toned and steady

Lips - Neither very thick nor very thin, adequate, capable of covering the mouth cavity and red in colour

Jaws - Large in size

Neck - Round in shape and not very large in size

Chest - Broad and plump

Clavicles and vertibral column - Not visible

Breasts - Having wide space in between them

Prarsva (sides of the chest) - Downwards and firm

Arms, thighs, fingers including toes - Round, full and extended

Hands and legs - Large in size and plump

Nails - Firm, round, unctuous, coppery coloured, properly elevated and convex like the back of a tortoise

Umbilicus - Whirled clock–wise and well depressed

Wait - Less than 3.4^{th} of the chest in circumference, even and plump with muscles

Buttocks - Round, firm, plump with muscles and neither excessively elevated nor excessively depressed

Thighs - Tapering downwards, round and plump

Calf region - Neither excessive plump nor excessively emaciated, having resemblance with that of a deer and having vessels, bones and joints well covered

Ankles - Neither excessively plump nor excessively emaciated

Feet - Having the characteristic features described above and having the shape like that of a tortoise.

To a child having a long span of a life is given to normal flatus, urine, stool, anus, sleep, vigil, fatigue, smiling, crying, sucking of milk and similar other factors/phenomena which are not described here, they are neither more nor less than the normal.

If the child is with the organs/ phenomena having attributes in contradiction with what is described above, then they are indicative of less span of life of the child.

Thus ends the signs and symptoms of a child having a long span of life. [51]

Selection of wet-nurse:

अतो धात्रीपरीक्षामुपदेक्ष्यामः।

अथ ब्रूयात्- धात्रीमानय समानवर्णां यौवनस्थां निभृतामनातुरामव्यङ्गामव्यसनामविरूपामजुगुप्सितां देशजातीयामक्षुद्रामक्षुद्रकर्मिणीं कुले जातां वत्सलामरोगां जीवद्वत्सां पुंवत्सां दोग्धीमप्रमत्तामनुच्चारशायिनीमनन्त्यावसायिनीं कुशलोपचारां शुचिमशुचिद्वेषिणीं स्तनस्तन्यसम्पदुपेतामिति॥५२॥

Now we shall describe the procedure to be adopted in selecting a wet-nurse. She is of the same caste, youthful (women before the attainment of youth have immature tissue elements and the tissue elements of old women had undergone destruction- hence they are not suitable to be employed as wet nurse), submissive, free from diseases, not deficient of limbs, not given to luxurious living, not ugly looking (because of deformity in her organs), not given to hateful disposition, born in the same locality, not mean minded, not hateful disposition, born in the same locality, not given to mean acts, born in a respectable family, having affection for children, free from illness, having living children, having sons, having plenty of milk, careful, not given to sleeping over clothes soiled with excreta, not having a husband of lower caste (e.g a sudra woman having a Candala Husband), skilful in service, observing cleanliness, having aversion for dirty things, having the excellence of breasts and milk. [52]

Excellence of breasts:

तत्रेयं स्तनसम्पत्- नात्यूर्ध्वौ नातिलम्बावनतिकृशावनतिपीनौ युक्तपिप्पलकौ सुखप्रपानौ चेति (स्तनसम्पत्)॥५३॥

The qualities of excellent breasts are as follows:
- They are situated at a very high level in the chest
- They should not hang very loose
- They should neither be very lean nor very plump
- They have nipples of proportionate size
- The child should find it easy to suckle them.

This is about the excellence of breasts. [53]

Excellence of breast- milk

स्तन्यसम्पतु प्रकृतिवर्णगन्धरसस्पर्शम्, उदपात्रे च दुह्यमानमुदकं व्येति प्रकृतिभूतत्वात्; तत् पुष्टिकरमारोग्यकरं चेति (स्तन्यसम्पत्)॥५४॥

अतोऽन्यथा व्यापन्नं ज्ञेयम्।

तस्य विशेषाः:- श्यावारुणवर्णं कषायानुरसं विशदमनालक्ष्यगन्धं रूक्षं द्रवं फेनिलं लघ्वतृप्तिकरं कर्शनं वातविकाराणां कर्तृ वातोपसृष्टं क्षीरमभिज्ञेयं ; कृष्णनीलपीततताम्रावभासं तिक्ताम्लकटुकानुरसं कुणपरुधिरगन्धि भृशोष्णं पित्तविकाराणां कर्तृ च पित्तोपसृष्टं क्षीरमभिज्ञेयम्, अत्यर्थशुक्लमतिमाधुर्योपपन्नं लवणानुरसं घृततैलवसामज्जगन्धि पिच्छिलं तन्तुमदुकपात्रेऽवसीदच्छ्लेष्मविकाराणां कर्तृ श्लेष्मोपसृष्टं क्षीरमभिज्ञेयम्॥५५॥

Milk of excellent quality should have natural colour, smell, taste and touch. When poured over the water in a pot, it gets mixed up with the water if it is endowed with natural qualities. This provides nourishment and maintains good health of the child.

If the qualities of milk do not conform to the above, then it is considered as vitiated. Characteristic features of the milk vitiated with Doshas are as follows:

Vitiating Dosa and Characteristic features of the vitiated milk

Vata - Blackish or reddish in colour, astringent in Anurasa (after taste), clear, absence of any conscious smell, unctuous, liquid, frothy, light, not satisfying and causing emaciation and Vatika diseases

Pitta - Blackish, bluish, yellowish or coppery in colour, bitter, sour or pungent in after-taste; having smell like that of a dead body or blood; excessively hot and causing Paittika diseases

Kapha - Exceedingly white in colour, excessively sweet in taste and having saline after taste; having the smell of ghee, oil, Vasa (Muscle fat) and bone marrow; slimy; thready; settling down at the bottom when poured into a vessel containing water and causing Slaismika type of diseases. [54-55]

Treatment of vitiated breast- milk

तेषां तु त्रयाणामपि क्षीरदोषाणां प्रतिविशेषमभिसमीक्ष्य यथास्वं यथादोषं च वमनविरेचनास्थापनानुवासनानि विभज्य कृतानि प्रशमनाय भवन्ति|

पानाशनविधिस्तु दुष्टक्षीराया यवगोधूमशालिषष्टिकमुद्गहरेणुककुलत्थसुरासौवीरकमैरेयमेदकलशुनकरञ्जप्रायः स्यात्|

क्षीरदोषविशेषांश्चावेक्ष्यावेक्ष्य तत्तद्विधानं कार्यं स्यात्|

पाठामहौषधसुरदारुमुस्तमूर्वागुडूचीवत्सकफलकिराततिक्तककटुकरोहिणीसारिवाकषायाणां च पानं प्रशस्यते, तथाऽन्येषां तिक्तकषायकटुकमधुराणां द्रव्याणां प्रयोगः क्षीरविकारविशेषानभिसमीक्ष्य मात्रां कालं च|

इति क्षीरविशोधनानि||५६||

When (breast) milk gets vitiated, the specific nature of the vitiation is ascertained, and depending upon the Doshas involved and the quantum of their vitiation, the mother is given Vamana (emetic therapy), Virechana (purgation therapy), asthapana (corrective enema) and Anuvasana (unctuous enema) whichever is found suitable, for the cure of the ailment.

The food and drink of the mother whose milk is vitiated should for the most part consist of barley, wheat, Shali (Oryza sativa Linn), Sasthika (a type of Shali), Mudga (Vigna radiata), harenuka (Lathyrus aphaca Linn), alcoholic preparations like Sura, Sauviraka Maireyaka and Medaka, Merr). Suitable regimens are advised to her depending upon the specific nature of the vitiation of milk.

Keeping in view the specific nature of the vitiation of milk, dose and time, it is beneficial to administer the decoction of Patha (Cissampelos pareira Linn), Mahausadha (Zingiber officinale Rosc), Suradaru (Cedrus deodara Loud), Musta (Cyperus rotundus Linn), Murva (Clematis triloba) Heyne ex Roth), Guduci (Tinospora cordifolia Miers), fruit of Vatsaka (Holarrhena antidysenterica wall) Kiratatikta (Swertia chirata Buch –Han), Katurohini (Picrorhiza kurroa Royle ex Benth) (Individually or all of them together) and Sariva (Hemidesmus indicus R.B) and such other drugs having bitter, astringent, pungent and sweet tastes.

Thus, the measures for the correction of the vitiation of milk are described. [56]

Promoters of Lactation:

क्षीरजननानि तु मद्यानि सीधुवर्ज्यानि, ग्राम्यानूपौदकानि च शाकधान्यमांसानि, द्रवमधुराम्ललवणभूयिष्ठाश्चाहाराः, क्षीरिण्यश्चौषधयः, क्षीरपानमनायासश्च, वीरणषष्टिकशालीक्षुवालिकादर्भकुशकाशगुन्द्रेत्कटमूलकषायाणां च पानमिति (क्षीरजननानि)||५७||

The following are the promoters of lactation:

Wines except Sidhu (a type of wine)

Vegetable, corns and meat of animals which are domesticated and which inhabit the marshy land and water.

Food having the predomience of liquid ingredients or ingredients having sweet, sour and saline tastes

Medicinal plants having milky juice like Dugdhika (Euphorbia microphylla Heyne) and Kalambika (Ipomea reptans Poir).

Intake of milk and carefree living

Intake of the decoction of the roots of Virana (Vetiveria zizanioides nash), Sasthika (a type of Shali) (Oryza sativa Linn), Iksuvalika (Asteracantha longifolia Nees), Darbha (a type of Kusa) Kusa (Demostachya bipinnata Stapf), Kasha (Saccharum spontaneum Linn).

These are the promoters of lactation. [57]

Procedure for feeding the child:

धात्री तु यदा स्वादुबहुलशुद्धदुग्धा स्यातदास्नातानुलिप्ता शुक्लवस्त्रं परिधायैन्द्रीं ब्राह्मीं शतवीर्यां सहस्रवीर्याममोघामव्यथां शिवामरिष्टां वाट्यपुष्पीं विष्वक्सेनकान्तां वा बिभ्रत्योषधिं कुमारं प्राङ्मुखं प्रथमं दक्षिणं स्तनं पाययेत्|

इति धात्रीकर्म||५८||

The milk of the wetnurse is sweet in taste, copious and pure. Such a wet-nurse should take her bath, use unction, wear white cloth as well as medicines like Aindri (Citrullus colocynthis Schard), Brahmi (Bacopa monnieri Pennel), Satavirya (Cynodon dactylon Pers), Sahasravirya (a type of satavirya), Amogha (Emblica officinalis Gaertn), Avyatha (Tinospora cordifolia Miers), Siva (Terminalia chebula Linn), Arista (Picrorhiza kurroa Royle ex Benth), Vatyapuspi (Sida rhombifolia Linn) and Visvaksenakanta (Callicarpa macrophylla Vahl). Thereafter, keeping the child facing towards the east, she should make him suckle her right breast first.

Thus, the duties of a wetnurse are described. [58]

Nursery:

अतोऽनन्तरं कुमारागारविधिमनुव्याख्यास्यामः- वास्तुविद्याकुशलः प्रशस्तं रम्यमतमस्कं निवातं प्रवातैकदेशं दृढमपगतश्वापदपशुदंष्ट्रिमूषिकपतङ्गं सुविभक्तसलिलोलूखलमूत्रवर्चःस्थानस्नानभूमिमहानसमृतुसुखं यथर्तुशयनासनास्तरणसम्पन्नं कुर्यात्; तथा सुविहितरक्षाविधानबलिमङ्गलहोमप्रायश्चित्तं शुचिवृद्धवैद्यानुरक्तजनसम्पूर्णम्।
इति कुमारागारविधिः॥५९॥

Now we shall describe the procedure for the construction of a nursery for the child. The nursery is constructed under the supervision of an expert architect. It should be
- A commendable one
- Beautiful
- Free from darkness
- Sheltered from drought
- Admitting air only from one side
- Sturdy
- Free from Svapada (animals in general), Damstrin (fanged creatures), Rats and moths
- Well planned places for water storage, grinding, lavatory, bathroom and kitchen
- Comfortable for living in all seasons (air conditioned) and
- Furnished with beds, seats and spreads in conformity with the needs of that particular season

There should be proper arrangements for the protection of the house from outside attacks. Sacrifices, auspicious rites, offering of oblations and recitation of verses are performed in the house. This house is kept crowded with persons who are clean, experienced physicians and those who have attachment with the family.

Thus, the procedure for the construction of the nursery is described. [59]

Cleanliness of beds etc:

शयनासनास्तरणप्रावरणानि कुमारस्य मृदुलघुशुचिसुगन्धीनि स्युः; स्वेदमलजन्तुमन्ति मूत्रपुरीषोपसृष्टानि च वर्ज्यानि स्युः; असति सम्भवेऽन्येषां तान्येव च सुप्रक्षालितोपधानानि सुधूपितानि शुद्धशुष्काण्युपयोगं गच्छेयुः॥६०॥

Beds, seats, spreads and apparel of the child should be soft, light, clean and fragrant. Those which are soiled with sweat, excreta, germs, urine and stool are discarded. If it is not possible to procure new ones, then the old ones should be well exposed to the sun after they are washed thoroughly. Thus, they can be used only after they are rendered clean and dry. [60]

Drugs for fumigation of cloths:

धूपनानि पुनर्वाससां शयनास्तरणप्रावरणानां च
यवसर्षपातसीहिङ्गुगुग्गुलुवचाचोरकवयःस्थागोलोमीजटिलापलङ्कषाशोकरोहिणीसर्पनिर्मोकाणि घृतयुक्तानि स्युः॥६१॥

Barley, mustard, Atasi (Linum usitatissimum Linn), Hingu (Ferula narthex Boiss), Guggulu (Commiphora mukul Engl), Vaca (Acorus calamus Linn), Coraka (Angelica glauca Edgew), Vayastha (Bacopa monnieri Pennel), Golomi (a type of Vaca), Jatila (Nardostachys jatamansi D. C), Palankasha (a type of guggulu), Asoka (Saraca indica Linn), Rohini (Picrorhiza kurroa Royle ex Benth) and slough of snake mixed with ghee is used for fumigation of clothes used for beds, spreads and apparel. [61]

Wearing talismans:

मणयश्च धारणीयाः कुमारस्य खड्गगरुरुगवयवृषभाणां जीवतामेव दक्षिणेभ्यो विषाणेभ्योऽग्राणि गृहीतानि स्युः; ऐन्द्र्याद्याश्चौषधयो जीवकर्षभकौ च, यानि चान्यान्यपि ब्राह्मणाः प्रशंसेयुरथर्ववेदविदः||६२||

The child is made to wear the following as talismans:

Jewels - like pearls etc (as prescribed in the Atharva Veda)

Tips of the right horns of rhinoceros, deer, gayal or bull collected when they are alive

Medicinal plants like Aindri etc. (vide para 58 of this chapter and sutra 4:18) Jivaka (?) and Rsabhaka (?)

Such other things as are praised and prescribed by the Brahmanas well versed with the AtharvaVeda. [62]

Toys:

क्रीडनकानि खलु कुमारस्य विचित्राणि घोषवन्त्यभिरामाणि चागुरूणि चातीक्ष्णाग्राणि चानास्य प्रवेशीनि चाप्राणहराणि चावित्रासनानि स्युः||६३||

Toys of the child is variegated, sound producing, beautiful, light, without sharp edge, incapable of being swallowed, fraught with no danger to life and un-frightening [63]

Child should not be frightened:

न ह्यस्य वित्रासनं साधु|

तस्मात्तस्मिन् रुदत्यभुञ्जाने वाऽन्यत्र विधेयतामगच्छति राक्षसपिशाचपूतनाद्यानां नामान्याह्वयता कुमारस्य वित्रासनार्थं नामग्रहणं न कार्यं स्यात्||६४||

One should not frighten the child (at any stage), therefore, whether he cries or does not eat or does not submit to discipline, he must not be frightened by calling the names of Raksasa, Pisaca, Putana etc. (all evil creatures). [64]

Management of Pediatric diseases:

यदि त्वातुर्यं किञ्चित् कुमारमागच्छेत् तत् प्रकृतिनिमित्तपूर्वरूपलिङ्गोपशयविशेषैस्तत्त्वतोऽनुबुध्य सर्वविशेषानातुरौषधदेशकालाश्रयानवेक्षमाणश्चिकित्सितुमारभेतैनं मधुरमृदुलघुसुरभिशीतशङ्करं कर्म प्रवर्तयन्|

एवंसात्म्या हि कुमारा भवन्ति|

तथा ते शर्म लभन्ते चिराय|

अरोगे त्वरोगवृत्तमातिष्ठेद्देशकालात्मगुणविपर्ययेण वर्तमानः, क्रमेणासात्म्यानि परिवर्त्योपयुञ्जानः सर्वाण्यहितानि वर्जयेत्|

तथा बलवर्णशरीरायुषां सम्पदमवाप्नोतीति||६५||

एवमेनं कुमारमायौवनप्राप्तेर्धर्मार्थकौशलागमनाच्चानुपालयेत्||६६||

If the child gets afflicted with any disease, it should be properly diagnosed, with due regard to the specific nature of the etiology, premonitory symptoms, symptoms and Upashaya (homologatory signs) of the disease. Simultaneously, characteristic features of the patient, drugs, locality, season and physical constitution of the child is examined.

Thereafter, he should be treated by administering therapies which are sweet, soft, light, fragrant, cold and comfortable and those which yield long standing effects. If he is free from any disease whatsoever, the child should be made to resort to regimens which are opposite in quality to the locality, time and bodily constitution for the maintenance of positive health. Unwholesome regimens should gradually be avoided. By doing so, the child gets endowed with excellent strength, complexion, physical constitution and span of life.

In this manner, from childhood to youth, the child is brought up till he is competent to perform religious rites and earn wealth. [65-66]

इति पुत्राशिषां समृद्धिधिकरं कर्म व्याख्यातम्|

तदाचरन् यथोक्तैर्विधिभिः पूजां यथेष्टं लभतेऽनसूयक इति||६७||

Thus the measures for the fulfillment of desire to have progeny are described. By taking recourse to these factors in the prescribed manner, one who is free from envy is blessed (with progeny) according as he wishes. [67]

तत्र श्लोकौ-
पुत्राशिषां कर्म समृद्धिकारकं यदुक्तमेतन्महदर्थसंहितम्‌|
तदाचरन्‌ ज्ञो विधिभिर्यथातथं पूजां यथेष्टं लभतेऽनसूयकः||६८||

To sum up:-

Measures described here fulfill the desire of the individual to obtain a son and they are of great importance. By taking recourse to these measures in a prescribed manner, wise man free envy is blessed (with a child) according as he wishes. [68]

शरीरं चिन्त्यते सर्वं दैवमानुषसम्पदा|
सर्वभावैर्यतस्तस्माच्छारीरं स्थानमुच्यते||६९||

This section is known as "Sharirasthana" because it deals with the description of the knowledge which is conducive to be understanding of all the godly and human aspects of the phenomena in the individual's body. [69]

इत्यग्निवेशकृते तन्त्रे चरकप्रतिसंस्कृते शारीरस्थाने जातिसूत्रीयं शारीरं नामाष्टमोऽध्यायः||८||
इति चरकसंहितायां चथुर्थं शारीरस्थानं सम्पूर्णम्‌|

Thus ends the eighth chapter of the Sharira section dealing with the description of the method of procreation as conducive to the understanding of the human body, of Agnivesha's work as redacted by Charaka. [8]

Thus ends the Sharira Section.

इन्द्रियस्थानम् Indriya Sthanam

25

Indriyasthana Chapter 1 Varna Swareeyam Indriyam

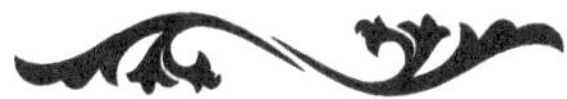

IndriyaSthana (Section on the Symptoms of Imminent Death)

अथातो वर्णस्वरीयमिन्द्रियं व्याख्यास्यामः||१||

इति ह स्माह भगवानात्रेयः||२||

Now we shall expound the chapter on "Signs and Symptoms of Imminent Death as Indicated by complexion and Voice". Thus said Lord Atreya [1-2]

Factors to be examined to determine residual span of life:

इह खलु वर्णश्च स्वरश्च गन्धश्च रसश्च स्पर्शश्च चक्षुश्च श्रोत्रं च घ्राणं च रसनं च स्पर्शनं च सत्त्वं च भक्तिश्च शौचं च शीलं चाचारश्च स्मृतिश्चाकृतिश्च प्रकृतिश्च विकृतिश्च बलं च ग्लानिश्च मेधा च हर्षश्च रौक्ष्यं च स्नेहश्च तन्द्रा चारम्भश्च गौरवं च लाघवं च गुणाश्चाहारश्च विहारश्चाहारपरिणामश्चोपायश्चापायश्च व्याधिश्च व्याधिपूर्वरूपं च वेदनाश्चोपद्रवाश्च च्छाया च प्रतिच्छाया च स्वप्नदर्शनं च दूताधिकारश्च पथि चौत्पातिकं चातुरकुले भावावस्थान्तराणि च भेषजसंवृत्तिश्च [१] भेषजविकारयुक्तिश्चेति परीक्ष्याणि प्रत्यक्षानुमानोपदेशैरायुषः प्रमाणावशेषं जिज्ञासमानेन भिषजा||३||

Below mentioned are the important factors which needs to be examined by the physician who wishes to know and ascertain the residual life span of the patient by means of direct observation, inferential knowledge and scriptural testimony :

Varna – colour / complexion

Svara – voice

Gandha - smell

Rasa – taste

Sparsha –touch

Chakshu – eyes

Shrotram – ears

Ghrana – nose

Rasanam – tongue

Sparshanam – skin

Sattvam – mind

Bhaktim – desire

Shaucham – purity

Shilam – conduct

Achara - refined behaviour

Smrti – memory

Aakrti – shape

Prakrti – nature

Vikrti – morbidity

Bala – strength

Glani – exhaustion

Medha – intelligence

Harsha – exhilaration

Rauskyam – dryness

Sneha – unctuousness

Tandra - drowsiness (sleep)

Aarambha – onset of diseases

Gauravam – heaviness

Laghavam – lightness

Guna – qualities / attributes

Aahara – diet

Vihara – regimens

Aahara parinama – transformation / digestion of food

Upaya – collection of diseases (many diseases manifesting at the same time, syndrome)

Apaya - disappearance of the disease suddenly, without any reason

Vyadhi purvarupam – premonitory features of the disease

Vedana – pain

Upadrava - complications

Chaya – luster

Pratichaya – shadow

Svapna – dreams

Dutadhikara darshanam - bad omens visualised by the physician

Pathi cha utpatikam - bad omens seen by the doctor on his way to the patient's house

Aatura kule bhavaavasthaantarani - Bad omens at the residence of the patient

Bheshaja samvrti – obstruction / concealing of medicines

Bheshaja vikarayukti – defective medicines / absence of effects of medicine [3]

Out –line of the method of examination:

तत्र तु खल्वेषां परीक्ष्याणां कानिचित् पुरुषमनाश्रितानि, कानिचिच्च पुरुषसंश्रयाणि|
तत्र यानि पुरुषमनाश्रितानि तान्युपदेशतो युक्तितश्च परीक्षेत, पुरुषसंश्रयाणि पुनः प्रकृतितो विकृतितश्च||४||

Among some of the factors described in the above verse some of them relate to the patients and some other factors do not relate to them. Scriptural inscriptions and inference are the two tools which help in ascertaining the factors which do not relate to the patients. The factors which are related to patients should be ascertained from their natural and unnatural (morbid) dispositions. [4]

Various types of prakriti (natural disposition):

तत्र प्रकृतिर्जातिप्रसक्ता च, कुलप्रसक्ता च, देशानुपातिनी [१] च,
कालानुपातिनी च वयोऽनुपातिनी च, प्रत्यात्मनियता चेति|
जातिकुलदेशकालवयःप्रत्यात्मनियता हि तेषां तेषां पुरुषाणां ते ते भावविशेषा भवन्ति||५||

Depending on the distinct features of the below mentioned, the natural disposition is of six categories :

1. Caste e.g., purity among Brahmanas

2. Family e.g., purity with regard to character and conduct in a good family

3. Geography e.g., manifested due to being born in a specific locality, country or geographical region e.g., people living in Banga / Vanga region are intellectual.

4. Time factor e.g., purity in the Satya Yuga i.e., the first epoch / good strength in visarga kala i.e., in the monsoon,

autumn and early winter seasons and deficit strength in adana kala i.e., late winter, spring and summer

5. Age factor e.g., predominance of kapha in childhood, predominance of pitta in the adolescence and adulthood and predominance of vata in old age

6. Individuality / personal factor – depends on the physique, mind and sense organs of an individual and is different in different individuals [5]

Various types of Vikrti (unnatural disposition):

विकृतिः पुनर्लक्षणनिमित्ता च, लक्ष्यनिमित्ता च, निमित्तानुरूपा च||६||

The morbid condition is of three types, viz

Lakshana nimitta - caused by bodily marks

Lakshya nimitta - caused by etiological factors and

Nimittanurupa - caused by such factors which resemble the etiological factors [6]

Bodily marks as indicative of unnatural disposition:

तत्र लक्षणनिमित्ता नाम सा यस्याः शरीरे लक्षणान्येव हेतुभूतानि भवन्ति दैवात्; लक्षणानि हि कानिचिच्छरीरोपनिबद्धानि भवन्ति, यानि हि तस्मिंस्तस्मिन् काले तत्राधिष्ठानमासाद्य तां तां विकृतिमुत्पादयन्ति|७|

If the bodily marks indicate certain morbid conditions as a result of past actions they are called as Lakshana Nimitta. There are certain bodily marks / signs / symptoms which during the maturation of good or bad deeds get settled in some parts of the body and give rise to morbidities in due course of time. [7-i]

Etiological factors as indicative of unnatural disposition:

लक्ष्यनिमित्ता तु सा यस्या उपलभ्यते निमित्तं यथोक्तं निदानेषु|७|

If the morbid conditions are caused by etiological factors as described in Nidana section they will be known as Lakshya nimitta e.g., aggravation of Vata due to the intake of dry food etc etiological factors. Example – there are four causes / etiological factors of rajayakshma i.e., excessive indulgence in herculean activities, forcible withholding of natural urges, depletion of body tissues and eating foods in erratic / erroneous ways. [7-ii]

Factors resembling aetiological factors:

निमित्तानुरूपा तु निमित्तार्थानुकारिणी या, तामनिमित्तां निमित्तमायुषः प्रमाणज्ञानस्येच्छन्ति भिषजो भूयश्चायुषः क्षयनिमित्तां प्रेतेलिङ्गानुरूपां, यामायुषोऽन्तर्गतस्य ज्ञानार्थमुपदिशन्ति धीराः| यां चाधिकृत्य पुरुषसंश्रयाणि मुमूर्षतां लक्षणान्युपदेक्ष्यामः| इत्युद्देशः|तं विस्तरेणानुव्याख्यास्यामः||७||

These are the deformities / premonitory symptoms which serve the function (objective, purpose) of etiological factors i.e., producing a disease and giving the knowledge of the disease. Such unnatural situations i.e., symptoms are known as Nimittanurupa.

In a real sense they are not causative factors. But they definitely serve as yardsticks in measuring the lifespan of individuals. Apart from this they are also indicators of death resulting from diminution of life span. Therefore, the knowledge of these unnatural situations (symptoms) is of utmost importance. They help the physicians in ascertaining the lifespan of an individual which cannot be determined or confirmed by other tools of examination.

We shall describe such symptoms which are manifested in a person who is in very close proximity to death (death is almost ascertained). In this instance it is stated briefly but shall be explained in greater detail in the later contexts of the section. [7]

Normal and abnormal complexion:

तत्रादित एव वर्णाधिकारः तद्यथा- कृष्णः, श्यामःश्यामावदातः, अवदातश्चेति प्रकृतिवर्णाः शरीरस्य भवन्ति; यांश्चापरानुपेक्षमाणो विद्यादनूकतोऽन्यथा वाऽपि निर्दिश्यमानांस्तज्ज्ञैः||८||

a. Natural complexions:
To start with, complexion is being described. There are four types of natural complexions :

- black
- bluish
- bluish white
- white

There are also some other types of natural complexions. They need to be ascertained by similarities (colours similar to the above mentioned) or from the instructions of experts (experts who can demarcate normal and abnormal complexions / colours with authenticity.

b. Unnatural complexions:
नीलश्यावताम्रहरितशुक्लाश्च वर्णाः शरीरस्य वैकारिका भवन्ति; यांश्चापरानुपेक्षमाणो विद्यात् प्राग्विकृतानभूत्वोत्पन्नान् |
इति प्रकृतिविकृतिवर्णा भवन्त्युक्ताः शरीरस्य|
There are five types of unnatural complexions. They are:

- blue
- grey
- coppery
- green and
- albino (abnormally white)

Similarly, there are some other unnatural types of complexions which are produced anew. They too need to be understood on the basis of their similarity with the above-mentioned abnormal complexions. Similarly, if the natural complexion which was bestowed at birth changes in later part of one's life, that complexion too shall be considered as abnormal. Thus, the normal (natural) and abnormal (unnatural) complexions in the body are described. [8]

Combination of normal and abnormal complexions indicating imminent death:
तत्र प्रकृतिवर्णमर्धशरीरे विकृतिवर्णमर्धशरीरे, द्वावपि वर्णौ मर्यादाविभक्तौ दृष्ट्वा; यद्येवं सव्यदक्षिणविभागेन, यद्येवं पूर्वपश्चिमविभागेन, यद्युत्तराधरविभागेन, यद्यन्तर्बहिर्विभागेन, आतुरस्यारिष्टमिति विद्यात्; एवमेव वर्णभेदो मुखेऽप्यन्यत्र वर्तमानो मरणाय भवति||९||
It may so happen that half of the body may have natural complexion and the other half of the body would have unnatural complexion and both these complexions are demarcated by an even demarcating line. These normal and abnormal complexions simultaneously appearing in right and left sides, front and back sides, upper and lower parts or internal and external parts of the body should be considered as signs of imminent death for a given individual. Natural and unnatural complexions may simultaneously appear in the face and other parts of the body; they also indicate imminent death of the individual. [9]

Similar other factors:
वर्णभेदेनेति यथा वर्णविभागेन रिष्टं, तथा ग्लान्यादिविभागेनापीत्यर्थः|
हर्ष इहोपचयो ज्ञेयः, मानसहर्षस्येह चाक्षुषाधिकारेऽसङ्गतत्वात्||१०||
The description pertaining to the complexion also applies to other signs like emaciation and plumpness as well as dryness and unctuousness. [10]

Other morbid signs indicating imminent death:
तथा पिप्लुव्यङ्गतिलकालकपिडकानामन्यतमस्यानने जन्मातुरस्यैवमेवाप्रशस्तं विद्यात्||११||

Similarly, the appearance of any one of the below mentioned on the face of the patient is indicative of imminent death :

- Piplu (port- wine mark)
- Vyanga (freckles)
- Tilakalaka (black mole)
- Pidaka (Pimple) [11]

Morbid complexions:

नखनयनवदनमूत्रपुरीषहस्तपादौष्ठादिष्वपि च वैकारिकोक्तानां वर्णानामन्यतमस्य प्रादुर्भावो हीनबलवर्णेन्द्रियेषु लक्षणमायुषः क्षयस्य भवति॥१२॥

Appearance of any one of the abnormal colours in nails, eyes, urine, stool, hands, legs and lips (as described in Para 9 of this chapter) is indicative of imminent death if it is associated with diminution of :

- strength
- complexion
- sensory perception [12]

Other morbid conditions:

यच्चान्यदपि किञ्चिद्वर्णवैकृतमभूतपूर्वं सहसोत्पद्येतानिमित्तमेव हीयमानस्यातुरस्य शश्वत्, तदरिष्टमिति विद्यात्।

इति वर्णाधिकारः॥१३॥

Sudden and accidental appearance of any other unusual morbid complexion is always indicative of growing weakness of the patient. They therefore appear in the form of premonitory signs of imminent death. [13]

Normal and abnormal voice:

स्वराधिकारस्तु- हंसक्रौञ्चनेमिदुन्दुभिकलविङ्ककाककपोतजर्जरानुकाराः प्रकृतिस्वरा भवन्ति;

यांश्चापरानुपेक्षमाणोऽपि विद्यादनूकतोऽन्यथा वाऽपि निर्दिश्यमानांस्तज्ज्ञैः।

एडककलग्रस्ताव्यक्तगद्गदक्षामदीनानुकीर्णास्त्वातुराणां स्वरा वैकारिका भवन्ति; यांश्चापरानुपेक्षमाणोऽपि

विद्यात् प्राग्विकृतानभूत्वोत्पन्नान् ।

इति प्रकृतिविकृतिस्वरा व्याख्याता भवन्ति॥१४।

The normal human voice resembles the voice of one or more of the below mentioned:

Hamsa (swan),

Kaauna (demoiselle crane),

Nemi (wheel),

Dundubi (Kettle drum),

Kalavinka (house sparrow),

Kaka (crow),

Kapota (dove)

Jarjara (a type of drum)

There are some other types of natural voices which can be ascertained by similarities or from the instructions of experts. The voice of moribund patients resembles that of sheep (wild Goat) and is feeble, inaudible, indistinct, choked, hoarse, and painful and unclear (not clearly manifested). Similarly, there are some other unnatural types of sounds which are produced anew.

Thus, the normal and abnormal types of voice of the individual are explained. [14]

Morbidity in voice indication imminent death:

तत्र प्रकृतिवैकारिकाणां स्वराणामाश्वभिनिर्वृत्तिः स्वरानेकत्वमेकस्य चानेकत्वमप्रशस्तम्‌|

इति स्वराधिकारः||१५||

The below mentioned types of voice related abnormalities too indicate imminent death :

if the abnormal type of voice manifest spontaneously or

in an individual there are many such abnormal types of voices or

if only one abnormal voice in the individual appears to be of diverse types

Thus, the morbidity pertaining to voice is explained. [15]

इति वर्णस्वराधिकारौ यथावदुक्तौ मुमूर्षतां लक्षण ज्ञानार्थमिति||१६||

So, the topics on complexion and voice are properly described with a view to provide knowledge regarding moribund persons. [16]

Recapitulation:

भवन्ति चात्र-

यस्य वैकारिको वर्णः शरीर उपपद्यते|

अर्धे वा यदि वा कृत्स्ने निमित्तं न च नास्ति सः||१७||

नीलं वा यदि वा श्यावं तामं वा यदि वाऽरुणम्‌|

मुखार्धमन्यथा वर्णो मुखार्धेऽरिष्टमुच्यते||१८||

स्नेहो मुखार्धे सुव्यक्तो रौक्ष्यमर्धमुखे [१] भृशम्‌|

ग्लानिर्धे तथा हर्षो मुखार्धे प्रेतलक्षणम्||१९||

तिलकाः पिप्लवो व्यङ्गा राजयश्च पृथग्विधाः|

आतुरस्याशु जायन्ते मुखे प्राणान् मुमुक्षतः||२०||

पुष्पाणि नखदन्तेषु पङ्को वा दन्तसंश्रितः|

चूर्णको वाऽपि दन्तेषु लक्षणं मरणस्य [२] तत्‌||२१||

ओष्ठयोः पादयोः पाण्योरक्ष्णोर्मूत्रपुरीषयोः|

नखेष्वपि च वैवर्ण्यमेतत् क्षीणबलेऽन्तकृत्||२२||

यस्य नीलावुभावोष्ठौ पक्वजाम्बवसन्निभौ|

मुमूर्षुरिति तं विद्यान्नरो धीरो गतायुषम्||२३||

एको वा यदि वाऽनेको यस्य वैकारिकः स्वरः|

सहसोत्पद्यते जन्तोर्हीयमानस्य नास्ति सः||२४||

यच्चान्यदपि किञ्चित् स्याद्वैकृतं स्वरवर्णयोः|

बलमांसविहीनस्य तत् सर्वं मरणोदयम् [३] ||२५||

तत्र श्लोकः:-

इति वर्णस्वरावुक्तौ लक्षणार्थं मुमूर्षताम्‌|

यस्तौ [४] सम्यग्विजानाति नायुर्ज्ञाने स मुह्यति||२६||

Thus, it is said:

The following are the symptoms of moribund persons:

- Appearance of abnormal complexion in the entire or half of the body of the individual without any (visible) cause;
- If in half of the face there is blue, blackish, coppery or tawny colour and the colour of the remaining half is otherwise.
- Manifestation of unctuousness in one half of the face and roughness in the other half
- Appearance of plumpness in one half of the face and emaciation in the other half
- Spontaneous appearance of various types of Tila (black Mole), Piplu (Port wine mark), Vyanga (freckles) and Raji (spots like Mustard) in the face of the patient

- Appearance of flower life spots in nails and teeth, and sticky and powder like substance in the teeth;
- Discolouration of lips, legs, heels, eyes, urine, stool and nails of the patient when he is diminished of strength
- When both the lips become bluish like the rip fruits of Jambu (Syzygium Cumini Skeels)
- Sudden manifestation of single or multiple morbidities in the voice in a weak patient.

Such other abnormalities in the voice and complexion of an individual who is devoid of strength and flesh also indicate imminent death. [17-25]

तत्रश्लोकः-
इतिवर्णस्वरावुक्तौलक्षणार्थमुमूर्षताम्|
यस्तौसम्यग्विजानातिनायुर्ज्ञानेसमुह्यति||२६||
To sum up:
Various types of morbidity pertaining to complexion and voice are described here with a view to ascertaining in the signs and symptoms of moribund patients one who knows this does not tumble in ascertaining the span of life. [26]

इत्यग्निवेशकृते तन्त्रे चरकप्रतिसंस्कृते इन्द्रियस्थाने वर्णस्वरीयमिन्द्रियं नाम प्रथमोऽध्यायः||१||
Thus ends the first chapter on signs and symptoms of Imminent Death as indicated by complexion and voice of Indriya section of Agnivesha's work as redacted by Charaka.

26

Indriyasthana Chapter 2
Pushpitakam Indriyam

अथातः पुष्पितकमिन्द्रियं व्याख्यास्यामह||१||

इति ह स्माह भगवानात्रेयः||२||

We shall now expound the chapter on "The exhalation of odour indicative of imminent Death". Thus said Lord Atreya [1-2]

A simile:

पुष्पं यथा पूर्वरूपं फलस्येह भविष्यतः|

तथा लिङ्गमरिष्टाख्यं पूर्वरूपं मरिष्यतः||३||

Just like flowers appear before the production of fruits, the fatal symptoms and signs appear before the death of a person (as premonitory symptoms). [3]

अप्येवं तु भवेत् पुष्पं फलेनाननुबन्धि यत्|

फलं चापि भवेत् किञ्चिद्यस्य पुष्पं न पूर्वजम् ||४||

न त्वरिष्टस्य जातस्य नाशोऽस्ति मरणादृते|

मरणं चापि तन्नास्ति यन्नारिष्टपुरःसरम्||५||

All flowers do not eventually shape up into fruits in the future. Certain flowers may be devoid of fruition. Similarly, sometimes even fruits may be produced without any flowers i.e., there are no flowers before the fruits are produced. But once the fatal symptoms appear they wouldn't disappear without having caused death. This means to tell that once these symptoms are produced, they will definitely cause (result into) death. Conversely there isn't any death without being preceded by its premonitory symptoms i.e., fatal signs and symptoms. [4-5]

Inability to comprehend signs of imminent death because of Intellectual blasphemy:

मिथ्यादृष्टमरिष्टाभमनरिष्टमजानता|

अरिष्टं वाऽप्यसम्बुद्धमेतत् प्रज्ञापराधजम्||६||

An ignorant person sometimes wrongly views pseudo symptoms as real premonitory symptoms. Sometimes he does not even recognise the real premonitory symptoms as such. All this is the result of intellectual blasphemy. [6]

ज्ञानसम्बोधनार्थं तु लिङ्गैर्मरणपूर्वजैः|

पुष्पितानुपदेक्ष्यामो नरान् बहुविधैर्बहून् ||७||

With a view to explaining the several premonitory symptoms preceding death as indicative of its imminence, we now illustrate the various persons with such manifestations. [7]

Characteristic smell of moribund persons:

नानापुष्पोपमो गन्धो यस्य भाति दिवानिशम्‌|
पुष्पितस्य वनस्येव नानाद्रुमलतावतः||८||
तमाहुः पुष्पितं धीरा नरं मरणलक्षणैः|
स ना संवत्सराद्देहं जहातीति विनिश्चयः||९||
एवमेकैकशः पुष्पैर्यस्य गन्धः समो भवेत्‌|
इष्टैर्वा यदि वाऽनिष्टैः स च पुष्पित उच्यते||१०||
समासेनाशुभान्‌ गन्धानेकत्वेनाथवा पुनः|
आजिघ्रेद्यस्य गात्रेषु तं विद्यात्‌ पुष्पितं भिषक्‌||११||
आप्लुतानाप्लुते काये यस्य गन्धाः शुभाशुभाः|
व्यत्यासेनानिमित्ताः स्युः स च पुष्पित उच्यते||१२||
तद्यथा- चन्दनं कुष्ठं तगरागुरुणी मधु|
माल्यं मूत्रपुरीषे च मृतानि कुणपानि च||१३||
ये चान्ये विविधात्मानो गन्धा विविधयोनयः|
तेऽप्यनेनानुमानेन विज्ञेया विकृतिं गताः||१४||
इदं चाप्यतिदेशार्थं लक्षणं गन्धसंश्रयम्‌|
वक्ष्यामो यदभिज्ञाय भिषङ्मरणमादिशेत्‌||१५||
वियोनिर्विदुरो गन्धो यस्य गात्रेषु जायते|
इष्टो वा यदि वाऽनिष्टो न स जीवति तां समाम्‌||१६||
एतावद्गन्धविज्ञानं,...|१७|

A person whose body emits fragrance similar to that of many flowers, as if the smell is coming from a garden in which many types of fragrant flowers and creepers (trees and creepers bearing fragrant flowers) are grown, is called as pushpita i.e., the person's body is flowering / flowered. This is because these are the symptoms of impending death (fatal signs and symptoms). Thus, such manifestations are indicative of imminent death. Any person presenting with such signs and symptoms is sure to die within a span of one year. A body of the person which emits the fragrance of only one flower be it fragrant or foul smelling is also considered as pushpita.

If the body is of a person is emitting many unpleasant odours at a time or even if unpleasant / foul smell of different flowers (flowers having unpleasant smell) is emitted at different times which can be perceived by the organ of smell i.e., nose, the person will be regarded as being pushpita.

Even if the smell of the body resembles the fragrance of different pleasant and unpleasant flowers, one by one, a person with such manifestation is also regarded as "Puspita". Here a variety of unpleasant odours are emitted simultaneously from the body of the patient which indicates fatal signs or symptoms of impending death.

If the body emits unpleasant odour even when covered with fragrant unguents and pleasant odour when no unguents are applied, if the unpleasant unguents emit pleasant odour and pleasant odours emit unpleasant odour or when pleasant and unpleasant odours are emitted alternatively from the body of the same person, he is known to be pushpita.

Odour of Chandana (Santalum album Linn), Kustha (Saussurea lappa G.B Clarke), Tagara (Valeriana wallichi Dc), Aguru (Aquilaria agallocha Roxb), honey and garland are pleasant. Odour of urine, faeces and dead bodies (of human beings or animals) are unpleasant. According to this analogy, odour from similar other sources is also to be considered as premonitory symptoms by inference.

We shall further explain as examples, the premonitory symptoms based on olfactory perception in order to facilitate general appreciation of such symptoms by knowing which a physician can predict imminent death. Ex - the individual whose body emits pleasant or unpleasant smell continuously without any appreciable cause cannot survive for more than a year.

This is all about premonitory symptoms based on the smell of the body of the individual. [8-17]

Taste of moribund persons:

...रसज्ञानमतः परम्।
आतुराणां शरीरेषु वक्ष्यते विधिपूर्वकम्।।१७।।
यो रसः प्रकृतिस्थानां नराणां देहसम्भवः।
स एषां चरमे काले विकारं भजते द्वयम्।।१८।।
कश्चिदेवास्यवैरस्यमत्यर्थमुपपद्यते।
स्वादुत्वमपरश्चापि विपुलं भजते रसः।।१९।।
तमनेनानुमानेन विद्यादि्वकृतिमागतम्।
मनुष्यो हि मनुष्यस्य कथं रसमवाप्नुयात्।।२०।।
मक्षिकाश्चैव यूकाश्च दंशाश्च मशकैः सह।
विरसादपसर्पन्ति जन्तोः कायान्मुमूर्षतः।।२१।।
अत्यर्थरसिकं कायं कालपक्वस्य मक्षिकाः।
अपि स्नातानुलिप्तस्य भृशमायान्ति सर्वशः।।२२।।

Now we shall appropriately describe the signs of imminent death, as indicated by the taste in the patient's body. The normal bodily taste of human beings undergoes two types of modification in the event of death. This modification may be either in the form of an extremely abnormal taste (in the mouth) or in the form of extreme sweetness. Morbid conditions of taste can only be inferred. One cannot otherwise have a direct perception of such conditions (one cannot lick or taste the body of the patient to access the taste of the body).

In the case of the first types of morbidity, flies, lice, wasps and mosquitoes get away from the body of a moribund person having an abnormal taste. On the other, hand, flies repeatedly surround the body of a moribund person having extremely sweet taste (of the body) even after he has taken bath or has applied unguents. [17-22]

तत्र श्लोकः:-
सामान्येन मयोक्तानि लिङ्गानि रसगन्धयोः।
पुष्पितस्य नरस्यैतत्फलं मरणमादिशेत्।।२३।।

To sum up: Symptoms of imminent death of the individual (Puspita) relating to the taste and smell in his body are described here in general. Such symptoms lead to death of the individual. [23]

इत्यग्निवेशकृते तन्त्रे चरकप्रतिसंस्कृते इन्द्रियस्थाने पुष्पितकमिन्द्रियं नाम द्वितीयोऽध्यायः।।२।।

Thus ends the second chapter on the "Exhalation of Odour Indicative of Imminent Death" of Indriya section of Agnivesha's work as redacted by Charaka.

27

Indriyasthana Chapter 3
Parimarshaneeyam Indriyam

अथातः परिमर्शनीयमिन्द्रियं व्याख्यास्यामः||१||

इति ह स्माह भगवानात्रेयः||२||

Now we shall expound the chapter on the signs of imminent death as indicated by touch. Thus, said lord Atreya. [1-2]

वर्णे स्वरे च गन्धे च रसे चोक्तं पृथक् पृथक्|

लिङ्गं मुमूर्षतां सम्यक् स्पर्शेष्वपि निबोधत||३||

Signs of imminent death as indicated by complexions, voice, smell, and taste are already subscribed separately. Those indicated by touch are being described now. [3]

Examination of moribund persons by touch:

स्पर्शप्राधान्येनैवातुरस्यायुषः प्रमाणावशेषं जिज्ञासुः प्रकृतिस्थेन पाणिना शरीरमस्य केवलं स्पृशेत्, परिमर्शयेद्वाऽन्येन|

परिमृशता तु खल्वातुरशरीरमिमे भावास्तत्र तत्रावबोद्धव्या भवन्ति|

तद्यथा- सततं स्पन्दमानानां शरीरदेशानामस्पन्दनं, नित्योष्मणां शीतीभावः, मृदूनां दारुणत्वं, श्लक्ष्णानां खरत्वं, सतामसद्भावः, सन्धीनां स्रंसभ्रंशच्यवनानि; मांसशोणितयोर्वीतीभावः, दारुणत्वं, स्वेदानुबन्धः, स्तम्भो वा; यच्चान्यदपि किञ्चिदीदृशं स्पर्शानां लक्षणं भृशविकृतमनिमित्तं स्यात्| इति लक्षणं स्पृश्यानां भावानामुक्तं समासेन||४||

A physician who is desirous of ascertaining the lifespan of a given patient just on the basis of touch should touch the entire body of the patient with his hand (palm). His hands should neither be too cold nor too hot and should have normal temperature.

If the hands of the physician are not healthy, he shall get the patient touched and examined by some other person (in whom he trusts). Even if the patient's social customs do not permit the physician to touch the body of the patient or if the patient is of such status that the physician cannot touch the body of the patient (example – preceptor's wife being a patient) he should get the patient touched and examined by some other person.

While touching the body of the patient, the below mentioned points need to be observed:

- Absence of movements (pulsation) in such of the organs of the body which move or pulsate constantly
- Coldness in organs which are normally (almost always) warm
- Hardness in soft organs
- Roughness in smooth organs
- Absence of organs which are normally present
- Major or minor dislocation of joints- downwards or sidewards
- Excessive diminution of muscle tissue and blood

• 303 •

- Appearance of hardness in body parts
- Persistent sweating or its total absence

The above-mentioned symptoms or similar other symptoms which reflect abnormal tactile / touch conditions without any appreciable cause are indicative of imminent death. Thus, the tactile symptoms indicative of imminent death is briefly described. [4]

Details of examination:

तद्व्यासतोऽनुव्याख्यास्यामः- तस्य चेत् परिमृश्यमानं पृथक्त्वेन पादजङ्घोरुस्फिग्गुदरपार्श्वपृष्ठेषिकापाणिग्रीवाताल्वोष्ठललाटं स्विन्नं शीतं स्तब्धं दारुणं वीतमांसशोणितं वा स्यात्, परासुरयं पुरुषो न चिरात् कालं मरिष्यतीति विद्यात्।

तस्य चेत् परिमृश्यमानानि पृथक्त्वेन गुल्फजानुवङ्क्षणगुदवृषणमेढ्रनाभ्यंसस्तनमणिकपर्शुकाहनुनासिकाकर्णाक्षिभ्रूशङ्खादीनि स्रस्तानि व्यस्तानि च्युतानि स्थानेभ्यः स्कन्नानि वा स्युः, परासुरयं पुरुषोऽचिरात् कालं मरिष्यतीति विद्यात्।।५।।

We shall now expound such symptoms in greater detail. If the feet, knees, buttocks, abdomen, sides of the chest, vertebral column, hands, neck, palate, lips and forehead of the patient are touched separately and if they are found wet, cold, rigid, hard or devoid of flesh and blood, it should be inferred that the life span of that individual has come to an end and he will die soon.

If in any person the ankles, knees, hips, anus, testicles, pains, umbilicus, shoulder, breasts, wrist joints, ribs, jaws, nose, ears, eyes, eyebrows and temples have become loose, scattered, displaced, dislocated or have become stiff and hard, then it should be predicted that the individual might face instantaneous death. [5]

Details of examination:

तस्य चेन्मन्ये परिमृश्यमाने न स्पन्देयातां, परासुरिति विद्यात्।

तस्य चेद्दन्ताः परिकीर्णाः श्वेता जातशर्कराः स्युः, परासुरिति विद्यात्।

तस्य चेत् पक्ष्माणि जटाबद्धानि स्युः, परासुरिति विद्यात्।

तस्य चेच्चक्षुषी प्रकृतिहीने, विकृतियुक्ते- अत्युत्पिण्डिते, अतिप्रविष्टे, अतिजिह्मे, अतिविषमे, अतिमुक्तबन्धने, अतिप्रसुते, सततोन्मिषिते, सततनिमिषिते, निमिषोन्मेषातिप्रवृत्ते, विभ्रान्तदृष्टिके, विपरीतदृष्टिके, हीनदृष्टिके, व्यस्तदृष्टिके, नकुलान्धे, कपोतान्धे, अलातवर्णे, कृष्णपीतनीलश्यावताम्रहरितहारिद्रशुक्लवैकारिकाणां वर्णानामन्यतमेनातिप्लुते वा स्यातां, तदा परासुरिति विद्यात्।

अथास्य केशलोमान्यायच्छेत्, तस्य चेत् केशलोमान्यायम्यमानानि प्रलुच्येरन् न चेद्वेदयेयुस्तं परासुरिति विद्यात्।

तस्य चेदुदरे सिराः प्रकाशेरञ् श्यावताम्रनीलहारिद्रशुक्ला वा स्युः, परासुरिति विद्यात्।

तस्य चेन्नखा वीतमांसशोणिताः पक्वजाम्बववर्णाः स्युः, परासुरिति विद्यात्।

अथास्याङ्गुलीरायच्छेत्; तस्य चेदङ्गुलय आयम्यमाना न स्फुटेयुः, परासुरिति विद्यात्।।६।।

The physician should carefully examine the exhalation, manya (region of carotid arteries, nape of the neck), teeth, eyelashes, eye, hair (of the head), loman (short hairs of the remaining parts of the body of the individual), abdomen, nails and fingers of the patients. The following conditions are indicative of imminent death of the patient:

- too long (deep) or short (shallow) breathe (exhalation)
- absence of pulsation in his manya (nape of the neck / region of carotid arteries) when touched;
- teeth covered and adhered with dirt, is excessively white and covered with sugary particles
- matting of eyelashes
- If his eyes are devoid of natural characteristics and endowed with unnatural ones e.g. if they are
- excessively projected
- excessively withdrawn
- excessively slanted;
- excessively uneven
- excessively loose
- have excessive secretions

- perpetually open
- perpetually closed
- very quick, frequent and continuous blinking (increased frequency in opening and closure)
- rolling, reverted, deficient or scattered vision
- with morbidity of nakulandhya (or blindness of mongoose) i.e. they view everything as white during day time
- with morbidity of kapotandhya (or the blindness of pigeon) i.e. they view everything as black during day time
- fiery eyes – eyes look red like burning coal
- endowed with excessively black, yellow, blue, darkish brown, coppery, green, turmeric, yellow or white colour;
- if the hair (of the head) and loman (short hair of the remaining parts of the body of the individual) of the patient are pulled they come out easily with roots but do not cause pain.
- if the veins on the abdomen are visible and have darkish brown, coppery, blue, turmeric, yellow or white colours or similar such colours.
- If his nails are devoid of flesh and blood and black like ripe fruit of jambu (Syzygium cuminin skeels)
- if finger joints do not produce cracking sound even when bent and pressed [6]

तत्र श्लोकः-

एतान् स्पृश्यान् बहून् भावान् यः स्पृशन्नवबुध्यते|

आतुरे न स सम्मोहमायुर्ज्ञानस्य गच्छति||७||

To sum up:

The physician who can understand all the various tactile sensations by touch will seldom fail to ascertain the life span of the patient. [7]

इत्यग्निवेशकृते तन्त्रे चरकप्रतिसंस्कृते इन्द्रियस्थाने परिमर्शनीयमिन्द्रियं नाम तृतीयोऽध्यायः||३||

Thus ends the third chapter on "the signs of imminent death as indicated by touch" of the Indriya section of Agnivesa's work as redacted by Charaka.

28

Indriyasthana Chapter 4
Indriyaneekam Indriyam

अथात इन्द्रियानीकमिन्द्रियं व्याख्यास्यामः||१||

इति ह स्माह भगवानात्रेयः||२||

We shall expound the chapter on the signs and symptoms of imminent death as indicated by the characteristic features of sense organs. Thus said Lord Atreya [1-2]

Role of inference in the examination:

इन्द्रियाणि यथा जन्तोः परीक्षेत विशेषवित्|

ज्ञातुमिच्छन् भिषङ्मानमायुस्तन्निबोधत ||३||

अनुमानात् परीक्षेत दर्शनादीनि तत्त्वतः|

अद्धा हि विदितं ज्ञानमिन्द्रियाणामतीन्द्रियम्||४||

We shall now explain as to how an expert physician desirous of ascertaining the span of life of patients should examine the sense organs of a patient. The knowledge of sense organs is always beyond the purview of perception; this is the ultimate truth. Therefore the examination of sense organs shall be done with inference. [3-4]

Specific features of signs of imminent death:

स्वस्थेभ्यो विकृतं यस्य ज्ञानमिन्द्रियसंश्रयम् [१] |

आलक्ष्येतानिमित्तेन लक्षणं मरणस्य तत्||५||

इत्युक्तं लक्षणं सम्यगिन्द्रियेष्वशुभोदयम्|

तदेव तु पुनर्भूयो विस्तरेण निबोधत||६||

If any morbidity develops in the healthy sense organs without any visible cause this is indicative of imminent death. The signs and symptoms of imminent death pertaining to sense organs are explained in general in this context. They will be further elaborated in subsequent paragraphs. [5-6]

Characteristic features of vision indicative of imminent death:

घनीभूतमिवाकाशमाकाशमिव मेदिनीम्|

विगीतमुभयं ह्येतत् पश्यन् मरणमृच्छति||७||

If a patient views the sky as something solid (or like the earth) and the earth as something void (or like the sky), he is sure to die soon as these symptoms are inauspicious. [7]

यस्य दर्शनमायाति मारुतोऽम्बरगोचरः|

अग्निर्नायाति चादीप्तस्तस्यायुःक्षयमादिशेत्||८||

One who views the wind blowing in the sky in a corporeal form but does not see the flame of kindled fire, should be considered as a moribund person. [8]

जले सुविमले जालमजालावतते नरः।
स्थिते गच्छति वा दृष्ट्वा जीवितात् परिमुच्यते॥९॥

If a person happens to see (hallucination) a net being spread out in clean water, stagnant or moving one in spite of no net being present there, then this constitutes the premonitory symptoms of imminent death. [9]

जाग्रत् पश्यति यः प्रेतान् रक्षांसि विविधानि च।
अन्यद्वाऽप्यद्भुतं किञ्चिन्न [१] स जीवितुमर्हति॥१०॥

If one, even while awake, perceives Pretas (ghosts) and various types of Raksasas (demons) or any other supernatural elements, he will not live long [10]

योऽग्निं प्रकृतिवर्णस्थं नीलं पश्यति निष्प्रभम्।
कृष्णं वा यदि वा शुक्लं निशां व्रजति सप्तमीम्॥११॥

When the fire is viewed as blue, lustreless, black or white in spite of it being in its natural colour i.e., yellowish or reddish, this is indicative of the death of the patient after the seventh night. [11]

मरीचीनसतो मेघान्मेघान् वाऽप्यसतोऽम्बरे।
विद्युतो वा विना मेधैः पश्यन् [१] मरणमृच्छति॥१२॥

If one sees Marichi (cloud- light), or cloud or lightning when there is no cloud in the sky, this is indicative of imminent death. [12]

मृन्मयीमिव यः पात्रीं कृष्णाम्बरसमावृताम्।
आदित्यमीक्षते शुद्धं चन्द्रं वा न स जीवति॥१३॥
अपर्वणि यदा पश्येत् सूर्याचन्द्रमसोर्ग्रहम्।
अव्याधितो व्याधितो वा तदन्तं तस्य जीवितम्॥१४॥
नक्तं सूर्यमहश्चन्द्रमनग्नौ धूममुत्थितम्।
अग्निं वा निष्प्रभं रात्रौ दृष्ट्वा मरणमृच्छति॥१५॥
प्रभावतः प्रभाहीनान्निष्प्रभांश्च प्रभावतः।
नरा विलिङ्गान् पश्यन्ति भावान् भावाञ्जिहासवः॥१६॥
व्याकृतीनि विवर्णानि विसङ्ख्योपगतानि च।
विनिमितानि पश्यन्ति रूपाण्यायुःक्षये नराः॥१७॥
यश्च पश्यत्यदृश्यान् वै दृश्यान् यश्च न पश्यति।
तावुभौ पश्यतः क्षिप्रं यमक्षयमसंशयम्॥१८॥

The following symptoms relating to the visual sense indicate imminent death of the person:

- clear sun or the moon (unobstructed by the cloud) appear like an earthen plate covered with a black cloth seeing lunar or solar eclipse when there is no full moon of new moon respectively (seen by both normal and abnormal persons)
- seeing sun in the night, the moon in the day, the smoke when there is no fire or fire without flame in the night;
- appearance of bright things as devoid of lustre, the ones having no luster as bright – i.e., view things devoid of their real characteristics;
- to have visual perception in a distorted from i.e., to view things appearing as having multiple forms, devoid of complexion and inaccurate numbers without any reason
- to visualise the invisible ones and not to visualise the visible ones [13-18]

Hearing:

अशब्दस्य च यः श्रोता शब्दान् यश्च न बुध्यते।
द्वावप्येतौ यथा प्रेतौ तथा ज्ञेयौ विजानता॥१९॥
संवृत्याङ्गुलिभिः कर्णौ ज्वालाशब्दं य आतुरः।

न शृणोति गतासुं तं बुद्धिमान् परिवर्जयेत्॥२०॥

The following symptoms relating to the auditory sense organ indicate imminent death of the person:

- Hearing inaudible sounds and not to hearing the audible ones;
- Inability to hear the internal (astral) sound after closing ears with fingers; [19-20]

Smell:

विपर्ययेण यो विद्याद्गन्धानां साध्वसाधुताम्।
न वा तान् सर्वशो विद्यात्तं विद्यादिवगतायुषम्॥२१॥

If the olfactory sense of a person fails to distinguish between good and bad smells or is not responsive to any smell at all, he is considered as a moribund person. [21]

Taste:

यो रसान्न विजानाति न वा जानाति तत्त्वतः।
मुखपाकादृते पक्वं तमाहुः कुशला नरम्॥२२॥

If a person free from Mukhapaka (stomatitis and glossitis) does not perceive taste (does not have the gustatory sensation) at all nor can identify the exact tastes, he is also ripe for death. [22]

Touch:

उष्णाञ्छीतान् खराञ्छलक्ष्णान्मृदूनपि च दारुणान्।
स्पृश्यान् स्पृष्ट्वा ततोऽन्यत्वं मुमूर्षुस्तेषु मन्यते॥२३॥

If one has the tactile sensation of coldness in heat, of smoothness in coarseness, of softness in hardness and vice versa, he is to be considered as a moribund one. [23]

Supra-sensory perception:

अन्तरेण तपस्तीव्रं योगं वा विधिपूर्वकम्।
इन्द्रियैरधिकं पश्यन् पञ्चत्वमधिगच्छति॥२४॥
इन्द्रियाणामृते दृष्टेरिन्द्रियार्थानदोषजान्।
नरः पश्यति यः कश्चिदिन्द्रियैर्न स जीवति॥२५॥

Supra-sensory perception not preceded by austere penances or due yogic practices is indicative of imminent death. If one perceives things in an infallible manner in spite of the impairment of the respective sensory faculties, this is also indicative of imminent death [24-25]

Wrong perception:

स्वस्थाः प्रज्ञाविपर्यासैरिन्द्रियार्थेषु वैकृतम्।
पश्यन्ति येऽसद्बहुशस्तेषां मरणमादिशेत्॥२६॥

If a healthy person perceives things wrongly in contravention of the normal relationship between the sense organs and their objects as a result of mental perversion, he is sure to die soon. [26]

तत्र श्लोकः-

एतदिन्द्रियविज्ञानं यः पश्यति यथातथम्।
मरणं जीवितं चैव स भिषक् ज्ञातुमर्हति॥२७॥

To sum up:-

A physician who knows the science of premonition of death as indicated by the characteristic features of the sense organs can readily distinguish between life and death. [27]

इत्यग्निवेशकृते तन्त्रे चरकप्रतिसंस्कृते इन्द्रियस्थाने इन्द्रियानीकमिन्द्रियं नाम चतुर्थोऽध्यायः||४||

Thus ends the fourth chapter on the signs and symptoms of imminent death as indicated by the characteristic features of sense organs of Indriya Section of Agnivesha's work as redacted by Charaka.

29

Indriyasthana Chapter 5
Purvaroopeeyam Indriyam

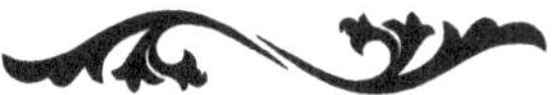

अथातःपूर्वरूपीयमिन्द्रियंव्याख्यास्यामः||१||

इतिहस्माहभगवानात्रेयः||२||

Now, we shall expound the chapter on the signs and symptoms of imminent death as indicated by the premonitory symptoms of diseases. Thus said Lord Atreya [1-2]

Premonitory symptoms indicative of imminent death:

पूर्वरूपाण्यसाध्यानां विकाराणां पृथक् पृथक्|

भिन्नाभिन्नानि वक्ष्यामो भिषजां ज्ञानवृद्धये||३||

पूर्वरूपाणि सर्वाणि ज्वरोक्तान्यतिमात्रया|

यं विशन्ति विशत्येनं मृत्युर्ज्वरपुरःसरः||४||

अन्यस्यापि च रोगस्य पूर्वरूपाणि यं नरम्|

विशन्त्यनेन कल्पेन तस्यापि मरणं ध्रुवम्||५||

We shall now separately explain the premonitory symptoms- general as well as specific –relating to the incurable diseases as a means to promote the knowledge of the physician. If in a patient of fever all the premonitory symptoms of fever manifest themselves excessively it shall be considered as sure signs of death. Similarly, all the premonitory symptoms of other diseases manifesting themselves excessively are sure signs of imminent death of the patient. [3-5]

पूर्वरूपैकदेशांस्तु वक्ष्यामोऽन्यान् सुदारुणान्|

ये रोगाननुबध्नन्ति मृत्युर्यैरनुबध्यते [१] ||६||

बलं च हीयते यस्य प्रतिश्यायश्च वर्धते|

तस्य नारीप्रसक्तस्य शोषोऽन्तायोपजायते||७||

श्वभिरुष्ट्रैः खरैर्वाऽपि याति यो दक्षिणां दिशम्|

स्वप्ने यक्ष्माणमासाद्य जीवितं स विमुञ्चति||८||

प्रेतैः सह पिबेन्मद्यं स्वप्ने यः कृष्यते शुना|

सुघोरं ज्वरमासाद्य जीवितं स विमुञ्चति||९||

We shall explain some other premonitory symptoms of the most fatal type which follow the various diseases and are in turn followed by death. If a patient of consumption indulging in sex suffers from diminution of strength and aggravation of Pratishyaya (Coryza) he is sure to die. If a person travels towards the south riding a dog, camel or ass in his dreams, he gets affected with tuberculosis which consequently leads to his death.

If a person drinks wine in the company of ghosts or gets dragged by dogs in a dream, he gets afflicted with a serious type of fever leading to his death. Such diseases as follow the premonitory symptoms described above must result in death. Riding a dog, camel, pig and ass in a dream is already described in Nidana 6:13 as premonitory symptoms of

Rajayakshma (Tuberculosis). The same dream is regarded as a premonitory symptom of death if the travel is towards the south. [6-9]

लाक्षारक्ताम्बराभं यः पश्यत्यम्बरमन्तिकात्।
स रक्तपित्तमासाद्य तेनैवान्ताय नीयते॥१०॥
रक्तस्रग्रक्तसर्वाङ्गो रक्तवासा मुहुर्हसन्।
यः स्वप्ने ह्रियते नार्या स रक्तं प्राप्य सीदति॥११॥

If the sky appears to be red like a cloth smeared with lac from a nearby distance, the patient falls victim to raktapitta (a disease characterised by bleeding from different parts of the body) leading to his death. If a person in his dreams wears red garlands and apparel with his entire body looking red (smeared with red colour), laughs frequently and is dragged by a woman, he falls victim to Raktapitta leading to his death. [10-11]

शूलाटोपान्त्रकूजाश्च दौर्बल्यं चातिमात्रया।
नखादिषु च वैवर्ण्यं गुल्मेनान्तकरो ग्रहः॥१२॥
लता कण्टकिनी यस्य दारुणा हृदि जायते।
स्वप्ने गुल्मस्तमन्ताय क्रूरो विशति मानवम्॥१३॥

Colic pain, meteorism (swelling of the abdomen caused by gas in the intestines or peritoneal cavity), gurgling sound in the intestine and excessive weakness, discolouration of nails etc. results in Gulma (a disease characterised by a growth in the abdomen) leading to death of the patient. If in a dream one has the growth of spiky creeper on his chest, he falls a victim to fatal type of Gulma, [12-13]

कायेऽल्पमपि संस्पृष्टं सुभृशं यस्य दीर्यते।
क्षतानि च न रोहन्ति कुष्ठैर्मृत्युर्हिनस्ति तम्॥१४॥
नग्नस्याज्यावसिक्तस्य जुह्वतोऽग्निमनर्चिषम्।
पद्मान्युरसि जायन्ते स्वप्ने कुष्ठैर्मरिष्यतः॥१५॥

If even the slightest injury gives rise to excessive wounds in the body and the wounds do not heal up, the patient dies of skin disease / leprosy. If in a dream, a person naked, anointed with ghee, offering oblations to the fire without flame has growth of lotus flower on his chest, he would die of leprosy. [14-15]

स्नातानुलिप्तगात्रेऽपि यस्मिन् गृध्नन्ति मक्षिकाः।
स प्रमेहेण संस्पर्शं प्राप्य तेनैव हन्यते॥१६॥

If the flies get attracted towards an individual even after he has taken bath and used unguents, he falls victim to Prameha (obstinate urinary disorders including diabetes). This Prameha would eventually prove fatal for him. [16]

Dream:

स्नेहं बहुविधं स्वप्ने चण्डालैः सह यः पिबेत्।
बध्यते स प्रमेहेण स्पृश्यतेऽन्ताय मानवः॥१७॥

If a person in his dreams drinks various types of unctuous substance in accompaniment with the Chandalas (a person born from a Shudra father and a Brahmin mother MW), he also falls victim to Prameha which will be fatal to him. [17]

Premonitory symptoms of Psychic diseases:

ध्यानायासौ तथोद्वेगौ मोहश्चास्थानसम्भवः।
अरतिर्बलहानिश्च मृत्युरुन्मादपूर्वकः॥१८॥
आहारद्वेषिणं पश्यन् लुप्तचित्तमुदर्दितम्।
विद्याद्धीरो मुमूर्षुं तमुन्मादेनातिपातिना॥१९॥
क्रोधनं त्रासबहुलं सकृत्प्रहसिताननम्।
मूर्च्छापिपासाबहुलं हन्त्युन्मादः शरीरिणम्॥२०॥
नृत्यन् रक्षोगणैः साकं यः स्वप्नेऽम्भसि सीदति।

स प्राप्य भृशमुन्मादं याति लोकमतः परम्||२१||
असतमः पश्यति यः शृणोत्यप्यसतः स्वनान्|
बहून् बहुविधान् जाग्रत् सोऽपस्मारेण बध्यते||२२||
मतं नृत्यन्तमाविध्य प्रेतो हरति यं नरम्|
स्वप्ने हरति तं मृत्युरपस्मारपुरःसरः||२३||

The symptoms which are indicative of imminent death preceded by insanity are mental wandering, exertion, bewilderment, illusion in inopportune situations, indifference and loss of strength. The person will definitely die in quick time due to a strong attack of insanity if he is found to have aversion to food, if he has diversion of mind / absentmindedness, and suffers from udarda i.e., urticaria.

Extreme irritation, frightfulness, continued smile on his face after its onset, excess of fainting and thirst are indicative of imminent death due to insanity.If one gets drowned in water while dancing with the demons in his dream, he succumbs to an acute attack of insanity. A person who in his wakeful state sees darkness wherein there is no darkness and listens to all types of sounds even though there are no such sounds, will soon succumb to Apasmara (epilepsy).

One is sure to succumb to an attack of apasmara if he while dancing in an intoxicated state is caught by Preta (soul of a dead person) with his face downwards. [18-23]

स्तभ्येते प्रतिबुद्धस्य हनू मन्ये तथाऽक्षिणी|
यस्य तं बहिरायामो गृहीत्वा हन्त्यसंशयम्||२४||
शष्कुलीर्वाऽप्यपूपान् वा स्वप्ने खादति यो नरः|
स चेतादृक् छर्दयति प्रतिबुद्धो न जीवति||२५||

A person definitely succumbs to bahirayama (a condition characterized by opisthotonus of the body) if his jaw bone (lower), manya (nape of the neck / the region of carotid artery) and the two eyes become stiff while awake. If one takes saskuli (a large round cake prepared of ground rice, sugar and sesame, and cooked in oil MW) and Apupa (cake of flour MW) in his dreams and vomits similar substance while being awake cannot live long. [24-25]

एतानि पूर्वरूपाणि यः सम्यगवबुध्यते|
स एषामनुबन्धं च फलं च ज्ञातुमर्हति||२६||

If one is conversant with these premonitory symptoms, he can very well comprehend the consequential developments and final results thereof. [26]

Dreams indicative of imminent death:

इमांश्चाप्यपरान् स्वप्नान् दारुणानुपलक्षयेत्|
व्याधितानां विनाशाय क्लेशाय महतेऽपि वा||२७||
यस्योतमाङ्गे जायन्ते वंशगुल्मलतादयः|
वयांसि च विलीयन्ते स्वप्ने मौण्ड्यमियाच्च यः||२८||
गृध्रोलूकश्वकाकाद्यैः स्वप्ने यः परिवार्यते|
रक्षःप्रेतपिशाचस्त्रीचण्डालद्विडान्ध्रकैः ||२९||
वंशवेत्रलतापाशतृणकण्टकसङ्कटे|
संसज्जति हि यः स्वप्ने यो गच्छन् प्रपतत्यपि||३०||
भूमौ पांशूपधानायां वल्मीके वाऽथ भस्मनि|
श्मशानायतने श्वभ्रे स्वप्ने यः प्रपतत्यपि [४] ||३१||
कलुषेऽम्भसि पङ्के वा कूपे वा तमसाऽऽवृते|
स्वप्ने मज्जति शीघ्रेण स्रोतसा ह्रियते [५] च यः||३२||
स्नेहपानं तथाऽभ्यङ्गः प्रच्छर्दनविरेचने|
हिरण्यलाभः कलहः स्वप्ने बन्धपराजयौ||३३||

उपानद्युगनाशश्च प्रपातः पादचर्मणोः।
हर्षः स्वप्ने प्रकुपितैः पितृभिश्चावभर्त्सनम्॥३४॥
दन्तचन्द्रार्कनक्षत्रदेवतादीपचक्षुषाम्।
पतनं वा विनाशो वा स्वप्ने भेदो नगस्य वा॥३५॥
रक्तपुष्पं वनं भूमिं पापकर्मालयं चिताम्।
गुहान्धकारसम्बाधं स्वप्ने यः प्रविशत्यपि॥३६॥
रक्तमाली हसन्नुच्चैर्दिग्वासा दक्षिणां दिशम्।
दारुणामटवीं स्वप्ने कपियुक्तेन याति वा॥३७॥
काषायिणामसौम्यानां नग्नानां दण्डधारिणाम्।
कृष्णानां रक्तनेत्राणां स्वप्ने नेच्छन्ति दर्शनम्॥३८॥
कृष्णा पापा निराचारा दीर्घकेशनखस्तनी।
विरागमाल्यवसना स्वप्ने कालनिशा मता॥३९॥
इत्येते दारुणाः स्वप्ना रोगी यैर्याति पञ्चताम्।
अरोगः संशयं गत्वा कश्चिदेव प्रमुच्यते॥४०॥

The following are the other dreams of the most dangerous types which indicate either the death of the patient or affliction of individuals with serious types of diseases:

- Growth of Bamboo, shrubs, creepers etc., in the head
- Birds make nest in one's hairs
- Loss of hairs of the scalp
- The person is surrounded (and attacked by) by vultures, owls, dogs, crows etc
- The person is surrounded by Rakshas (demons), Preta (soul of dead persons), Pisaca (evil spririts), women, Candala (a person born of Sudra father and Brahmin mother M.W), Dravidas and Andhras.
- The person gets trapped in the forests of bamboos, Vetra (Salix caprea Linn), creeper, snare, grass and thorny trees.
- Falling down while walking in the above-mentioned types of forests
- Falling down on the ground with dust, ant-hill or ashes or cemetery or ditch while walking;
- Drowning in dirty water, mud or the well covered with darkness
- Being carried away by the rapidly flowing stream of water, rivers etc
- Intake of fatty substance, anolntment, emesis or purgation of fats
- Receipt of gold
- Quarreling with someone, getting arrested and getting defeated
- Losing or forgetting both the shoes, peeling of the skin out of feet
- Exhilaration
- Getting yelled at and insulted by angry forefathers
- Fall or extinction / destruction of teeth, moon, sun, stars, the gods, lamp and eyes
- Hills crack / break down into pieces and keep falling;
- Entering into a forest full of red flowers, the earth wherein red flowers are grown, the places of sinful acts, funeral pyre or a cave dense with darkness or filled with shrubs and creepers
- Moving southwards by wearing red garlands, laughing out loudly and being naked
- Going into frightful forests along with monkeys / on a chariot yoked by monkeys.
- Seeing people who are dark in complexion having red eyes, wearing ochre coloured cloth, of terrific appearance, naked, with a stick in hand.
- Seeing a sinful woman of black colour devoid of conduct with long hair, nails and breasts, wearing garlands and apparel of awkward colours / devoid of colour.

These are the dangerous types of dreams which indicate the death of patients. If an individual not afflicted with any disease sees such dreams, he is also likely to succumb to diseases. Instances of such persons surviving after such dreams are very rare. [27-40]

Process of manifestation of dreams:

मनोवहानां पूर्णत्वाद्दोषैरतिबलैस्त्रिभिः।
स्रोतसां दारुणान् स्वप्नान् काले पश्यति दारुणे॥४१॥
नातिप्रसुप्तः पुरुषः सफलानफलांस्तथा।
इन्द्रियेशेन मनसा स्वप्नान् पश्यत्यनेकधा॥४२॥

When the Manovaha srotas (vessels attached to the heart, channels of mind) are filled with the exceedingly aggravated three Doshas, one sees terrific dreams in ominous situations. It is only in a half-awakened state that a person is enabled by his mind which controls the sense organs, to have the diverse types of dreams meaningful or meaningless. [41-42]

Types of dream:

दृष्टं श्रुतानुभूतं च प्रार्थितं कल्पितं तथा।
भाविकं दोषजं चैव स्वप्नं सप्तविधं विदुः॥४३॥

The dream relates to the following seven factors in wakeful state:

- Visual perception
- Auditory perception
- Experiences though other means
- One's own desire;
- Imaginary as premonitions;
- Futuristic
- Caused by the aggravations of Doshas [43]

Results of various types of dream:

तत्र पञ्चविधं पूर्वमफलं भिषगादिशेत्।
दिवास्वप्नमतिह्रस्वमतिदीर्घं च बुद्धिमान्॥४४॥
दृष्टः प्रथमरात्रे यः स्वप्नः सोऽल्पफलो भवेत्।
न स्वपेद्यं पुनर्दृष्ट्वा स सद्यः स्यान्महाफलः॥४५॥
अकल्याणमपि स्वप्नं दृष्ट्वा तत्रैव यः पुनः।
पश्येत् सौम्यं शुभाकारं तस्य विद्याच्छुभं फलम्॥४६॥

The first five types of dreams listed in the previous paragraph, dreams experienced during the day time, those which are either too short or too long are not meaningful for a physician (that is to say such dreams cannot be regarded as having any premonitory value). Dreams experienced in the first part of the night are less meaningful. If one does not get sleep after experiencing a dream, then that dream is highly meaningful. Even if one experiences an inauspicious dream but thereafter again if he experiences an auspicious one, this is indicative of auspicious results. [44-46]

तत्र श्लोकः:-

पूर्वरूपाण्यथ स्वप्नान् य इमान् वेत्ति दारुणान्।
न स मोहादसाध्येषु कर्माण्यारभते भिषक्॥४७॥

To sum up: -The physician who is acquainted with these premonitory symptoms and dreams indicative of imminent death will not be trapped in ignorance and will also not initiate the treatment of these patients who are incurable. [47]

इत्यग्निवेशकृते तन्त्रे चरकप्रतिसंस्कृते इन्द्रियस्थाने
पूर्वरूपीयमिन्द्रियं नाम पञ्चमोऽध्यायः||५||

Thus ends the fifth chapter on the "Signs and symptoms of imminent death as indicated by the premonitory symptoms of diseases" of Indriya section of Agnivesha's work as redacted by Charaka.

30

Indriyasthana Chapter 6 Katamani Shareereeyam Indriyam

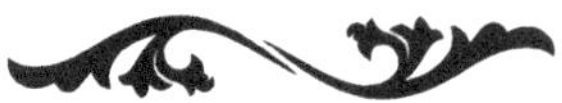

अथातः कतमानिशरीरीयमिन्द्रियं व्याख्यास्यामः||१||

इति ह स्माह भगवानात्रेयः||२||

Now we shall expound the chapter on the signs and symptoms of imminent death as indicated by the characteristic physical features of the patient. Thus said Lord Atreya [1-2]

Physical symptoms indicative of imminent death:

कतमानि शरीराणि व्याधिमन्ति महामुने!|

यानि वैद्यः परिहरेद्येषु कर्म न सिद्ध्यति||३||

इत्यात्रेयोऽग्निवेशेन प्रश्नं पृष्टः सुदुर्वचम्|

आचचक्षे यथा तस्मै भगवांस्तन्निबोधत||४||

यस्य वै भाषमाणस्य रुजत्यूर्ध्वमुरो भृशम्|

अन्नं च च्यवते भुक्तं स्थितं चापि न जीर्यति||५||

बलं च हीयते शीघ्रं तृष्णा चातिप्रवर्धते|

जायते हृदि शूलं च तं भिषक् परिवर्जयेत्||६||

O! Great sage, who are the ailing persons for whom treatment is of no avail and to whom the physician must not provide treatment?

Atreya answered this question as follows: The patient with the below mentioned symptoms should not be treated by the physician :

- feeling of excruciating pain in the upper part of the chest while speaking
- vomiting out food
- indigestion of food even if it is retained in the stomach
- sudden diminution of strength
- excessive increase of thirst
- pain a in the heart [3-6]

हिक्का गम्भीरजा यस्य शोणितं चातिसार्यते|

न तस्मै भेषजं दद्यात् स्मरन्नात्रेयशासनम्||७||

The patient suffering from bloody diarrhoea and hiccup originating from a deeply located organ should not be administered any medicine remembering the instructions of Atreya. [7]

आनाहश्चातिसारश्च यमेतौ दुर्बलं नरम्‌।
व्याधितं विशतो रोगौ दुर्लभं तस्य जीवितम्‌||८||

A weak patient afflicted with painful conditions like Anaha (distension of abdomen) and diarrhoea will not survive. [8]

आनाहश्चातितृष्णा च यमेतौ दुर्बलं नरम्‌।
विशतो विजहत्येनं प्राणा नातिचिरान्नरम्‌||९||

A weak patient afflicted with Anaha (distension of abdomen) and excessive thirst will surely die soon. [9]

ज्वरः पौर्वाह्णिको यस्य शुष्ककासश्च दारुणः।
बलमांसविहीनस्य यथा प्रेतस्तथैव सः||१०||

A person is as good as dead if he is deficient in strength and flesh and also suffers from morning fever along with severe dry cough. [10]

यस्य मूत्रं पुरीषं च ग्रथितं सम्प्रवर्तते।
निरूष्मणो जठरिणः श्वसनो न स जीवति||११||
श्वयथुर्यस्य कुक्षिस्थो हस्तपादं विसर्पति।
ज्ञातिसङ्घं स सङ्क्लेश्य तेन रोगेण हन्यते||१२||
श्वयथुर्यस्य पादस्थस्तथा स्रस्ते च पिण्डिके।
सीदतश्चाप्युभे जङ्घे तं भिषक् परिवर्जयेत्‌||१३||
शूनहस्तं शूनपादं शूनगुह्योदरं नरम्‌।
हीनवर्णबलाहारमौषधैर्नोपपादयेत्‌||१४||

The person will not survive if he is suffering from dyspnoea, abdominal disease, and lack of power of digestion and also passes hard stool and urine in condensed form.

The person will die after a prolonged illness if the abdominal oedema of the patient spreads to hands and feet.

The patient should not be administered any kind of medicine if he is suffering from diminution in the complexion, strength, capacity for the intake of food and is also suffering from oedema in hands, legs, genitals / perineum and abdomen. [11-14]

उरोयुक्तो बहुश्लेष्मा नीलः पीतः सलोहितः।
सततं च्यवते यस्य दूरात्तं परिवर्जयेत्‌||१५||
हृष्टरोमा सान्द्रमूत्रः शूनः कासज्वरार्दितः |
क्षीणमांसो नरो दूराद्वर्ज्यो वैद्येन जानता||१६||
त्रयः प्रकुपिता यस्य दोषाः कष्टाभिलक्षिताः |
कृशस्य बलहीनस्य नास्ति तस्य चिकित्सितम्‌||१७||
ज्वरातिसारौ शोफान्ते श्वयथुर्वा तयोः क्षये।
दुर्बलस्य विशेषेण नरस्यान्ताय जायते||१८||
पाण्डुरश्च कृशोऽत्यर्थं तृष्णयाऽभिपरिप्लुतः।
डम्बरी कुपितोच्छ्वासः प्रत्याख्येयो विजानता||१९||

The physician should discard the patient from a distance if he has copious expectoration of phlegm having blue, yellow or red colour.

If an emaciated person gets horripilation, passes condensed urine and suffers from oedema, cough and fever, a wise physician should discard him from a distance.

A person should not be treated if he is emaciated and weak, and all the three Doshas in him get (simultaneously) aggravated to such an extent that they are incapable of being corrected.

If fever and diarrhoea occur after oedema or vice versa, the patient suffering from such ailments, especially the weaker ones, succumb to death.

A patient having pallor, excessive emaciation, excessive thirst, rigid and fixed vision, and difficult expiration, should be discarded by an enlightened physician. [15-19]

हनुमन्याग्रहस्तृष्णा बलह्लासोऽतिमात्रया।
प्राणाश्चोरसि वर्तन्ते यस्य तं परिवर्जयेत्॥२०॥

If a person having lockjaw and rigidity in the nape of the neck / carotid region of the neck also suffers from thirst and excessive diminution of strength and the signs of life confined to the chest only, such a patient should be discarded. [20]

ताम्यत्यायच्छते शर्म न किञ्चिदपि विन्दति।
क्षीणमांसबलाहारो मुमूर्षुरचिरान्नरः॥२१॥
विरुद्धयोनयो यस्य विरुद्धोपक्रमा भृशम्।
वर्धन्ते दारुणा रोगाः शीघ्रं शीघ्रं स हन्यते॥२२॥
बलं विज्ञानमारोग्यं ग्रहणी मांसशोणितम्।
एतानि यस्य क्षीयन्ते क्षिप्रं क्षिप्रं स हन्यते॥२३॥
आरोग्यं हीयते यस्य प्रकृतिः परिहीयते।
सहसा सहसा तस्य मृत्युर्हरति जीवितम्॥२४॥

If a person with emaciation, diminished strength and lack of digestive power gets attacks of fainting and violent movement of the organs of the body and is difficult to manage with any measures, he succumbs to death immediately. If serious diseases of mutually contradictory etiological factors and lines of treatment get suddenly aggravated in a person, he succumbs to death in quick time.

A person having sudden diminution of strength, intellect, health, flesh, blood and functions of grahani (duodenum and the upper part of small intestine which are responsible for digestion and absorption of food) succumbs to death soon.

If there is sudden deterioration of health and change in the physical constitution of the individual, such a patient succumbs to death immediately. [21-24]

तत्र श्लोकः-
इत्येतानि शरीराणि व्याधिमन्ति विवर्जयेत्।
न ह्येषु धीराः पश्यन्ति सिद्धिं काञ्चिदुपक्रमात्॥२५॥

Ailing persons of these (above mentioned) types should be discarded. The wise physician should not anticipate success of his treatment in such cases. [25]

इत्यग्निवेशकृते तन्त्रे चरकप्रतिसंस्कृते इन्द्रियस्थाने कतमानिशरीरीयमिन्द्रियं नाम षष्ठोऽध्यायः॥६॥

Thus ends the sixth chapter on the signs and symptoms of imminent death as indicated by the characteristic features of the patient of Indriya section of Agnivesha's work as redacted by Charaka.

31

Indriyasthana Chapter 7
Pannaroopeeyam Indriyam

अथातः पन्नरूपीयमिन्द्रियं व्याख्यास्यामः||१||

इति ह स्माह भगवानात्रेयः||२||

Now we shall expound the chapter on the signs of imminent death as indicated by the distortion of the image reflected in the pupil. Thus said lord Atreya[1-2]

Shadow image in pupil:

दृष्ट्यां यस्य विजानीयात् पन्नरूपां कुमारिकाम्|

प्रतिच्छायामयीमक्ष्णोर्नैनमिच्छेच्चिकित्सितुम्||३||

The physician should not treat the patient if any distortions are found in the shadow image in the pupil of the patient. [3]

Other types of shadow:

ज्योत्स्नायामातपे दीपे सलिलादर्शयोरपि|

अङ्गेषु विकृता यस्य च्छाया प्रेतस्तथैव सः||४||

The patient is considered as good as dead if there is any distortion in any part of the shadow of the body caused by moon- light, sunlight or the light of a lamp and of the image as reflected in the water or mirror. [4]

Distortions in shadow:

छिन्ना भिन्नाऽऽकुला च्छाया हीना वाऽप्यधिकाऽपि वा|

नष्टा तन्वी द्विधा च्छिन्ना विकृता विशिरा च या||५||

एताश्चान्याश्च याः काश्चित् प्रतिच्छाया विगर्हिताः|

सर्वा मुमूर्षतां ज्ञेया न चेल्लक्ष्यनिमित्तजाः||६||

Persons having shadows which are broken, split, hazy, devoid of certain organs, added with certain more organs, not conspicuous, bifurcated, deformed and without the head, and similar other shadows, without any visible cause, may be considered as moribund. [5-6]

संस्थानेन प्रमाणेन वर्णेन प्रभया तथा|

छाया विवर्तते यस्य स्वस्थोऽपि प्रेत एव सः||७||

A person whose shadow or reflected image changes in shape, measurement, colour and luster, he is as good as dead even if he appears to be healthy. [7]

संस्थानमाकृतिर्ज्ञेया सुषमा विषमा च सा|

मध्यमल्पं महच्चोक्तं प्रमाणं त्रिविधं नृणाम्||८||

प्रतिप्रमाणसंस्थाना जलादर्शातपादिषु|

छाया या सा प्रतिच्छाया च्छाया वर्णप्रभाश्रया||९||

The term "samsthana" stands for shape. It might be even or uneven. Similarly, measurement may be of three kinds - medium, short or large. The image reflected in water, mirror, sun etc. corresponding to the measurement and shape of the body of the individual is known as praticchaya. Pratichchaya is nothing but reflected shadow based on the colour and lustre of the individual. [8-9]

Mahabhutas and shadow:

खादीनां पञ्च पञ्चानां छाया विविधलक्षणाः|
नाभसी निर्मला नीला सस्नेहा सप्रभेव च||१०||
रूक्षा श्यावारुणा या तु वायवी सा हतप्रभा|
विशुद्धरक्ता त्वाग्नेयी दीप्ताभा दर्शनप्रिया||११||
शुद्धवैदूर्यविमला सुस्निग्धा चाम्भसी मता|
स्थिरा स्निग्धा घना श्लक्ष्णा श्यामा श्वेता च पार्थिवी||१२||
वायवी गर्हिता त्वासां चतस्रः स्युः सुखोदयाः |
वायवी तु विनाशाय क्लेशाय महतेऽपि वा||१३||

The following are the distinctive features of shadows relating to each of the five mahabhutas.
1. Akasa - Clear, blue, unctuous and lustrous
2. Vayu - Dry, brown, and aruna (reddish)
3. Agni - Pure red, brilliant and pleasing to the eyes.
4. Jala - Clear like vaidurya (cat's eye) and excessively unctuous.
5. Prthvi - Stable, unctuous, compact, smooth, black and white.
The shadow pertaining to vayu is of inferior category whereas the remaining four are indicative of happiness. The former is indicative of great calamities and miseries. [10-13]

Various types of luster:

स्यातैजसी प्रभा सर्वा सा तु सप्तविधा स्मृता|
रक्ता पीता सिता श्यावा हरिता पाण्डुराऽसिता||१४||
तासां याः स्युर्विकासिन्यः स्निग्धाश्च विपुलाश्च याः|
ताः शुभा रूक्षमलिनाः सङ्क्षिप्ताश्चाशुभोदयाः ||१५||

All types of luster are constituted of tejas mahabhuta i.e. fire element. They are of seven types, viz, red, yellow, white, brown, green, pandura (pale yellow) and black. Of them those which are emanative, unctuous and dense are auspicious. On the other hand, those which are dry, dirty and thin are inauspicious. [14-15]

Shadow vis a vis luster:

वर्णमाक्रामति च्छाया भास्तु वर्णप्रकाशिनी|
आसन्ना लक्ष्यते च्छाया भाः प्रकृष्टा प्रकाशते||१६||
नाच्छायो नाप्रभः कश्चिदिवशेषाश्चिह्नयन्ति तु|
नृणां शुभाशुभोत्पत्तिं काले छायाप्रभाश्रयाः||१७||

The chaya (shadow) circumscribes the complexion of the body whereas the prabha (luster) illuminates the complexion. The shadow can be observed from nearby whereas the luster illuminates from a distance. There is nothing devoid of shadow or luster. Certain distinctive features of the shadow and the luster when mature indicate emergence of auspicious or inauspicious results in respect of human beings. [16-17]

Signs of imminent death:

कामलाऽक्ष्णोर्मुखं पूर्णं शङ्खयोर्मुक्तमांसता|

सन्त्रासश्चोष्णगात्रत्वं यस्य तं परिवर्जयेत्||१८||

उत्थाप्यमानः शयनात् प्रमोहं याति यो नरः|

मुहुर्मुहुर्न सप्ताहं स जीवति विकत्थनः ||१९||

संसृष्टा व्याधयो यस्य प्रतिलोमानुलोमगाः|

व्यापन्ना ग्रहणी प्रायः सोऽर्धमासं न जीवति||२०||

Yellowness of the eyes, swelling in the face, temples devoid of flesh, terrifying appearance and high temperature of the body (are the symptoms of imminent death) Patients with such symptoms must not be treated. A patient who faints again and again while being taken out of the bed cannot survive even for a week. A patient who suffers from diseases caused by more than one dosha in which both the upward and downward tracks are afflicted and whose grahani (duodenum and other parts of small intestine) are deranged cannot survive longer than a fortnight. [18-20]

उपरुद्धस्य रोगेण कर्शितस्याल्पमश्नतः|

बहु मूत्रपुरीषं स्याद्यस्य तं परिवर्जयेत्||२१||

दुर्बलो बहु भुङ्क्ते यः प्राग्भुक्तादन्नमातुरः |

अल्पमूत्रपुरीषश्च यथा प्रेतस्तथैव सः||२२||

इष्टं च गुणसम्पन्नमन्नमश्नाति यो नरः|

शश्वच्च बलवर्णाभ्यां हीयते न स जीवति||२३||

प्रकूजति प्रश्वसिति शिथिलं चातिसार्यते|

बलहीनः पिपासार्तः शुष्कास्यो न स जीवति||२४||

ह्रस्वं च यः प्रश्वसिति व्याविद्धं स्पन्दते च यः|

मृतमेव तमात्रेयो व्याचचक्षे पुनर्वसुः||२५||

ऊर्ध्वं च यः प्रश्वसिति श्लेष्मणा चाभिभूयते|

हीनवर्णबलाहारो यो नरो न स जीवति||२६||

An emaciated patient, who takes very little food but passes urine and stool in large quantities, should not be treated. A weak patient who takes food which is more in quantity than his previous meal(s) but passes urine and stool in small quantities should be considered as already dead. If a person who is weak, thirsty and has dryness of mouth, suffers from groaning, dyspepsia and diarrhea, then he does not survive. If the person is short of breath and there are irregular movements in his body, then according to Punarvasu Atreya, he does not survive. If a person, whose complexion, strength and capacity of intake of food are diminished, develops respiratory dyspnoea and gets afflicted with kapha, then he does not survive. [21-26].

ऊर्ध्वाग्रे नयने यस्य मन्ये चारतकम्पने|

बलहीनः पिपासार्तः शुष्कास्यो न स जीवति||२७||

यस्य गण्डावुपचितौ ज्वरकासौ च दारुणौ|

शूली प्रद्वेष्टि चाप्यन्नं तस्मिन् कर्म न सिध्यति||२८||

व्यावृत्तमूर्धजिह्वास्यो भ्रुवौ यस्य च विच्युते|

कण्टकैश्चाचिता जिह्वा यथा प्रेतस्तथैव सः||२९||

शेफश्चात्यर्थमुत्सिक्तं निःसृतौ वृषणौ भृशम्|

अतश्चैव विपर्यासो विकृत्या प्रेतलक्षणम्||३०||

निचितं यस्य मांसं स्यात्त्वगस्थिष्वेव दृश्यते|

क्षीणस्यानशनतस्तस्य मासमायुः परं भवेत्||३१||

- If a person who is weak, thirsty and having dryness of mouth suffers from rigid and upward look of the eyes and constant throbbing of the carotid region of the neck. He does not survive.
- If a person is having swollen cheeks from high fever and severe cough, cough, colicky pain and aversion for food, then no treatment will succeed in curing him.

- If there is distortion of the head, tongue and face, drooping of the eyebrows and appearance of thorny coating over the tongue, then such a person should be considered as already dead.
- If phallus gets excessively shrunken and the testicles hang excessively loose or vice versa, then the person having such abnormal signs should be considered as already dead.
- If an emaciated person who has wasting of muscle and who is reduced to skin and bones does not take food, his residual span of life is not more than one month. [27-31]

तत्र श्लोकः-

इदं लिङ्गमरिष्टाख्यमनेकमभिजज्ञिवान्‌|

आयुर्वेदविदित्याख्यां लभते कुशलो जनः||३२||

To sum up: - a wise person who is well versed with these various types of signs indicative of imminent death, is entitled to be called Ayurvedavit (knower of the "science of medicine"). [32]

इत्यग्निवेशकृते तन्त्रे चरकप्रतिसंस्कृते इन्द्रियस्थाने पन्नरूपीयमिन्द्रियं नाम सप्तमोऽध्यायः||७||

Thus ends the seventh chapter on the signs if imminent death as indicated by the "distortion of images reflected in the pupil" of the Indriya section of Agnivesha's work as redacted by Charaka.

32

Indriyasthana Chapter 8 Avak Shiraseeyam Indriyam

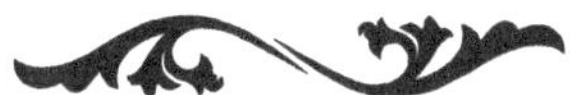

अथातोऽवाक्शिरसीयमिन्द्रियं व्याख्यास्यामः||१||

इति ह स्माह भगवानात्रेयः||२||

We shall now expound the chapter on imminent death as indicated by signs like distortion of the shadow of the individual viz. the inversion of the shadow of the head. Thus said Lord Atreya[1-2]

Signs of Imminent death:

अवाक्शिरा वा जिह्मा वा यस्य वा विशिरा भवेत्|

जन्तो रूपप्रतिच्छाया नैनमिच्छेच्चिकित्सितुम्||३||

जटीभूतानि पक्ष्माणि दृष्टिश्चापि निगृह्यते |

यस्य जन्तोर्न तं धीरो भेषजेनोपपादयेत्||४||

यस्य शूनानि वर्त्मानि न समायान्ति शुष्यतः|

चक्षुषी चोपदिह्येते यथा प्रेतस्तथैव सः||५||

भ्रुवोर्वा यदि वा मूर्ध्नि सीमन्तावर्तकान् बहून्|

अपूर्वानकृतान् व्यक्तान् दृष्ट्वा मरणमादिशेत्||६||

त्र्यहमेतेन जीवन्ति लक्षणेनातुरा नराः|

अरोगाणां पुनस्त्वेतत् षड्रात्रं परमुच्यते |३| ||७||

In the shadow of an individual if the head is found to be inverted (head pointing downwards and legs pointing upwards), is irregular or without the head, that individual should not be treated.

A person should also not be treated if in a person there is matting of eyelashes or absence of vision (because of the matting of eye-lashes of both lids together).

If in an emaciated person, there is swelling of the eyelids, if both the eyelids do not meet each other (due to swelling), if there is accumulation of dirt in the eyes and also if there is burning sensation in the eyes he is considered as equal to being dead.

If in a person, there are many well manifested simantas (lines formed by the parting of hair to each side) without them being made and Avartakas (whirls of hairs) in the eyebrows or in the hairs of the head which were neither found earlier nor made artificially, he is sure to die soon.

If the above-mentioned signs appear in individuals suffering from diseases, they survive for three days only. If they appear in persons who are not suffering from any diseases, such individuals may live for a maximum duration of six days. [3-7]

आयम्योत्पाटितान् केशान् यो नरो नावबुध्यते।
अनातुरो वा रोगी वा षड्रात्रं नातिवर्तते॥८॥
यस्य केशा निरभ्यङ्गा दृश्यन्तेऽभ्यक्तसन्निभाः।
उपरुद्धायुषं ज्ञात्वा तं धीरः परिवर्जयेत्॥९॥

If a person with or without a disease does not survive for more than six nights if he does not have any sensation when his hairs are pulled out and uprooted.If the hair of the individual appears to be greasy even when no unctuous substances (like oil) has been applied, he is considered to be at the end point of his life and hence should not be treated. [8-9]

ग्लायते नासिकावंशः पृथुत्वं यस्य गच्छति।
अशूनः शूनसङ्काश प्रत्याख्येयः स जानता॥१०॥
अत्यर्थविवृता यस्य यस्य चात्यर्थसंवृता।
जिह्मा वा परिशुष्का वा नासिका न स जीवति॥११॥
मुखं शब्दश्रवावोष्ठौ शुक्लश्यावातिलोहितौ।
विकृत्या यस्य वा नीलौ न स रोगाद्विमुच्यते॥१२॥

If there is depression and thickening / separation of the ridge of the nose, if the nose appears swollen in spite of it not being swollen up, the patient having these signs should not be treated by the wise physician.
Excessive enlargement or constriction of the nasal orifices, distortion in shape and extreme dryness of the nose indicate that the individual will not survive. If the face, ears and lips become abnormally white, brown, excessively red or blue without any obvious cause, then such a patient seldom recovers from the disease. [10-12]

अस्थिश्वेता द्विजा यस्य पुष्पिताः पङ्कसंवृताः।
विकृत्या न स रोगं तं विहायारोग्यमश्नुते॥१३॥
स्तब्धा निश्चेतना गुर्वी कण्टकोपचिता भृशम्।
श्यावा शुष्काऽथवा शूना प्रेतजिह्वा विसर्पिणी॥१४॥
दीर्घमुच्छ्वस्य यो ह्रस्वं नरो निःश्वस्य ताम्यति।
उपरुद्धायुषं ज्ञात्वा तं धीरः परिवर्जयेत्॥१५॥
हस्तौ पादौ च मन्ये च तालु चैवातिशीतलम्।
भवत्यायुःक्षये क्रूरमथवाऽपि भवेन्मृदु॥१६॥
घट्टयञ्जानुना जानु पादावुद्यम्य पातयन्।
योऽपास्यति मुहुर्वक्रमातुरो न स जीवति॥१७॥
दन्तैश्छिन्दन्नखाग्राणि नखैश्छिन्दन्छिरोरुहान्।
काष्ठेन भूमिं विलिखन्न रोगात् परिमुच्यते॥१८॥
दन्तान् खादति यो जाग्रदसाम्ना विरुदन् हसन्।
विजानाति न चेद्दुःखं न स रोगाद्विमुच्यते॥१९॥
मुहुर्हसन् मुहुः क्ष्वेडन् शय्यां पादेन हन्ति यः।
उच्चैश्छिद्राणि विमृशन्नातुरो न स जीवति॥२०॥

A patient having morbid conditions like:
Teeth getting white like the colour of the bone, appearance of white spots (Puspa-lit, meaning flower) over teeth and adhesion of slush / dirt / muddy substance (material) over them cannot recover from the disease.

If the tongue becomes rigid, senseless, heavy, excessively coated with a thorn like fur, brown in colour, dry or swollen and constantly mobile, then the patient having such signs is considered as good as dead.
If a person faints after a short expiration followed by a long inspiration, then considering that his end is near he should not be treated.

Excessive coldness, roughness and softness in hands, legs and nape of the neck indicate the end-of-life span of that person.

A person, who strikes one knee with the other, throws down legs after lifting them up and frequently turns the face to one or the other side, does not survive.

The patient who gnashes teeth while awake, cries and laughs loudly and does not have pain sensation, does not recover from the disease.

The patient, who frequently laughs, cries and shouts, keeps hitting the bed with his feet and puts finger into the nostrils, ears and eyes and does not survive for long. [13-20]

Need for immediate observation:
यैर्विन्दति पुरा भावैः समेतैः परमां रतिम्‌|
तैरेवारममाणस्य ग्लास्नोर्मरणमादिशेत्‌||२१||
न बिभर्ति शिरो ग्रीवा न पृष्ठं भारमात्मनः|
न हनू पिण्डमास्यस्थमातुरस्य मुमूर्षतः||२२||
सहसा ज्वरसन्तापस्तृष्णा मूर्च्छा बलक्षयः|
विश्लेषणं च सन्धीनां मुमूर्षोरुपजायते||२३||
गोसर्गे वदनाद्यस्य स्वेदः प्रच्यवते भृशम्‌|
लेपज्वरोपतप्तस्य दुर्लभं तस्य जीवितम्‌||२४||
नोपैति कण्ठमाहारो जिह्वा कण्ठमुपैति च|
आयुष्यन्तं गते जन्तोर्बलं च परिहीयते||२५||
शिरो विक्षिपते कृच्छ्रान्मुञ्चयित्वा प्रपाणिकौ|
ललाटसुप्रतस्वेदो मुमूर्षुश्च्युतबन्धनः ||२६||
If a debilitated patient develops disliking for the same factors (and things) by getting which he used to get extremely happy in the past, his death should be considered imminent.

If the neck of the patient is unable to support the weight of his head, the head gets tilted to one side, the back doesn't tolerate the weight of the body and the patient feels difficult / impossible to sit, and when his jaws cannot hold / support the morsel of food in the mouth – this indicates his imminent death.

If in a patient signs like fever, thirst, fainting, diminution of strength perspiration occurs in the face, there is little chance of his survival.

If the ingested food does not reach the throat, or the tongue falls back over the throat (thereby causing obstruction) and there is diminution of strength, then the death of the person is imminent.

If the person moves his head with difficulty by the help of the fore-arms and if there is sweating in the forehead and looseness of joints, he is moribund. [21-26]

तत्र श्लोकः:-
इमानि लिङ्गानि नरेषु बुद्धिमान्‌ विभावयेतावहितो मुमूर्षुषु|
क्षणेन भूत्वा ह्युपयान्ति कानिचिन्नचाफलं लिङ्गमिहास्ति किञ्चन||२७||
To sum up:
The wise physician should closely search for these signs repeatedly because some of them disappear in a short

moment after their manifestation. None of these signs remain without leading to the consequences already described i.e., all of them indicate imminent death. [27]

इत्यग्निवेशकृते तन्त्रे चरकप्रतिसंस्कृते इन्द्रियस्थानेऽवाक्शिरसीयमिन्द्रियं नामाष्टमोऽध्यायः ||८||

Thus ends the 'eight chapter' on imminent death as indicated by signs like the distortion of shadow of the individual, viz, the inversion of the shadow of the head, of the Indriya section of Agnivesha's work as redacted by Charaka.

33

Indriyasthana Chapter 9 Yasya Shyava Nimitteeyam Indriyam

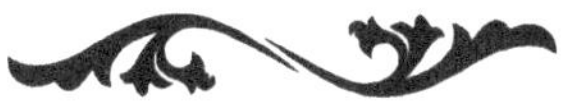

अथातो यस्यश्यावनिमित्तीयमिन्द्रियं व्याख्यास्यामः||१||

इति ह स्माह भगवानात्रेयः||२||

Now we shall explore the chapter on imminent death as indicated by signs like blackish brown coloration of the eyes. Thus said Lord Atreya [1-2]

Signs of imminent death:

यस्य श्यावे परिध्वस्ते हरिते चापि दर्शने|

आपन्नो व्याधिरन्ताय ज्ञेयस्तस्य विजानता||३||

निःसङ्गः परिशुष्कास्यः समृद्धो व्याधिभिश्च यः|

उपरुद्धायुषं ज्ञात्वा तं धीरः परिवर्जयेत्||४||

If the eyes of the patient appear blackish brown or green in colour and are devoid of vision, he is sure to die. Nonsensitiveness and dryness of the mouth of the patient associated with the aggravation of the diseases indicates the end of the span of his life. A wise physician should not treat such cases.

हरिताश्च सिरा यस्य लोमकूपाश्च संवृताः|

सोऽम्लाभिलाषी पुरुषः पित्तान्मरणमश्नुते||५||

शरीरान्ताश्च शोभन्ते शरीरं चोपशुष्यति|

बलं च हीयते यस्य राजयक्ष्मा हिनस्ति तम्||६||

A person having green coloration of veins, obstruction of hairs follicles and desire for sour foods / substances will die of disorders caused by aggravated pitta. A person whose hands and legs (limbs) look attractive, the other parts of the body are getting emaciated and his strength is getting diminished would die of tuberculosis.

अंसाभितापो हिक्का च छर्दनं शोणितस्य च|

आनाहः पार्श्वशूलं च भवत्यन्ताय शोषिणः||७||

Consumption associated with Amsabhitapa (burning sensation in the shoulder region), hiccup, haemoptysis (lit vomiting of blood), anaha (constipation along with distension of stomach) and parsvasula (pain in the sides of the chest) leads to the death of the patient.

वातव्याधिरपस्मारी कुष्ठी शोफी तथोदरी|

गुल्मी च मधुमेही च राजयक्ष्मी च यो नरः||८||

अचिकित्स्या भवन्त्येते बलमांसक्षये सति|

अन्येष्वपि विकारेषु तान् भिषक् परिवर्जयेत्||९||

The patients suffering from the below mentioned diseases should not be treated when they have diminution of strength and muscles / flesh (because they do not yield to any treatment) :

- Vatavyadhi (diseases caused by the vitiation of Vata)
- Apasmara (epilepsy)
- Kustha (obstinate skin diseases including leprosy)
- Sopha (oedema)
- Udara (obstinate type of abdominal diseases)
- Gulma (phantom tumour)
- Madhumeha (obstinate urinary disorders including diabetes mellitus)
- Rajayakshma (tuberculosis, wasting diseases)

Similarly other patients in such conditions (suffering from diseases associated with depletion of strength and muscles) should also be rejected (should not treat) by the physician.

विरेचनहृतानाहो यस्तृष्णानुगतो नरः।
विरिक्तः पुनराध्माति यथा प्रेतस्तथैव सः॥१०॥

If a person suffering from Anaha (constipation associated with distension in abdomen) is relieved by purgation but subsequently develops thirst and suffers from Anaha again in spite of the purgation having been given, he should be considered as good as dead.

पेयं पातुं न शक्नोति कण्ठस्य च मुखस्य च।
उरसश्च विशुष्कत्वाद्यो नरो न स जीवति ॥११॥

If a person is unable to drink liquid substances due to the dryness of throat, mouth and the chest, he does not survive.

स्वरस्य दुर्बलीभावं हानिं च बलवर्णयोः।
रोगवृद्धिमयुक्त्या च दृष्ट्वा मरणमादिशेत्॥१२॥

Weakness in the voice, diminution of the strength and complexion and aggravation of the disease without any reasons / causes indicate the imminent death of the patient.

ऊर्ध्वश्वासं गतोष्माणं शूलोपहतवङ्क्षणम्।
शर्म चानधिगच्छन्तं बुद्धिमान् परिवर्जयेत्॥१३॥

A patient having dyspnoea, absence of heat in the body, affliction with pain in the groins and absence of any response to the treatment should not be treated by the physician. [3-13]

Exploratory therapy:

अपस्वरं भाषमाणं प्राप्तं मरणमात्मनः।
श्रोतारं चाप्यशब्दस्य दूरतः परिवर्जयेत्॥१४॥
यं नरं सहसा रोगो दुर्बलं परिमुञ्चति।
संशयप्राप्तमात्रेयो जीवितं तस्य मन्यते॥१५॥
अथ चेज्ज्ञातयस्तस्य याचेरन् प्रणिपाततः।
रसेनाद्यादिति ब्रूयान्नास्मै दद्यादिवशोधनम्॥१६॥
मासेन चेन्न दृश्येत विशेषस्तस्य शोभनः।
रसैश्चान्यैर्बहुविधैर्दुर्लभं तस्य जीवितम्॥१७॥

A patient who makes a statement in a choked voice about the advent of his own death and hears sounds / words which are indicative of inauspicious (reveal bad news) things / events, should be discarded from a distance (not be treated). According to Master Atreya, if a weak patient gets rid of a disease all of a sudden, his life should be considered as in danger. If his relatives approach the physician in all humanity for help, he should prescribe food with meat-soup and must not administer any kinds of elimination therapies. If specific improvement in his health is not observed within one month in spite of the administration of various types of meat soup, the patient is sure to die. [14-17]

निष्ठ्यूतं च पुरीषं च रेतश्चाम्भसि मज्जति|
यस्य तस्यायुषः प्राप्तमन्तमाहुर्मनीषिणः||१८||
निष्ठ्यूते यस्य दृश्यन्ते वर्णा बहुविधाः पृथक्|
तच्च सीदत्यपः प्राप्य न स जीवितुमर्हति ||१९||
पित्तमूष्मानुगं यस्य शङ्खौ प्राप्य विमूर्च्छति [२] |
स रोगः शङ्खको नाम्ना त्रिरात्राद्धन्ति जीवितम्||२०||
सफेनं रुधिरं यस्य मुहुरास्यात् प्रसिच्यते|
शूलैश्च तुद्यते कुक्षिः प्रत्याख्येयस्तथाविधः||२१||
बलमांसक्षयस्तीव्रो रोगवृद्धिररोचकः|
यस्यातुरस्य लक्ष्यन्ते त्रीन् पक्षान्न स जीवति||२२||

If the sputum, stool and semen of a person sink when placed on water, he should be considered as moribund. If several colours appear in the sputum of a person and it sinks in water, he cannot survive. A morbid condition caused by the interaction of the vitiated pitta with agni (bodily heat) in the temporal region is known as Sankhaka which kills the patient in three nights. If a person suffering from pain in the lower abdomen frequently vomits blood along with foam like substance, then he should not be treated. If there is sudden diminution in strength and flesh of the patient and aggravation of the disease associated with arocaka (anorexia), the patient cannot survive for more than three fortnights. [18-22]

तत्र श्लोकौ-
विज्ञानानि मनुष्याणां मरणे प्रत्युपस्थिते|
भवन्त्येतानि सम्पश्येदन्यान्येवंविधानि च||२३||
तानि सर्वाणि लक्ष्यन्ते न तु सर्वाणि मानवम्|
विशन्ति विनशिष्यन्तं तस्माद्बोध्यानि सर्वतः||२४||

To sum up: -The above are the signs indicative of imminent death of a person. These and such others should be observed by the physician. All of them are manifested in moribund persons. All of them, however, do not appear in the same moribund person. The physician should be conversant with these signs in their entity. [23-24]

इत्यग्निवेशकृते तन्त्रे चरकप्रतिसंस्कृते इन्द्रियस्थाने यस्यश्यावनिमित्तीयमिन्द्रियं नाम नवमोऽध्यायः||९||

Thus ends the ninth chapter on imminent death as indicated by signs like black-brown coloration of the eyes of the Indriya section of Agnivesha's work as redacted by Charaka.

34

Indriyasthana Chapter 10 Sadyo Maraneeyasm Indriyam

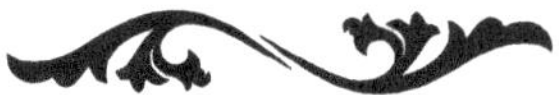

अथातः सद्योमरणीयमिन्द्रियं व्याख्यास्यामः||१||

इति ह स्माह भगवानात्रेयः||२||

We shall now explore the chapter on the "Signs indicative of Impending sudden Death".Thus said Lord Atreya[1-2]

Premonitory signs of Sudden death:

सद्यस्तितिक्षतः प्राणॉल्लक्षणानि पृथक् पृथक्|

अग्निवेश! प्रवक्ष्यामि संस्पृष्टो यैर्न जीवति||३||

O! Agnivesha, I shall describe separately the signs indicative of sudden death. The patient afflicted with these signs does not survive. They are as follows:

वाताष्ठीला सुसंवृद्धा तिष्ठन्ती दारुणा हृदि|

तृष्णयाऽभिपरीतस्य सद्यो मुष्णाति जीवितम्||४||

Intense thirst in a patient suffering from a painful and fully manifested Vatasthila (hard tumour caused by vitiated Vata) in the cardiac region will take away life immediately.

पिण्डिके शिथिलीकृत्य जिह्मीकृत्य च नासिकाम्|

वायुः शरीरे विचरन् सद्यो मुष्णाति जीवितम्||५||

Movement of the vitiated Vayu all over the body after producing laxity in the calf muscles and irregularity in the structure of the nose will cause immediate death.

भ्रुवौ यस्य च्युते स्थानादन्तर्दाहश्च दारुणः|

तस्य हिक्काकरो रोगः सद्यो मुष्णाति जीवितम्||६||

Development of hiccup in a patient who has dropping of the eyebrows and excessive burning sensation in the body will take away his life almost immediately.

क्षीणशोणितमांसस्य वायुरूर्ध्वगतिश्चरन्|

उभे मन्ये समे यस्य सद्यो मुष्णाति जीवितम्||७||

Distension of the nape of the neck on both sides (carotid regions of the neck) by the aggravated Vayu moving upwards in a patient having diminution of blood and flesh will cause immediate death of the patient.

अन्तरेण गुदं गच्छन् नाभिं च सहसाऽनिलः|

कृशस्य वङ्क्षणौ गृह्णन् सद्यो मुष्णाति जीवितम्||८||

Affliction of the groins of a weak / emaciated patient by the sudden aggravation of vayu between the anus and the umbilicus; will cause immediate death.

वितत्य पर्शुकाग्राणि गृहीत्वोरश्च मारुतः|
स्तिमितस्यायताक्षस्य सद्यो मुष्णाति जीवितम्||९||

Stretching of the tips of ribs by the aggravated Vayu afflicting the chest of a patient whose eyes are dilated and who feels Staimitya (as if covered with a wet cloth) will die immediately.

हृदयं च गुदं चोभे गृहीत्वा मारुतो बली|
दुर्बलस्य विशेषेण सद्यो मुष्णाति जीवितम्||१०||

Seizure (affliction) of both heart and anus by strongly aggravated Vayu in a patient who is exceedingly weak will cause death instantaneously.

वङ्क्षणं च गुदं चोभे गृहीत्वा मारुतो बली|
श्वासं सञ्जनयञ्जन्तोः सद्यो मुष्णाति जीवितम्||११||

Dyspnoea caused by the strongly aggravated Vayu after having afflicted (seized) both the groin regions and the anus will cause immediate death of the patient.

नाभिं मूत्रं बस्तिशीर्षं पुरीषं चापि मारुतः|
प्रच्छिन्नं जनयञ्छूलं सद्यो मुष्णाति जीवितम्||१२||

Production of cutting-pain by Vayu as a result of the affliction of umbilicus, urine, Bastishira (kidneys) and faeces will cause instantaneous death.

भिद्येते वङ्क्षणौ यस्य वातशूलैः समन्ततः|
भिन्नं पुरीषं तृष्णा च सद्यः प्राणाञ्जहाति सः||१३||

A patient whose entire body has been pervaded by aggravated vata, if severe blasting kind of pain manifests in both the groins and if the person also has diarrhea and thirst he will die immediately.

आप्लुतं मारुतेनेह शरीरं यस्य केवलम्|
भिन्नं पुरीषं तृष्णा च सद्यो जह्यात् स जीवितम्||१४||

Occurrence of diarrhoea and thirst in a patient whose entire body is pervaded by aggravated Vata will die soon.

शरीरं शोफितं यस्य वाताशोफेन देहिनः|
भिन्नं पुरीषं तृष्णा च सद्यो जह्यात् स जीवितम्||१५||

Occurrence of diarrhoea and thirst in a patient whose body is swollen because of Sotharoga of Vatika type will die almost immediately.

आमाशयसमुत्थाना यस्य स्यात् परिकर्तिका|
भिन्नं पुरीषं तृष्णा च सद्यः प्राणाञ्जहाति सः||१६||

Diarrhea and thirst occurring in a patient suffering from tearing (cramp like) pain originating from stomach and intestines will kill the patient immediately.

पक्वाशयसमुत्थाना यस्य स्यात् परिकर्तिका|
तृष्णा गुदग्रहश्चोग्रः सद्यो जह्यात् स जीवितम्||१७||

Thirst and acute spasm in the anal region occurring in a patient suffering from cutting / tearing type of pain (cramp like) originating from colon almost kills the patient immediately.

पक्वाशयमधिष्ठाय हत्वा सञ्ज्ञां च मारुतः|
कण्ठे घुर्घुरकं कृत्वा सद्यो हरति जीवितम्||१८||

If in a patient the aggravated vata getting localized in the colon causes unconsciousness and also produces gurgling or murmuring sounds in the throat, it causes immediate death of the patient.

दन्ताः कर्दमदिग्धाभा मुखं चूर्णकसन्निभम्|
सिप्रायन्ते च गात्राणि लिङ्गं सद्यो मरिष्यतः||१९||

Appearance of teeth as if adhered with mud, face as if covered with ashes and excessive perspiration all over the body as if the body is sprinkled with water of sipra river and the body is also cold due to sweating, the patient will die immediately.

तृष्णाश्वासशिरोरोगमोहदौर्बल्यकूजनैः|
स्पृष्टः प्राणाञ्जहात्याशु शकृद्भेदेन चातुरः||२०||

If diarrhoea, thirst, dyspnoea, headache, unconsciousness, debility and groaning sound from the throat occur simultaneously in a patient he is sure to die immediately. [3-20]

तत्र श्लोकः:-
एतानि खलु लिङ्गानि यः सम्यगवबुध्यते|
स जीवितं च मर्त्यानां मरणं चावबुध्यते||२१||

To sum up: The physician who perfectly comprehends these signs can very well anticipate the survival or death of the patient. [21]

 इत्यग्निवेशकृते तन्त्रे चरकप्रतिसंस्कृते इन्द्रियस्थाने सद्योमरणीयमिन्द्रियं नाम दशमोऽध्यायः||१०||

Thus ends the tenth chapter on the "Signs Indicative of Impending Sudden Death" of the Indriya Section of Agnivesha's work as redacted by Charaka.

35

Indriyasthana Chapter 11 Anu Jyoteeyam Indriyam

अथातोऽणुज्योतीयमिन्द्रियं व्याख्यास्यामः||१||

इति ह स्माह भगवानात्रेयः||२||

We shall now explore the chapter on "Imminent Death as indicated by Signs like the Diminution of Bodily Heat". Thus said Lord Atreya [1-2]

Signs of imminent death:

अणुज्योतिरनेकाग्रो दुश्छायो दुर्मनाः सदा|

रतिं न लभते याति परलोकं समान्तरम्||३||

The below mentioned indicate that the person is going to die within one year time:

diminution of the bodily heat

absence of the power of concentration of mind

loss of complexion

weakness of mind

absence of attachment for life [3]

बलिं बलिभृतो यस्य प्रणीतं नोपभुञ्जते|

लोकान्तरगतः पिण्डं भुङ्क्ते संवत्सरेण सः||४||

सप्तर्षीणां समीपस्था यो न पश्यत्यरुन्धतीम्|

संवत्सरान्ते जन्तुः स सम्पश्यति महत्तमः||५||

विकृत्या विनिमित्तं यः शोभामुपचयं धनम्|

प्राप्नोत्यतो वा विभ्रंशं समान्तं तस्य जीवितम्||६||

The birds (crow) refusing to eat bali i.e., offering of a part of the daily meal to all creatures offered by an individual would indicate that he would die within one year time and also that he would partake the manes offered by his relatives (offering given for the dead persons) being in the world beyond death within a year thereafter. If a person is not able to see the "Arundhati" star situated adjacent to the saptarshi constellation (the Great Bear), he is said to succumb to death after one year thereafter. Sudden gain or loss of luster, plumpness or wealth without any appreciable reason indicates the death of the person one year thereafter. [4-6]

भक्तिः शीलं स्मृतिस्त्यागो बुद्धिर्बलमहेतुकम्|

षडेतानि निवर्तन्ते षड्भिर्मासैर्मरिष्यतः||७||

Cessation of desire, conduct, and memory, sense of sacrifice, intellect and strength without any appreciable reason indicates the death of the person within six months. [7]

धमनीनामपूर्वाणां जालमत्यर्थशोभनम्|

ललाटे दृश्यते यस्य षण्मासान्न स जीवति||८||
लेखाभिश्चन्द्रवक्राभिर्ललाटमुपचीयते|
यस्य तस्यायुषः षड्भिर्मासैरन्तं समादिशेत्||९||

Appearance of an exceedingly shining network of blood vessels which were not there before, on the forehead of the individual indicates that he will not survive beyond six months. If there is an increase in the plumpness of the forehead of the individual because of the development of crescent shaped furrows, his life span is bound to come to an end within six months. [8-9]

शरीरकम्पः सम्मोहो गतिर्वचनमेव च|
मत्तस्येवोपलभ्यन्ते यस्य मासं न जीवति||१०||
रेतोमूत्रपुरीषाणि यस्य मज्जन्ति चाम्भसि|
स मासात् स्वजनद्वेष्टा मृत्युवारिणि मज्जति||११||

If there are tremors in the body and fainting (losing consciousness), if the movements of the body parts (gait disorders) and speech (delirium) are abnormally disturbed just like in an intoxicated person (mad person) the person will not live for even one month. If a person who hates (developed aversion) his own relatives and friends the semen, urine and faeces sink when placed on water, he succumbs to death within one month. [10-11]

हस्तपादं मुखं चोभे विशेषाद्यस्य शुष्यतः|
श्यूयेते वा विना देहात् स च मासं न जीवति||१२||
ललाटे मूर्ध्नि बस्तौ वा नीला यस्य प्रकाशते|
राजी बालेन्दुकुटिला न स जीवितुमर्हति||१३||
प्रवालगुटिकाभासा यस्य गात्रे मसूरिकाः|
उत्पद्याशु विनश्यन्ति न चिरात् स विनश्यति||१४||
ग्रीवावमर्दो बलवाञ्जिह्वाश्वयथुरेव च|
ब्रध्नास्यगलपाकश्च यस्य पक्वं तमादिशेत्||१५||
सम्भ्रमोऽतिप्रलापोऽतिभेदोऽस्थ्नामतिदारुणः [३] |
कालपाशपरीतस्य त्रयमेतत् प्रवर्तते||१६||
प्रमुह्य लुञ्चयेत् केशान् परिगृह्णात्यतीव च|
नरः स्वस्थवदाहारमबलः कालचोदितः||१७||

If there is emaciation of the hands, feet and face of the individual, with the body without undergoing any such change, or if there is swelling of hands, feet and face and absence of swelling in the middle part of the body, he does not survive for one month. Appearance of crescent shaped blue lines on the forehead, head and pelvic region indicates that the person will not survive. If eruptions of Masurika (pox) / eruptions resembling masura (lentil) having the appearance of coral beads (reddish in colour) manifest in an individual and immediately disappear, he will die immediately. A person having acute squeezing-pain in the neck, swelling of the tongue, inguinal lymphadenitis and inflammation (ulcers, sores) of mouth and throat should be considered as ripe for death i.e., that person will die soon. Excessive giddiness, extreme delirium and severe acute breaking pain in bones - these three symptoms will lead the patient to the noose of death i.e., he will not survive for long. A weak person, who pulls out his hair in a state of unconsciousness and in spite of having less strength - eats food in excessive quantities just like a healthy person, is as good as dead. [12-17]

समीपे चक्षुषोः कृत्वा मृगयेताङ्गुलीकरम्|
स्मयतेऽपि च कालान्ध ऊर्ध्वगानिमिषेक्षणः ||१८||
शयनादासनादङ्गात् काष्ठात् कुड्यादथापि वा|
असन्मृगयते किञ्चित् स मुह्यन् कालचोदितः||१९||

A person whose vision is fixed and directed upwards as he gazes in shock / bewilderment, who searches for his hands and fingers which are placed in front of his eyes (is not sure if he has hands and fingers) and smiles while doing so, succumbs to death immediately. If because of hallucination, a person tries to search for something which does not exist in the beds, seats, limbs of the body, wooden blocks or walls, he is as good as dead. [18-19]

अहास्यहासी सम्मुह्यन् प्रलेढि दशनच्छदौ|
शीतपादकरोच्छ्वासो यो नरो न स जीवति||२०||
आह्वयंस्तं समीपस्थं स्वजनं जनमेव वा|
महामोहावृतमनाः पश्यन्नपि न पश्यति||२१||

A person who out of delusion laughs in circumstances where there is no cause for laughter, who licks his own lips and whose feet, hands and breath are cold does not survive. A person who keeps calling out for his relatives and other people who are in his vicinity (in the range of his visual field) and with his mind surrounded and clouded by immense delusion (indicative of immediate death) does not see people or things though his eyes who are closer to him should be considered to be nearer to death. [20-21]

अयोगमतियोगं वा शरीरे मतिमान् भिषक्|
खादीनां युगपद्दृष्ट्वा भेषजं नावचारयेत्||२२||

Persons who are unable to perceive objects of senses which are existent and simultaneously perceives the objects of senses which are non-existent, should not be treated [22]

अतिप्रवृद्ध्या रोगाणां मनसश्च बलक्षयात्|
वासमुत्सृजति क्षिप्रं शरीरी देहसञ्ज्ञकम्||२३||
वर्णस्वरावग्निबलं वागिन्द्रियमनोबलम्|
हीयतेऽसुक्षये निद्रा नित्या भवति वा न वा||२४||

Excessive aggravation of the disease and diminution of strength of mind (will power) results in the soul departing from its physical abode (body) i.e. will die. When the span of life comes to an end there is diminution of complexion, voice and the power of digestion, speech, senses and the mind and the person either sleeps always or does not get sleep at all. [23-24]

भिषग्भेषजपानान्नगुरुमित्रद्विषश्च ये|
वशगाः सर्व एवैते बोद्धव्याः समवर्तिनः||२५||
एतेषु रोगः क्रूगते भेषजं प्रतिहन्ग्रते|
नैषामन्नानि भुञ्जीत न चोदकमपि स्पृशेत्||२६||

A person having aversion for physicians, medicine, drinks, foods, preceptors and friends should be considered as already under the grip of the "God of Death". Diseases of these persons will continue existing and medicines do not produce any beneficial effect on them. One should never take anything from them, neither the food nor water from their home (offered by them). [25-26]

पादाः समेताश्चत्वारः सम्पन्नाः साधकैर्गुणैः|
व्यर्था गतायुषो द्रव्यं विना नास्ति गुणोदयः||२७||

The four factors essential for the treatment, i.e., the physician, the drug, the attendant and the patient along with their excellent attributes are of no avail in the cases where the span of life has come to an end. When there is no balance of life span where will the effects (attributes) of the medicines manifest i.e., how does the disease get cured? This is because without Dravya (or cause) i.e., lifespan there is no possibility of the manifestation of the Guna (effect) i.e., 'cure from the disease'. [27]

परीक्ष्यमायुर्भिषजा नीरुजस्यातुरस्य च|
आयुर्ज्ञानफलं कृत्स्नमायुर्ज्ञे ह्यनुवर्तते||२८||

The physician should examine the span of life of a healthy person as well as patients because the entire treatment is dependent upon this knowledge. [28]

तत्र श्लोकः-

क्रियापथमतिक्रान्ताः केवलं देहमाप्लुताः|

चिह्नं कुर्वन्ति यद्दोषास्तदरिष्टं निरुच्यते||२९||

To sum up: -Signs produced by the vitiated Doshas which have transcended the sphere of treatment and pervaded all over the body, are known as Aristas (signs of imminent death). [29]

इत्यग्निवेशकृते तन्त्रे चरकप्रतिसंस्कृते

इन्द्रियस्थानेऽणुज्योतीयमिन्द्रियं नामैकादशोऽध्यायः||११||

Thus ends the eleventh chapter on the "Imminent Death as Indicated by Signs like Diminution of Bodily Heat" of Indriya Section of Agnivesa's work as redacted by Caraka.

36

Indriyasthana Chapter 12 Gomaya Choorneeyam Indriyam

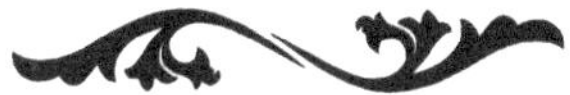

अथातो गोमयचूर्णीयमिन्द्रियं व्याख्यास्यामः||१||

इति ह स्माह भगवानात्रेयः||२||

We shall now explore the chapter on "Imminent Death as indicated by signs like the appearance of a Substance resembling Cow dung powder in the Head". Thus said Lord Atreya [1-2]

Signs of imminent Death:

यस्य गोमयचूर्णाभं चूर्णं मूर्धनि जायते|

सस्नेहं भ्रश्यते चैव मासान्तं तस्य जीवितम्||३||

If an unctuous powder resembling that of cow dung appears in and falls down from the head. The patient may live for one month only.

निकषन्निव यः पादौ च्युतांसः परिधावति|

विकृत्या न स लोकेऽस्मिंश्चिरं वसति मानवः||४||

Morbid conditions like the rubbing of legs on the round and drooping of the shoulders of an individual while running indicate his imminent death.

यस्य स्नातानुलिप्तस्य पूर्वं शुष्यत्युरो भृशम्|

आर्द्रेषु सर्वगात्रेषु सोऽर्धमासं न जीवति||५||

One would not live for more than a fortnight if after bath or application of unction, his chest gets dried up while the rest of the body remains wet.

यमुद्दिश्यातुरं वैद्यः संवर्तयितुमौषधम् |

यतमानो न शक्नोति दुर्लभं तस्य जीवितम्||६||

If the physician is very keen to administer a therapy to the patient, but does not succeed in preparing the medicines for the same (in spite of all the efforts to do so) or provide the treatment, such a patient hardly survives.

विज्ञातं बहुशः सिद्धं विधिवच्चावचारितम्|

न सिध्यत्यौषधं यस्य नास्ति तस्य चिकित्सितम्||७||

If a drug which is well known for its therapeutic effects, which has been successfully tried in many other cases and which is administered according to the prescription in the scriptures, fails to produce the desired effect on a particular patient, he should be considered as beyond treatment i.e., his death is assured.

आहारमुपयुञ्जानो भिषजा सूपकल्पितम्|

यः फलं तस्य नाप्नोति दुर्लभं तस्य जीवितम्||८||

If the diet prepared under the supervision of an experienced physician properly administered to a patient does not produce the desired effect, the patient succumbs to death. [3-8]

Characteristic features of messenger:

दूताधिकारे वक्ष्यामो लक्षणानि मुमूर्षताम्|
यानि दृष्ट्वा भिषक् प्राज्ञः प्रत्याख्यायादसंयमम्||९||
मुक्तकेशेऽथवा नग्ने रुदत्यप्रयतेऽथवा|
भिषगभ्यागतं दृष्ट्वा दूतं मरणमादिशेत्||१०||
सुप्ते भिषजि ये दूताश्छिन्दत्यपि च भिन्दति|
आगच्छन्ति भिषक् तेषां न भर्तारमनुव्रजेत्||११||
जुह्वत्यग्निं तथा पिण्डान् पितृभ्यो निर्वपत्यपि|
वैद्ये दूता य आयान्ति ते घ्नन्ति प्रजिघांसवः||१२||
कथयत्यप्रशस्तानि चिन्तयत्यथवा पुनः|
वैद्ये दूता मनुष्याणामागच्छन्ति मुमूर्षताम्||१३||
मृतदग्धविनष्टानि भजति व्याहरत्यपि|
अप्रशस्तानि चान्यानि वैद्ये दूता मुमूर्षताम्||१४||
विकारसामान्यगुणे देशे कालेऽथवा भिषक्|
दूतमभ्यागतं दृष्ट्वा नातुरं तमुपाचरेत्||१५||
दीनभीतद्रुतत्रस्तमलिनामसतीं स्त्रियम्|
त्रीन् व्याकृतींश्च षण्डांश्च दूतान् विद्यान्मुमूर्षताम्||१६||
अङ्गव्यसनिनं दूतं लिङ्गिनं व्याधितं तथा|
सम्प्रेक्ष्य चोग्रकर्माणं न वैद्यो गन्तुमर्हति||१७||
आतुरार्थमनुप्राप्तं खरोष्ट्ररथवाहनम्|
दूतं दृष्ट्वा भिषग्विद्यादातुरस्य पराभवम्||१८||
पलालबुसमांसास्थिकेशलोमनखद्विजान्|
मार्जनीं मुसलं शूर्पमुपानच्चर्म विच्युतम्||१९||
तृणकाष्ठतुषाङ्गारं स्पृशन्तो लोष्टमश्म च|
तत्पूर्वदर्शने दूता व्याहरन्ति मुमूर्षताम्||२०||
यस्मिंश्च दूते ब्रुवति वाक्यमातुरसंश्रयम्|
पश्येन्निमित्तमशुभं तं च नानुव्रजेद्भिषक्||२१||
तथा व्यसनिनं प्रेतं प्रेतालङ्कारमेव वा|
भिन्नं दग्धं विनष्टं वा तद्वादीनि वचांसि वा||२२||
रसो वा कटुकस्तीव्रो गन्धो वा कौणपो महान्|
स्पर्शो वा विपुलः क्रूरो यद्वाऽन्यदशुभं भवेत्||२३||
तत्पूर्वमभितो वाक्यं वाक्यकालेऽथवा पुनः|
दूतानां व्याहृतं श्रुत्वा धीरो मरणमादिशेत्||२४||
इति दूताधिकारोऽयमुक्तः कृत्स्नो मुमूर्षताम्|२५|

Now we shall explain the signs of imminent death as indicated by characteristic features of the messenger who comes to take the physician to the patient's house. If such signs are observed, the wise physician should reject the patient (should not treat) without hesitation (because his death would be confirmed)-

- If the messenger arrives at the physician's house when the latter is dishevelled (has not combed his hairs or kept them open), naked, crying or unclean, the patient should be considered as moribund.

- If the messenger arrives at the physician's house when the latter is sleeping, is cutting something, or is breaking open something, the physician should not go towards the patient's house or attempt to treat him or her.
- If the messenger arrives at the physician's house while the latter is offering oblations to the fire or Pinda (balls of food) to his ancestors (as oblation) then the patient for whom the messenger was sent would succumb to death.
- The messenger of the patient who is about to die will come to the door of the physician who is hearing or speaking something inauspicious.
- If the messenger approaches the physician when the latter is talking about a dead, burnt or destroyed / mutilated thing or person or is speaking / discussing inauspicious tasks or news, the patient for whom the messenger has come will die soon.
- If the messenger comes to the physician's house or place which has attributes similar to those of the disease from which the patient is suffering, he should be considered as moribund. Example - If the patient is suffering from Raktapitta (a condition characterised by bleeding from various parts of the body) and the messenger sent by him arrives at the physician's house when fire is burning nearby (desa) or burning mid-day (Kala), both of which have attributes similar to those of Rakthapitta, the patient is sure to die.
- If the messenger is in a miserable condition, frightened, hurried, terrified and unclean or if the messenger happens to be a woman without chastity who has worn unclean clothes, or if three messengers come at a time, or if he has deformed organs (handicap) or if the messenger is a eunuch, the patient for whom such a messenger is sent is to be considered as moribund.
- If the messenger is deficient in any organs of his body, if his limbs, nose or ears have been cut (mutilated, damaged), is an ascetic, is the one who is observing chastity, or if he is indulged in cruel actives the physician should not attend the patient for whom such a messenger has come (because the patient is anyhow going to die).
- If the messenger comes in a vehicle carried by a donkey of camel (or riding a donkey or camel) or a chariot, the patient for whom he has been sent succumbs to death.
- When the physician sees the messenger for the first time, if the latter is found to be touching either straw, chaff, flesh, bone, hair of the head, small hairs of the body, nails, teeth, broom, rod meant for pounding grains, tray used for winnowing, leather pieces from shoes, grass, wood pieces, husk, charcoal, lump of earth / clay, or stone, the patient for whom he has been sent should be considered as moribund.
- If the physician sees bad omens while the messenger describes the condition of the patient, he should not accompany such a messenger to the patient's house i.e., such an incident indicates imminent death of the patient.
- Similarly, if the physician comes across a sorrowful person, dead body or Pretalankara (adornments of dead persons) he should not attend the patient.
- If the physician happens to see someone (something) being cut, burnt or dead (destroyed) or the sound of statement describing such incident, or tastes which are acute and pungent, or smell which is exceedingly stinky like that of a corpse, or touch of things which are exceedingly harsh or such other sensory objects which are considered inauspicious, immediately before or during the receipt of the message or after hearing the call of the messenger, the patient for whom the messenger is sent should be considered as nearing death.

Thus, all about the signs of imminent death as indicated by the characteristic features of the messenger who comes from the patient's house to the physician is described [9-25]

An incident in physician's way to patient's house:

पथ्यातुरकुलानां च वक्ष्याम्यौत्पातिकं पुनः||२५||
अवक्षुतमथोत्क्रुष्टं स्खलनं पतनं तथा|
आक्रोशः सम्प्रहारो वा प्रतिषेधो विगर्हणम्||२६||
वस्त्रोष्णीषोत्तरासङ्गश्छत्रोपानद्युगाश्रयम्|
व्यसनं दर्शनं चापि मृतव्यसनिनां तथा||२७||
चैत्यध्वजपताकानां पूर्णानां पतनानि च|

हतानिष्टप्रवादाश्च दूषणं भस्मपांशुभिः||२८||
पथच्छेदो बिडालेन शुना सर्पेण वा पुनः|
मृगद्विजानां क्रूराणां गिरो दीप्तां दिशं प्रति||२९||
शयनासनयानानामुत्तानानां च दर्शनम्|
इत्येतान्यप्रशस्तानि सर्वाण्याहुर्मनीषिणः||३०||
एतानि पथि वैद्येन पश्यताऽऽतुरवेश्मनि|
शृण्वता च न गन्तव्यं तदागारं विपश्चिता||३१||
इत्यौत्पातिकमाख्यातं पथि वैद्यविगर्हितम्|३२|

Now we shall discuss the signs of imminent death as indicated by the characteristic features of incidents in the physicians' way to the patient's house or at the time of arrival at his (patient's) house:

- Sneezing, sounds of someone crying out of fear or screaming, stumbling, falling, hearing someone crying / yelling out of anger or disappointment, vision of people quarrelling or beating each other, someone preventing from going ahead or hearing of abuses.
- Some abnormalities suddenly seen in the clothes, turban, shawl, umbrella or pair of shoes such that they cannot be worn or carried or vision of relatives of the dead person who are grieving or vision of dead or grieving persons on the pathway to patient's house.
- Falling or Caitya (religious Fig tree), flag staff, flag or pitcher filled with water, arrival of information regarding death or other inauspicious things, body getting covered or polluted by ashes or dust.
- Cats, dogs or snakes crossing the path, or hearing wild animals like jackals, vultures etc crying loudly facing southwards.
- Vision of beds, seats, vessels and vehicles which are turned upside down—all these are considered to be inauspicious by the wise.
- A wise physician who comes across these auspicious and ominous signs or hears about them in his way to the patient's house or at the time of arrival at his (patient's) house should not proceed further (to the patient's house).

Thus, the signs of imminent death as indicated by the characteristic features of the physician's way to the patient's house are described. The physician should avoid treating the patient in such situations. [25-31]

Indications while entering and inside the patient's house:

इमामपि च बुध्येत गृहावस्थां मुमूर्षताम्||३२||
प्रवेशे पूर्णकुम्भाग्निमृद्बीजफलसर्पिषाम्|
वृषब्राह्मणरत्नान्नदेवतानां च निर्गतिम्||३३||
अग्निपूर्णानि पात्राणि भिन्नानि विशिखानि च|
भिषङ् मुमूर्षतां वेश्म प्रविशन्नेव पश्यति||३४||
छिन्नभिन्नानि दग्धानि भग्नानि मृदितानि च|
दुर्बलानि च सेवन्ते मुमूर्षोर्वेश्मिका जनाः||३५||
शयनं वसनं यानं गमनं भोजनं रुतम्|
श्रूयतेऽमङ्गलं यस्य नास्ति तस्य चिकित्सितम्||३६||
शयनं वसनं यानमन्यं वाऽपि परिच्छदम्|
प्रेतवद्यस्य कुर्वन्ति सुहृदः प्रेत एव सः||३७||
अन्नं व्यापद्यतेऽत्यर्थं ज्योतिश्चैवोपशाम्यति|
निवाते सेन्धनं यस्य तस्य नास्ति चिकित्सितम्||३८||
आतुरस्य गृहे यस्य भिद्यन्ते वा पतन्ति वा|
अतिमात्रममत्राणि दुर्भं तस्य जीवितम्||३९||

The characteristic features of the house of the moribund patient are as follows:

- At the time of entrance into the house of the moribund patient, if the physician observes the exit (from the patient's house) of pitcher filled with water, fire, earth, seeds, fruit, ghee, a bull, a Brahmin, precious stones, prepared food or idols of the Gods it should be considered as ominous
- Inside such a patient's house he may see the broken vessels filled with fire (in which fire is lit) or the fire without flame and only smoke arising from the fire (extinguished fire)
- Things that are broken, cracked, burnt, split or crushed are used by important persons residing in the house of the patient who is moribund
- If inauspicious and unpleasant things are being said about the bed, cloth, vehicle, gait / journey and food etc of the patient (inside patient's house) the treatment of such a patient will not become successful (the patient will surely die)
- If the relatives of the patient arrange for his bed, cloth, vehicle and other apparel which are befitting for dead bodies, then the patient should be considered as already dead.
- No treatment would become fruitful in curing the patient if the food given to him becomes exceedingly rotten and the fire for him gets extinguished in spite of it being supplied with fuel in adequate quantity and the place wherein the fire is lit is devoid of wind.
- If saucers and plates often fall down and get broken in the house of a patient then his life can hardly be saved. [32-39]

Need and scope of repetition:

भवन्ति चात्र-

यद्द्वादशभिरध्यायैर्व्यासतः परिकीर्तितम्|
मुमूर्षतां मनुष्याणां लक्षणं जीवितान्तकृत्||४०||
तत् समासेन वक्ष्यामः पर्यायान्तरमाश्रितम्|
पर्यायवचनं ह्यर्थविज्ञानायोपपद्यते||४१||
अत्यर्थं पुनरेवेयं विवक्षा नो विधीयते|
तस्मिन्नेवाधिकरणे यत् पूर्वमभिशब्दितम्||४२||

Thus, it is said:

Signs of imminent death of moribund persons described in detail in the twelve chapters will now be described in brief in a different way which elucidates their inherent meaning. It is of course not the intention to go into the subject again in detail because such details are already described in the respective chapters. [40-42]

Signs of impending death:

वसतां चरमं कालं शरीरेषु शरीरिणाम्|
अभ्युग्राणां विनाशाय देहेभ्यः प्रविवत्सताम्||४३||
इष्टांस्तितिक्षतां प्राणान् कान्तं वासं जिहासताम्|
तन्त्रयन्त्रेषु भिन्नेषु तमोऽन्त्यं प्रविविक्षताम्||४४||
विनाशायेह रूपाणि यान्यवस्थान्तराणि च|
भवन्ति तानि वक्ष्यामि यथोद्देशं यथागमम्||४५||
प्राणाः समुपतप्यन्ते विज्ञानमुपरुध्यते|
वमन्ति बलमङ्गानि चेष्टा व्युपरमन्ति च||४६||
इन्द्रियाणि विनश्यन्ति खिलीभवति चेतना |
औत्सुक्यं भजते सत्त्वं चेतो भीराविशत्यपि||४७||
स्मृतिस्त्यजति मेधा च ह्रीश्रियौ चापसर्पतः|
उप्प्लवन्ते पाप्मान ओजस्तेजश्च नश्यति||४८||
शीलं व्यावर्ततेऽत्यर्थं भक्तिश्च परिवर्तते|
विक्रियन्ते प्रतिच्छायाश्छायाश्च विकृतिं प्रति||४९||

शुक्रं प्रच्यवते स्थानादुन्मार्गं भजतेऽनिलः|
क्षयं मांसानि गच्छन्ति गच्छत्यसृगपि क्षयम्||५०||
ऊष्माणः प्रलयं यान्ति विश्लेषं यान्ति सन्धयः|
गन्धा विकृतिमायान्ति भेदं वर्णस्वरौ तथा||५१||
वैवर्ण्यं भजते कायः कायच्छिद्रं विशुष्यति|
धूमः सञ्जायते मूर्ध्नि दारुणाख्यश्च चूर्णकः||५२||
सततस्पन्दना देशाः शरीरे येऽभिलक्षिताः|
ते स्तम्भानुगताः सर्वे न चलन्ति कथञ्चन||५३||
गुणाः शरीरदेशानां शीतोष्णमृदुदारुणाः|
विपर्यासेन वर्तन्ते स्थानेष्वन्येषु तद्विधाः||५४||
नखेषु जायते पुष्पं पङ्को दन्तेषु जायते|
जटाः पक्ष्मसु जायन्ते सीमन्ताश्चापि मूर्धनि||५५||
भेषजानि न संवृतिं प्राप्नुवन्ति यथारुचि|
यानि चाप्युपपद्यन्ते तेषां वीर्यं न सिध्यति||५६||
नानाप्रकृतयः क्रूरा विकारा विविधौषधाः|
क्षिप्रं समभिवर्तन्ते प्रतिहत्य बलौजसी||५७||
शब्दः स्पर्शो रसो रूपं गन्धश्चेष्टा विचिन्तितम्|
उत्पद्यन्तेऽशुभान्येव प्रतिकर्मप्रवृत्तिषु||५८||
दृश्यन्ते दारुणाः स्वप्ना दौरात्म्यमुपजायते|
प्रेष्याः प्रतीपतां यान्ति प्रेताकृतिरुदीर्यते||५९||
प्रकृतिर्हीयतेऽत्यर्थं विकृतिश्चाभिवर्धते|
कृत्स्नमौत्पातिकं घोरमरि(नि)ष्टमुपलक्ष्यते||६०||
इत्येतानि मनुष्याणां भवन्ति विनशिष्यताम्|
लक्षणानि यथोद्देशं यान्युक्तानि यथागमम्||६१||

The soul who is spending his final moments in the present body in which he is located, who is enthusiastic to leave this body and travel further ahead, who is ready to get detached from the life elements which he had liked them earlier and migrate to yet another body before this body succumbs to final darkness in the form of death, the process of destruction in the body is initiated in the person who is about to enter the darkness called death after he getting detached and separated from the instruments (organs) of the body.

As proposed earlier the signs which are manifested and the modifications which take place in the individual and his soul during this time will now be described. This is based upon the scriptural authority. They are as follows:

- Affliction of Prana i.e., vital breath, clouding of understanding, the parts of the body become weak and there is drainage of strength from limbs (they become less active as their functions are impaired), and there is cessation of movements.
- Destruction of sensory and motor functions (due to impairment of activities in sensory organs and motor organs)
- Impairment of consciousness
- Restlessness and anxiety in the mind about life
- Affliction of the mind with fear
- Deprivation of memory and retention power, intellect, natural modesty and luster of the body
- Aggravation of diseases caused by sinful acts
- Destruction of Ojas and complexion
- Radical change in the conduct and character of the person
- Changes in what he likes
- Perversion and abnormality in the reflected image and luster of the individual

- Expulsion (ejaculation) of the semen takes place even when the person is sexually not provoked or not in the sexual act
- Upward movement of Vayu
- Wasting of muscle tissue and blood
- Diminution of the warmth and heat (in places wherein it should naturally be present) and development of coldness in those parts of the body
- Dislocation / laxity of joints
- Foul smell emanated from the body
- Hoarseness of voice
- Impairment of complexion / discoloration of the body
- Dryness of the orifices of the body
- Appearance as if smoke is coming from the head
- Appearance of substance like the power of cow dung in the head which is indicative of imminent death
- Complete cessation of pulsation / movements in the parts (organs) of the body which usually pulsate constantly in normal conditions
- Manifestation of attributes of opposite nature in those parts of the body which are either cold, hot, soft, or rough; and similar other features
- Appearance of flower like signs of white spots in nails and adherence of mud like substance in teeth
- Matting of eye-lashes and manifestation of Simantas i.e. lines caused by parting of hair in the head (in spite of not being manually parted)
- Difficulty in obtaining the desired drugs for preparing the medicines towards the patient and even if such drugs are obtained, their actions (and the action of the medicines made by those drugs) are not manifested in consonance with their potency.
- Sudden manifestation and worsening of serious diseases of diverse types and requiring different types of treatment by overpowering the strength and Ojas (power of resistance to diseases and decay).
- Manifestation of inauspicious sound, touch, taste, vision, smells, action and thoughts in the physician while treating such patients.
- Appearance of cruel dreams and manifestation of evil disposition for the patient and the people closer to him become his rivals.
- Hostility of the messenger and change in complexion to that of a dead person.
- Diminution of the normal characteristic features of the body, abnormality in the health status and aggravation of the morbid conditions.
- Manifestation of all the inauspicious signs all of a sudden

As proposed earlier, the signs of imminent death based on scriptural authority are described. [43-61]

Information on impending death to be kept secret:

मरणायेह रूपाणि पश्यताऽपि भिषग्विदा।
अपृष्टेन न वक्तव्यं मरणं प्रत्युपस्थितम्॥६२॥
पृष्टेनापि न वक्तव्यं तत्र यत्रोपघातकम्।
आतुरस्य भवेद्दुःखमथवाऽन्यस्य कस्यचित्॥६३॥
अब्रुवन्मरणं तस्य नैनमिच्छेच्चिकित्सितुम्।
यस्य पश्येद्विनाशाय लिङ्गानि कुशलो भिषक्॥६४॥

In spite of being aware of the onset of the bad prognostic signs of impending death, the physician should not announce the imminence of death without being specially requested for that. If the announcement of a bad prognosis is likely to cause collapse of the patient or distress of others (relatives and friends around), the physician should not announce anything about the approaching death (of the patient) in spite of being specially requested for. The wise physician should however refrain from treating patients having signs of imminent death without making an announcement of the approaching death. [62-64]

Good prognostic signs should be disclosed:
लिङ्गेभ्यो मरणाख्येभ्यो विपरीतानि पश्यता|
लिङ्गान्यारोग्यमागन्तु वक्तव्यं भिषजा ध्रुवम्||६५||
दूतैरौत्पातिकैर्भावैः पथ्यातुरकुलाश्रयैः|
आतुराचारशीलेष्टद्रव्यसम्पत्तिलक्षणैः||६६||

If the physician comes across auspicious signs of recovery (opposite to the inauspicious signs of approaching death) of the patient as indicated by:

- characteristic features of the messenger
- sudden manifestation of certain auspicious signs
- signs in the physician's way to patient's house
- characteristic features of the patient's residence
- manner and conduct of the patient
- availability of drugs at ease
- He should make this announcement positively. [65-66]

Messengers indicating good prognosis:
स्वाचारं हृष्टमव्यङ्गं यशस्यं शुक्लवाससम्|
अमुण्डमजटं दूतं जातिवेशक्रियासमम्||६७||
अनुष्ट्रखरयानस्थमसन्ध्यास्वग्रहेषु च|
अदारुणेषु नक्षत्रेष्वनुग्रेषु ध्रुवेषु च||६८||
विना चतुर्थीं नवमीं विना रिक्तां चतुर्दशीम्|
मध्याह्नमर्धरात्रं च भूकम्पं राहुदर्शनम्||६९||
विना देशमशस्तं चाशस्तौत्पातिकलक्षणम्|
दूतं प्रशस्तमव्यग्रं निर्दिशेदागतं भिषक्||७०||

The following types of messengers are to be considered as auspicious that is – messenger indicative of favourable prognosis:

- he would have good conduct and pleasant behaviour
- he is not devoid of any organ of his body;
- he is of good repute and clad with white cloths;
- he has not completely shaved, he has a tuft of hair in the crown of his head and his hairs are not matted,
- he is similar in caste, dress and action to the patient,
- he has not arrived in a vehicle carried by camel or donkey
- he has not come at the time of Sandhya i.e., morning or evening twilight
- he has not come during inauspicious planetary positions
- he has come at a time when cruel stars are present or during presence of dhruva star (he has come at a time when the Uttaraphalguni, Uttarasadha, Uttarabhadrapada and Rohini stars are auspicious and on auspicious Tithis i.e., dates)
- he has not come on 4th, 9th, and 14th days or rikta tithi (date) of the lunar fortnight
- he has come at a time other than the noon or midnight, when there is no earthquake and when there is no eclipse
- he has come to a place which is not defamed and which is devoid of inauspicious characteristics
- he is not perturbed [67-70]

Incident on the way or while entering patient's house indicating good prognosis:

दध्यक्षतद्विजातीनांवृषभाणांनृपस्यच॥७१॥
रत्नानांपूर्णकुम्भानांसितस्यतुरगस्यच।
सुरध्वजपताकानांफलानांयावकस्यच॥७२॥
कन्यापुंवर्धमानानांबद्धस्यैकपशोस्तस्था।
पृथिव्याउद्धृतायाश्चवह्ने:प्रज्वलितस्यच॥७३॥
मोदकानांसुमनसांशुक्लानांचन्दनस्यच।
मनोज्ञस्यान्नपानस्यपूर्णस्यशकटस्यच॥७४॥
नृभिर्धन्वा:सवत्सायावडवाया:स्त्रियास्तथा।
जीवञ्जीवकसिद्धार्थसारसप्रियवादिनाम्॥७५॥
हंसानांशतपत्राणांचाषाणांशिखिनांतथा।
मत्स्याजदि्वजशङ्खानांप्रियङ्गूनांघृतस्यच॥७६॥
रुचकादर्शसिद्धार्थरोचनानांचदर्शनम्।
गन्ध:सुरभिर्वर्णश्चसुशुक्लोमधुरोरस:॥७७॥
मृगपक्षिमनुष्याणांप्रशस्ताश्चगिर:शुभा:।
छत्रध्वजपताकानामुत्क्षेपणमभिष्टुति:॥७८॥
भेरीमृदङ्गशङ्खानांशब्दा:पुण्याहनिस्वना:।
वेदाध्ययनशब्दाश्चसुखोवायु:प्रदक्षिण:॥७९॥
पथिवेश्मप्रवेशेतुविद्यादारोग्यलक्षणम्।८०।

If while entering or on his way to the patient's house, the physician comes across the following, then he can predict the recovery of the patient:

- Curd
- Aksata (grains of intact rice)
- Brahmanas
- Bulls
- King
- Gems
- Pitchers filled with water
- White horse
- Flags and banners dedicated to Lord Indra
- Fruits
- Grains of barley
- Boys and girls seated on the lap (or boys, girls and earthen plate)
- An animal of good breed tied to a rope
- Cultivated land
- Kindled fire
- Sweets
- White coloured flower
- Sandal paste
- Delicious food articles and drinks
- A cart fully loaded with human beings
- A cow together with a calf
- A mare with her calf
- A woman with her child

- Cakora (cukor)
- Siddhartha
- Sarasa (crane)
- Oataka (sparrow)
- Swan
- Satapatra (parrot)
- Casa (blue joy)
- Peacock
- Fish
- Goat
- Elephant tusk
- Priyangu (Callicarpa macrophyla Vahl)
- Ghee
- Rucaka (ornaments of horses)
- Mirror
- White mustard
- Gorocana (bile of cow)
- Fragrance
- Things having white colour
- Sweet taste
- Sweet and auspicious voices of animals, birds and human beings
- Unfolding of umbrellas, flags and banners
- Prayers
- Sound of cattle drums, drums and conches
- Punyaha (auspicious sounds)
- Sounds of vedic recitations and soothing wind from the South direction. [71-80]

Signs of good prognosis:

मङ्गलाचारसम्पन्नःसातुरोवैशिमकोजनः||८०||
श्रद्दधानोऽनुकूलश्चप्रभूतद्रव्यसङ्ग्रहः|
धनैश्वर्यसुखावाप्तिरिष्टलाभःसुखेनच||८१||
द्रव्याणांतत्रयोग्यानांयोजनासिद्धिरेवच|
गृहप्रासादशैलानांनागानामृषभस्यच||८२||
हयानांपुरुषाणांचस्वप्नेसमधिरोहणम्|
सोमार्काग्निद्विजातीनांगवांनृणांपयस्विनाम्||८३||
अर्णवानांप्रतरणंवृद्दिधःसम्बाधनिःसृतिः|
स्वप्नेदेवैःसपितृभिःप्रसन्नैश्चाभिभाषणम्||८४||
दर्शनंशुक्लवस्त्राणांह्रदस्यविमलस्यच|
मांसमत्स्यविषामेध्यच्छत्रादर्शपरिग्रहः||८५||
स्वप्नेसुमनसांचैवशुक्लानांदर्शनंशुभम्|
अश्वगोरथयानंचयानंपूर्वोत्तरेणच|
रोदनंपतितोत्थानंद्विषतांचावमर्दनम्||८६||

The following are the auspicious signs indicative of a sure success in the treatment of a patient:
Engagement in auspicious acts, faithfulness and favourable disposition of the patient and his kinsmen;
Collection of adequate funds and other accessories
Attainment of wealth, power and happiness

Easy availability of desired things
Easy availability of drugs in abundance and availability of different methods of preparing medicines from them and using them, favourable effect of these drugs when administered and
Dreams like (a) climbing on the roof of the house, palace, hill, elephant, bull, horse and human being (b) vision of the moon, the sun, fire, Brahmana, cow and man of repute, (c) swimming in the ocean; (d) improvement of health, (e) end of sufferings, (f) dialogue with the gods and forefathers in their pleasing mood (g) vision of white garments and a clean lake, (h) obtaining of meat, fish, poison, unclean objects umbrella and mirror (i) vision of white flowers (j) riding of horses, bulls and chariots and moving towards the north-east, (k) weeping; (l) rising after fall and (m) subjugation of enemies [80-86]

सत्त्वलक्षणसंयोगोभक्तिर्वैद्यद्विजातिषु।
साध्यत्वंनचनिर्वेदस्तदारोग्यस्यलक्षणम्॥८७॥
आरोग्याद्बलमायुश्चसुखंचलभतेमहत्।
इष्टांश्चाप्यपरान्भावान्पुरुषःशुभलक्षणः॥८८॥

Moreover, appearance of noble qualities, faithfulness, devotion to physicians and Brahmana, subjective feeling of curability of diseases, freedom from anxiety constitutes the signs and symptoms of quick recovery from illness. A man of auspicious characteristics attains strength, longevity, happiness and other desirable objects only when he possesses good health. [87-88]

तत्रश्लोकौ-
उक्तंगोमयचूर्णीयेमरणारोग्यलक्षणम्।
दूतस्वप्नातुरोत्पातयुक्तिसिद्धिव्यपाश्रयम्॥८९॥

To sum up: -In this chapter on "Imminent death as indicated by signs like the appearance of substance resembling cow dung powder in the head", signs and symptoms of imminent death, accidental happenings, reasoning and accomplishments of success are described. [89]

Utility of the knowledge:
इतीदमुक्तंप्रकृतंयथातथंतदन्ववेक्ष्यंसततंभिषग्विदा।
तथाहिसिद्धिंचयशश्चशाश्वतंससिद्धकर्मालभतेधनानिच॥९०॥

Signs and symptoms described in this chapter should always be properly studied by the physician. It is only then that a physician can attain success, fame and wealth as well as accomplishment through treatment. [90]

इत्यग्निवेशकृते तन्त्रेचरकप्रतिसंस्कृते इन्द्रियस्थाने गोमयचूर्णीयमिन्द्रियं नाम द्वादशोऽध्यायः॥१२॥
इति चरकसंहितायां पञ्चममइन्द्रियस्थानं सम्पूर्णम्।

Thus ends the 12th chapter on "Imminent death as indicated by signs like the appearance of a substance resembling cow-dung powder in the head" of the Indriya Section of Agnivesha's work as redacted by Charaka.

Easy Ayurveda Publications

All our book publications are available at
www.EasyAyurveda.com/Books

English Books:
Charaka Samhita Volume 1,2,3 and 4 - English Translation
Ashtanga Hrudayam Sutrasthanam - English Translation
Living Easy With Ayurveda
Easy Ayurveda Home Remedies
Tridosha Made Easy
Ayurveda Tarka

Hindi Books:
Ayurved Samadhan

Kannada Books:
Sugama Jivanakkagi Ayurveda
Ayurveda Santvana

Malayalam Books
Ayurveda Asvasam
Jeevitha Soukhyathinu Ayurvedam

All our book publications are available at
www.EasyAyurveda.com/Books